DIMENSIONS OF NURSING ADMINISTRATION

DIMENSIONS OF NURSING ADMINISTRATION

Theory, Research, Education, Practice

Edited by

Beverly Henry, R.N., M.S.N., Ph.D.
James R. Dougherty, Jr. Centennial Professor in Nursing Service Administration, The University of Texas, Austin, Texas

Clara Arndt, R.N., Ph.D.
Consultant and Instructor, Continuing Education of Nursing Services, Wadsworth Veterans Administration Medical Center, Los Angeles, California

Marie Di Vincenti, R.N., Ed.D.
Director, Graduate Nursing Program, Louisiana State University Medical Center, New Orleans, Louisiana

Ann Marriner-Tomey, R.N., Ph.D.
Professor, Graduate Department of Nursing Administration and Teacher Education, Indiana University School of Nursing, Indianapolis, Indiana

BLACKWELL SCIENTIFIC PUBLICATIONS

Boston   Oxford   London   Edinburgh   Palo Alto   Melbourne

Blackwell Scientific Publications

Editorial Offices:
Three Cambridge Center, Suite 208, Cambridge, Massachusetts 02142, USA
Osney Mead, Oxford OX2 0EL, England
8 John Street, London, WC1N 2ES, England
23 Ainslie Place, Edinburgh, EH3 6AJ, Scotland
107 Barry Street, Carlton, Victoria 3053, Australia
667 Lytton Avenue, Palo Alto, California 94301, USA

Blackwell Scientific Publications, Inc.
Copyright © 1989 by Blackwell Scientific Publications, Inc.
Printed in the United States of America
89 90 91 92 5 4 3 2 1
Typeset by The William Byrd Press, Inc.
Printed and bound by Haddon Craftsmen, Inc.

Library of Congress Cataloging-in-Publication Data

Dimensions of nursing administration.

Includes bibliographies and index.
1. Nursing services—Administration. I. Henry,
Beverly, 1939– . [DNLM: 1. Administrative
Personnel. 2. Nursing, Supervisory. 3. Nursing
Theory. WY 105 D582]
RT89.D56 1988   362.1′73′068   88-26259
ISBN 0-86542-051-3

Contents

Contributors

Judith W. Alexander, R.N., Ph.D.
Assistant Professor, College of Nursing, University of South Carolina, Columbia, South Carolina

Martha Raile Alligood, Ph.D., R.N.
Associate Professor and Chair, Department of Nursing Practice, College of Nursing, University of South Carolina, Columbia, South Carolina

Ruth A. Anderson, Ph.D., R.N.
Assistant Professor, School of Nursing, University of Texas at Austin, Austin, Texas

James H. Anway, M.S.N., R.N.
Pittsburgh, Pennsylvania

Clara Arndt, R.N., Ph.D.
Consultant and Instructor, Continuing Education of Nursing Services, Wadsworth Veterans Administration Medical Center, Los Angeles, California

Sister Rose Therese Bahr, Ph.D., R.N., F.A.A.N.
Professor of Nursing; Associate Director, Life Cycle Institute; Director, Gerontology Center, The Catholic University of America, Washington, DC

E. Kathryn Barnett, R.N., Ph.D.
Professor of Nursing and Dean, School of Nursing, Auburn University at Montgomery, Montgomery, Alabama

Barbara Stevens Barnum, Ph.D., R.N.
Adjunct Professor of Nursing, Teachers College, Columbia University, New York, New York

Mary L. Botter, M.S.N., R.N.
Assistant Professor, La Salle University, Philadelphia, Pennsylvania

Judy L. Luckenbill Brett, R.N., M.S.N., Ph.D.
Director, Nursing Systems, Robert Wood Johnson University Hospital; Assistant Professor, Rutgers, The State University of New Jersey, New Brunswick, New Jersey

Joan Burritt, D.N.Sc., R.N.
Assistant Clinical Director, Obstetrics, Gynecology and Pediatrics Nursing, Yale–New Haven Hospital, New Haven, Connecticut

Theresa L. Carroll, R.N., Ph.D.
Associate Dean, Graduate Program, School of Nursing, Duquesne University, Pittsburgh, Pennsylvania

John D. Crossley, M.B.A., M.S.N., R.N.
Senior Associate Director of Nursing, University of Iowa Hospitals and Clinics, Iowa City, Iowa

Jacqueline Dienemann, R.N., Ph.D.
Coordinator Nursing Administration and Assistant Professor, School of Nursing, George Mason University, Fairfax, Virginia

Colleen K. DiIorio, Ph.D., R.N., C.N.R.N.
Director, Center for Nursing Research; Associate Professor, Nell Hodgson Woodruff School of Nursing, Emory University, Atlanta, Georgia

Marie Di Vincenti, R.N., Ed.D.
Director, Graduate Nursing Program, Louisiana State University Medical Center, New Orleans, Louisiana

Barbara A. Donaho, R.N., M.A., F.A.A.N.
Vice President for Nursing and Patient Services, Shands Hospital, Gainesville, Florida

Sandra R. Edwardson, Ph.D., R.N.
Associate Professor, School of Nursing, University of Minnesota, Minneapolis, Minnesota

Karen L. Elberson, M.S.N., R.N.
Assistant Professor, Nell Hodgson Woodruff School of Nursing, Emory University, Atlanta, Georgia

Jacqueline Fawcett, Ph.D., F.A.A.N.
Associate Professor and Section Chairperson, Science and Role Development, University of Pennsylvania School of Nursing, Philadelphia, Pennsylvania

Helen M. Ference, Ph.D., F.N.S.
Director, Nightingale Society, Carmel, California

Ruth Barney Fine, R.N., M.N., F.A.A.N.
Associate Professor and Director, Graduate Program Nursing Administration, School of Nursing, University of Washington, Seattle, Washington

H. George Frederickson, Ph.D.
Edwin O. Stein Distinguished Professor of Public Administration, University of Kansas, Lawrence, Kansas

Cynthia M. Freund, Ph.D., R.N., B.S.N.
Associate Professor and Chair, Department of Core Studies, The School of Nursing, University of North Carolina at Chapel Hill, Chapel Hill, North Carolina

Barbara B. Frink, M.S., R.N.
Doctoral Candidate, Nursing Administration, University of Pennsylvania, Philadelphia, Pennsylvania; Assistant Director of Nursing Research, Children's Hospital National Medical Center, Washington, DC

Doris J. Froebe, R.N., Ph.D.
Chairman, Nursing Administration, Teacher Education; Acting Associate Dean, Graduate Program, Indiana University School of Nursing, Indianapolis, Indiana

Barbara Fuszard, Ph.D., R.N.
Professor, Nursing Administration, School of Nursing, Medical College of Georgia, Augusta, Georgia

Cecilia Gibbons, R.N., M.S.N., C.N.A.
Chief, Nursing Service, Veterans Administration Medical Center, Sioux Falls, South Dakota

Gina Giovinco, R.N., Ph.D., Ed.D.
Associate Professor, Department of Nursing, College of Health, University of Central Florida, Orlando, Florida

Mary Alice Green, B.S.N., R.N.
Director, Continuing Education, Shands Hospital at the University of Florida; Graduate Student in Nursing Administration, Gainesville, Florida

Nannette L. Goddard, R.N., M.S.
Senior Partner, Consulting, Goddard Management Resources, Houston, Texas; Assistant Professor, Graduate Management Program, The University of Texas School of Nursing at Galveston, Galveston, Texas

Sarah Hall Gueldner, D.S.N., R.N.
Associate Professor, Department of Adult Nursing, School of Nursing, Medical College of Georgia, Augusta, Georgia

Elizabeth A. Hefferin, D.P.H., R.N., F.A.A.N.
Associate Chief, Nursing Service for Research, Wadsworth Division, West Los Angeles Veterans Administration Medical Center, Los Angeles, California

Beverly Henry, R.N., M.S.N., Ph.D.
James R. Dougherty, Jr. Centennial Professor in Nursing Service Administration, The University of Texas, Austin, Texas

Ada Sue Hinshaw, Ph.D., R.N., F.A.A.N.
Director, National Center for Nursing Research, Bethesda, Maryland

Patricia Hinton-Walker, Ph.D., R.N.
Associate Dean and Professor, Nell Hodgson Woodruff School of Nursing, Emory University, Atlanta, Georgia

Loucine M. D. Huckabay, R.N., C.P.N.P., Ph.D., F.A.A.N.
Professor of Nursing, Department of Nursing, California State University, Long Beach, Long Beach, California

Bonnie Mowinski Jennings, R.N., D.N.Sc., LTC, A.N.
Nurse Researcher, U.S. Army Health Care Studies and Clinical Investigation Activity, Health Services Command, Fort Sam Houston, Texas

Katherine R. Jones, R.N., Ph.D.
Associate Professor, Graduate Program in Health and Hospital Administration, University of Florida, Gainesville, Florida

Barbara Anne Keddy, R.N., B.Sc.N., M.A., Ph.D.
Associate Professor, School of Nursing and Department of Sociology and Social Anthropology, Dalhousie University, Halifax, Nova Scotia, Canada

Jean A. Kelley, Ed.D., R.N., F.A.A.N.
Assistant Dean, Graduate Programs in Nursing, School of Nursing, University of Alabama at Birmingham, Birmingham, Alabama

Karlene Kerfoot, Ph.D., R.N.
Senior Vice President, Nursing, St. Luke's Episcopal Hospital, Houston, Texas

Imogene M. King, Ed.D., R.N.
Professor, College of Nursing, University of South Florida, Tampa, Florida

Sharon B. Krajnak, R.N., M.S.N., C.N.A.
Associate Chief, Nursing Service/Education, Veterans Administration Medical Center, Nashville, Tennessee

Diane R. LaRochelle, Ph.D., R.N.
Professor, College of Nursing, University of Florida, Gainesville, Florida

Madeleine M. Leininger, Ph.D., L.H.D., F.A.A.N.
Professor of Nursing, College of Nursing; Professor of Anthropology, College of Liberal Arts; Director, Transcultural Nursing Program, Wayne State University, Detroit, Michigan

Arlene Lowenstein, R.N., Ph.D.
Associate Professor and Chairperson, Department of Nursing Administration, School of Nursing, Medical College of Georgia, Augusta, Georgia

Lois C. Malkemes, R.N., Ph.D.
Technical Advisor, Ernst & Whinney, Dallas, Texas

Barbara A. Mark, R.N., Ph.D.
Chairman, Department of Nursing Administration and Information Systems; Director, Doctoral Program in Nursing Administration, School of Nursing, Medical College of Virginia, Virginia Commonwealth University, Richmond, Virginia

Ann Marriner-Tomey, R.N., Ph.D.
Professor, Graduate Department of Nursing Administration and Teacher Education, Indiana University School of Nursing, Indianapolis, Indiana

John McConnell, R.N., M.S.
President, National Gerontological Nursing Association, New Carrollton, Maryland

Afaf Ibrahim Meleis, Ph.D., F.A.A.N.
Professor and International Kellogg Fellow, Department of Mental Health, Community and Administrative Nursing, School of Nursing, University of California, San Francisco, San Francisco, California

Peggy Nazarey, R.N., M.S.N.
Director of Nursing, Harbor-UCLA Medical Center; Assistant Dean for Clinical Affairs, School of Nursing, University of California, Los Angeles, Los Angeles, California

Audrey L. O. Nelson, R.N., M.N.
Rehabilitation Nursing Care Coordinator, James A. Haley Veterans' Hospital, Tampa, Florida; Doctoral Student, College of Nursing, University of Florida, Gainesville, Florida

Barbara A. Norton, B.S., M.P.H., R.N.
Associate Professor, Indiana University School of Nursing, Indianapolis, Indiana

Dorothy W. Nunn, R.N., B.S.N.
Quality Assurance Coordinator, Veterans Administration Medical Center, Indianapolis, Indiana

Dorothea E. Orem, M.A.N.Ed., D.Sc.
Savannah, Georgia

Rosemarie Rizzo Parse, R.N., Ph.D.
Professor of Nursing and Coordinator, Center for Nursing Research, Hunter College of the City University of New York, New York, New York

Ellen Tate Patterson, D.S.N., R.N.
Coordinator, Nursing Research, University of Alabama Hospital, Birmingham, Alabama

Jane F. Pendergast, Ph.D.
Division of Biostatistics, Department of Statistics, University of Florida, Gainesville, Florida

Sydney H. Pendleton, R.N., Ed.D.
Prairie Village, Kansas

Gaye W. Poteet, R.N., Ed.D.
Professor and Assistant Dean of Graduate Program, School of Nursing, East Carolina University, Greenville, North Carolina

Mona Raborn, R.N., C.N.A.
Director of Nursing, Jefferson Davis Memorial Hospital, Natchez, Mississippi

Mary Jane Reinhart, R.N.C., M.S.N.
Doctoral Candidate, School of Nursing, Indiana University, Indianapolis, Indiana; Instructor, School of Nursing, Wright State University–Miami Valley, Dayton, Ohio

Rachel Rotkovitch, R.N., M.S.
Consultant in Nursing Management, Branford, Connecticut

Sister Callista Roy, R.N., Ph.D., F.A.A.N.
Professor/Nurse Theorist, School of Nursing, Boston College, Chestnut Hill, Massachusetts

Cynthia C. Scalzi, Ph.D., R.N.
Associate Professor, Program Director, Nursing Administration, School of Nursing, University of Pennsylvania, Philadelphia, Pennsylvania

Lillian M. Simms, Ph.D., R.N.
Associate Professor of Nursing Administration, School of Nursing, The University of Michigan, Ann Arbor, Michigan

Enrica Kinchen Singleton, R.N., Dr.P.H.
Professor and Coordinator, Nursing Service Administration, Graduate Program, School of Nursing, Louisiana State University Medical Center, New Orleans, Louisiana

Kathleen A. Smyth, Ed.D., F.A.A.N.
Professor of Nursing, College of Nursing, University of Florida, Gainesville, Florida

Myrtis J. Snowden, Dr.P.H., F.A.A.N., R.N.
Professor/Coordinator, Public Health/Community Health Nursing, Graduate Program in Nursing, School of Nursing, Louisiana State University Medical Center, New Orleans, Louisiana

Mary Lou Steedley, B.S.N., M.S., R.N.
Administrator, Touro At Home (Hospital-Based Home Care Program), Touro Infirmary; Adjunct Assistant Professor, Department of Applied Health Sciences, School of Public Health and Tropical Medicine, Tulane University, New Orleans, Louisiana

Russell C. Swansburg, Ph.D., R.N., C.N.A.A.
Professor, School of Nursing, Medical College of Georgia, Augusta, Georgia

Terry Throckmorton, R.N., Ph.D.
Associate Professor, Texas Woman's University, Houston, Texas

Linda L. Tilby, R.N., M.S.N.
Assistant Administrator, Patient Services, St. Joseph Hospital, Augusta, Georgia

Marjorie A. White, Ph.D., F.A.A.N.
Professor, College of Nursing; Affiliate Professor, Sociology, University of Florida, Gainesville, Florida

Sandy Wisener, R.N., M.S.N.
Principal, Ernst & Whinney, Dallas, Texas

Foreword

THIS BOOK has three major virtues. First, contributions by leading scholars and practitioners of nursing and nursing administration are collected under one cover. Second, the timing of the volume is superb: the coalescence of contemporary thought in a single volume is needed by educators, practitioners, and researchers in 1988 through the year 2000. Third, the contents represent thinking at the forefront of this dynamic nursing specialty—a wide range of selections reflecting the intellectual roots of nursing administration are carefully included. The result is a comprehensive perspective of knowledge and practice.

Recognition of nursing administration as a nursing specialty for master's-level preparation has gained considerable momentum in recent years. The initiation of curriculums and approval of master's programs for nursing administration by accrediting agencies has fostered the development of new programs: enrollments have increased almost too rapidly!

Nursing administration as a major focus is also prominent in many doctoral programs: administration of nursing services is an extremely popular choice of students. Consequently, the history and suggestions for curriculum content made in the book will be especially useful for planning future programs.

In the middle 1970s, explorations of library holdings revealed that few graduate-level publications were available focusing on problems encountered by nurses in administrative positions. Still less information was available about theory and inquiry in the field. While a growing body of research is available in nursing and management science, relatively little information is available addressing the science of administrative nursing. Books like this one, plus the growing fund of useful data generated by dissertations and faculty doing their own research, will go far toward facilitating scholarly development of both the discipline of nursing and the subdiscipline of nursing administration.

Stronger and stronger alliances of educators and practicing nurse administrators are being forged to develop nursing administration as a key element in the profession. These alliances are nowhere more apparent than in this volume, where editors, advisors, and authors describe the viewpoints of both academics and practitioners. Pooling the talents of faculty and practitioners enriches the education students receive and broadens the opportunities for research and the development of new, useful knowledge. The fruits of these alliances will increase the cogency of future instruction. And more importantly, the outcomes of these cooperative efforts will improve the quality of patient care.

We think this volume is especially important because of the extent to which it reflects the combined thinking of educators and practicing nurse administrators. Leadership for research in the practice arena is most often provided by service agency-based nurses. Pragmatic, reliable information flows from the settings where nursing services are provided and augments previously generated knowledge in nursing and management science. The synthesis of knowledge described in this volume demonstrates the mutuality of interdisciplinary practice and thinking.

As seen in the selections, at least two levels

of analysis are pivotal in nursing administration: the individual or group level, and the organizational level. For nurse administrators, individuals may be consumers or populations of nurses and other workers employed in health-care agencies. Organizations are conceived of as service agencies in single and multi-institutional configurations, and the variety of professions having an effect on health-care services. The humanistic orientation in nursing theory, which nurses bring to practice and research promotes investigations that aim to enhance, sustain, and encourage the performance of all members of a nursing organization—clients and professionals alike. An emphasis on health and individualism, as well as on environmental forces, ensures improved organization behavior and cost-effective services. For nurse administrators, as many of the authors in this volume suggest, issues related to humanism in health care are juxtaposed with the economic realities of health-care costs.

Significant changes in health-care financing in recent years have altered the mechanisms for delivering nursing services. Assessment and analysis of policies have become more and more essential for strategic planning. And careful, orderly data collection for quality assurance and budget analysis have come to be an increasingly important function. The problems in nursing administration require modification of standard research techniques and the application of findings of investigations conducted by scientists both in nursing and in related fields.

The contributions to this volume demonstrate that empirical data on which to base decisions are increasingly available and that methods for collecting new data are on the horizon. Moreover, the well-known authors who have contributed suggest that research in nursing administration within naturalistic settings is valuable, as are more controlled studies in which variables are manipulated to improve understanding of the outcomes of nursing interventions. Research involving qualitative approaches has gained considerable currency in management: through qualitative studies the most important variables for future experimental investigations will be identified and defined.

It is exciting to examine the contents of this book. So much of what is described is new information for the field. Knowledge in nursing administration is accumulating at an accelerating pace. Readers will have the opportunity, as we have, to examine the progress to date and to reflect on the events and knowledge that will mold the future of the administration of nursing services.

Lois Malasanos, Ph.D., R.N., F.A.A.N.
Dean and Professor

Molly Dougherty, Ph.D. R.N.
Professor and Director of Research

College of Nursing
University of Florida
Gainesville, FL

Preface

THE FOCUS of this volume is on four dimensions of nursing administration—its theory, research, education and practice. The purpose of the anthology is to provide sixty-five authors with a forum to discuss varying aspects of the four dimensions, some of which have been only briefly touched on elsewhere. Our aim overall has been to suggest how the integration of theory and research from nursing and management science pertains to the inquiry and practice of nursing administration.

The book is organized in five sections devoted to nursing and organization theory, and to research, education and practice. The sections open with an introduction written by one of the editors who first provides the rationale for the content in the section and second, provides a summary of each chapter. The introductions stand alone. For the reader who is interested in an overview of the entire volume, reading the introductions to the sections will be worthwhile.

For all the sections, each of the contributing authors was asked to do the following: address the dimensions of a complex problem in nursing administration; elucidate state-of-the-art knowledge in nursing and cognate fields; suggest how research and theory can bring about new, useful ways of addressing the problem; and propose new mechanisms and strategies to help resolve the problem.

Contributors, it should be noted, were selected based on the strength of their existing stature and well-established national reputations or because they were known to the editors, had given important presentations at the National Council on Graduate Education for Administration in Nursing (CGEAN), and had a message about nursing administration the editors thought deserved to be widely considered.

Analysis of nursing models and theoretical perspectives in management science is the starting point of the book. There is more and more information in the existing literature that describes generating and testing hypotheses derived from nursing models for clinical practice. Little information is available, however, describing nursing theory for nursing service administration. A goal of the book is to begin to fill this gap in nursing knowledge. In addition, perspectives in public and business administration which have been given little attention in nursing are analyzed for their potential usefulness to nursing administration.

The goal in each section is to stimulate thinking about the dimensions of complex problems in the field and how they are being or can be tackled by academicians and administrators at work in health service organizations. To keep the ideas developed throughout the book based in the realities of the workplace, one-third of the contributing authors are practicing nurse executives. Moreover, academicians were sought who had worked as administrators for a significant time during their careers. And four of the nation's finest nurse executives, Rowena Bishop, Barbara Donaho, Sally Knox, and Linda Sims served as advisors to the editors.

The book is intended for master's and doctoral students in nursing administration; practicing nurse executives; faculty at all levels who teach theory, research, and nursing administration; and senior-level baccalaureate students interested in careers in complex organizations. The heavy emphasis on theory and research, and on merging nursing and organization theory for applications in practice, should prove especially useful to academicians and to nurse executives who are responsible for using and testing theory in the workplace.

Throughout the book, our intent has been to address a number of topics in depth. But we have *not* tried to provide a complete compendium of theories, or research methods, or suggestions for education and practice. Our goal, rather, has been to focus on topics related to each of the four themes which are not addressed in other texts. For example, we know of few places where one can find discussions about how to think about integrating nursing and management theory. That such an integration should take place, however,

has been talked about since the 1950s. We have found little information about the research methodologies that may be best for investigations focusing on problems in nursing administration. Yet research, not only to solve problems in organizations but to build knowledge, is a central function of the effective nurse executive. There are over 70 graduate programs in the country with a major or minor focus of study in nursing administration. The chapters in the education section will provide the faculty who are responsible for these programs with useful information about the structure, content, and articulation of graduate and undergraduate curriculums. And we hope that the topics addressed in the practice section about the management of home and long-term care, about executive succession, and about values in organizations will be of immediate use.

Acknowledgments

M ANY have contributed to this book: some directly, others indirectly, some recently, others historically. As a master's student, I was impressed forever by Dorothy Johnson and her emphasis on theories and science. Talk in the 1960s of models of nursing was new. But it was challenging, and it was from these early conversations over two decades ago that subsequent discussion of theory for nursing administration was derived. I am indebted to other faculty at the University of California (UCLA)—to Dean Lulu Hassenpflug, professor Donna Vredevoe, and Clara Arndt, especially, for their long-standing contributions to nursing and nursing administration.

From the more recent past, many, many words of appreciation are warranted for the support and contributions of the Council on Graduate Education for Administration in Nursing (CGEAN). Members have provided valuable insights about education and research to enhance the practice of nursing administration.

The ideas for the content are also a result of the *National Nursing Administration Research Priorities Study*, which was supported by a grant from the Division of Nursing, Bureau of Health Professions, Health Resources and Services Administration, Public Health Service, and the National Center for Nursing Research, the National Institutes of Health, between 1984 and 1986. The suggestions and conclusions expressed by the authors and editors, however, are their own and do not necessarily represent the views of the support groups and funding agencies cited.

Each of the universities where the editors work—the University of Florida, Indiana University, and Louisiana State University—also deserve sincere acknowledgment. Developing a publishable document takes time and resources. Students in our schools, our deans, and coworkers have been tolerant and helpful. We are in their debt.

We are indebted too, to the nurse executives who served as advisors: Rowena Bishop, chief of nursing at the Wadsworth Division of the Veterans Administration Medical Center in Los Angeles; Barbara Donaho, vice-president for nursing and patient services, Shands Hospital, Gainesville, Florida; Sally Knox, associate director of hospitals for nursing, Indiana University Hospitals, Indianapolis; and Linda Sims, associate hospital director, Ochsner Foundation Hospital, Jefferson, Louisiana.

Speaking for all the editors and advisors, we have benefited greatly from the thinking that has gone into the manuscripts included in the volume. To each of the contributing authors, we say a special thank you for your many ideas and valuable suggestions. As editors who value diversity, we are grateful and we anticipate that readers too, will be appreciative.

Last but not least, the generous assistance and the enduring patience of the editors and staff at Blackwell Scientific Publications, especially Richard Zorab and Susan Van Dam, are heartily acknowledged.

B. H.

DIMENSIONS OF NURSING ADMINISTRATION

Introduction: Nursing Theory for Nursing Administration

Beverly Henry
Clara Arndt

THEORETICAL frameworks where logic is clear and relationships are testable are superior, for the most part, to the individual, largely intuitive theories we all develop about how the world works. Good theories which provide us with a way to categorize events and activities and to relate those categories to what we see in everyday life make human existence in a society as complex as ours far more palatable. People search for knowledge to help make sense of what occurs. Theory is an important form of knowledge: good theories help us make important choices and undertake critical tasks to help individuals and organizations grow and succeed.

The purpose of this opening section is to provide a number of nurse theorists with the opportunity to describe nursing theory for building knowledge and improving practice in nursing administration. As editors, we talked at some length about which of the themes in the book—theory, research, education, or practice—should be emphasized to illustrate the integration of nursing and management knowledge for improved inquiry and practice. Those in academe will find the emphasis on nursing and organization theory useful. Readers who are practicing managers, however, may wish our emphasis had been otherwise: because of the extremely complex problems at work, they may wonder why we did not emphasize more pressing, immediate concerns. It should be noted at this point that all four editors have worked both as nurse administrators and as educators. Each of us has one foot in the world of education and the other in service. We know only too well how demanding the activities of everyday operations can be. And we understand too, how highly essential deciding and doing is. But we also think that Lewin hit the nail on the head when he said, "Nothing is as practical as a good theory."

Because we believe so strongly that theory makes life easier—because we agree with Lewin that good theory is highly practical—we settled on emphasizing theory by placing manuscripts addressing both nursing and organization theory first, then integrating theory throughout the subsequent chapters focusing on research and education for practice.

To reiterate, our primary reason for focusing on theory was this: as educators, we are committed to using, disseminating, and developing knowledge. As educators, we are committed most of all to the generation and dissemination of knowledge that is intelligent and useful in the workplace. We realize full well that if education for nursing administration is to be more than the puny weed of both nursing and management, then the knowledge that is unique to nursing in the administration nurses do, needs to be elucidated.

A place to begin in our theory-finding endeavor is with existing nursing and organization theory—the organized knowledge of nursing and management. Hence the distinctive content of this book—so unlike that of others, where nursing theory, many organization theories, and the integration of knowledge from the two fields are not dealt with as seriously or by as wide a range of authors.

To summarize Section I, authors approach theory for nursing administration in three ways. Meleis, Pendleton, Scalzi, and Fawcett, and their coauthors analyze theories and the contribution of nursing administration to nursing's body of knowledge. Seven theorists—King, Leininger, Orem, Parse, Roy, and Alligood and Gueldner (for Rogers)—extend theories of nursing to nursing administration. In four chapters, by Elberson, Nunn and Marriner, DiIorio, and Ference, the authors describe ways to apply a particular nursing theory to the practice of nursing administration.

Meleis and Jennings open with a discussion of the importance of theoretical nursing. After reviewing state-of-the-art nursing theory, these authors describe the problems—as challenges—of the existing relationship between nursing theory and nursing administration. They cite three: the use of non-nursing theories, the education of nurse administrators, and the influence of research in nursing administration. They express concern about the heavy reliance that nurse administrators place on management theory; about educational programs for nursing administration in which nursing theory is rarely emphasized; and about the paucity of research in nursing administration. The authors then propose four strategies to tackle these challenges: creating a culture in organizations where nursing knowledge is valued and used; implementing nursing theories using new structures, processes, and languages; finding

ways of contributing to the growth of nursing knowledge; and developing analogues for nursing administration that use the domains of nursing theory.

In Chapter 2, "Cultural Care Theory and Nursing Administration," Leininger builds a strong case for the importance of care and caring as understood by various societies around the world. Leininger develops an equally sound argument supporting the importance of the idea of care for nursing administration. She says that contemporary organizations in American society are multicultural and that individuals with varying cultural perspectives conceive of organizations, management, and health services differently; therefore, alternative organizational forms are needed that are aligned with varying cultural perspectives and that satisfy the varying expectations of the consumers and professionals involved. She continues by pointing out that more and more health service organizations are becoming multisystem corporations with international holdings, a factor that adds to the need for transcultural knowledge based on research and on understanding of care as the central and unique element of nursing.

Leininger provides a succinct overview of her theory of culture care diversity and universality with reference to nursing administration. She identifies the values and assumptions of her theory and provides the reader with a number of research questions.

In Chapter 3 King provides an overview of general systems theory—cast against the backdrop of trends in organization theory—and descriptions of her systems framework and theory of goal attainment. Taking as a starting point the issue of how to provide nursing services where resources are constrained, she raises two questions: How can effective nursing care be provided where there is a decrease in staffing ratios? And how can nurse administrators organize to maintain standards in the face of rapidly expanding technologies and the concomitant emphasis on cost controls? She responds to these questions by suggesting that nurse administrators cope by fostering theory-based practice and by using theoretically sound administrative approaches. A number of strategies are described including restructuring the functions of professional nurses and implementing goal-oriented record systems.

Elberson describes how nurse administrators can use King's theory to understand and analyze nursing administrative practice. She describes the similarities between King's conceptual framework and the theory of nursing administration developed by Arndt and Huckabay. The concepts of goal setting, organizations as open systems, and roles are central ideas. Elberson also provides a useful discussion of interaction and transaction at the personal, interpersonal, and social-system levels.

Orem, in Chapter 5, "Nursing Administration, A Theoretical Approach," begins by providing a definition of "nursing administration." She differentiates practicing nurses managing the work of patient care because of care deficits, and nurses managing nursing services for organizational enterprises. She raises five critical questions—about the domain and boundary of nursing, the populations served by nursing and the rules to ensure the provision of care, the courses of action to manage the provision of nursing, and the context and domain over which nursing administration has authority. Next, Orem describes a general theory of nursing administration deriving from the question of what nursing adds to the word "administration" when the two are conjoined. The presuppositions on which she bases her theory are explicated for the reader; managerial responsibilities for nurse administrators are described.

Nunn and Marriner-Tomey, in Chapter 6, discuss applying Orem's model to nursing administration. Describing experiences at the Indianapolis Veterans Administration Medical Center, these authors explain how they gained administrative support, gathered information from other agencies, conducted conferences with key individuals in their organization, developed training programs, and used consultants.

Parse, in Chapter 7, first describes her man-living-health (MLH) theory, then provides readers with suggestions for the management of a nursing service where the theory is implemented. A philosophy of nursing, standards of practice, and criteria for evaluation provide readers with specifics relative to the use of the MLH model.

In Chapter 8, entitled "Roy's Adaptation Model: Theories for Nursing Administration," Roy and Anway propose a theory of organizations as adaptive systems using Roy's adaptation model as a framework. The authors make a number of the assumptions in systems and adaptation theory explicit, then discuss the consequences of these for a new perception of nursing administration.

DiIorio, in Chapter 9, entitled "Application of the Roy Model to Nursing Administration," systematically describes ways to extend Roy's adaptation model of nursing to nursing administration. She begins by providing readers with a detailed overview of the central elements of Roy's theory. In the remainder of the chapter, she extends the components of Roy's model—person, health, environment, and nursing—to the administration of nursing services. DiIorio's careful uses of cases and examples to illustrate the points she makes, and her reflections based on conversations with Roy make this comprehensive essay an especially important contribution.

Alligood, in Chapter 10, entitled "Rogers's Theory and Nursing Administration: A Perspective on Health and Environment," provides the reader with useful explanations of the building blocks and basic principles of Rogers's theory of unitary human beings. She describes Rogers's perceptions of health and environment and compares the Nightingale and Rogers emphases on environment. Alligood suggests that perhaps the most fruitful area for future investigations will be environment, one of nursing's more strongly agreed-on paradigm concepts. Citing the empirical investigations of nurses who have tested and extended Rogers's theory—Ference, Cowling, Barrett, Rawnsley, McDonald, and Gueldner—Alligood describes how principles of the theory have been operationalized and how they can be analyzed for nursing administration.

In Chapter 11, Gueldner discusses "Applying Rogers's Model for Nursing Administration: Emphasis on Client and Nursing." Gueldner suggests that in practice, using Rogers's perspective, all nurses "increase the capacity of each individual in a system to participate knowingly in change." The author provides readers with diagrams depicting nursing situations and suggests ways of understanding clients, nursing and the environment of nursing administration using Rogers's theory.

Ference describes how to use nursing science theories based on Rogers's work to administer nursing services in Chapter 12. She discusses the implications for organizational structures, communication, and power. In this chapter there is also a section on quality assurance in the nursing science perspective which readers interested in implementing a nursing service based on Rogers's theory will find interesting.

The essays up to this point focus primarily on the first element of nursing administration—nursing. All of the authors share their ideas about how to think of nursing with respect to nursing administration. In Section II, the focus is on the second element of nursing administration—on administration. However, before proceeding, three essays provide a transition from nursing to management and conclude Section I.

In Chapter 13, Pendleton provides us with a succinct explanation of the relationship of models and theories to the development of science. Moreover, she addresses how disciplines use knowledge from other fields. Pendleton then takes the position that many theories of nursing are not designed to build a body of nursing science per se. Instead, what exist are theories of nurses and the nursing profession. In a later chapter, I will argue that existing nursing theories, for the most part, are actually individual-level theories of how nurses manage care. Said in slightly different ways, this, too, is Pendleton's position. She argues that two of the profession's overarching ideas or metaparadigm concepts—nursing and health—describe the profession but are not capable of explaining interventions and outcomes of care. Pendleton continues by stating that just as physicists, for example, are not part of theories of physics, nurses should not be part of the theories intended as building blocks of nursing science. She states that Rogers's theory most nearly parallels the development of theory in other scientific fields.

Chapter 14 was developed by Scalzi and Anderson. These authors perceive nursing administration in terms of a dominant theoretical model from the social sciences—one in which vital, effective organizations are viewed as open biological systems. They conceive of the development of theory for nursing administration in three stages: the single domain, interface, and systems view. In the single domain perspective, nursing alone is the concern; where the single perspective dominates thinking, the goal of the nurse administrator is restricted to the production of quality nursing products. In the interface model, both nursing and organization are domains. The nurse administrator in this perspective is positioned at the interface of the two domains and is confronted with two sets of goals, often in conflict, deriving from the two parts of the system. In the organismic systems model, nursing administration is viewed as a whole—that is, nursing and the organization are viewed as two interdependent domains forming a total entity. In the systems perspective, nurse managers take as their goal both quality care and organizational effectiveness to achieve total system vitality.

Fawcett and graduate students at the University of Pennsylvania wrote Chapter 15, the final chapter in Section I, entitled "Conceptual Models of Nursing and Organization Theories." First the authors describe the central elements of Roy's adaptation model and Neuman's systems model of nursing. They then discuss ways to modify these for nursing administration. The authors take the position that because the theories derived from nursing models have not been sufficiently developed, construction of conceptual-theoretical systems of knowledge for nursing administration must begin with management science. Contingency, role, and marketing theories are cited as examples of theories in management that may be congruent with Roy's and Neuman's theories of nursing.

1

Theoretical Nursing Administration: Today's Challenges, Tomorrow's Bridges

Afaf Ibrahim Meleis
Bonnie Mowinski Jennings

THEORETICAL nursing constitutes the premises on which the domain of nursing is formulated, the concepts that preoccupy members of the discipline, the outcomes that nurses wish to achieve, and the theories that guide nursing research and practice. During the past three decades, nursing theories have evolved from ideals to realities and from dreams to tangible resources. This evolution, however, has not been consistent among all nursing practice specialties.

Nursing administration, for example, has not attended to nursing theory as fundamental to its scientific growth. This is a serious omission because nurse administrators are in positions that determine the parameters of nursing practice and patient care. Nurse administrators are also valuable resources and can contribute to developing theories that represent the nursing domain.

Therefore, the threefold purpose of this chapter is to: (1) briefly review the state of the art of nursing theory; (2) consider the challenges posed by the present relationship between nursing theory and nursing adminis-

tration; and (3) propose the bridges necessary for future advances in the development and use of nursing theory by nurse administrators.

NURSING THEORY: THE STATE OF THE ART

Defining nursing theory has preoccupied nurses for at least two decades. The complexity of definition emanates both from the terms that have been used interchangeably with theory, such as conceptual framework and model, as well as from the focus of the definitions themselves, which range from structure to the domain concepts. Definitions cover the gamut from confirmed hypotheses to a medium by which hypotheses are generated to the utility of theory for practice. To simplify things, nursing theory can be defined as a coherent, communicable articulation and conceptualization of responses to health and illness by human beings in their environments.[1]

Although the purpose of nursing theory is to describe, explain, predict, or prescribe nursing care, it is neither an end result nor an outcome. It is a cyclical, ongoing process that is combined with philosophical premises, practice, results of research, scientific state-

The opinions or assertions in this chapter are the private views of the authors and are not to be construed as official or as reflecting the views of the Department of the Army or the Department of Defense.

ments, experiences, and history. Nursing theory not only guides the development of questions and the formulation of answers, it accommodates the discovery of multiple realities.

As the 1980s stretch toward the end of the decade, it has become more readily accepted that nursing theory is both a means and a goal for nursing knowledge development. Such acceptance is manifested in the renaissance of the nursing theories developed by Nightingale, Johnson, and Travelbee, among others. The numerous educational programs, workshops, courses, and seminars built around nursing theory are additional indicators that theory in nursing has been accepted as central to nursing's development as a discipline. In addition, theoretical nursing has been in the spotlight nationally and internationally; its influence is also visible in publications that address research and practice. Despite its widespread appeal, however, the connections between theoretical nursing and nursing administration are not readily observable.

NURSING THEORY AND NURSING ADMINISTRATION: THE CHALLENGES

Placed in historical perspective, the state of theory development in nursing administration and use of a theoretical nursing perspective by nurse administrators is not dissimilar to conditions found previously in other areas of nursing specialization. Three overriding constraints help to account for the paucity of use and development of nursing theory in nursing administration. These are: (1) the use of nonnursing theories, (2) the education of nurse administrators, and (3) the influence of research in nursing administration.

The Use of Nonnursing Theory

The phenomenon of "what is imported is superior"[1] (p. 44)—or valuing and using theories developed in other disciplines without question—is equally applicable to nursing administration, nursing research, and nursing practice. This phenomenon is expressed in nursing's tradition of looking outside the discipline for frameworks and paradigms to guide practice—of borrowing from other fields. Knowledge development in nursing practice was constrained because of our depending exclusively on theories external to nursing. Development of knowledge for nursing administration has been similarly deterred.

More than 10 years ago, Jacox[2] noted that the theoretical basis of nursing administration was derived largely from other disciplines. A current appraisal of theory in nursing administration indicates that managerial, sociological, and psychological theories are still the dominant frameworks from which nursing administration is practiced. From the literature, it is apparent that nurse administrators use and apply organizational theory,[3] role theory,[4-6] social exchange theory,[7] change theory,[8] social theory,[9] motivational theory,[10] and general systems theory.[11-12]

The current practice of nursing administration is also guided largely by theories used in the business world. Health care is a hugh industry that has taken on an increasingly businesslike demeanor since the early 1980s, when economic developments radically altered the nation's health policy.[13-16] It is therefore not entirely surprising that nurse administrators have turned to business and management models as a basis for their thinking. The use of management by nurse administrators is analogous to the way nurses have used the medical model to shape clinical practice.

But just as the medical model alone is not suited to the clinical practice of nursing, the sole reliance on management and administrative theories from other disciplines is not suitable to the practice of nursing administration. In fact, the service orientation and centrality of human beings to health care organizations have been cited as overriding reasons that preclude the mere transplanting of ideologies from other disciplines to nursing administration.[17–20]

"The nurse managers . . . must . . . synthesize two disciplines—nursing and management"[20] (p. 775). Nurse managers are challenged not only to join knowledge of management with their nursing acumen, but to blend, transform, and balance the two sources of knowledge so as to keep nursing care the focus of their management. Synthesis is not only the critical concept in fusing nursing with management, it is also the critical connection between nursing theory and nursing administration.

A decade ago, Dimond and Slothower[17] asserted that the lack of a firm cognitive base for the practice of nursing administration suggested that "Nursing administration is functioning from an atheoretical (or untested theoretical) base" (p. 3). Although organizational, business, and financial theories are now common to the contemporary practice of nursing administration, a theoretical deficit remains. As Trandel-Korenchuk[21] points out, there are no well-developed theories of nursing administration. This insight is particularly significant when the centrality of theory to science is considered.

Education for Nurse Administrators

The second major constraint faced by nurse administrators in using a theoretical nursing perspective originates from nursing education. Education has been identified as the common denominator of scholarship, with doctoral preparation being the vehicle for socializing individuals into the roles of scientist and scholar.[22–24] Consequently, Gortner[25] suggests that nursing's service heritage stifled the development of an appreciation for what constitutes science. The educational base for nursing has only recently moved into the

university,[26–27] and doctoral education in nursing itself did not appear until the mid-1960s.[28–29]

Although university-based education is becoming the norm for nurses in general and preparation at the graduate level is increasingly common, until 1980 university-based nursing education for nursing administration was limited.[30–33] The thrust to increase clinical knowledge made advanced preparation for practice the rewarded route in graduate education.[20,31–32] Therefore, knowledge for clinical practice grew, while knowledge and scholarly development in nursing administration did not. The impact of these tendencies is vividly reflected in the fact that less than 25% of nurses in administrative positions (i.e., administrators, supervisors, head nurses) have a baccalaureate degree, and less than 1% of nurses in administrative positions have a master's degree in nursing.[34]

The significance of this situation is underscored when one considers that nurse administrators are responsible for the nursing care provided to all patients and families in their respective institutions. Further, nurse administrators must grapple with the recent economic and technologic developments in health-care that pose a multitude of challenges for contemporary nursing practice.[13–16,35–36] Although McClure[31] notes that there are harbingers of improvements in the educational preparation for nurse administrators, it is essential to assess that trend.

Perhaps because nursing was remiss in providing education for administration, many nurses, feeling a need for more knowledge and skills, turned to management programs offered by other disciplines. Because nurse administrators need to be educated in both nursing and management, it is clear that graduate education external to nursing does not foster advanced knowledge of the mother discipline. It is also possible that nonnursing programs promote one's allegiance with management at the expense of the nurse administrator's identity as nurse. It is the identity as nurse that is the source of professionalism; it is the salient identity that unites the discipline.[37]

Another concern surfaces as well. Examining the curricula designed to prepare nurse administrators reveals an absence of education in nursing theory. In two studies that evaluated master's programs in nursing administration, it was apparent that traditional management courses were the prevailing focus of the curricula.[32,38] In fact, Duffy and Gold[38] concluded that nursing and nonnursing master's administration programs prepared graduates at a similar level. However, it was not evident that nursing theory occupied a place in the nursing administration programs.

Although Cleland[39] espouses developing and including nursing theory courses in master's and doctoral programs in nursing, it is not evident that this goal has been reached. Nurse educators may have become so intent on preparing administrators in a managerial sense that the nursing perspective in nursing administration may have been inadvertently omitted. The nursing administration curriculum may have become crowded with management and administrative courses, leaving no room for studying nursing theories. This omission is serious. To reiterate Stevens's[19-20] perspective, the nurse manager must synthesize both nursing and management. This blend and balance may be lacking in programs that prepare nurse administrators.

Research in Nursing Administration

It has been noted that there is a paucity of substantive nursing administration research.[17,33] This dearth of research can be traced to the early 1970s when developing knowledge for nursing practice became a major goal in nursing. As clinical research became the valued pursuit, the study of nursing administration was neglected. According to McClure,[31] "the denigration of the study of nursing administration has taken its toll. . . . [There are] very few individuals who are real scholars, able to develop new knowledge in the area" (p. 69).

It is time to reconsider the place of nursing administration in developing knowledge for the practice of nursing. As already stated, the lack of research specific to nursing administration cannot be excused by pointing to the availability of relevant knowledge from other disciplines. A product-line orientation that is not adjusted for the human beings central to health care will not be as effective for nursing. It is essential to manage nursing's unique problems and rewards by viewing situations and people through nursing's unique spectacles.

Further, according to Gortner,[40] research is a tool of science. While Ziman[41] points to the difficulty of defining science, it can be simplistically viewed as principles, ideas, and empirically derived knowledge. Theory gives order and continuity to science; it enhances meaning, defines nursing's body of knowledge, and directs research and practice.[1,42-44]

It is apparent that theory, practice, and research are inextricably intertwined. Any one part of the triad independent of the other two is diminished in relevance and meaning.[45] Thus, research is needed to develop theory and guide practice; practice helps to develop theory, modify theory, and pose questions for research; and theory guides and influences practice.

The void created by the dearth of nursing administrative research needs to be filled for another reason. Specifically, most nursing practice and patient care occur in institutions. Conway[46] underscores the importance of this condition by adducing that nurse administrators are accountable "to safeguard and extend the specialized knowledge that is nursing to those clients who are in need of it" (p. 30). Conway goes on to emphasize that only nurse administrators can bring a nursing perspective to the organizational management group. Nurse administrators are in a position to establish policy, influence decision making, advance clinical practice, and influence the destiny of nursing.

NURSING ADMINISTRATION VIA THEORETICAL NURSING: THE BRIDGES

Seeing a phenomenon from the perspectives of different disciplines and domains shapes the kinds of research questions asked and the types of answers obtained. A domain also provides a framework for analyzing problems and devising solutions. To confine administrators to the use of organizational, sociological, and psychological theories limits their ability to view the client as central in every administrative situation they encounter.

For example, if health is defined from the perspective of the biomedical domain, then desired outcomes might be limited to the absence of disease or diminution of unwanted symptoms. Such an orientation may dictate a certain period of recovery and time of discharge, according to biomedically oriented parameters. These parameters might differ if the view were one that encompassed individuals as whole persons and included their perceptions of a sense of well-being. This latter view focuses on health, while the former emphasizes disease.[47] Subscribing to a model based on health rather than disease influences the number of staff, the mix of personnel, job descriptions, standards of care, and how quality of care is defined. Such differences may even be reflected in the total organizational goals.

To transcend the gap between nursing theory and nursing administration, bridges can be built to connect theories of the discipline to this specialty. Fundamental to these bridges is the synthesis of a nursing perspective with organizational, financial, psychological, and sociological theories that are relevant to nursing administration. Any perspective alone leaves the nurse administrator with less power than do the views combined. Further, a nursing perspective is central to mobilizing nurse administrators' contributions to a coherent knowledge base that will be useful to the nursing discipline.

There are four general strategies that a nurse administrator might adopt to promote the use of a nursing perspective. These are: (1) creating a culture for theoretical nursing, (2) empowering nurses to use a nursing perspective, (3) valuing and acknowledging nurses' potential contributions to expand knowledge and develop theory, and (4) unifying knowledge common to both nursing practice and nursing administration.

Creating a Culture

Nurse administrators are responsible for the external organizational environment in which employees practice and they are role models for the staff. Therefore, if nurses are expected to use a nursing perspective to guide their practice, and if nurses are expected to use nursing theory and nursing research as the basis for their interventions, then cultural milieu that values science needs to be developed.

A culture consists of values, norms, sanctions, rewards, and behaviors that are shared by a group of people. Nurse administrators are in a position to define and shape the culture that envelops the nurse clinician, the client, and the nurse administrator as well. Cultural values and behaviors are not confined to one situation, to one incident of leadership, or to one event. They are manifested in themes and patterns that cross time and events.[48–50]

A culture that addresses a nursing domain and helps to actualize the use of nursing theory occurs, for example, because the nurse manager considers nursing care outcomes that are patient-focused whenever staffing is discussed. A theoretically sound culture is manifested when the nurse administrator finds opportunities to speak about the central assumptions, concepts, and goals of nursing; when the nurse administrator understands and helps others appreciate the differences between models of clinical excellence in nursing as compared with those in other fields. For example, nursing actions may take more time than medical actions because the technologies nurses use in their practice are different. These include interactions, use of self, and evaluating the whole patient situation rather than focusing solely on presenting problems.[51]

When nurse administrators create a culture that respects, ratifies, and rewards values that emanate from using both the nursing domain and its theories in order to guide action, members of the culture are more likely to adopt such values. To create such cultures, nurse administrators must let nursing values guide their actions in recruiting and hiring nurses, in granting rewards, in developing in-service education, in addressing budgetary needs, and in discussing needs for patient care as well as staffing. Further, nurse administrators can use nursing theory to evaluate patterns in problems, and as a resource for finding resolutions. A culture that respects theoretical nursing exists only when nurse administrators genuinely understand and are thoroughly familiar with linkages between nursing theory, nursing practice, and nursing administration.

Empowering Nurses

As the culture that uses theoretical nursing as the basis for nursing practice evolves, nurse administrators also develop methods for empowering nurses to use nursing theory in their daily work. An impressive accumulation of evidence demonstrates nurse administrators' involvement in implementing nursing theories as frameworks for the delivery of patient care. Along with general guidelines for nursing theory implementation,[52] reports also reflect how various institutions have operationalized models by Johnson,[53–54] Neuman,[55–56] Orem,[57] and Roy.[58]

One indicator of a cultural identity is the use of unique language, symbols, and syntax. The language, symbols, and syntax common to the process of using nursing theories to guide patient care may help to create a theoretical nursing culture. Implementing nursing theory to guide patient-care delivery and clinical nursing practice, however, is not exactly the same as using nursing theory as the basis of nursing administrative practice. Nevertheless, operationalizing and implementing nursing theory indicates that nurse administrators acknowledge the need for theory in the nursing discipline.

Further, nurse administrators' existing familiarity with nursing theory can be used as a catalyst and positive force to help transform nursing theory into a sturdy pylon from which future bridges can be built. Perhaps the challenge for nurse administrators is not only to use nursing theory to guide their administrative practice, but to synthesize it in their work.

In addition to adopting nursing models to guide practice, there are other tactics for empowering nurses to use theories from the nursing domain. First, nursing rounds could be conducted with a focus on the mission of nursing, central concepts of the domain, and nursing theories. These rounds might explore hunches and problems of an administrative nature as well as those that are rooted in clinical challenges. Second, the nurse administrator might articulate and implement standards of practice and role expectations derived from a nursing perspective. For example, change-of-shift report could be guided by a nursing analysis of the patient condition rather than a biomedical approach. This orientation could also be instituted as a standard and framework for nursing notes. A third strategy of empowerment could be for the nurse administrator to argue in favor of staffing resources that enable nurses to focus on human beings and interactions.

In the fourth and final approach to be considered here, clinical and administrative decisions would be expected to reflect nursing theories. Blenner's work, derived from Rogerian theory, provides an exemplar of this tactic in describing how people process environmental stimuli.[59] Blenner's research indicates that people tend to be dominant in one of two processing methods: augmenters are people who are sensitive to stimuli, while reducers dampen stimuli. A patient with a reducer personality will be distressed in situations with limited stimulation, while the augmenter personality may be stressed by excessive input.

Therefore, such theory could be used to direct both patient placement on units as well as the plans for nursing therapeutics. The augmenter in critical care will benefit from a different nursing approach than the reducer in critical care. The same theory may help to account for determining the patient environment that is most congruent with nurses' stimuli-processing methods. Some nurses may thrive in a hectic patient-care arena, while others may be adversely affected by the excessive stimulation. The use of such theory could conceivably provide different explanations and possible solutions for such phenomena as attrition and turnover among nurses.

Valuing Theory Development

Clinical nurses and nurse administrators are not only the reservoirs for theory use, they are also resources for theory development. This duality is essential because theory development and use are dialectically related; one cannot contribute as effectively without the other, to knowledge development. The nature of nursing practice, the intensity of nurses' association with their clients, and the

wisdom they gain from their clinical work could be the genesis for theory development. Acknowledging and valuing the rich potential nurses have to contribute to the growth of nursing knowledge and theory may help them articulate and share their insights and ideas with others. Such an opportunity for exchange is the essence of theory development.

Theory development is a process that involves a variety of techniques, among which are self-reflection, dialoguing with colleagues, collating nursing notes, observing, writing, and presenting.[1,44] The process of theory development is a time-consuming, ongoing activity, but a necessary one for knowledge development. It is also a process that is more suitable to some nurses than others. To demonstrate that this process is valued, nurse administrators may sanction and recognize the role of the nurse in discovering knowledge for patient care.

There is another dimension to valuing theory. Along with encouraging practitioners to develop theory, nurse administrators themselves can contribute to theory development by identifying and developing theory relevant to the phenomena of nursing administration. Many of the phenomena of nursing administration share a heritage with other disciplines; these include power, conflict, decision making, negotiation, communication, and leadership. For nursing administration, however, the phenomena would be developed from the unique perspective of nursing. Power, for example, would not merely be a general sociological concept. From the stance of nursing theory development it would instead be advanced with consideration of not only what power is but how power is used by women and by nurses.

Power is a catalyst, according to Styles,[60] the consequence of which is to bring about desired outcomes.[61] What are the exemplars of effective and ineffective use of power? How do these compare between the genders?

How are the dynamics of power affected when men and women are juxtaposed in their various roles in the health-care system? What are the positive features of power, and how can nurse administrators mobilize them to achieve *nursing's* desired outcomes? These are only a few of the innumerable questions that could be explored by nurse administrators in the process of developing the phenomenon of power into a theory of power in nursing.

In sum, valuing the process of theory development is modeled by nurse administrators in their attempts to build knowledge on which their administrative practice is based. Phenomena unique to clinical practice and nursing administration that require description and explanation form the core of involvement in theory development. Some of the phenomena that are related to both administrative and clinical practice, such as the health of employees, benefit from collaborative attempts between clinicians and administrators to develop theory. This aspect of valuing is further elucidated by the final strategy for promoting the use of a nursing perspective.

Unifying Practice and Administration Through Theory

The domain concepts, which represent the boundaries of the nursing discipline, have traditionally been defined and used in a manner congruent with clinical practice. By refocusing the definitions, nursing's theoretical heritage becomes relevant to administrative practice and knowledge. This adjustment is not as complicated as it initially appears. As Meleis[62] articulates, "nursing phenomena are human phenomena. They represent the experiences of nurses and clients; both are human beings and participants in the health-care system" (p. 12).

An effort at this redefinition has been made by Chaska,[63] who suggests that the concept of person, when extended, includes individuals working in the health-care organization (e.g., nurses); a redefined concept of nursing refers to the practice of administration; a redefined concept of health reflects the organizational state of well-being; and a redefined concept of environment is society. Chaska's vision can be modified slightly. For example, persons could include practitioners as well as clients. In this domain nurse administrators could consider a wide spectrum of issues from evaluating professional practice to assessing job satisfaction and turnover. Nursing, as an administrative domain, would not only refer to the practice of administration but also to actualizing the synthesis of nursing and management acumen.

Health might be redefined to embrace not only the well-being of the organization, but the health of care providers. It is paradoxical that while promoting health and well-being is the goal of health-care organizations, the health of employees may be in jeopardy.[64] The thrust of the occupational stress movement is the deleterious effects of work stress on employee health.[65–66] It is plausible that the work environment, as experienced by nurses, also has an effect on the therapeutic milieu as experienced by patients. The reciprocal effects of worker and organizational health might be addressed as well.

Another possible modification of Chaska's[63] suggestions concerns the environment. Rather than considering the concept of environment only as society at large, environment could be defined in terms of some of its dimensions: macro, micro, internal, and external. For example, the macrodimension of environment might concern the total health-care institution, while the microdimension might focus on a particular nursing unit or the nursing department. Similarly, the dimension of internal environment could embrace the arena in which nursing is practiced, where nurse-client-administrator interactions occur. Administrators can strive to establish the physical, psychological, sociological, and nursing climate that maximizes benefits to all persons and minimizes detrimental effects. The external dimension of the environment might be explored by assessing the effects of prospective payment, federal policies and legislation, and legal matters.

Studies designed to develop knowledge for nursing administration have the particular potential to contribute to nursing-theory development regarding the domain of environment. Nightingale, a visionary nurse administrator par excellence,[27,67–68] recognized the importance of environment to patient care.[69–70] Yet, environment has been studied less extensively than nursings' other domain concepts.[1,71–73] Developing the domain concept of environment through nursing administrative research is an important goal, since nursing administrators are largely responsible for creating the environment in which nursing is practiced.

In addition to extending the definitions of the traditional domain concepts, nursing practice and administration could be unified by another central concept—transition.[1,74] "Role transition denotes a change in role relationships, expectations, or abilities. Role transitions require persons to incorporate new knowledge, alter their behavior, and thus change their definitions of themselves in their social context"[75] (p. 265). The shift from clinician to head nurse fits the description of role transition.

There are many similarities between the transition from clinician to manager[5,76–77] and the transition from inpatient to outpatient roles. Both situations raise a number of relevant questions, typified by the following: How might the transition from clinician to manager be facilitated? What eases the transition? What makes it more difficult? Which is better in the long run—a well-planned transition or one that is initially ambivalent and ambiguous? How does one make the transition from clinician to manager, while still retaining "nurse" or "well person" as the salient identity?

Further, although the concepts of role insufficiency and supplementation were developed to explain potential nursing problems with clients undergoing a transition,[75] the framework is equally relevant to the transition from provider of care to manager of care. As nurses enter the realm of management, they may experience a sense of role insufficiency, or a difficulty in performing the new role. Role supplementation is a nursing therapeutic for preventing or reducing role insufficiency. Developing such concepts could demonstrate their centrality to both clinical and administrative nursing.

Another possible benefit of using the domain concepts to focus administrative nursing practice is that these common referents can help unify nurse clinicians and nurse administrators. In the innumerable studies of stress among nurses, administrators are frequently mentioned as a source of stress. The behavior of nurse administrators tends to be perceived in a somewhat unfavorable light by nurse clinicians because of their obligation to uphold the highest standards of care and base decisions on the needs of the larger organization.

However, some of the tension between nurse administrators and nurse clinicians can be reduced by using nursing theory as a common framework for both. Nurse administrators will always have a management tint to the lenses through which they view their responsibilities. But if the lenses for practice and administration are ground with the correction for nursing, then a sense of unity may begin to prevail.

In conclusion, knowledge unique to the discipline of nursing is beginning to evolve, and the process of nursing-knowledge development is moving at an accelerated speed. Many milestones reflect these achievements—increasing reports of research, presentations, proliferation of scientific nursing journals, scholarly debates, and a growing cadre of nurses prepared at the graduate level. The challenge that continues to confront the discipline is developing theoretical foundations in nursing that can be used as frameworks for nursing research and practice. Nowhere is such a challenge more apparent than in nursing administration.

Clinicians, researchers, and theoreticians have been working diligently to build bridges between practice, research, and theory. The decade of the 1990s is the time to begin building similar bridges between theoretical nursing and nursing administration. As Jennings[78] asserts, "Scientific foundations are equally germane to nurse administrators . . . administrative knowledge should develop in a manner congruent with the rest of the discipline" (p. 67). However, scholars, by definition, are thinkers. Administrators, by necessity, are doers. The contemplation and action involved in these two roles may seem antithetical. In reality, the situation is not unlike the clinicians' milieu, which is also action-oriented. It is no less possible to unite nursing theory and administration than to fuse nursing theory and clinical practice. In both cases, the task is difficult but not impossible. In either case, the patient is the ultimate beneficiary.

REFERENCES

1. Meleis AI. Theoretical nursing: Development and progress. Philadelphia: JB Lippincott, 1985.
2. Jacox A. The research component in the nursing service administration masters program. J Nurs Adm 1974;4(2):35–39.
3. Smith D. Organizational theory and the hospital. J Nurs Adm 1972;2(3):19–24.
4. Carter KA. Managerial role development in the nursing supervisor. Superv Nurse 1980;11(7):26–28.
5. Gambacorta S. Head nurses face reality shock, too! Nurs Manage 1983;14(7):46–48.
6. Hardy ME, Conway ME, eds: Role theory. Perspectives for health professionals. Norwalk, CT: Appleton-Century-Crofts, 1978.
7. Chapman CM. The use of sociological theories and models in nursing. J Adv Nurs 1976;1:111–127.
8. Spicer JG, Lewis EM. Using theory to promote change. Nurs Adm Q 1981;5(2):53–57.
9. Goldstein JR. Nursing stations design using a social theory model. J Nurs Adm 1979;9(4):21–25.
10. Cleland VS. The use of existing theories. Nurs Res 1967;16:118–121.
11. Arndt C, Huckabay LMD. Nursing administration. Theory for practice with a systems approach. St. Louis: CV Mosby, 1980.
12. Gaynor AK, Berry RK. Observations of a staff nurse: An organizational analysis. J Nurs Adm 1973;3(3):43–49.
13. Aiken L. The practice setting: An overview of health policy issues. In: Aiken L, ed. Health policy and nursing practice. New York: McGraw-Hill, 1981, pp. 3–16.
14. Davis CK. The Federal role in changing health care financing: Parl 1. Nurs Economics 1983;1:10–17.
15. Davis CK. The Federal role in changing health care financing: Part 2. Nurs Economics 1983;1:98–104, 146.
16. Shaffer FA. DRG's: History and overview. Nurs Health Care 1983;4:388–396.
17. Dimond M, Slothower L. Research in nursing administration: A neglected issue. Nurs Adm Q 1978;2(4):1–8.
18. McClure ML. The administrative component of the nurse administrator's role. Nurs Adm Q 1979;3(4):1–17.
19. Stevens BJ. Nursing theory. Analysis, application, evaluation. Boston: Little, Brown, 1979, pp. 103–111, 113–127.
20. Stevens BJ. Improving nurses' managerial skills. Nurs Outlook 1979;27:774–777.
21. Trandel-Korenchuk DM. Concept development in nursing research. Nurs Adm Q 1986;11(1):1–9.
22. Armiger B. Scholarship in nursing. Nurs Outlook 1974;22:160–164.
23. May KM, Meleis AI, Winstead-Fry P. Mentorship for scholarliness: Opportunities and dilemmas. Nurs Outlook 1982;30:22–28.
24. Merton RK. The sociology of science. Chicago: University of Chicago Press, 1973, pp. 452–455, 500.
25. Gortner SR. Researchmanship: Structures for research productivity. West J Nurs Res 1982;4:119–123.
26. Nahm HE. History of nursing—a century of change. In: McCloskey JC, Grace HK, eds. Current issues in nursing. Boston: Blackwell Scientific Publications Inc, 1981, pp. 14–26.
27. Palmer IS. From whence we came. In: Chaska N, ed. The nursing profession. A time to speak. New York: McGraw-Hill, 1983, pp. 3–28.
28. Grace HK. The development of doctoral education in nursing: In historical perspective. J Nurs Educ 1978;17:17–27.
29. Matarazzo JD, Abdellah FG. Doctoral education for nurses in the United States. Nurs Res 1971;20:404–414.
30. Blair E. Needed: Nursing administration leaders. Nurs Outlook 1976;24:550–558.

31. McClure ML. Promoting practice-based research: A critical need. J Nurs Adm 1981;11(11, 12):66–70.
32. Price SA. Master's programs preparing nursing administrators? What are the essential components? J Nurs Adm 1984;14(1):11–17.
33. Stevens BJ. Education in nursing administration. Superv Nurse 1977;8(3):19–23.
34. American Nurses' Association. Facts about nursing 84–85. Kansas City, MO: American Nurses' Association, 1984/85, p. 27.
35. Naisbitt J, Elkins J. The hospital and megatrends. Hosp Forum 1983;26(3):9, 11–12, 17.
36. Naisbitt J, Elkins J. Part 2. The hospital and megatrends. Hosp Forum 1983;26(4):52–56.
37. Jennings BM, Rogers S. Merging research and practice: A case of multiple identities. J Advanced Nurs (in press)
38. Duffy ME, Gold NE. Education for nursing administration: What investment yields highest returns? J Nurs Adm 1980;10(9):31–38.
39. Cleland V. An articulated model for preparing nursing administrators. J Nurs Adm 1984;14(10):23–31.
40. Gortner SR. Nursing science in transition. Nurs Res 1980;29:180–183.
41. Ziman J. What is science? In: Klemke ED, Hollinger R, Kline AD, eds. Introductory readings in the philosophy of science. Buffalo, NY: Prometheus Books, 1980, pp. 35–54.
42. Chinn PL Jacobs MK. Theory and nursing. A systematic approach. St. Louis: CV Mosby, 1983, pp. 2–12.
43. Menke EM. Critical analysis of theory development in nursing. In: Chaska N, ed. The nursing profession. A time to speak. New York: McGraw-Hill, 1983, pp. 416–426.
44. Walker LO, Avant KC. Strategies for theory construction in nursing. Norwalk, CT: Appleton-Century-Crofts, 1983.
45. Fawcett J. A declaration of nursing independence: The relation of theory and research to nursing practice. J Nurs Adm 1980;10(6):36–39.
46. Conway ME. Knowledge generation and transmission: A role for the nurse administrator. Nurs Adm Q 1979;3(4):29–44.
47. Shaver JF. A biophysical view of human health. Nurs Outlook 1985;33:186–191.
48. Deal T, Kennedy A. Corporate cultures. Menlo Park, CA: Addison Wesley, 1982, pp. 3–36.
49. Ouchi W, Price R. Hierarchies, clans, and theory Z: A new perspective on organization development. In: Hackman J, Lawler E, Porter L, eds. Perspectives on behavior in organizations. New York: McGraw-Hill, 1983, pp. 564–577.
50. Peters T, Waterman R. In search of excellence. New York: Harper & Row, 1983, pp. 279–291.
51. Masson V. Nurses and doctors as healers. Nurs Outlook 1985;33:70–73.
52. Capers CF. Using nursing models to guide nursing practice: Key questions. J Nurs Adm 1986;16(11):40–43.
53. Auger JA, Dee V. A patient classification system based on the behavioral systems model of nursing: Part 1. J Nurs Adm 1983;13(4):38–43.
54. Dee V, Auger JA. A patient classification system based on the behavioral systems model of nursing. Part 2. J Nurs Adm 1983;13(5):18–23.
55. Capers CF, O'Brien C, Quinn R, Kelly R, Fenerty A. The Neuman systems model in practice. Planning phase. J Nurs Adm 1985;15(5):29–38.
56. Ross MM, Bourbonnais FF. The Betty Neuman systems model in nursing practice: A case study approach. J Adv Nurs 1985;10:199–207.
57. Anna DT, Christensen DG, Hohon SA, Ord L, Wells SR. Implementing Orem's conceptual framework. J Nurs Adm 1978;8(11):8–11.
58. Mastal MF, Hammond H, Roberts MP. Theory into hospital practice: A pilot implementation. J Nurs Adm 1982;12(6):9–15.
59. Two researchers awarded grants. Calif Nurse 1987;83(2):12.
60. Styles MM. On nursing: Toward a new endowment. St. Louis: CV Mosby, 1982, pp. 213–223.
61. Salancik GR, Pfeffer J. Who gets power—and how they hold onto it: A strategic contingency model of power. In: Hackman J, Lawler E, Porter L, eds. Perspectives on behavior in organizations. New York: McGraw-Hill, 1983, pp. 417–429.
62. Meleis AI. Theory development and domain concepts. In: Moccia P, ed. New approaches to theory development. New York: NLN Pub. No. 15-992, 1986, pp. 3–21.
63. Chaska N. Theories of nursing and organizations: Generating integrated models for administrative practice. In: Chaska N, ed. The nursing profession. A time to speak. New York: McGraw-Hill, 1983, pp. 720–730.
64. Jennings BM. Social support: A way to a climate of caring. Nurs Adm Q 1987;11(4):63–71.
65. Holt RR. Occupational stress. In: Goldberger L, Breznitz S, eds. Handbook of stress. Theoretical and clinical aspects. New York: The Free Press, 1982, pp. 419–444.
66. Pelletier KR. Healthy people in unhealthy places. New York: Delacorte Press, 1984.
67. Dennis KE, Prescott PA. Florence Nightingale: Yesterday, today, and tomorrow. ANS 1985;7(2):66–81.
68. Parker P. Florence Nightingale: First lady of administrative nursing. Superv Nurse 1977;8(3):24–25.
69. Nightingale F. Notes on nursing. What it is, and what it is not. New York: Dover Publications, Inc, 1860/1969.
70. Torres G. Florence Nightingale. In: George JB, Chairperson, the nursing theories conference group. Nursing theories. The base for professional nursing practice. Englewood Cliffs, NJ: Prentice-Hall, 1980, pp. 27–38.
71. Chopoorian TJ. Reconceptualizing the environment. In: Moccia P, ed. New approaches to theory development. New York: NLN Pub. No. 15-1992, 1986, pp. 39–54.
72. Flaskerud JH, Halloran EJ. Areas of agreement in nursing theory development. ANS 1980;3(1):1–7.

73. Kim HS. The nature of theoretical nursing. Norwalk, CT: Appleton-Century-Crofts, 1983. pp. 79–115.
74. Chick N, Meleis AI. Transitions: A nursing concern. In: Chinn PL, ed. Nursing research methodology. Issues and implementation. Rockville, MD: Aspen, 1986, pp. 237–257.
75. Meleis AI. Role insufficiency and role supplementation: A conceptual framework. Nurs Res 1975;24: 264–271.
76. Darling LW, McGrath LG. The causes and costs of promotion trauma. J Nurs Adm 1983;13(4):29–33.
77. Dooley SL, Hauben J. From staff nurse to head nurse: A trying transition. J Nurs Adm 1979;9(4): 4–7.
78. Jennings BM. Nursing theory development: Successes and challenges. J Adv Nurs 1987;12:63–69.

2

Cultural Care Theory and Nursing Administration

Madeleine M. Leininger

DURING the past three decades, several theorists, researchers, and scholars in the field of nursing have actively developed and systematically examined nursing's distinct domains of knowledge. A number of conceptual and theoretical perspectives have become evident with different research paradigms to explicate the phenomena of nursing. These developments have been encouraging, as nursing delineates what constitutes its distinct focus to guide nursing education and practice. It has been a challenge to explicate nursing knowledge because of the complex and embedded ideas that characterize it, but also because of different theoretical interests and positions taken by nurses of what constitutes nursing's unique perspective as a discipline and profession.

Unquestionably, there is no right or wrong theory of nursing; rather, there are theories that have a lesser or greater potential to explain, describe, interpret, and predict nursing from a local to a worldwide, or universal perspective. It is academically and theoretically healthy to see nurses deliberate about different theories and concepts and not close the door to theories that show some of the greatest potential to explain nursing, especially worldwide. It is therefore encouraging to see different theories systematically examined or tested to determine what characterizes the essence of nursing.

Some nurses have already been "fixed on" a few concepts, such as man (or person), health, environment, and nursing as the central concepts of the metaparadigm of nursing.[1] As I have stated in other publications, these four concepts need to be reconsidered because of their major limitations as central or unique to nursing.[2-3] There are several major limitations of these four concepts. First, *man* as a generic concept is not distinct to nursing, as practically all humanistic and scientific fields focus on generic man. Moreover, some disciplines, such as anthropology, have been involved in studying man intensively and extensively through time and place for more than a century. Second, one cannot use *nursing* as a distinct concept and then attempt to *explain* the same phenomenon by the same term. Third, *environment* and *health* have possibilities for explaining nursing, but further refinements and more specificity are needed to show nursing's unique focus, in contrast with other disciplines, that claims these concepts as central to the field. Currently, very few nurses have been doctorally prepared in the environmental sciences, such as ecology or geography and human environments, and other similar fields in which environmental scientists integrate these dimensions with social, cultural, and ecological environmental data. While some nurses have demonstrated a historical interest in health since the Nightingale era, most nurses have not focused in depth on health *per se*, but rather on medical illnesses, diseases, and disabilities. Granted, more nurses are interested in and are studying health today, as central to nursing, but much knowledge based on research is needed to establish the epistemological base of health as unique to nursing.

The most neglected and most central historic concept in nursing is "human care." This concept, I hold, is what has made nursing distinct since its beginning, and will continue into the future if nurses study it in depth and systematically. Interestingly, the public has viewed nursing with care acts and decisions for many years. Care is, indeed, the essence of, and the major concept to explain nursing. As I have stated in several works, care is *the unique, dominant, and unifying factor of nursing*, and the most powerful concept for explaining, interpreting, and predicting nursing outcomes.[4–7] Care as a noun is the phenomenon to be explained; caring is the action component.

It is ironic that so many nurse-scholars and theoreticians have not considered care to be the central concept or phenomenon of nursing until the author focused on the concept in the early 1960s. Several resistance factors have been identified in publications.[8–9] With my theory of "Cultural Care Diversity and Universality," which began to be developed in the late 1950s, the concept of care and transcultural care became meaningful to nurses. Transcultural care is now seen as an important and essential domain of study. Earlier resistance, to study and theorize about care as the unique and central concept of nursing, was characterized by such statements by nurses as, "Care is too soft and insignificant to explain nursing"; "Care is 'too female' and is a demeaning concept to nursing"; "Care has no power for nurses to explain nursing"; and "Care is only an action or task concept and not a phenomenon to explain nursing"[10] (pp. 13, 14, 16). Conceptualization and systematic study of care has been evident in the work of care theorists such as Gaut, Reiman, Roy, Leininger, Watson, Gardner and other participants in the National Research Care Conference. These nurse theorists and research-

ers are making care visible as a central and distinct concept of nursing.[11–13] Nurses have often used care as a cliché; today it is a major concept to be fully studied, known, valued and used in client care, and in administrative practices. Nurses are now discovering how much there is to know about human care as the epistemological and ontological base of nursing knowledge and practice.

In this chapter, I will present my "Cultural Care Diversity and Universality" theory of nursing and discuss its relevance and usefulness to academic and clinical nursing administration. The importance of administrative care from a comparative cultural stance is a new area of study and practice for many nurse administrators.

RATIONALE FOR CARE THEORY IN NURSING ADMINISTRATION

Before presenting the theory, a few preliminary reasons for focusing on care theory in nursing administration and from the viewpoint of cultural diversity and universality, will be highlighted.

First, our world of nursing is multicultural and administrators must accommodate to diverse needs and patterns of people. Nurse administrators in education and service are faced with the growing importance to understand and work effectively with people of different cultures within and outside their countries. Likewise, administrative structures, functions, and processes need both to reflect changes to accommodate diversity and to consider the universal features and components of administration. The importance for nurse administrators to make their practices *fit with* changing cultural values, beliefs, and lifeways in their own country, and to articulate these changes with worldwide nursing services is a major challenge for nurses today, and will be a greater challenge in the future. If nursing service and education are to be relevant, effective, and satisfying to the diverse people nurses serve, then nurse administrators need to give far more thought to the idea of cultural diversity and universal aspects of nursing administration. Most important, nurse administrators need a theory (or several theories) to conceptualize their administrative activities and systematically study outcomes. My theory offers an important means to achieve this goal.[14]

Second, as diverse cultural systems are recognized with their varying values and practices worldwide, nurse administrators will no longer be able to think and function from a *unicultural* perspective. The needs of clients, staff, and students in different institutions, cultures, and subcultures will require that nursing education and service change. In 1987, it is estimated that less than 50% of all cultural minorities in the United States receive nursing care services; this is especially true for mental health services.[15] In many USA schools of nursing, the population tends to be more unicultural (Anglo-American) than multicultural, but changes must occur as minorities enroll from many different cultures. More thought should be given to ways to attract and retain clients, clinical staff, and students from many diverse cultures and subcultures in our institutions. New administrative structures, values, and processes that support and enrich multicultural realities in which nursing exists are needed. Individuals, families, or groups from diverse cultures are often neglected or avoided in nursing service and education, mainly because most administrative philosophies have failed to address cultural diversity, except as problems or for minority representation. Misunderstanding, ineffective communication, cultural shock, and cultural imposition of practices can reduce the desire for clients, staff, faculty, and students to enter our service or educational systems. Moreover, the high costs of nursing service and education limit future enriching experiences for culturally diverse people. The theory of cultural care diversity and universality provides a means to identify and study such factors, and then to develop appropriate nursing administration goals and action plans to accommodate human diversities.

Third, nurse administrators need to consider role differentiation and gender value differences in future organizational structures and functions as they apply to a worldwide different cultural values in nursing. Recognition of these differences is essential for effective future administrative practices and for program development, implementation, and evaluation. In clinical settings, more and more nurses from unknown cultures will be providing care to clients in the future. Nurse administrators and clinicians will need to know the cultural values, beliefs, and practices of nurses and clients to ensure safe, quality care. Nurses from Egypt, Iraq, the Philippines, Mexico, China, Japan, Korea, and virtually every nation in the world will be giving care to clients, not only in their own countries, but throughout the world. Differences in gender and role expectations and differences in values and in expressions of beliefs will affect nursing practices and the quality of care given. Cultural stresses and conflicts between nursing staff and clients are already evident; discord will become more evident by the year 2000. Nurse administrators, therefore, will need to know, understand, and plan for these changes in their administrative plans and structures to reduce interstaff conflicts and problems related to client care, and improve multicultural employee care services.

In nursing education, deans, associate deans, and other administrators will be faced with similar problems. They must realize that different teaching and learning methods and theories will be essential to understand and help students from different cultures. Faculty and staff problems related to multicultural differences in students' values and lifeways are already a major factor in faculty and student shortage and satisfaction. Administrative organizational structures with a caring ethos are needed to establish schools of nursing to help students and faculty deal with differences in cultural values and practices. As of 1987, there have been virtually no studies in nursing education and service to vestige changing values, role and gender differences from a transcultural administrative perspective. Far more culture-specific services to staff, clients, and others appear to be needed to reduce nurse turnover in service and educational settings. Moreover, the cultures of nursing education and service have not been limitedly studied, yet these cultures influence organizational structures and management modes in decision-making and care practices. Since 1970, I provided a beginning for the study of the culture of nursing and leadership styles.[16-17] My theory of cultural care diversity and universality can provide or stimulate further knowledge in this area related to role management, cultural structures and multicultural organization practices in nursing education and clinical services. It should stimulate new ways to deal with current administrative concerns.

Fourth, my theory has great possibilities for examining different types of professional and academic administrative organizations. There is a cultural movement to develop alternatives to traditional bureaucratic structures that are congruent with a greater variety of social structures, world views, values, and environmental contexts.[18] Assessing differences and similarities among organizational structures and their functions is essential to render quality nursing services. What types of organizational structures are most effective to achieve desired goals? What are the major characteristics of alternative and traditional nursing organizational structures? How are organizations similar or different in their cultural values, practices, and effectiveness? What are the strengths and limitations

of the various types of organizations that could successfully advance nursing education and services worldwide?

There is evidence that nursing faculty favor a *collegial type of academic administrative organization* in contrast to the traditional *rational-legal bureaucratic organization. Collegial* type refers to participatory management decisions and actions made in a spirit of collegial respect with participants who are informed on the subject; whereas *rational legal bureaucratic* type refers to decisions and actions that tend to be coercive, and are mandated from legal or rational stances. Most hospitals and clinics, however, tend to be tightly bound to the more bureaucratic structure due to medical historical dominance, and political and economic pressures. As nurses increasingly move between academic and clinical settings, they become dissatisfied with nondemocratic or bureaucratic structures; they are often unable to recognize and understand existing structures and how to change them. More and more professional nurses need autonomy in order to establish nursing as a discipline and profession, and to regulate and control professional affairs. Tightly controlled bureaucratic organizations in education or service settings limit nurses' abilities to achieve these goals. More collegial rather than legal-bureaucratic organizations are needed for the new culture of nursing administration.

According to the author's observations and experiences in five major academic institutions over the past three decades, rational-legal bureaucratic types of organizations prevail. Faculty in progressive schools and service institutions, however, are seeking collegial and other alternative types of organizations. Since nursing education has moved into institutions of higher learning, this trend has been evident. But there are education and service administrators who value functioning with the cult of efficiency using rational-legal bureaucratic style and fail to value collegial administration. This has led to dissatisfactions with employees, frustration, and resignations by nurses with doctoral preparation who value democratic collegial work relations. In nursing service, professionals prepared in alternative democratic types of organizations are quick to express their dissatisfaction with an administrator whose philosophy, leadership style, and organization are oppressive or too controlling. In both nursing service and education, there have been very few alternative organizational models that accommodate cultural differences in management, human needs and conditions. In anthropology, ethnoadministrative models that accommodate different corporate and business groups as cultural values have been studied since the 1930s.

The theory of cultural diversity and universality can be used to study different types of organizational structures in education and nursing service to fulfill nursing needs, conditions and interests of faculty, students, clinical staff and clients. Similarities and differences in new culturally based organizations are providing promising directions for nursing's future. The cultural perspective can be used to assess the current "unification model" of organizational fit with nursing education and service in accommodating culturally diverse needs and values of people, in similar and different organizational structures.

A related and extremely relevant area that merits immediate study is the growing trend toward the *corporatization of nursing education and health care services*. What are the actual or potential benefits, the differences and similarities between corporate and noncorporate cultural nursing systems? How do nursing systems interface and function with larger organizations? Comparative studies of corporate cultural nursing systems as independent or interfacing systems could yield valuable data. Such studies might well prevent unfa-

vorable short- and long-term organizational consequences. I predict an increase in corporate structures in institutions of higher education for nursing and in all universities in the next decade that will be modeled after business management rather than academic goals. What will be the effect of these corporate structures on the quality of nursing education?

Unquestionably, nursing schools and services will merge with larger educational institutions in the very near future for economic and other reasons. What types of nursing organizational structures will be congruent with parent and larger institutions? Culturally congruent structures with similar philosophies may have a better chance of surviving than those with highly dissimilar philosophies and modes of functioning based on political and economic factors.

In general, nursing is entering a new and challenging era, not only in our country, but worldwide. Nursing will need to deal directly and knowledgeably with diverse cultures and institutions to establish itself as a relevant and viable profession and discipline. Nurse administrators will find the theory of diversity and universality helpful to study different organizations and to think openly, and comparatively about different societies and cultural systems. Unquestionably, nursing administrators must be futuristic and think about ways to develop alternative types of administrative structures with concomitant functions that may change over time to meet society needs and conditions. Most assuredly, the cultures of nursing service and education need to be studied from a theoretical perspective. The theory of cultural care diversity and universality provides one of the broadest and most relevant frameworks for such investigations because it focuses on the central essence of nursing and is a worldwide theory. Let us now turn to some essentials of the theory.

AN OVERVIEW: THEORY OF CULTURAL CARE DIVERSITY AND UNIVERSALITY

There are different ways to define, construct, and systematically examine (or test) theories. I have defined *theory* as a creative and systematic means to describe, interpret, and explain a domain(s) of inquiry, or some phenomenon under consideration, in order to gain new insights, different viewpoints, or acquire substantive knowledge about the domain or phenomenon under study. A theory can range from describing, to explaining, or interpreting a concrete or abstract idea or phenomenon. Most theories, to be viable over time need to be grounded in concepts that are congruent with cultural and social realities. Even the most abstract theory needs to have some reality. In general, theories are directed toward explaining, interpreting, and predicting phenomena that may often be vague, imprecise, or limited ways. Theories are never complete. But often theorists seek to understand some phenomena as fully and widely as possible in order to increase or expand explanatory knowledge about the subject, or to substantiate a position. Nursing theories have this characteristic plus others, depending on the interests and experiences of the theorists.

My theory holds that there are cultural care diversities and universalities of human care and nursing care among all cultures in the world, and these differences and similarities of generic care provide the epistemological and ontological explanations for establishing a body of nursing care knowledge and practices. I have further theorized that if nurses know the cultural meanings, patterns, expressions, structure, and functions of human care among different cultures in the world, they can explain, interpret, and predict the activities and outcomes of generic care and provide desired professional nursing-care that is congruent with individual, family, community, or societal needs. I have also predicted that shared meanings of care patterns, and lived-through experiences are related to transcultural explanations of worldview, social structure, cultural values, beliefs, language, and the environment of human beings.[19–20] Based upon my anthropological and ethnonursing research experiences, I predicted that most generic care values and expressions are embedded in, or are an integral part of social structures, cultural values, and worldviews which nurse researchers need to study as ethnographic dimensions of specific cultures to obtain accurate and reliable care findings.

The theory of cultural care diversity and universality is based on the central assumption and belief that human care is the essence of nursing and the distinctive component that differentiates nursing contributions to humanity from other disciplines or professions. My theory has an anthropological base in that all homo sapiens are born, live, and die within the context of particular cultural worldviews, cultural values, and social structure contexts, which give meaning and relevance to care. Accordingly, human care is part of the cultural context of humans and must be studied to discover the way cultures express, know, give meaning to, and practice care. In order to determine what is universal or different about human care, nurses need to study various cultures in depth, and then use this knowledge to help clients in times of health, illness, and death. I contend that a transcultural approach is essential to provide professional nursing care that is culturally congruent to clients. It supports the maintenance of health or well-being, supports recovery, and provides meaningful living and dying experiences for individuals, families, and groups from diverse or similar cultures. Thus, nurses need to know and understand different cultures to gain a comparative nursing perspective on what constitutes meaningful and satisfying care. If nurses discover the shared meanings, values, beliefs, and practices of different cultures, then they will be able to identify ways to provide culturally congruent care. I also predict that if care is fully known and understood, one will discover the meaning of health or well being. Moreover, by focusing on the phenomenon of care transculturally, nurses will have a sound and reliable foundation for establishing nursing care knowledge and practice. Most important, I contend that knowledge of care derived from diverse cultures provides the broadest epistemological and ontological basis for knowing the essence, nature, and characteristics of care worldwide. From this knowledge, one will not only serve people in culture-specific ways, but he or she will also understand institutions—such as hospitals, clinics, and other agencies—as cultural institutions with their own unique care values, norms, and practices. Thus, one can predict the health of an institution by its care beliefs, values, and practices. I also predict that there are variations among folk and professional health systems that influence human care processes and administrative structures and functions.

Finally, according to my theory, I predict that three intervention modes guide nursing care decisions, judgments, and actions and that these modes are based on social structures, cultural values, worldviews, environmental factors, folk and professional care systems. The three intervention modes are: (1) cultural care maintenance or preservation; (2) cultural care accommodation or negotiation; and (3) cultural care repatterning or restructuring.[15] A data base to guide these interventions will be developed after identifying and establishing cultural care knowledge from the above dimensions.

The purpose of my cultural care theory is to describe, interpret, explain, and predict the diversity and universality of the meanings, processes, and structures of human care to determine what is universal and nonuni-

versal about human care, in order to guide effective and satisfying nursing practices. The ultimate goal of the theory is to provide culturally congruent care that is acceptable, meaningful, and satisfying to individuals, families, communities, and institutions so that health or well being will be promoted, and to facilitate healing and recovery through professional nursing practices. From an institutional perspective, it provides a theoretical framework to study how institutions use, interpret, and predict goals that fit with the communities they serve. The theory can be used to get an institutional view to study how individuals, families, groups, cultures, and institutions reflect care values, norms, and practices that fit with social structure and other structural elements of the theory. Findings from the theory will be essential to guide nursing administration decisions and actions, and to assess care outcomes from the three modes of intervention.

Cultural care theory is derived from both anthropology and nursing, and is based on my 35 years of research, education, and clinical experiences in the two disciplines, and with many different cultures worldwide. The theory has been developed, refined, and used over a period of twenty-five years using mainly ethnography, ethnoscience, and ethnonursing research methods to study care and nursing phenomena. It was also influenced by social scientists' thinking and research in the construction of this complex, holistic, and culturally based theory of nursing care to fit nursing's distinct perspective. Particularly important were the writings of anthropologists Spradley and Malinowski on ethnographic work, and Geertz on interpretive analysis of cultural values, experiences, symbols, and other cultural media.[21–23] I used Pikes's ideas of *emic* (local viewpoints) and *etic* (outsider viewpoints) linguistic terms for naturalistic studies of ethnocare and ethnohealth; but I always added life experiences of the people I studied as essential to the ethnonursing method.[24] The ideas of Redfield, the originator of the worldview concept in anthropology, also influenced my theory.[25] From these scholars and creative thinking I formulated ideas relevant to nursing and a model to depict the essential components of care phenomena.

During the past decade, dialogue and research findings generated in studies by several nurses studying the phenomenon of care have provided findings to support and refine my theory. Drs. Gaut, nurse-philosopher; Watson, nurse-phenomenologist; Aamodt, nurse-anthropologist; as well as many students have provided invaluable related care insights.[26–27] The National Research Care Conferences, held annually since 1976, have been valuable in refining and further developing the theory. The development of the Sunrise visual-conceptual model has been most helpful to those using the theory.

PROPOSITIONAL ASSUMPTIONS OF THE THEORY

The following propositional assumptions are used in the care theory:

1. Care is essential for human growth, development, survival, and facing death.
2. Universal and diverse concepts, forms, expressions, patterns, and processes of human care exist among all cultures in the world.
3. Care is the essence of nursing and the distinct, dominant, and unifying component of nursing as a profession and discipline.
4. Care is essential to curing processes; there can be no curing without caring.
5. All human cultures have folk and professional care values, beliefs, and practices that influence human care practices.
6. Cultural care values and patterns

differ in Western and nonWestern societies.
7. Every nursing situation or event is transcultural which needs to be identified and understood to provide meaningful and congruent care decisions and actions.
8. Generic and professional care are essential as effective healing and caring forces to promote health and well-being.
9. Culturally based care can reduce cultural conflicts, stresses, and problems.
10. Nursing is a culture with its own cultural care values that influences caregiving and care-receiving behaviors.

Definition of Key Terms Used in the Theory

In the development of the theory, the following terms and their definitions were used.[28]

1. *Culture* refers to the shared values, beliefs, norms, and lifeway practices of a particular group that are learned, used, and transmitted, and which guides individual and group thinking, decisions, and actions in patterned ways.
2. *Care* (noun) refers to abstracted behaviors or *phenomena* that reflect assistive, supportive, or facilitative expressions toward or for another individual or group to ameliorate or improve a human condition or lifeway. *Caring* (verb) refers to *actions* that are assistive, supportive or facilitative toward or for another individual or group with evident or anticipated needs to ameliorate or improve a human condition or lifeway.
3. *Cultural Values* refers to the highly desired or preferred ways of acting or thinking that are retained over time and that govern actions and decisions within a given culture or subculture.

4. *Cultural Care Diversity* refers to the variability of meanings, patterns, values, or symbols of care that are culturally derived and shared to improve or ameliorate a human condition or lifeway.
5. *Cultural Care Universality* refers to similar, common, or more uniform meanings, patterns, values, or symbols of care that are culturally derived and shared to improve or ameliorate a human condition or lifeway.
6. *World View* refers to the way people view or look at their world (or the universe) to form a picture or value stance as their perspective of life.
7. *Social Structure* refers to the different structural (or organizational) elements of a society (or culture) such as religion, kinship, political, economic, educational, technologic, and cultural dimensions that give order, meaning and constancy to people, and yet are dynamic and change over time.
8. *Folk Context* refers to the traditional nonprofessional, local, or indigenous services that provides home remedies or folk-care (or -cure) services to people.
9. *Professional Context* refers to the organized care (or cure) services that are offered by health personnel who have been formally prepared in a professional field or area.
10. *Cultural Care Preservation (or Maintenance)* refers to those culturally congruent, assistive, facilitative, or enabling ways to help individuals or groups retain or maintain a healthy, favorable, or satisfying lifeway.
11. *Cultural Care Accommodation (or Negotiation)* refers to those culturally congruent, assistive, facilitative, accommodating, or negotiable ways that help individuals or groups adapt to, adjust to, or cope with a health condition in a

favorable, beneficial, or satisfying lifeway.
12. *Cultural Care Repatterning* (or restructuring) refers to those culturally congruent ways that reflect ways in which an individual's or group's lifeway(s) have been significantly changed or altered so that a beneficial, favorable, or satisfying health pattern can be established.
13. *Cultural Care Congruence* refers to a meaningful fit or a similarity in correspondence with the care patterns, values, or lifeways between or among individuals, groups, or institutions to support beneficial outcomes.
14. *Cultural Context* refers to the *totality* of a particular situation, event, or designated lifeway that gives meaning to the people involved because of the inherent values, symbols, language, expressions, social structure, physical environment, and other factors known and recognized in the setting or situation.
15. *Health* refers to a state of *well-being* that is culturally defined, valued, and practiced, and reflects the ability of individuals (or groups) to perform their daily role activities in a culturally satisfying way.

THE CONCEPTUAL AND THEORETICAL SUNRISE MODEL

While conceptualizing and theorizing about cultural care, the Sunrise Model in Figure 2.1 was developed and refined.[29,30] The Sunrise Model symbolizes the "rising of the sun" to represent care as "light to the world" and to present culture care as a full and total perspective of the essense of nursing. As one can see from the model, several factors have the potential to influence human care and health (or well being). In this visual model, the arrows are used to show influences, and indicate the multiple forces influencing care of individuals, families, groups and institutions

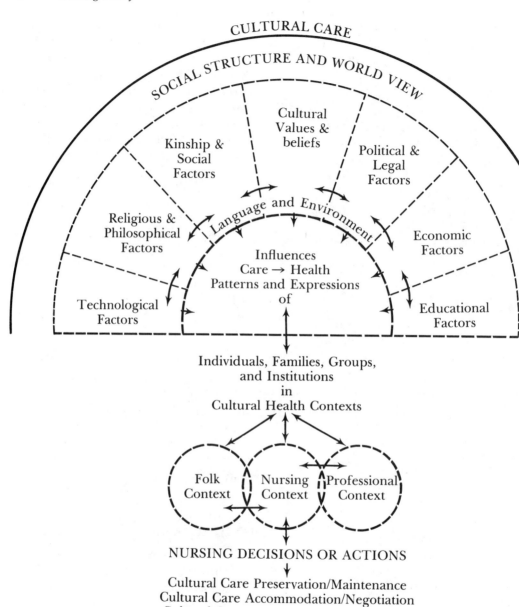

Figure 2.1 Leininger Sunrise Model of Cultural Care Diversity and Universality. Arrows indicate influence.

of diverse cultural backgrounds. The upper part of the model shows the world view and social structure (religious, political, economic, kinship, education, technology, and cultural values) as important components to be systematically examined through the language and environmental context of the people under study.

In the lower part of the Sunrise Model, the folk and professional contexts are depicted in which nursing is a large part of the professional context. Individuals, families, and groups are influenced by these health contexts which need to be examined to determine appropriate nursing decisions and actions that would provide congruent care to clients in institutions.

From a systematic analysis of all the components depicted in the model—from social structure and world view, to folk and professional contexts through the language and environment, one can arrive at cultural congruent nursing care decisions and actions that are satisfying and meaningful to the individual or group which reflect decisions as: (1) cultural care preservation or maintenance; (2) cultural care accommodation or negotiation; and (3) cultural care repatterning or restructuring.[30] While it is also possible to study particular components of theory in relation to care, one needs to consider the total dimensions or components of the theory to get a full and comprehensive picture. In some cultures, aspects of the social structure factors receive more emphasis than in other cultures, which is an interesting discovery in itself. For example, the Gadsup people of New Guinea (whom I studied for nearly two years) emphasized their kinship, religious and cultural values, but not technology nor education.

The researcher may use the qualitative or quantitative paradigms to study the theory. I have used primarily the qualitative paradigm in order to study inductively cultural care aspects as they have been largely unknown to

nurses worldwide. I also used ethnography and ethnonursing methods with an *emic* focus with the theory with fifteen cultures since 1960. Ethnomethods (or people-centered focus) is extremely valuable to obtain grounded data *directly* from people about care. The results from the use of theory and model have been highly rewarding; I have identified 84 care constructs from the cultures studied. Moreover, a wealth of substantive data have been obtained from informants who have provided many new insights about the meaning, forms and expressions of care and health in different folk and professional contexts. Differences and similarities among cultures have been identified. The results are presented in other publications which the reader may want to review.[32,33]

Of special significance is the fact that there are no universal or worldwide ethnocare concepts, but there are some recurrent care concepts such as (1) concern for, (2) attention to, (3) respect for, and (4) helping. More diversity in human care forms, meanings, processes and uses was found than universalities or similarities. Interestingly, the critical care concepts that have been identified in specific cultures were not known to nurses. Thus, many individuals and families have not received professional care that fits with their cultural care values, beliefs and lifeways. By not using culture specific care, one can predict (and often see) cultural conflicts, dissatisfaction, and sometimes resistance to nursing care practices, especially where major differences exist between the client and professional nurses' values. Readers interested in more of the specific care findings are referred to other publications as cited in the references.

To date, the theory and ethnomethods have been limitedly used to study specifically administrative care constructs in different nursing contexts except by the theorist. Thus there are great opportunities to use this theory in the future. Let us turn to some of the potential uses of the theory for ethnoadministrative studies in this last section.

AREAS OF INQUIRY AND RESEARCH QUESTIONS FOR NURSING SERVICE AND EDUCATION ADMINISTRATORS

In considering the use of my theory of cultural care, a number of inquiry care areas and research questions can be offered, especially with thought to Western and non-Western cultures. These questions should stimulate the nurse administrator to explore what is universal or non-universal about nursing administration with a care perspective, and to consider ways to generate theoretical statements related to comparative ethnoadministration. Research findings from the questions could well provide some new and different perspectives about nursing care administration. The use of qualitative research methods such as ethnography, ethnonursing, audio-visuals, and oral life histories are recommended to document, describe and interpret vague and unknown aspects of care. A search for in-depth meanings and comparative data should bring some promising data not yet known nor being investigated by nurse administrators.

A. **Research Queries for Nursing Service Administrators in Using the Cultural Care Theory**
   1. What are the comparative meanings and manifest expression of cultural care to nurse administrators in the United States, Canada, and in other countries?
   2. How can nurse administrators make human care a more visible and central focus of nursing services?
   3. What attributes or characteristics constitute universal and nonuniversal features of nursing care service administration in Western and non-Western cultures?

4. What alternative types of nursing organization and management services show the greatest potential to serve people of different cultures?
5. What are the strengths and limitations of a *collegial* type of organizational structure versus a *legalistic bureaucratic* organization for Western and non-Western nursing service administration?
6. What types of cultural stresses and conflicts do clients of diverse cultural backgrounds experience with administrators who espouse cultural values that are clearly different from those of the client or staff nurses?
7. What innovative approaches can nursing service administrators use to accommodate cultural care differences in nursing care practices, and provide congruent care practices for clients?
8. What features of social structure in American nursing services tend to have the most significant impact upon nursing care of different cultural groups such as North American Indian, Amish, African, Anglo, Mexican, Haitian, and other clients?
9. What steps could be taken to help nursing service administrators to shift from the current norm of preoccupation with resource reallocation, efficiency and cost effectiveness to that of quality care services for diverse cultures in any society as a major goal for the future?
10. Given the fact that many cultural minorities do not utilize or seek professional nursing and other health-care services for many reasons, what creative approaches or

strategies could be used to attract people of these diverse cultures to use hospital or community-based nursing services using care as the major focus?

11. What are some diverse or universal ethical and clinical problems of providing care to clients of different cultures whose values, beliefs, and practices differ considerably from the philosophy and values of nursing service administrators?

12. As of 1987, nursing service administrators limitedly know and incorporate folk health-care practices into professional nursing services, yet folk practices are important to clients and should be made congruent with professional care practices. What can be done to facilitate the incorporation of folk and professional care practices into nursing by administrators?

13. Since Western nursing care values and practices tend to contrast sharply with many non-Western cultural values, what could nursing service administrators do to prepare or help nurses deal with such differences and reduce client noncompliances?

14. What can nurse administrators do to reduce serious and largely unrecognized cultural imposition practices as nurses work with clients, nurses, educators and practitioners of different cultures?

15. What nursing management processes are more or similar or common in public and private nursing services in Western and non-Western cultures?

16. How could nursing service managers market quality of care in a cost effective way to the public?

17. In what ways could nursing service administrators establish care as the central focus of nursing with a highly favorable public care image of nursing worldwide?

18. What are some of the major resistance factors why nurse administrators have not focused on comparative cultural care, and what can be done to alleviate this problem?

19. What research methods show the greatest promise for accurately explicating, describing, and interpreting care phenomena from the perspective views of diverse cultures and nursing service practices?

20. Given the litigious nature of U.S. clients, what could nurse administrators do now to decrease the likelihood of clients suing nurses because of inadequate, negligent or non-culturally based care?

21. With the predicted future trend toward extensive home care services and to accommodate clients of different cultures in their natural home setting, what can be done now to provide culturally congruent home care?

B. Research Questions for Nurse Educators Using Cultural Care Theory

1. What are the common meanings of cultural care to nurse educators?

2. With the cyclical shortage of nurses, what universal and diverse administrative care approaches could be used to recruit and retain people in nursing education, especially cultural minorities that are still underrepresented in schools of nursing?

3. What types of organizational

structures and role changes are needed to establish and promote a caring and collegial ethos in schools of nursing, thus replacing some non-caring and authoritarian structures?

4. What nursing administration and faculty resistance factors or theories can explain the lack of focus on human or cultural care still evident in schools of nursing?

5. In view of the fact that today less than 1% of nurse administrators, 20% of undergraduate and 14% of graduate students have any formal preparation in transcultural care and nursing practices, what steps should be taken to change this situation so that nurse administrators, faculty and students will be prepared to care for people of different cultural backgrounds?

6. How might cultural care diversity and universality theory become a dominant means to influence the philosophy, organizational structure and curricula of schools of nursing in the future as a caring profession?

7. What innovative strategies and theories could nursing deans use to develop faculty to function with a multicultural care perspective for local, national, and international nursing?

8. Given the fact that faculty and student cultural conflicts prevail in most schools of nursing, how can cultural care theory be used to study such conflicts using the three types of nursing care modes in Leininger's theory to deal with the recurrent cultural conflicts?

9. How could the theory be used by nurse administrators to recruit and retain transcultural nursing faculty to teach and do research with undergraduate and graduate nursing students, and thus alleviate the critical deficit of transcultural nursing knowledge in schools of nursing?

10. What creative uses of the Theory of Cultural Care Diversity and Universality could be used by nurse administrators to shift past philosophical and educational perspectives from a unicultural to a multicultural perspective and to establish organizational structures and roles to support the changes?

11. In light of the need to establish transcultural education and research centers (or institutes) in the United States and worldwide, what new roles should nurse administrators in collaboration with nursing services take to support the preparation of nurses to be knowledgeable and skilled when caring for people of different cultures?

12. How can the theory be used to help academic nurse administrators reduce the cultural gaps of faculty as they work with nursing service staff who may have different care values from those of nurse educators and top administrators?

13. What are the universal and diverse administrative practices of deans in schools of nursing worldwide?

14. What explains the cultural variabilities on university campuses in the way different policies and management practices are used by nursing administrators in schools of nursing?

15. What is the meaning of "corporate cultures" to deans of schools of nursing, and how do they envision they will influence academic management in the future?

16. What are the differences and similarities among disciplines in the health sciences regarding cultural care values in administration, education, and research?
17. What has been the cultural impact of high technology on administration, teaching, and research in schools of nursing that support a human care focus?
18. What universal and non-universal ethical care problems are nursing education administrators facing with students and faculty as they work with clients of strange or unknown cultures?
19. What are some of the contemporary cultural incongruities and ethical concerns between administrators and faculty that lead to less confidence in deans' administrative leadership?
20. What are some of the common and different cultural care concepts, principles and practices taught in baccalaureate, master's, and doctoral nursing programs, which support congruent quality nursing care practices of diverse cultures?

In summary, there are many rich and diverse possibilities for using my theory of "Cultural Care Diversity and Universality" for nurse administrators in academic and service settings. Administrators are facing a growing number of diverse cultural and social forces that influence nursing decisions, finances, and effectiveness in their work. A host of critical administrative problems related to functioning in a rapidly changing society and world culture need to be studied to prevent future serious problems. Increased cultural demands from clients, students and faculty bring to nurse administrators' attention that they are functioning in a rapidly changing world and need transcultural care knowledge

to help them in their work. The long delay in dealing with the cultural dimensions of nursing education and service has necessitated the need for us to "catch up" to fulfill societal requirements of the nursing profession. With this need has come the need for theories that are not culture bound.

Nurse administrators need to prepare themselves in transcultural nursing with their cognates in anthropology to develop a broad and comparative understanding of administration. They need a theory such as Cultural Care Diversity and Universality to gain a worldwide view of people and nursing for the twenty-first century. Indeed, nurse administrators should be thinking, acting, and researching problems from a worldwide perspective rather than a local view in order to discover new approaches to old problems. The cultural perspective helps one to think broadly and to critically re-examine ethnocentric tendencies.

One of the most exciting possibilities in the future is to establish transcultural nursing administrative courses and institutes so that nurse administrators could study in depth common and diverse worldwide care philosophies, theories, and practices. Ethnoadministration with a transcultural care focus will be the new approach by the year 2010. Now is the time to consider this new direction for top and middle level nurse administrators. They will also be learning from managers worldwide and will travel to function in different nursing and health care services that they barely know today. Nursing practices need to be studied that reflect nursing's distinct contribution to the care of humanity. Nurse administrators can make these changes if they will take risks and envision future types of diverse roles in a changing multicultural world. I firmly believe that nurse administrators will discover and value more fully the significance and importance of human care and will make it the essence of nursing. When this occurs, public and private research monies and other resources will be forthcoming to continue in the discovery of care as the epistemological and practice base of nursing. For the first time in nursing, nurses will have identifiable and distinct knowledge to practice and support their actions and decisions. The future looks promising. However, it is contingent on nurse leaders who are willing to grasp a comparative care worldview and to develop care patterns that accommodate cultural diversities. I believe nursing education and nursing service leaders must provide culturally based care as the new direction in nursing so that professional nurses can ultimately care for all people in the world based on substantive (research based) comparative knowledge and exquisite nursing care skills. This goal is what the public seeks now from nursing.

REFERENCES

1. Fawcett J. The metaparadigm of nursing: present status and future refinements. Images: Nurs Scholarship 1984;16(3):84–86.
2. Leininger M. Care: The essence of nursing and health. In: Leininger M., ed. Care: the essence of nursing and health. Thorofare, NJ: Slack Inc, 1984, pp. 1–16.
3. Leininger M. Care: an essential human need. Thorofare, NJ: Slack Inc, 1981, pp. 1–20.
4. Ibid.
5. Leininger M. Caring: the essence and central focus of nursing. American Nurses Foundation. Nursing Research Report. 1976 February. 12(1), pp. 2, 14.
6. Leininger M. Caring: the essence and central focus of nursing. American Nurses Foundation. Nursing Research Report. 1976 February. 12(1), pp. 2, 14.
7. Leininger M. Transcultural nursing: concepts, theories and practices. New York: John Wiley & Company, 1978.
8. Leininger M. Care: discovery and uses in clinical and community nursing. Detroit: Wayne State University Press, 1987, pp. 1–30.
9. Leininger M. Care facilitating and resistance factors on the culture of nursing. In Wolf Z., ed. Clinical care in nursing. MD: Aspen Publication, 1986, pp. 1–23.
10. Ibid.
11. Ibid.
12. Leininger M. 1984, pp. 1–20.
13. Leininger M, 1981, pp. 17–24; 25–36; 61–69; 70–82.
14. Leininger M. Transcultural care diversity and universality: A theory of nursing. Nursing and health care; 1985; 6(4):209–212.
15. Miranda M, Kitano H, eds: Mental health research and practice in minority communities: development of culturally sensitive training programs. 1986 U.S. Department of Health and Human Services, MD, pp. xv–xxi.
16. Leininger M. The culture concept and American culture values in nursing. In: Nursing and Anthropology: Two worlds to blend. New York: John Wiley & Sons, 1970, pp. 45–52.
17. Leininger M. The leadership crisis in nursing: a critical problem and challenge. J Nurs Adm 1974; 4(2):28–34.
18. Rothschild J, Russell R. Alternatives to bureaucracy: democratic participation in economy. In: Turner R, Short Jr, J, eds. Annual Review of Sociology. Vol. 12. Palo Alto: Annual Reviews, 1986, pp. 307–345.
19. Leininger M. Towards conceptualization of transcultural health care systems: concepts and a model. In: Leininger M, ed. Human care issues, Transcultural health care issues and conditions. Philadelphia: FA Davis Co, 1974, pp. 3–23.
20. Leininger M, 1981, pp. 209–211.
21. Spradley JE. Ethnographic interview. New York: Holt, Rinehart & Winston, 1979.
22. Malinowski B. Field method. In Argonauts of the Western Pacific people. New York: Dutton, 1922/1963.
23. Geertz C. Interpretation of cultures. New York: Basic Books, 1973.
24. Pike K. Language in relation to a unified theory of the structure of human behavior. Glendale, CA: Summer Institute of Linguistics, 1954, Vol. 1.
25. Redfield R. The little community. Chicago: University of Chicago Press, 1957.
26. Gaut D. Conceptual analysis of caring: research method. In Leininger M, ed. Caring: An essential human need. Thorofare, NJ, 1981, pp. 17–25.
27. Watson J. Human science and human care. Norwalk, CN: Appleton-Century-Crofts, 1985.
28. Leininger M, 1985, p. 210.
29. Leininger M. Care: the essence of nursing and health. Thorofare, NJ: Slack Inc, 1984, pp. 137–145.
30. Leininger M. 1985, pp. 209–212.
31. Leininger M. Qualitative research methods in nursing. Orlando, FL: Grune and Stratton Company, 1985, pp. 33–73.
32. Leininger M. Ethnocare, ethnohealth and ethnonursing of selected urban cultures. Detroit: Wayne State University (in press).
33. Leininger M. Southern Rural Black and White American Lifeways on Care and Health Phenomena. In: Leininger M, ed. *Qualitative Research Methods in Nursing*, Orlando: Grune & Stratton, 1985, pp. 195–216.
34. Leininger M. Cultural care diversity and universality: a theory of nursing with research methods and findings, 1988 (in press).

3

King's Systems Framework for Nursing Administration

Imogene M. King

THE PURPOSE of this chapter is to suggest new and creative ways to implement strategies in nursing administration that address selected dimensions of certain critical issues. A few historical highlights related to organizations, management, and general systems theory are mentioned. An overview of King's systems framework, from which a theory of goal attainment was derived, is discussed. The basic concepts of a new theory of administration for nursing, formulated from King's conceptual framework, are presented. Use of the two theories leads to new strategies for organizing the delivery of nursing services, coping with issues, and resolving problems.

Nursing service administration does not exist in a vacuum; rather, it is one aspect of complex interactions in organizations and in society. Several historical elements in the development of scientific management are highlighted to place nursing administration in the context of the social systems in which nurses function.

HISTORICAL HIGHLIGHTS IN ADMINISTRATION

In the early 1900s, industrial engineering introduced wage and incentive plans to the workplace. In the 1930s and 1940s, the idea of quality and production control was related to task performance. Time and motion studies were done on specific tasks.[1,2] Operations research—the design and operations of sys-tems—began in Great Britain during the 1940s.[3] Systems analysis involved studies of resource allocation and programming to attain goals in a cost-effective way.[4,5] In the 1950s, statistical models were used to develop procedures for decision making.

Changes in administrative and organization theories can be divided into four schools of thought. The first school of thought was the traditional staff-and-line hierarchic organization. Major concepts of this school of thought were authority, power, status, control, communication, and responsibility. The second school of thought introduced human relations to management thinking and resulted in a behavioral approach to administration that focused on personal influence. The concepts were values and facts, values and goals, perception, communication, and decision making. A third school of thought combined the traditional and behavioral approaches to management. This perspective focused on the hierarchic organizational structure and considered the goals of the worker and the goals of the organization. The concepts included status, authority, control, power, motivation, interpersonal competence, and individual and organization goals. A fourth school, the systems approach, included concepts of structure, function, resources, goals, decision making, environment, information, communication, growth, feedback and provided substantive knowledge for use in organizations.[6–8] Several major differences between the first 3 schools of

Table 3.1 Organizational Approaches

Traditional Approach	Systems Approach
1. Emphasize the design of the organizational structure, and then think about the communication needed to implement it	1. Emphasize the design of communication structure, and then think about the organization needed to implement it
2. Emphasize chain of command, lines of authority and responsibility	2. Emphasize channels of communication, information flow, and decisions
3. Provide compartments of authority and responsibility	3. Provide networks between question and answer points

thought, a traditional approach, and a systems approach are listed in Table 3.1.[9]

Modern organization theory blends some of the concepts of the traditional approach with new concepts of systems to attain goals, one of which is worker satisfaction.[10] Organizations are an integral part of every human being's environment. In the systems approach, managers identify the mission of the organization, clarify goals, and provide for a flow of information through clear lines of communication.[11-13] Decision making is a key element in allocation and use of resources—both human and material.[14-18]

GENERAL SYSTEMS THEORY

Von Bertalanffy (1968) proposed general systems theory to give scientists and managers an approach to study the organized complexity of systems. General systems theory concepts of organization, wholeness, control, self-regulation, and purposiveness, are different from classical science of the past, which dealt with cause and effect relations. General systems theory was created for sciences concerned with "organized wholes." Von Bertalanffy[19] noted that general systems theory is a general science of "wholeness . . . in itself purely formal but applicable to the various empirical sciences" (p. 37).

General systems theory is defined as a "complex of elements standing in interactions"[19] (p. 33). Distinguishing characteristics of systems are goals, structure, functions, resources, and decision making. Organizations

are social systems with specific goals. Social units within organizations also have specific goals. Goal attainment is one of the important outcomes for the social units that comprise the formal and informal structure of an organization. The structure and functions of systems are formed to achieve goals. Resources—human and material—are identified in relation to the goals of systems. In decision making the human element is a critical dimension in any organization. King's conceptual framework provides a structure for nursing service administrators to examine the relationships of nursing to health-care organizations, to clients, to health care in the community, and to the larger environment of society.[20] Before presenting a general systems framework and theory for nursing that is useful for planning new strategies, selected issues in nursing service administration will be discussed.

CRITICAL ISSUES IN NURSING

Organizations have existed since human beings first formed groups for survival. They are formed to coordinate human and material resources to achieve goals. Nursing is an organized profession in a highly technological and complex society. The delivery of direct nursing care to the public is a major function in health care systems.[21]

A critical issue that has demanded the attention of nurse administrators is helping to maintain a cost-effective health care system. One dimension of this issue is the role of professional nurses and their scope of practice. The scope of practice, expanded during the 1980s, has seen an emphasis on independent and collaborative functions of nurses. The need for professional nurses has increased without a concomitant increase in the supply. Is there an inadequate utilization of nursing personnel according to education and experience? What innovative approaches can be identified to utilize knowledge and skills of professional nurses in their expanded role?

A second dimension is the shortage of professional nurses, which means a decrease in human resources even as technologic complexity continues to increase. The number of professional nurses engaged actively in practice has decreased in recent years. Newspapers, radio, and television have highlighted the nursing shortage. How can nurse administrators organize nursing care systems to maintain standards in health care organizations? How can nurse administrators and practitioners assure effectiveness of nursing care with increased technology and decreased human resources? Strategies for organizing nursing care delivery systems need to be identified and used in addressing these questions.

One function of administrators is to collaborate with nurses in formulating a nursing care delivery system in an organization. This function includes identifying and disseminating the philosophy and conceptual framework of the nursing system. If a systems approach is used, goals will be clearly stated and a communication system will be designed to facilitate the flow of information vertically, horizontally, and across structural units. Decisions need to be made on matters involving legal and ethical aspects of nursing and health care.

Evaluation of the effectiveness of nursing care provided to clients is one of the most relevant administrative functions and is related to a key issue in nursing practice: the measurement of effective nursing care. Nursing care must not only be effective for the clients served, but it must be cost effective for the institution. Each professional group must recognize its dependent role and functions in the system. A collaborative role among all health professionals is essential to attain the common goal—care of clients. The expanded role of professional nurses implies that they will function more independently; this presents another issue for nurse administrators. Prior to discussing strategies for addressing these issues, such as the usefulness of theory-based practice and theory-based nursing administration, an overview of King's general systems framework and theory is presented.

KING'S GENERAL SYSTEMS FRAMEWORK AND THEORY

Human beings do not function in a vacuum. Individuals are influenced by their interactions with the environment, and they in turn influence the environment. The three dynamic interacting systems illustrated in Figure 3.1 show the interrelationships between individuals, called personal systems, who function in a variety of social systems through interpersonal systems. In decision making and problem solving, it is essential that the interaction of the three systems be considered.[22]

The practicing nurse functions in several interpersonal systems such as those comprised of nurse and patient, nurse and family, nurse and nurse, nurse and physician, and nurse and nurse administrator, nurse and allied professionals. However, the central focus is care of individuals at the level of personal systems. Exchange of information links the three systems. Understanding the intricate interplay of these systems is essential for nurse administrators if they are to focus on total patient requirements, as well as on the functional efficiency of departments and

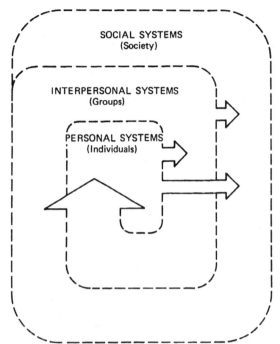

Figure 3.1 Dynamic Interacting Systems (Reproduced by permission from King, IM. A theory for nursing. N.Y.: Wiley & Sons, Inc., p. 11, 1981.)

their personnel. If nurse administrators use this general systems framework, designed by a nurse for nurses, to organize nursing-care delivery systems, decision making will be facilitated and allocating resources to achieve effective nursing care can be efficient and economical.[23]

In the 1980s, a systems approach has emerged as one way to cope with continuous change and to achieve goals. The conceptual systems[24] shown in Figure 3.1, demonstrate "wholeness" in that the three levels of functions in society are dynamic interactions of individuals as persons, individuals in groups, and individuals in society. To visualize these functions and interactions, think of nurses as individuals and of clients as individuals who make up a major component of the concrete level of function in health-care systems. If one thinks of one type of social system as the

hospital, then one can identify all of the interpersonal systems in that organization and see the need for an open communication system. Nurses are the key human resources in hospital systems, and whether they are aware of it or not, to a large extent they control the flow of information in these systems.

OVERVIEW OF KING'S CONCEPTUAL FRAMEWORK AND THEORY

The conceptual framework is called a general systems framework because it describes the characteristics of general systems. Again, these characteristics are goals, structure, functions, resources, and decision making. The goal of the nursing system is health for individuals, health for groups—such as the family, and health for communities within a society. The means to attain goals at each level of the organization are different. Nurses are in a position to identify the goals and specific means of achieving them at each level of function.

"Goals" are a major characteristic of a general system. The concept of health as the goal includes health promotion, health maintenance, and regaining a functional state of health. In working to attain this goal, nurses provide care for the ill, and the disabled, as well as those who are dying. King's framework demonstrates a goal—health—which meets one of the characteristics of a general systems framework.

The conceptual framework in Figure 3.1 demonstrates structure, a second characteristic of a general system. "Structure" can be viewed as the semipermeable boundaries between individuals, groups, and society. Within this broad structure, more specific units are designed to carry out the functions of the systems. Structure is the way of organizing individuals, objects, and things to attain goals. Structure provides for the allocation of resources to individuals in specific positions to enable them to perform functions in specific roles. Structure provides for information flow through communication channels for decision making.[25]

A third characteristic of general systems is the action element in an organization, the "functions." Functions flow from structure and goals. In the nursing profession, a license gives one the legal right to perform professional nursing functions. In addition, a code of ethics provides guidelines for professional nurses' decision making in specific situations. Functions are carried out by individuals to attain goals. Resources are allocated to perform functions.

"Resources," a fourth characteristic of general systems, are essential to perform functions within a structure to attain goals. One dimension of an issue in nursing administration mentioned previously is the decrease in human resources due to a shortage of professional nurses. How can human resources be acquired and allocated to fulfill the functions of an organization? As new technologies increase, will every health-care organization have the resources to acquire the new technologies? Two elements in decision making in health-care systems are the acquisition and allocation of resources.

"Decision making" is a fifth characteristic of general systems. How can nurse administrators make decisions about allocation of human resources when professional nurses are not available? How can this vital human resource—the professional nurse—function in a nursing-care delivery system to assure effective nursing? Decisions are made after considering alternatives and consequences relative to goals of individuals, groups, and society. Decision making is a process and a skill that is required at each level of the three dynamic interacting systems shown in Figure 3.1. Decisions at one level influence the behavior of individuals at all levels.

King's general systems framework was designed to provide a holistic view of the complexities of nursing within the larger environment of multiple groups within social systems. The concepts identified at the social-systems level of the framework are organization, power, authority, status, and control. In addition, role is an important concept that begins with knowledge of self. A concept of role implies self in relation to another as well as a position in an organization. Knowledge of these concepts is essential for nurses to understand self and interactions with relevant others, the environment, and the variety of interpersonal and social systems in which individuals grow, develop, work, live, and die. This general systems framework suggests that students in professional education programs should have opportunities to learn about these concepts and develop skill in decision making based on the collection of reliable facts and consideration of the alternatives and consequences of decisions.

Major Concept of the Framework

The major concepts in the three interacting systems shown in Figure 3.1 have been identified as perception, interaction, and organization[21] (p. 21). For example, the concept of perception has been identified in personal systems as knowledge that is essential to nurses if they are to understand themselves and others. Perceptions vary from one individual to another because of differences in backgrounds, knowledge, abilities, needs, values, and goals. Perceptions influence communications—the information component of interactions. The valuation component has been identified as transactions. Perceptual congruence between nurse and client, or nurse and supervisor, facilitates communication and goal attainment.

Interaction is a comprehensive concept which has been identified in interpersonal systems as knowledge that is essential for nurses to function in groups. Interaction is a process used to gather relevant information about human beings. Perception and communication are characteristics of interactions. Knowledge of these three concepts helps nurses set goals with clients or with nurse administrators and engage in transactions that lead to goal attainment.

A comprehensive concept in social systems is organization. Knowledge of organization provides information about power, authority, status, control, and communication in an organization. Decision making is the key activity in any organization. Decisions are made by individuals and by group consensus. Knowledge of the major concepts at each level of function in the three systems identified in King's framework facilitates goal attainment. Knowledge of self and perception in personal systems is related to communication, interaction, and transaction in the interpersonal systems, and all are related to roles in organizations.

The conceptual framework is a system of processes, including those of perception, communication, purposeful interactions, information, and decision-making. Specific skills are inherent in these processes.

The value of viewing nursing within a general systems framework is that it provides a way of looking at nursing phenomena holistically, yet with a focus on a specific situation. One way this framework helps nurses in hospitals and community health agencies is that it provides a focus for the delivery of nursing services to individuals in families and in specific communities.

In nursing education and in nursing practice, acceptance of the nursing process as a scientific method is self-evident. From King's conceptual framework, a theory of goal attainment was derived. This theory identified process and outcome variables.

Major Concepts of the Theory of Goal Attainment

The major concepts of the theory are perception, communication, self, interaction, transaction, role, growth and development, stress, time, and space[24] (pp. 145–149). These concepts are interrelated in any directly observable dyadic interaction such as nurse and client interaction or nurse and nurse administrator interaction. The concepts of the theory relate primarily to the interpersonal systems of the conceptual framework.

Nursing is defined in the theory as a process of action, reaction, and interaction whereby nurse and client share information about their perceptions in a nursing situation and through purposeful communication identify specific goals, concerns, and/or problems. Nurses and clients explore and agree to the means to attain a goal[24] (p. 2). In viewing this process as a system, nurses collect data about nurse variables, patient or client variables, and situation variables. Skills in observation and measurement are essential in using this process in nursing situations. The same process can be used to describe the interactions of the staff nurse, clinical specialist, supervisor, and administrator. It is a human process of interactions that leads to transactions and to goal attainment.

Nursing process as theory (shown in Figure 3.2) described in the theory of goal attainment, provides the knowledge needed to accompany the nursing process as scientific method. Nursing process as method and nursing process as theory are outlined in Table 3.2.

Nurses help individuals attain and maintain their health, and if there is some disturbance, such as illness or disability, nurses' actions are goal-directed to help individuals regain health or live with a chronic illness or a disability. This implies that health is a dynamic state of an individual in which constant change occurs. This explanation of health rejects a linear continuum of wellness-illness and identifies health as a dynamic state in which individuals are able to function in their usual roles.

Decision making is essential in applying

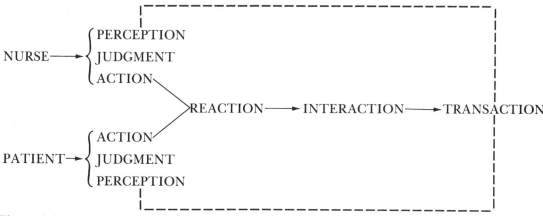

Figure 3.2 Nursing Process as Theory (Reproduced by permission from King, IM. A theory for nursing: Systems, concepts, process. N.Y.: Wiley and Sons, Inc., p. 63, 1981.)

knowledge in nursing-care delivery systems. In the theory of goal attainment, decision making is a shared collaborative process in which client and nurse give information to each other, identify goals, explore means to attain goals, and move toward goal attainment. This collaboration is identified in the theory as a critical independent variable called mutual goal setting. This is a process variable. The process of interactions that leads to transactions has been verified in a descriptive study[24] (p. 145). Transactions cannot be defined as such; rather, they are said to exist when the six elements in the interactions are present, as described in a model of transactions[24] (p. 156). This transaction model is useful in goal attainment in social systems such as health-care systems and nursing-care systems. Wherever human interactions take place in a specific structure and decisions are made to attain specific goals, the transaction model is useful. For example, it is useful in explaining interactions between employees and employers and between managers and workers.

STRATEGIES FOR COPING WITH PROBLEMS

How can the conceptual framework and the theory be used to identify strategies to cope with problems in nursing administration? The critical issues described earlier demand attention at the local, state, and national level

Table 3.2 Relation between Theory and Method

Nursing Process as Method*	Nursing Process as Theory[†]
A system of interrelated actions	A system of interrelated concepts
...Assess	...Perception of nurse and client
	...Communication of nurse and client
	...Interaction of nurse and client
...Plan	...Decision making about goals
	...Agree to means to attain goals
...Implement	...Transactions made
...Evaluate	...Goal attained (if not, why?)

* Yura, Helen and Walsh, M. The Nursing Process. Conn: Appleton Century Crofts, 1983.)
[†] King, IM. A theory for nursing: Systems, Concepts, Process. N.Y.: Wiley & Sons, Inc., 1981.)

of society. The delivery of direct nursing care to the public is a major component of health-care systems, and nurses comprise the largest group of health professionals. In this section strategies are discussed to help nurse administrators address the two questions mentioned previously: First, can effective nursing care be provided in complex health-care organizations, given existing cost containment programs and the expanded role of professional nurses? Second, how can nurse administrators organize nursing-care systems in health-care organizations to maintain standards and to assure effectiveness of nursing care, as well as contain costs?

These questions cannot be answered with specific formulas, but strategies for organizing nursing-care delivery systems can be provided for individuals who would like to try innovative and creative approaches.

Nurses are expected to function at a high level of performance every day and every hour in the concrete world of health-care systems. No other professional group is expected to be as intensely involved with human beings and groups. Historically, a philosophy has pervaded nursing that nurses provide individualized care for patients in hospitals, for families in homes, and for people in communities. This philosophy implies that human beings are the focus of direct and indirect nursing care. However, human beings are not isolated individuals. They are members of groups, beginning with the family into which they are born, grow, and develop. They are members of groups, joined during a lifetime, such as peers in school, associates in the workplace, and friends at the club. These groups make up communities. Individuals, groups, and communities all influence the behaviors of the other; the three levels of functioning are interrelated, and together they comprise a society.

One approach for coping with the problems in nursing is to use theory-based practice and theory-based administration. A the-ory of goal attainment at the interpersonal level has been published from King's general systems framework of three dynamic interacting systems[24] (pp. 141–161). Hypotheses derived from the theory are being tested in several studies. Recently a theory of administration for nursing has been developed from the social systems level of function in this framework. The major concepts of this new theory of administration are: organization, power, authority, status, role, control, decision making, perception, communication, interaction, and transaction.

This theory, when published in detail, will be useful in nursing service administration and in nursing education administration. King's theories will help nurse administrators and nurses cope with some important issues. Knowledge of the concepts of the new theory of administration can be used to analyze one's current organizational structure. The criteria for assessing an organization include the following: (1) the philosophy of the organization; (2) the goals of the health-care system; (3) the structure of the organization; (4) the functions of the organization; (5) the resources available to accomplish the goals; (6) the constraints in the organization; (7) the clarity of the lines of communication and responsibility; (8) and who makes the decisions about what.

An assessment using these kinds of criteria provides the information needed to make decisions for action relative to the issue of the expanded role of the professional nurse. For example, if the assessment data indicate that one of the contraints is related to the utilization of nurses according to their ability to function, as when there is no differentiation in function among graduates of baccalaureate, associate, diploma, and licensed practical nurses, this information can be used to state the problem and organize a plan to resolve the problem. In this case, licensing laws provide guidelines for practice and differentiate between professional and nonprofessional nursing functions. One of the functions of the registered nurse, according to law, is to observe, record, and report information about patients or clients, including any change in their status. This involves such tasks as measuring pulse and respiration rate, blood pressure, and body temperature. If these tasks are delegated to someone who is not a registered nurse, the R.N. is responsible for the accuracy of the measurements, for interpreting their meaning, and for initiating nursing actions.

Many tasks may be delegated, but a function can not be delegated. For years, nurses have taught patients and families to care for their skin, to take their pulse and blood pressure, to give insulin injections, and to plan special diets. These are tasks that are essential to implement the function of teaching patients and families about how to maintain their health. The function involves analysis and interpretation of data, to making decisions with and for patients through interactions and transactions. These professional functions require a broad base of knowledge, skills, and professional values that cannot be learned in two or three years in formal educational programs, or with two or three years of experience. A combination of both education and experience is necessary to perform the functions of a professional nurse.

One strategy a nurse administrator can use is to restructure job descriptions to reflect differentiation in roles and functions of all nursing personnel. Use of knowledge of the concepts of power, authority, status, and role in planning for this change will prevent resistance. Participation in decision making about the changes in job descriptions will provide input from those whom the change will affect. Restructuring the functions of nursing personnel can be one approach that will lead to increased performance on the part of the staff, which will in turn lead to efficiency and satisfaction. Another strategy might be to change the organizational chart to clearly

show the lines of communication and responsibility for each level of nursing personnel. Goals for individuals and for all departments in nursing administration will be attained when personnel have a part in setting goals.

A second issue has to do with measuring effective nursing care. The use of King's theory of goal attainment is offered as a strategy to address this issue by resolving a major problem of documentation. A Goal-Oriented Nursing Record System has been operationalized for renal dialysis units.[26] This system provides a way for nurses to document their care and to measure the effectiveness of the care provided to each individual. The major components of this documentation system are:

Data base
Nursing diagnosis
Goal list
Nursing orders
Flow sheets
Progress notes
Discharge summary

The data base provides information that is relevant for decision making. It begins with a nursing history. A form should be organized to assess activities of daily living. If possible, a reliable and valid instrument should be used to gather data. An interview guide is useful for gathering information about roles, stressors in the environment, patient perceptions of what is happening, and patients' values, goals, and learning needs.

From the assessment data, nursing diagnoses are made. For example, a patient with a myocardial infarction may indicate his or her fear of dying, or alterations in role in the family. Goals are formulated from the nursing diagnosis. The goals are written to show outcome behaviors in patients, such as "patient discusses fear of dying with nurses." Nursing orders are written by the professional nurse only, to provide consistency in care to help patients attain goals. For example, a nursing order related to the diagnosis of fear of dying might be "Purposeful interactions with patient every four hours or two times in a.m. and two times in p.m."

Flow sheets are used in most hospitals to record routine information required on all patients, such as pulse, temperature, respiration, and body temperature. In special care units, flow sheets are designed for special groups of patients with similar medical diagnoses. The purpose of a flow sheet is to save time and energy but provide essential data about the patient.

Progress notes help the professional nurse document the nursing care provided as it relates to goals and to legal and ethical aspects of care. For example, the "Patient called the nurse to his room at 9 a.m. to talk about his fear of dying." Another notation may indicate "Patient transported to Cardiac Catheter Laboratory on a stretcher at 10 a.m. Returned to room at 11:30 a.m." This is relevant information about the patient in that actual facts rather than inferences are recorded.

A discharge summary lists the nursing diagnoses and the goals by numbers. A notation at discharge might be as follows:

10-5-88 Discharge summary
  Nursing Diagnosis 1. Goal 1, 2, 3 identified and attained.
  Nursing Diagnosis 2. Goal 1, 2, 3 identified and attained.
    Goal 4 partially attained—to return to physical therapy two times week.

Goal attainment recorded in this manner demonstrates a measure of effective care. For example, if all the goals identified are attained, care is effective. When goals are not attained during hospitalization, this should be noted, the reasons given, and continuity of care recommended.

The economics in society, in health-care systems, and in health professions make it imperative to document the effectiveness of care. An information system called a Goal-Oriented Nursing Record System, based on the theory of goal attainment, was designed for nursing's use. This system, when implemented, provides a systematic way for nurses to document their care and measure its effectiveness. This system is helpful for documentation required in a quality assurance program: it provides a way to retrieve data for retrospective studies. The use of a documentation system based on a theory of goal attainment for nursing will help nurse adminstrators resolve major problems related to a major issue—measurement of the effectiveness of care.

In summary, a general systems framework reflects the nature of three dynamic interacting systems that influence the behavior of individuals and systems. A theory of goal attainment as process and outcome was explained, as was a new theory of administration for nursing derived from the social systems part of the framework. Suggestions were made to select a nursing framework that meets with one's individual and organizational philosophy to implement change. Remember, frameworks are designed to serve as guidelines, and are implemented differently in different organizations based on philosophies, goals, structures, and functions.

REFERENCES

1. Etzioni A. Modern organizations. Englewood Cliffs, NJ: Prentice Hall, 1964.
2. Meyer MW Structures, symbols, and systems. Boston, Mass: Little, Brown & Co, 1971.
3. Beer S. Decision and control. New York: Wiley & Sons, Inc, 1966.
4. Churchman CW. The systems approach. New York: Dell, 1968.
5. Simon HA. Administrative behavior. 2nd ed. New York: Free Press, 1965.
6. Baker F. General systems theory, research, and medical care. In: Sheldon A, ed. Systems and medical care. Cambridge: MIT Press, 1971.
7. Emery FE, ed: Systems thinking. Baltimore: Penguin Books, 1974.
8. Howland D, A hospital systems model. Nurs Res 1963;232–235.

9. McDonough AM, Garrett RJ. Management systems. Homewood, IL: Richard Irwin Publishers, 1965.

10. Fink SL, Jenks R, Willits JD. Designing and managing organizations. Homewood IL: Richard D Irwin Inc, 1983.

11. Griffiths D. Administrative theory. Englewood Cliffs, NY: Prentice Hall, 1959.

12. Hyman HH. Health planning—A systems approach. Germantown, MD: Aspen Systems Corp, 1976.

13. Kast FE, Rosenweig JE. Organization and management: a systems approach. New York: McGraw-Hill, 1974.

14. Grier MR. Decision making about patient care: Nurs Res 1976;76(2), 105–110.

15. Hansen AC. Professionalization of priority decision judgments. Nurs Res 1970;19(4):343–48.

16. King, IM. The decision makers perspective: patient aspects. In: Schuman L et al, eds. Operations research in health care. Baltimore: Johns Hopkins University Press, 1975.

17. LeMonica E, Finch FE. Managerial decision making. JONA 1977;7(5):20–28.

18. Sumidal SW. A computerized test for clinical decision making. Nurs Outlook 1972;20:458–61.

19. Von Bertalanffy L. General systems theory. New York: Braziller, Inc, 1968.

20. King IM. Toward a theory for nursing. New York: John Wiley & Sons, 1971.

21. Arndt C, Huckabay L. Nursing administration: theory for practice. St. Louis: CV Mosby, 1980.

22. King, IM. The health care system: nursing intervention subsystem. In: Werley H et al, eds. Health research: the systems approach. New York: Springer Publishing Co, 1976.

23. Howland D, McDowell WE. The measurement of patient care: a conceptual framework. Nurs Res 1964;4–7.

24. King IM. A theory for nursing: systems, concepts, process. New York: John Wiley and Sons, Inc, 1981.

25. Daubenmire JM, King IM. Nursing process models: A systems approach. Nurs Outlook, 1973;512–517.

26. King IM. Effective measure of nursing: use of King's goal oriented nursing record in renal dialysis units. AANT Journal, April, 1984.

27. Yura H, Walsh M. The nursing process. Norwalk. Conn: Appleton-Century-Crofts, 1983.

4

Applying King's Model to Nursing Administration

Karen Elberson

THE CONCEPTUAL framework developed by Imogene King for nursing serves as a practical guide for many nurses as they provide patient care.[1-5] Testing the applicability of this framework for the provision of direct patient care has begun, as has applying the framework to nursing education.[6] Less evident, yet of equal importance, is understanding the applicability of King's perspective for the administration of nursing services.

The definition of nursing formulated by King, and the definition of nursing administration developed by Arndt and Huckabay[7] are similar, suggesting the feasibility of adapting King's framework to nursing administration. The purpose of this chapter is to provide a brief overview of King's conceptual framework and to identify the similarities in King's and Arndt and Huckabay's models. In this chapter I emphasize interactive activities—the communication, collaboration, and mutual goal-setting of nurse administrators as suggested by King's model. In my conclusions I provide readers with information about related research and potential directions for future research where King's theory is tested and extended.

OVERVIEW OF KING'S CONCEPTUAL FRAMEWORK

Four concepts in King's theory are social systems, health, perception, and interpersonal relations. King defines nursing as "a process of human interactions between nurse and client whereby each perceives the other and the situation; and through communication, they set goals, explore means, and agree on means to achieve goals."[2] This definition incorporates three key elements of interaction, namely communication, collaboration, and goal setting.

King identifies three interacting systems—the personal, interpersonal, and social.[2] For the personal system, the ideas of perception, self, growth, image, time, and space are defined. The interpersonal system incorporates interaction, communication, transaction, roles, and stress. And the social system includes organization, authority, power, status, and decision making. According to King, through dynamic interactions among these three systems, nurses initiate the activities necessary to establish and meet goals relevant to the health and well-being of individuals and groups.

Perception refers to an individual's sense of reality. Life experiences and biological make-up are key elements of perception. The organization, interpretation, and transformation of information from sensory data and memory are the activities of perception.

Self is comprised of thoughts and feelings that contribute to one's awareness of individual existence. A person's total subjective environment—which includes ideas, attitudes, values, and commitments—are used to describe the self.

Growth and development, body image,

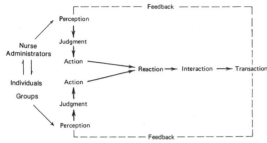

Figure 4.1   The Human Process—A Method for Study Nursing Administration

time, and space are ideas described by King.[2] Each has implications for interaction in terms of readiness, ability, reaction, timeliness, and territoriality. Interaction refers to the collaborative effort of two or more individuals directed toward achievement of a common goal. Action, reaction, interaction, transaction, and feedback are part of human interaction. This collaborative goal-oriented process, adapted to reflect nurse administrators, is illustrated in Figure 4.1.

Communication is also a major focus. Individuals communicate via interchange of thoughts and opinions. Communication is essential for the processing of information. Information transmission, interpretation of transmissions, and response to transmissions are all components of the communication process.

Transaction, role, and stress are additional concepts. Transaction facilitates goal achievement. Role refers to the expectations of individuals occupying certain positions in a social system. Stress creates the impetus for human interaction, the goal of which is the achievement of environmental balance or control.

The concepts of organization, authority, power, status, and decision making are also prominent in King's theory. Organizations are defined in terms of individuals in prescribed roles using resources to meet both personal and organizational goals.[2] Authority refers to legitimate power in an organization.

Superior-subordinate reciprocal relationships exist where superiors and subordinates are interdependent.

Power, a measure of the capacity to achieve goals in an organization, is needed for the generation of energy required in a dynamic, interactive social system. Status relates to power in an organizational position. In general, the higher the organizational position, the higher the status of the individual occupying that position.

Decision making, according to King, is goal-directed problem solving. The process of making decisions is viewed as dynamic and systematic.

King defines health as the "dynamic life experiences of a human being, which implies continuous adjustment to stressors in the internal and external environment through optimum use of one's resources to achieve maximum potential for daily living"[2] (p. 5).

LINKING KING'S CONCEPTUAL FRAMEWORK TO ARNDT AND HUCKABAY'S THEORY OF NURSING ADMINISTRATION

Arndt and Huckabay[7] developed a conceptual framework for nursing administration using a systems perspective. The model described by these authors focused on administrative processes and systems. In their model, administration is a means to accomplish objectives, to design organizations, to diagnose organizational problems, and to bring about change. Planning, organizing, directing, and controlling are the administrative processes that require interactions with the environment.

Arndt and Huckabay defined nursing service administration as "the process of setting and achieving objectives by influencing human behavior within a suitable environment."[7] The nurse administrator has the responsibility for creating an environment that is conducive to the achievement of mutually agreed on goals. These goals are set and agreed on in the context delimited by an organization's mission and philosophy.

Arndt and Huckabay, and King use open systems theory and draw heavily on communication theory. In open systems, inputs originate from external and internal environments. Understanding throughput or transformation involves analysis of organizational inputs within the boundaries defined by policies, procedures, and goals. Arndt and Huckabay refer to the transformation phase as a time for planning and implementing. Decision making is accomplished and objectives are achieved during transformation and collaborative efforts are involved. Outputs refer to the consequences or outcomes of patient care, which can be analyzed as objective data in the form, for example, of decreased hospital stay and reduced mortality, and as subjective data derived from patient satisfaction surveys.

As one reviews the terminology and relationships described by King and by Arndt and Huckabay, many similarities are found. Knowledge sources for the two theories in some instances are identical. Both focus on interaction, goal attainment through collaborative goal setting, and open systems. Both view organizations as open systems in which individuals, playing varying roles, interact with their environments. And both view humans as rational, goal-oriented makers of decisions. For King, the unit of analysis is the individual. The focus is the individual nurse managing care for patients and small groups of clients. For Arndt and Huckabay, the unit of analysis is also the individual, but in this case the focus is the individual nurse administrator managing the care provided by individual nurses and groups of nurses. Both perspectives are models of health-care management.

DYNAMIC INTERACTING SYSTEMS

In the section that follows, the key elements of King's framework discussed in the opening section of this chapter are adapted for nursing administration. I use examples of effective nursing administration practice to illustrate the relationships suggested by King's perspective.

Personal Systems

The element of King's framework that is especially useful for nursing administration is the notion of dynamic interacting systems. At a personal level, nurse administrators have perceptions of what is and what should be. These perceptions are based on their interpretation of information accumulated over time. Nurse administrators bring to any interaction a sense of themselves, their values, and commitments. Closely related to a sense of self is body image. Administrators develop an image of themselves based on the reactions of others. Nurses who are administrators have attained a level of maturity based on their genetic endowment, their perceptions, and previous experiences, all of which enhance or deter their interactions.

Nurse administrators also consider time and space when anticipating interactions. Effective managers understand that timing is a critical factor in the achievement of goals. Space, too, is a factor in goal achievement. Having space, giving others space, and creating attractive, appropriate office space are key factors in managerial success.

Interpersonal Systems

At the interpersonal level, nurse administrators organize information and communicate. The skills that effective nurse administrators possess include the ability to manage information. They determine the type of information that is needed, the best sources of information, optimal storage and retrieval methods, and how to analyze and disseminate the most useful information. Naisbitt[8] describes the latter part of the twentieth century as the information age. A caveat for nurse managers is to be aware of the danger of becoming data-rich but information-poor. The art of management involves efficiently identifying and using the most pertinent and the best information.

Interaction

Interaction may take place at any point relative to obtaining, storing, retrieving, and using information. Communication is an essential aspect of information processing. Effective nurse administrators using King's or Arndt and Huckabay's theories clarify their interpretation of information and ensure that those receiving new information have an accurate perception of the intent of communications. The ability of the nurse administrator to prioritize, summarize, and write and speak clearly and succinctly enhances interactions at the interpersonal and social-systems levels. Having a clear sense of organizational goals, and having congruent nursing department and individual goals also facilitate interactions, and ultimately results in the timely achievement of departmental and organizational goals.

Achievement of organizational goals may require planning for change. This planning requires communication, collaboration, and mutual goal setting to assure successful, satisfying change. Identifying those people who support a planned change, and those who do not, is viewed as helpful in establishing effective communication.

For communication to exist, the following are necessary: a sender or transmitter, a primary message, communication channels, receivers, and feedback. The nurse administrator, serving as a transmitter, has the responsibility for maintaining interactive relationships in which messages are timely and clear, channels are used appropriately, and feedback is identified and acted on.

Collaboration requires that participants approach one another with respect for each person's competence and with a sincere desire to maintain open and straight-forward communication.[9] From the perspectives of King, and Arndt and Huckabay, nurse administrators learn to react appropriately to a wide range of ideas and perceptions. Further, nurse administrators direct their energies toward the development of others for the achievement of agreed-on goals, and thus provide valuable input about the strategies that are useful for personnel development. In effective nursing organizations, measures are taken to ensure that staff nurses and nurse managers have the needed skills not only to solve problems but to plan for the future. Staff development programs are therefore designed to heighten nurses' awareness of an organization's history, its current status, operational trends, and strategic plans. Problem-solving exercises that use real-life problems can provide less experienced nurses with the opportunity to engage in critical thinking, thereby increasing the likelihood of their long-term success. When nursing staff and nurse managers are provided with development opportunities, the anticipated result, from King's perspective, is that more knowledgeable individuals interact more willingly and work more efficiently toward achieving organizational goals. The primary aim in these developmental transactions is to define objectives that are valued by both the individual and the organization.

Role

The concept of role is also prominent in King's framework. Nurse administrators occupy positions in health-care organizations and nursing departments. The responsibilities of people in these positions or roles are defined by each organization. Some organizations hold nurse administrators responsible for the department of nursing. Others give the nurse executive authority to control ancillary and medical services as well. Rules and procedures define the rights and obligations of the various roles played by nurse administrators. In some interactions, such as those engendered by ad hoc appointments, the usual bureaucratic role for the administrator is changed from manager to facilitator. Effective administrators are capable of identifying the more subtle role variations and playing the appropriate role, depending on the situation and purpose of an encounter.

Stress

Stress is a concept that can be viewed either positively or negatively depending on the circumstances. Organizations and individuals strive to survive by maintaining a relatively steady state. Occasional change in an organization or individual can be energizing. Too rapid or too much change creates excessive stress. Where stress is excessive, whether for individuals or groups, destruction ensues. In King's framework, nurse administrators can serve as gatekeepers, monitoring situations where change is warranted and slowing excessively rapid change. Knowledge of change theory and human behavior is crucial in administrative roles where it is necessary to create, maintain, or decrease stress to a point that is optimal for individuals and organizations.

An example of a needed change is the implementation of peer review for monitoring quality care. In many organizations, employees find that making judgments about their peers is stressful to the point of being debilitating. Intellectually, most nurses recognize the importance of democratized evaluative endeavors. But nurse administrators may have to assist their staffs to work through the emotional stress that accompanies increased individual responsibility. One of the ways of facilitating such a change, in King's view, is by setting mutually realistic goals for new undertakings in reasonable time frames.

Social Systems

At the social system level, the organization is the focus for nursing administration. From King's perspective, the purpose of organizations is to direct activities toward the achievement of goals. As a member of the management team in a health-care organization, the nurse administrator is expected to collaborate with managers in other departments and to compromise and change in ways that assure the integrity of the total organization. According to Drucker,[10] top managers who are willing and able to change themselves, their role, their relationships, and behavior are more likely to achieve organizational success. When change is being planned for the nursing department, the nurse administrator ensures that other departments are apprised of upcoming changes so that consideration can be given to such questions as, "How will this affect my department?" and "Have all alternatives been considered?" Theoretically, organizations that change in concert and move toward a prespecified set of goals have the vitality that is necessary for survival.

Authority and Power

Authority is granted by virtue of one's position in the hierarchy of an organization, by personal competency and skill, and by effective human relationship skills in leadership situations.[11] Power refers to the ability to allocate resources and to achieve specific goals. Nurse administrators who are knowledgeable about health-care finance, nursing care, and management increase the power of their position. The capacity to effect change in organizations is greatly enhanced by having a strong power base, and by using authority wisely in the achievement of individual and organizational objectives.

Status and Decision Making

Status refers to one's position in a group or organization. As nurse administrators become more proficient in the many aspects of management, their status is likely to be higher in organizations. The fact that nurse administrators represent the largest number of employees in the health-care work force will foster little status, however, if nurses in managerial positions are not competent in the execution of both their nursing and managerial responsibilities. Managerial changes are needed if organizations are to remain productive and viable.[12] Nurse administrators are expected to take an active role in defining medical as well as financial policy. Organizational governance is taking on new forms. Shared governance and participative management enhance interactive communication inside and outside of organizations. Planning for the long term has become as important as day-to-day operations. Proactive approaches to nursing management are becoming the norm. Ideally, nurse administrators determine which decisions must be made at the executive level of nursing and which can be made at other levels in the nursing organization. Mutual aims and goals are essential at all levels of decision making.

In summary, using King's systems framework, nurse administrators function in dynamic interacting systems at three levels—the personal, interpersonal, and social-system levels. Communication, collaboration and mutual goal setting are major activities. Understanding these ideas provides a useful way of thinking about managerial roles, decisions, and performance.

RELATED RESEARCH AND SUGGESTIONS FOR THE FUTURE

Swierczek conducted a study of 67 cases of organizational change. The findings of this survey provided strong support for King's framework. Collaboration was found in the phases of problem identification, goal setting, and intervention. Negotiation was identified as the key factor in problem determination. In goal setting, mutuality was uppermost. During the intervention phase, consensus was a prominent factor.[13]

The characteristics of collaboration described by Swierczek included shared power and mutual influence; high levels of cooperation and consensus; mutual goal setting and problem solving; and a compatibility of norms, values, and needs. Swierczek stated that although collaboration was important in achieving change, there should be more concern with defining goals for change where success is defined in terms of progress toward meeting predetermined goals.

In the future, qualitative and quantitative methodologies should be used to test and extend a theory as complex as King's. Observational studies of nurse administrators are needed to test the concepts and relationships in King's framework. Interviews could also be used to determine how nurses in administrative roles perceive goal-setting behavior. By combining observation and interview with the use of valid existing measures of satisfaction, role stress, and productivity a clearer understanding of the relationship of these factors to interaction and transaction can be formulated to guide the practice of nursing administration.

The following propositions generated by King and discussed by Fawcett can also be subjected to further scrutiny: (1) The nursing process will differ depending on contingencies in the environment. (2) The specific components of nursing are judgment, action, communication, evaluation, and coordination. (3) A relationship exists between nursing action and judgment, communication, evaluation, and coordination.[14]

Several conclusions can be drawn from this chapter. Nursing situations can be analyzed using the ideas in King's conceptual framework.[2] Nursing administration is one such situation. Nurse administrators, in their performance of expected duties, communicate, collaborate, and set goals. These activities are not carried out in isolation; they require interaction with other individuals, groups, and systems. Nurses managing health care are part of complex social systems. To make sense of their reality they must engage in systematic analyses when deciding among alternative strategies. The processing of information for the purposes of short-run problem solving, operations planning, and long-range strategic planning can be more clearly understood by using King's framework. In addition, by using King's goal-oriented nursing record, nurse administrators will have a systematic method for gathering information.[2] Nurses in managerial roles will also find King's conceptual framework of use when planning and implementing staff-development programs.

The need for people in nursing who possess high-level leadership and managerial skills is obvious; there are many organizations in existence today that are not healthy. And therein lies the challenge. Just as the health of individuals can be assessed in terms of their ability to adjust to stressors, the health of organizations can be assessed in terms of their ability to effectively meet goals. A healthy state for an organization presupposes that action, reaction, interaction, and transaction have taken place at the personal, interpersonal, and social-systems levels.

These processes can be likened to a concert created by a symphony. The maestro for nursing organizations is the nurse administrator. King's conceptual framework provides a useful guide for nurses as they strive to create the harmony necessary for effective health-care services.

REFERENCES

1. King IM. Toward a theory for nursing. New York: John Wiley & Sons, 1971.
2. King IM. A theory for nursing: systems, concepts, process. New York: John Wiley & Sons, 1981.
3. Daubenmire MJ, King IM. Nursing process models: a systems approach. Nurs Outlook 1973;21(8):512–517
4. King IM. Analysis and application of King's theory of goal attainment. In: Clements IW, Roberts FB eds. Family health: a theoretical approach to nursing care. New York: John Wiley & Sons, 1983.
5. Flynn J, Heffron PB. Nursing from concept to practice. Bowie, MD: Robert J. Brady, 1984.
6. Brown ST, Lee BT. Imogene King's conceptual framework: a proposed model for continuing education. J Adv Nurs 1980;5:467–473
7. Arndt C, Huckabay LMD. Nursing administration: theory for practice with a systems approach. 2nd ed. St. Louis: CV Mosby, 1980.
8. Naisbitt J. Megatrends. New York: Warner, 1983.
9. Lancaster J. Communication as a tool for change. In: Lancaster J, Lancaster W eds. The nurse as change agent. St. Louis: CV Mosby, 1982.
10. Drucker PF. The need to prepare for growth. In: Kotter J, Schlesinger L, Sathe V. Organization. Homewood, IL: Irwin, Inc, 1979.
11. Halal WE. The legitimacy cycle: long-term dynamics in the use of power. In: Kakabadse A, Parker C eds. Power, politics, and organizations. New York: John Wiley & Sons, 1984.
12. Keller G. Academic strategy. Baltimore: The Johns Hopkins University Press, 1983.
13. Swierczek, FW. Collaborative intervention and participation in organizational change. Group & Org Studies 1980;5(4):438–452.
14. Fawcett J. Analysis and evaluation of conceptual models of nursing. Philadelphia: F. A. Favis, 1984.

5

Nursing Administration, a Theoretical Approach

Dorothea Orem

THE PROCESS of scientific development of nursing administration necessarily begins with explication of the meaning of the term "nursing administration." The term combines the name for a specific form of health care, nursing, with the word administration. Administration connotes persons who through their actions within a defined situational context exercise the powers given them by legitimately constituted authorities of an enterprise to manage, that is, conduct and control the courses of affairs necessary to accomplish or contribute to the accomplishment of the enterprise's legitimate purpose(s) or mission.* When the words nursing and administration are conjoined in the compound noun, nursing administration, the connotation is that of persons whose managerial powers are specific to nursing viewed as a purpose-accomplishing service of an institution. At times the word administration is used to connote the actions of persons as described above. The individual with management power in this context is referred to as an administrator.

*This is a composite statement that adopts the meaning of administration as the body of persons who collectively manage an institution. This approach was taken to avoid the confusion that arises from efforts to distinguish the action word "administration" from the action word "management."

A TERM DEFINED

Definition

Nursing administration can be broadly defined as those persons who through their actions within a situational context manage courses of affairs specific to the provision of nursing now and at future times to described populations served by an institution, and in so doing exercise powers given them by the established authorities of the formally constituted enterprise, the purposes of which are accomplished in whole or in part through the provision of health care in the form of nursing. The term population is viewed as a class word and in this context the class is constituted from the individuals served or to be served by an organized enterprise.[1]

Nursing administration so defined, as well as the individual nursing administrator, is differentiated from persons qualified as nurses and authorized by some governmental body to practice nursing within its jurisdiction. Nursing administration within a formally constituted enterprise, such as a hospital, is considered as a managerial organ, a constituent part of its organizational structure.

Essential Distinctions

Qualified, legitimate nurses, that is, nursing practitioners, who produce a range of types of care systems in the form of nursing manage their own work operations, including the work of designing, planning for, and providing nursing to more than one person or group of persons during the same time and over some duration of time. Management by a nursing practitioner of the work of designing and providing systems of nursing care for a person or group, and management of nursing for a caseload of patients are conducting and controlling actions that are outside of the managerial actions of nursing administration. Nursing practitioners who are constituent members of organizations such as hospitals perform the operations specific to the professional practice of nursing. From an enterprise point of view they are production operators.

The critical differences between the actions of nurses and the actions of nursing administration can be viewed as a difference in their objects or foci. The object of the actions of nurses who engage in the practice of nursing is persons who seek and can benefit from nursing because of the presence of existent or predicted health derived or health related self-care or dependent-care deficits.[2] The object or focus of the actions of nursing administration is the definable but changing population of persons for whom a legally constituted enterprise ensures the continuing availability and actual provision of nursing.

The situational context for nurses engaged in nursing practice is wherever persons who seek and need nursing reside or where they come to receive nursing. Nurses may go to where patients are, in their homes, in hospitals, or other types of resident-care institutions. Or patients may come to clinics or other types of facilities where nurses are available to provide nursing. The situational contexts for the actions of nursing administration are broadly defined by positional locations of nursing administration in the organizational structure of enterprises and by the domain and boundaries of their vested managerial powers.

Residence services including lodging, food service, as well as housekeeping, laundry, and maintenance services provided by some health-service enterprises are outside the domain of both nursing practitioners and nursing administration. However, the boundaries of residence services and the boundaries of nursing often impinge heavily one upon the other. Nursing that contributes to the diagnosis and meeting of therapeutic self-care demands of individuals and to the diagnosis and regulation of the exercise or development of self-care and dependent-care capabilities of individuals occurs within the broader context of the daily living of these individuals.[3] Residence services of hospitals and other health-care institutions provide for persons served the essential and continuously required resources for daily living. This, also, is the purpose for making water, food, toilets, and waiting rooms available to persons who use clinics and other types of outpatient services.

Persons who constitute nursing administration should know and continuously develop insights about how residence services and nursing impinge as they serve one or more of the subpopulations of the enterprise. In some countries of the world residence services may be restricted to that of shelter.

The Definition Examined

The foregoing definition of nursing administration has identifiable elements or parts. These include the following:

1. Persons in situational contexts within institutions who "manage" courses of affairs specific to ensuring the continuous availability and provision of nursing.
2. Populations served by the institution that are in need of nursing now and at future times.
3. Established authorities of formally constituted institutions who give managerial power to nursing administration.

4. Purposes or missions of formally constituted enterprises.
5. Fulfillment in whole or in part of the purpose or mission of institutions through the provision of nursing to the populations served now and at future times.

The definition specifies both the human and the functional elements of nursing administration.

The named parts of the definition suggest that enlightened nursing administrators in health service enterprises or in other institutions with health service units, for example, as in colleges or industrial organizations, seek and use answers to the following critical questions:

1. What are the domain and boundaries of nursing as a form of health care?
   What is the nature of the points of articulation of nursing with other forms of health care?
2. How can populations to be provided with nursing be described from a nursing perspective in order to make judgments about nursing requirements?
   What are valid models and rules to ensure provision of nursing to each described subpopulation or sub-subpopulation?
3. What courses of action must be taken to conduct and control—that is, to manage—the availability and the provision of nursing to current and future populations served by the institutions?
4. What are the situational contexts within which nursing administration has the authority to exercise its power to manage courses of affairs specific to ensuring the provision of nursing to a population or subpopulation?
5. What are the defined and authorized domains and the boundaries of nursing administration in specific situational contexts to manage—that is, to conduct and

control—the affairs related to ensuring the continuing availability and provision of nursing to described populations?

Deepening understanding of the term nursing administration requires the resolution, the investigation, and the answering of the foregoing questions. The questions can be divided into those that have a nursing context, question 1; a combined nursing and institutional context, question 2; and those that have a nursing, a managerial, and an institutional context, question 3, 4 and 5. It is not the purpose of this chapter to provide answers to these questions. However, the questions as posed provide one road map for seeking understanding of nursing administration within health-care institutions and health-care units within other kinds of institutions.

A GENERAL THEORY

The foregoing exploration and exposition of the meaning of the term "nursing administration" lays out its essential elements and relationships in an explicit or implicit manner. The elements and relationships are more definitively expressed in the following descriptive explanation of nursing administration. This descriptive explanation may be considered as a general theory of nursing administration.

A Theory of Nursing Administration

All actions that are proper to nursing administration are actions that are produced by persons with foreknowledge of: (1) nursing as a field of knowledge and practice, (2) the purpose or mission of the institution of which they are an organic part, (3) how nursing contributes to mission fulfillment, and (4) the domain and boundaries of their received powers to manage courses of affairs that ensure the continuing provision of nursing to populations served. All actions that are proper to nursing administration regardless of situational location have a sequential order related to the purposes and the forms of the actions. Courses of action to provide continuous descriptions from a nursing perspective of populations to be provided with nursing are prior to courses of action to provide continuous calculation of what is required to provide nursing to the populations served at this time and at future times. These two courses of action are prior to and provide the substructure or foundation for as well as the linkages with the continuous management of all courses of affairs that ensure the continuing availability and provision of nursing to present and future populations served by the institution.

The foregoing theory, a theory about an organizational entity, namely, nursing administration, is expressed within an action frame reference. Actions proper to nursing administration are viewed (1) in relation to their performers who have four kinds of foreknowledge and (2) in relationship to the purposes or results of the actions. The expressed theory posits persons other than nursing practitioners as having roles in making nursing continuously available to persons served by the enterprise. The nursing focus of nursing administration is related to populations served through nursing. The managerial focus is on ensuring that nursing is continuously available and provided to persons with health derived or health related self-care or dependent care deficits. Deficit is a relational term that in nursing expresses the presence of a demand for continuing self-care that exceeds what individuals can do for themselves or their dependents.[4]

Analysis of the expressed theory of nursing administration will yield a set or sets of propositions which, upon further analysis will yield sets of propositions that are specific to real situations. Propositions expressed in terms of concrete realities specific to nursing administration in particularized situational contexts provide one basis for formulating testable hypotheses.

Formulation of the Theory

The general descriptive explanation of nursing administration resulted from investigation of two questions.

1. Does *nursing* make the managerial responsibilities of persons vested with such power and responsibilities specific?
2. If so, how does this come about?

The personal process of conceptualizing nursing administration was based on the understanding that both nursing and administration are entities in and of themselves. The critical question was: What does nursing add to the connotation of the word administration when the words are conjoined?

The process of conceptualizing was facilitated by common sense knowledge based on a variety of experiences in nursing administration as well as from an enabling level of achievement as a scholar in the fields of organization and administration. The process was reinforced by (1) dynamic knowing of the domain and boundaries of nursing as a field of knowledge and practice, (2) acceptance of nursing as a knowledge intensive field of practice, (3) acceptance that task-focused preparation and training is not enabling for the practice of nursing, and (4) by accepting nursing and other forms of health care as human services.

This general theory of nursing administration was formulated and expressed with the acceptance of a number of presuppositions, which include the following five major ones:

1. Health service institutions or health units of other types of institutions have purposes or missions that can be fulfilled at least in part through the provision of nursing to persons served by the institution.

2. Health service institutions or units serve persons who constitute describable changing populations.
3. Nursing administration is an organizational body, a component part of a health service institution or a unit of another type of institution.
4. Nursing administration in organized enterprises receives its managerial power from persons charged with institutional governance or with institutional administration.
5. Health-service institutions where nursing is provided as a continuously available service employ nursing practitioners or contract with them for their services, or grant them the privilege of practicing nursing within the institution.

These assumptions along with the general theory of nursing administration can serve as guides to persons who seek factual information about nursing administration in specific enterprises. Mastery of the theory and uncovering the substantive structure of each of its main elements will lead individuals to enhance their understanding of nursing administration.

SITUATIONAL CONTEXTS

A General Description

The term situational context used both in the definition and in the expressed general theory of nursing administration refers to the related and combined circumstances and facts that make or define a natural setting for the actions of persons who constitute nursing administration within the structures of organized institutions. It was previously stated that such natural settings are defined by positional locations of nursing administration in an organized structure of positions and by the domain and boundaries of nursing administration's vested managerial powers and

responsibilities. In existent institutions or units thereof, information to describe nursing administration's situational context would be specific to the institution. From a broader perspective, it is desirable to explore types of circumstances and kinds of facts and conditions that in general serve an investigator in describing and understanding nursing administration's action settings.

Positional Location

Positional location in an organizational structure is identified in terms of "distance," on the one hand, from existent governing and executive positions (e.g., governing boards and chief executive officers or institutional administrators) and on the other hand, from nursing production positions (positions of nursing practitioners and nurses who assist practitioners). There may be more than one nursing administration position at the same level in a structure of positions. This occurs as distance from institutional governing and executive positions increases and distance from production positions decreases. All nursing administration positions regardless of positional location carry responsibilities for functions that contribute to the effective performance of the entire enterprise. Together persons filling nursing administration positions constitute a management group with respect to ensuring the continuing availability and provision of nursing to populations served by institutions.

Nursing administration positions located in relation to the chief executive officer of an institution are more and more frequently identified as parts of an executive body concerned with institutional functioning now and in the future. Positions located in relationship to production units of an institution may combine the functions of nursing practitioner and operational unit administration. Vested managerial responsibilities, according to Drucker, are more appropriately understood in terms of functions than in terms of power over people.[5]

Domain and Boundaries

The managerial powers and responsibilities of nursing administration are restricted (1) by positional location in the organization, (2) by the nursing orientation of these powers and responsibilities, and (3) by the size and characteristics of the populations to be provided with nursing at this time and at future times.

The proposed general theory of nursing administration specifies two types of nursing administrators' actions that relate to the populations to be served. These are:

1. continuous descriptions of populations from the perspective of nursing, and
2. continuous calculation of what is required to provide nursing to populations served at this time and at future times.

These two courses of action and their results are initial means to describe and define the domain and boundaries of the managerial responsibilities of nursing administration within positional locations in the organization. However, it is the positional location of nursing administration in an organized structure of positions that initially limits nursing administration's managerial domain and boundaries by specifying extension of responsibility to the whole of the population served or to subpopulations from which it is constituted. For example, persons who receive managerial powers from governing boards or from chief executive officers have managerial responsibilities that extend to the whole of populations served.

Describing the managerial domain of nursing administration in terms of populations and subpopulations for which the continuing availability and production of nursing is to be ensured provides the means for giving specificity to functions that are generally recog-

nized as proper managerial functions. This approach also provides nursing administration with a basis for identifying boundary contacts of their managerial domains. Members of populations provided with nursing are also provided with other health and health-related services. This, as previously noted, holds for resident services as well. Boundary situations must be identified and needs for and processes and procedures for communication across boundaries established.

Knowing the domain and boundaries of managerial powers and responsibilities of nursing administration is viewed as both prior to and necessary for effectiveness in the performance of managerial functions. Since changes in the populations served may affect boundaries, such knowledge must be kept current.

MANAGERIAL RESPONSIBILITIES

Nursing administration has no meaning, function, or existence apart from formally organized enterprises. The work of this organ of an enterprise regardless of situational context is the work proper to managers. Managerial responsibilities vary by situational context. However, there are orientations, kinds of work and work operations that constitute common managerial responsibilities regardless of type of enterprise or positional location. The general or common responsibilities are described.

Orientations

The first essential work orientation of persons with managerial responsibilities is to the creation and maintenance of effective units of operation from which the enterprise is constituted and its mission is fulfilled. The second essential work orientation is toward knowing and maintaining the congruence of present decisions and courses of action with future demands for products or services and those internal and external factors that affect the enterprise as a whole or any of its units of operation. Drucker identifies these orientations as tasks to be done, namely, the creation of "a productive entity that turns out more than the sum of the resources put into it" and "to harmonize in every decision and action the requirements of the immediate and long-range future."[6]

Work Operations

The first managerial orientation and task is described as the proper ordering of persons and material resources so that a functioning whole is continuously created as organizational members fulfill their positional role responsibilities. The order to be brought about can be understood in terms of points of order in wholes with parts. There is the order of each part to its proper operations, the order of part to part, the order of each part to the perfection of the whole, and the order of the whole to an extrinsic end.[7]

Since enterprises are artificial, that is, created entities and not naturally existent ones, the whole that is an enterprise is continuously being made through the decisions and actions of people. This requires the managerial work operations of (1) objective setting, (2) analysis and organization of work and selection of people, (3) motivating and communicating, and (4) designing and ensuring the use of measurements of performance and results for the enterprise as a whole and for each of its unitary parts.[8]

The second managerial orientation and task is to ensure that the current decisions and actions incorporate or are in harmony with future requirements of the enterprise. Here the concern is for: the survival of the enterprise; its growth within the limits of its resources and the demands for its products or services; efficient use of resources; effectiveness of production; and capital for future

expenditures. Managerial responsibilities in this area are fulfilled when managers with knowledge of present operations and demands make decisions and take actions that look to ensuring future and continued operation of the enterprise.

What administration must know about the present and envision for the future relates to: the requirements for the performance of the essential institutional functions of production and distribution of products or services, and the financing of all current and future operations; and to the performance of functions to ensure the presence and effective action of people as well as to the continuing availability of material resources—equipment, supplies, and physical plant.

The managerial work operations associated with this orientation and task include: establishing and using standards and criteria for selection of people for operational and managerial positions; identification of costs of continuing operations and sources of capital to finance them; finding new operational methods or extension of methods presently in use in performance of the production or distribution or financing function; and, finally, in the development of self and others within the individual's managerial domain.

MANAGERIAL RESPONSIBILITIES AND NURSING

Nursing administration is enterprise oriented. The population to be served through the continuing availability and provision of nursing is a population first defined in its relationship to the enterprise. The actual availability and provision of nursing at this time or that time is a service that is justified in terms of its relationship and contribution to the purpose or mission of the enterprise. The three courses of action identified as specific to nursing administration in the foregoing expressed theory of nursing administration are enterprise oriented, since each is focused sequentially on the population to be served. It should be understood that all three courses of action or processes must be in continuous performance because of changes that occur in the populations served, as well as in theoretical and practical nursing knowledge and in prevailing social and economic conditions.

Nursing administration is nursing oriented. This occurs through nursing administrators' "dynamic knowing of nursing" and through their ability to think nursing. Nursing administrators' judgments and decisions cannot be practical and rational unless these persons know nursing as a discipline of knowledge and practice both in relationship to their own work and to the work of nursing practitioners.[9]

REFERENCES

1. Orem DE. Orem's conceptual model and community health nursing. In: Asay MK, Ossler CC, eds. Conceptual models of nursing, applications in community health nursing. Chapel Hill, NC: Department of Public Health Nursing, School of Public Health, University of North Carolina at Chapel Hill, May 1984, p. 48.
2. Orem DE. Nursing: concepts of practice. New York: McGraw-Hill, 1985, pp. 34–35.
3. Orem DE, 1985, pp. 37–38.
4. Orem DE, 1985, pp. 128–129.
5. Drucker PF. Management tasks, responsibilities, practices. New York: Harper & Row, 1985, pp. 48 and 394.
6. Drucker PF, 1985, pp. 398–399.
7. Niemeyer Sr MF. The one and the many in the social order according to Saint Thomas Aquinas. The Catholic University of America. Philosophical studies no. 130. Washington, DC: The Catholic University of America Press, 1951.
8. Drucker PF, 1985, pp. 399–401.
9. Van Eron M. Clinical application of self-care deficit theory. In: Riehl-Sisca J, ed. The science and art of self-care. Norwalk, CT: Appleton-Century-Crofts, 1985.

6

Applying Orem's Model in Nursing Administration

Dorothy Nunn
Ann Marriner-Tomey

D OES THEORY-BASED practice improve nursing care? An article reviewed by the Journal Club at Indianapolis Veterans' Administration Hospital said it did and stimulated an interest among the nurses in the club to find out for themselves. They added, "Explore existing nursing theories" to their nursing service goals, hired a consultant, examined various nursing theories, and implemented Orem's Self-Care Deficit Theory. The need for carefully planned change over a long period of time was also identified.

ADMINISTRATIVE SUPPORT

It is difficult to answer the questions: Does theory-based practice improve nursing care? What is a theory? What are nursing theories? Many nurses haven't studied nursing theory as part of their education. Just the mention of theory tends to be intimidating.

What hurdles, therefore, must be overcome in search of the answers to questions about nursing theory? The nurse administrators at the Indianapolis Veterans' Administration knew they must prepare themselves before they could lead staff to theory-based practice. They hired a consultant, studied theory development, and explored various theorists' work.

Orem's Self-Care Deficit Theory quickly emerged as a viable option. The concept of rehabilitation and self-care of the patient has been the focus of practice in the Veterans' Administration for years. This is reflected in the policy statement published by the Department of Medicine and Surgery, Washington, D.C., on April 21, 1975: "Nursing care will be an integral component of the total health care that will contribute to the promotion of health, the prevention of disease, health maintenance, supportive measures, and restoration to health." And again, on April 1, 1985: "Nursing Practice contributes to the promotion and maintenance of health, the prevention of disease, rehabilitation to optimal levels of functioning, and supportive measures for dignified death."

Orem's Self-Care Deficit Theory is consistent with the current mission and philosophy statements of nursing service. It seemed operational through the nursing process already in use in clinical practice.[1]

Next, the nurse administrators focused their efforts specifically on Orem's Self-Care Deficit Theory.[2–4,10] One nurse administrator, a head nurse, applied the model to real-life situations in clinical practice, and presented the following case on an ear, nose, throat (ENT) surgical unit to the executive group:

Mr. A., a 54-year-old white male, was a scheduled admission to the ENT unit. He told the head nurse on admission, "I have cancer of my voice box and I guess I'm going to die." The patient was ambulatory, clean and well-groomed, alert, and oriented. He was cooperative but very anxious. His chief complaint was that it was "hard to breathe." This resulted in difficulty in sleeping, orthopnea, and poor appetite. His voice was very hoarse. He stated he drank two or three beers and smoked two packs of cigarettes a day. He was taking no medication.

Further discussion revealed Mr. A. was self-employed. He was owner of a catfish restaurant on the Wabash River. His son was going to manage the restaurant, at least for awhile. Mr. A. was married and had a very concerned wife who had no documented health problems.

The head nurse and patient discussed the following philosophy and plan of care:

1. There would be changes in his life, but he wasn't going to die. Nurses would help him understand the changes and help him learn to adjust to these changes.
2. He was fortunate to be self-employed and given some time he would return to the restaurant.
3. He was moved to a private room where humidifying the room air would help his breathing.
4. Nurses planned teaching sessions for him and his wife the next day, which included meeting with the speech therapist and with a former patient with a laryngectomy.

The Figure 6.1 illustrates how this plan was compatible with the Self-Care Deficit Theory.[5–6]

The plan of care was initiated with the consensus of Mr. A. and his wife. He had his laryngectomy and right radical neck surgery. He was discharged approximately three weeks later as a self-care patient. The only follow-up of the patient was by the physician and the speech therapist. He no longer needed nursing care.

Outcome: He returned to manage his restaurant, with his son as assistant. He and his wife spent their winters in Florida.

They were very happy, close, and well adjusted.

Planned Change When Implementing a Nursing Theory

Education of key people was the first phase of the planned change. The nurse administrators had prepared themselves and demonstrated their support by hiring a consultant, allowing time for staff development, and sponsoring a retreat devoted to Orem's Self-Care Deficit Theory.

A telephone interview using a structured questionnaire of key people at Veterans' Administration Hospitals implementing Orem's Self-Care Deficit Theory revealed that the institutions that had made the most progress with the implementation had had structured courses over a prolonged period of time. One institution had developed work sheets for each major activity described by Orem. It is important to make bibliographies, selected articles related to the theory, and books available to key people in the organization. Those key people include nurses in administration, education, and quality assurance research who have the leadership expertise to bring about change. A series of conferences with this core group and a consultant knowledgeable about the theory are also helpful for assuring correct interpretation of a theory, as well as an agreement that a theory can be applied in nursing practice. This sound educational foundation is the first essential component for theory-based practice.

Using the key people for planning the implementation also is important. Activities include reviewing the philosophy and objectives of nursing service and changing them to reflect theory-based practice. Patient assessment instruments need to be revised to facilitate the collection of data necessary to apply the theory to practice. Care plans, standards of care, and evaluation mechanisms also need

A **Universal Self-Care**
   1. Adequate intake of air, water, nutrition
   2. Adequate elimination factors
   3. Activity and rest
   4. Solitude and social interaction
   5. Prevent hazards
   6. Promotion of human functioning (being normal)

Health Deviation Self-Care
   1. Changes in physical structure
   2. Changes in physical functioning
   3. Changes in behavior of habits of living

B **Self-Care Agency**
(capacity for self-care)

Causes for Deficit
   1. Knowledge
   2. Skills
   3. Motivation
   4. Unsafe to engage in self-care (not applicable to Mr. A.)
   5. Lack of potential for self care (not applicable to Mr. A.)

C **Deficits of Self-Care Actual**
   1. Airway clearance ineffective related to cancer of larynx
   2. Anxiety related to diagnosis
   3. Knowledge deficit related to surgical procedure and effects of surgery

Deficits Potential
   1. Alteration in physical structure related to laryngectomy
   2. Alterations in physical functioning related to:
   Air intake
   Inability to close airway
   Inability to smell
   Inability to speak in the normal manner

D **Nursing Agency**
Preoperative phase—Supportive-Educative
Immediate postoperative phase
   SICU · Wholly Compensatory
Transfer to ward · · · · · · · · · · · · Partially Compensatory
Week before discharge · · · · · · · · · Supportive-Educative

Figure 6.1 An illustration of the systematic assessment of self-care the nurse makes upon the admission of the client. This allows the determination of deficits in self-care to be identified (*A*), and an evaluation of the causes for the deficits (*B*). *C* describes the actual and potential deficits related to Mr. A. *D* illustrates the sequential changes in nursing care for Mr. A. from admission to discharge.

to be revised to assure that they are consistent with the theory.

Next, it is appropriate to select a pilot unit to begin the implementation of theory-based nursing. The survey of Veterans' Administration Hospitals using Orem's Self-Care Deficit Theory revealed that the majority of the agencies used long-term care units as pilot study units.[7]

An assessment of the organizing structure

for the delivery of nursing care on patient care units is important. A method of nursing-care delivery that has built in accountability of the professional nurse in clinical practice is critical. Accountability should be in place when an all resident nurse staff is implementing primary nursing. A modified primary nursing model can also support theory-based practice when the nurse is accountable for planning and goal setting with the patient, writing nursing orders, and evaluating progress even if he or she does not necessarily provide "hands on" care. Team nursing can support theory-based nursing if there is a permanent team leader who can assure continuity and accountability for care. Rotating staff nurses in and out of the team leader role does not facilitate the change to theory-based practice—nor does functional nursing.

Collaborative practice may also support theory-based practice. This may range from units with regularly scheduled multidisciplinary rounds to a hospital nurse practice committee that promotes and supports collaborative practice.

Next, the preparation of staff on the pilot units through structured classes, reading assignments, discussion groups, and evaluation of understanding is important. If there is an affiliation with a school of nursing, faculty and students need to be informed about the theory-based practice. Whether or not the school supports the theory-based practice will influence the continued use of the hospital

Implementation of Planned Change — Flow of Events

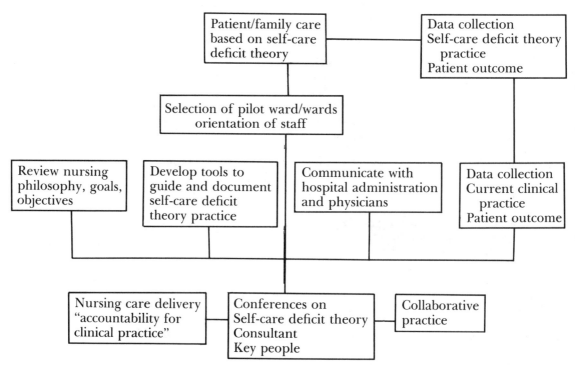

Figure 6.2 Illustration of the sequences of events necessary to implement change to theory based practice. The chart includes data collection related to quality of clinical practice and patient outcomes to make the determination if theory based practice improves nursing care.

facility for clinical practice for students. If the school faculty teach nursing theory and support the selected mode of theory-based practice, the preparation of new graduates and staff can be greatly enhanced. Conferences between clinical faculty, students, and staff are desirable. The hospital administrator, physicians, and family members will also need to be coached regarding the change to theory-based practice.[8] Figure 6.2 capsulizes these basic components of planned change.

EVALUATION

Nurses faced with cost containment, increased acuity of patients, reduced length of stay, and shifts to ambulatory care need to both ask and answer, "Does theory-based nursing practice make a difference?" Consequently, there needs to be a plan to evaluate care prior to implementation and periodically thereafter.[9]

Nursing monitors for the quality and appropriateness of care are already being used. The criterion for evaluating Orem's Self-Care Deficit Theory should include patient and family teaching, patient and family understanding, goal attainment, progress or lack of progress toward goals, and discharge planning to support continuing care after discharge where necessary. Patient and family satisfaction can be checked through the use of a questionnaire at the time of discharge. Patient outcomes need to be evaluated at the time of discharge and thereafter. Most Veterans Administration Hospital patients return to the Ambulatory Care Division for follow-up services and evaluation. Utiliza-

tion review reports can be used to identify the number and the reasons for readmissions.

It is also appropriate to check nurse and physician satisfaction. In one survey, 30 out of 39 nurses perceived that theory-based practice would increase their job satisfaction, five said it wouldn't, and four were uncertain.

After an Orem's Self-Care Deficit Theory retreat, attendants were asked, "Do you believe patients would benefit if you based your nursing practice on this model?" Thirty-four said yes, two said no, and three were uncertain. If evaluation demonstrates improved patient outcomes, and increased patient, family, physician, and nurse satisfaction, the credibility of theory-based nursing practice is enhanced.

REFERENCES

1. Joseph LS. Self-care and the nursing process. Nurs Clinics of North America 1980; 15(1):131–143.
2. Orem DE. Nursing: concepts of practice. 3rd ed. New York: McGraw-Hill Inc., 1985.
3. Calley JM et al. The Orem self-care nursing model. In: Riehl SP, Ray C, Conceptual models for nursing practice. New York: Appleton-Century-Crofts, 1980, pp. 302–314.
4. Herrington JV, Houston S. Using Orem's theory: a plan for all seasons. Nurs Health Care, 1984; pp. 45–47.
5. Aggleton P, Chalmers H. Orem's self-care model. Nurs Times 1986; 36–39.
6. Anna J et al. Implementing Orem's conceptual framework. J Nurs Adm 1978; 8–11.
7. Mullin VI. Implementing the self-care concept in the acute case setting. Nurs Clinics of North America 1980; 15(1):177–190.
8. Clinton JF et al. Developing criterion measures of nursing care: case study of a process. J Nurs Adm 1977; 7(7):41–45.
9. Gallant BW, McLane AM. Outcome criteria: a process for validation at the unit level. J Nurs Adm 1979;9(1):14–21.
10. Eben JD et al. Self-care deficit theory of nursing. In: Marriner A. Nursing theorists and their work. St. Louis: The CV Mosby Co, 1986 pp. 117–130.

7

Parse's Man*-Living-Health Model and Administration of Nursing Service

Rosemarie Rizzo Parse

HOW would nursing services be administered in a setting where the man-living-health theory is reflected in practice? This question, to be answered in this chapter, is based on the following assumptions:

1. Administration as a part of management science is a unique field, distinct from the discipline of nursing.
2. The principles of administration that govern a particular nursing service unit should be congruent with the theory guiding the nursing practice in that unit.

The purpose of this chapter is to set fourth some essentials about the administration of nursing services where Parse's theory is the theoretical base of nursing practice. Two major areas will be addressed: first, the man-living-health theory, and second, some essential aspects of nursing service administration of a man-living-health practice.

PARSE'S THEORETICAL BASE OF NURSING PRACTICE

The theory of man-living-health evolves from the simultaneity paradigm[1] and is based on

*The term "man" throughout this chapter refers to mankind in the generic sense, Homo sapiens.

beliefs about man, environment, and health that reflect noncausal transformation. Noncausal transformation is the continuously changing process coconstituted by the man-environment interrelationship; Man and environment evolve mutually and simultaneously. Man is viewed as an open being, different from the sum of parts, free to choose meaning in situations. Man and environment cocreate rhythmical patterns. Each pattern, man, and environment, is recognized as unique, yet each participates in cocreating the other. Man viewed from this perspective is not divided into "bio," "psycho," "socio," and spiritual components, but rather is viewed as unitary with unique patterns of relating. Man has the capacity to hope and dream and move beyond the "now" in experiencing various levels of the universe simultaneously.

Health, in the man-living-health theory, is viewed as a process of becoming, experienced by the person.[1,2] It is a nonlinear entity, a set of values cocreated in interrelationship with the environment and others. Health is man's lived experiences unfolding day to day, it is not the absence of disease nor is it man coping with the environment. "Man-living-health" is the central phenomenon of the theory. Man's patterns of relating manifest health from a personal perspective as mean-

69

TABLE 7.1   Principles of Man-Living-Health with Dimensions of the Practice Methodology

Principle I Structuring meaning multidimensionally is cocreating reality through the languaging of imaging and valuing.	**Dimension I** Illuminating meaning is shedding light in "explicating" the was, is, and will be as it appears now.
Principle II Cocreating rhythmical patterns of relating is living the paradoxical unity of revealing-concealing, enabling-limiting, while connecting-separating.	**Dimension II** Synchronizing rhythms happens in "dwelling with" the pitch, yaw, and roll of the interhuman cadence.
Principle III Cotranscending with the possibles is powering unique ways of originating in the process of transforming[2] (p. 41).	**Dimension III** Mobilizing transcendence happens in "moving beyond" the meaning moment to what is not yet[1] (p. 167).

ing is given through choices made in various situations. These choices incarnate man's intended hopes and dreams as reality is shaped on the basis of value priorities. In light of this, one is responsible for the cocreation of one's personal health.

These basic beliefs about man and health are the philosophical groundings of the theory of man-living-health. Nine specific assumptions form the foundation of the theory;[2] these have been synthesized into the following three (pp. 161-162):

1. Man-living-health is freely choosing personal meaning in situations through the intersubjective process of relating value priorities.
2. Man-living-health is cocreating rhythmical patterns of relating in open interchange with the environment.
3. Man-living-health is cotranscending multidimensionally with unfolding possibles.

These assumptions provide the philosophical framework for the theory; the principles and theoretical structures emerge from this framework. Three major ideas are emphasized in the theory: (1) man structures personal meaning from experiences at various levels of the universe simultaneously (multidimensionally); (2) man, with the environ-

ment and others, cocreates rhythmical patterns that are paradoxical in nature; (3) man cotranscends, moves beyond the "now," with envisioned dreams and hopes of what is not-yet. These three major ideas reflect the view of man as different from the sum of parts, free to choose, bearing full responsibility for choices, and living health as a process of becoming.

The three major principles of the theory and their exact formulation appear in Parse.[2] From these principles arise research and practice methodologies unique to the man-living-health theory.[1] The principles are specified in Table 7.1 and aligned with the coordinate dimensions and processes of practice.

MAN-LIVING-HEALTH PRACTICE METHODOLOGY

It is clear from Table 7.1 that the dimensions and processes of practice evolve directly from the principles of the theory.[1] Deriving the practice methodology directly from the theory is a concrete way to connect theory to practice. The goal of man-living-health practice is the enhancement of the quality of life as viewed by the person and family. The practice takes place in the context of nurse-person and nurse-group interrelationships.

The nurse and person or group engage in dialogue, and whatever other activities are essential in a particular situation, with a goal toward "explicating" the meaning of the situation. That meaning shows itself in the language, explicit and tacit, with which the person or family share thoughts and feelings. Sharing thoughts and feelings in speech and movement "illuminates meaning." Simultaneously, the nurse is "synchronizing rhythms" by giving self over to the rhythms of the person and family and dwelling with the thrusting and turning of interhuman encounters (the pitch, yaw, and roll). The nurse does not focus on changing the rhythms to fit his or her own value system, like some nursing theories would advocate, but rather goes with the person and family to reach the harmony they seek in the situation. "Mobilizing transcendence" occurs simultaneously with illuminating meaning and synchronizing rhythms. This is "moving with" the person and family beyond the moment to their dreams and hopes of what is not-yet.[1,3,4]

The beginning dialogue between nurse and person focuses on the meaning for the person of the present situation, how it changes personal life goals, who the most important people are to the person, who and what provide the most comfort, and the person's major hopes, dreams, and plans. Through this nurse-person dialogue, a personal description of health is written, along with emerging patterns of health, which are the major themes that surface in the dialogue. The descriptions of health and emerging patterns of health are directly elicited from the person experiencing the situation. The plans for change related to hopes and dreams are decided on by the person, and articulated in a plan of care by the nurse. The plan of care is from the person's own perspective and not necessarily consistent with societal beliefs about health.

The man-living-health theory espouses different beliefs from other extant theories; thus, the practice based on this theory is unlike traditional practice. This practice is not the offering of advice and opinions from the personal health-value system of the nurse nor is it a canned approach to care. It is a subject-to-subject interrelationship, a loving, true presence shared with the other, for the purpose of enhancing the quality of life for that person and family.[1] The dimensions and processes described above are the empirical life of the theory of man-living-health, and they incarnate the beliefs about man, environment, and health inherent in that theory. These dimensions and processes of practice are not congruent with the nursing process. The nursing process is the practice method widely used in the discipline. It has four major areas—assessment, planning, implementation, and evaluation—and is really the problem-solving process. In traditional nursing practice, the problem-solving process, called nursing process, is used in developing nursing care plans, which are based on an assessment by a nurse that includes information about a person's biopsychosocial and spiritual well-being. The planning phase of the process includes identification by the nurse of needs, diagnoses, or problems and prescriptions for nursing orders designed to meet these needs. Implementation is conducted by the nurse, who carries out the orders specified in the plan, and evaluation indicates whether the implementation was successful in meeting the person's needs as assessed by the nurse. This is how the problem-solving process is traditionally applied to nursing. It is a systematized method congruent with totality paradigm theories and frameworks. It is not a practice methodology evolving from a belief system in the discipline of nursing.

Mature disciplines have their own research and practice methodologies generated from the ontologies in the discipline.[1] There are no alternative practice methodologies articulated yet for other theories in the discipline of nursing.

NURSING SERVICE ADMINISTRATION AND PARSE'S THEORY

When the practice methodology of man-living-health exists in a health-care setting, administration of nursing services is not traditional. The leadership process of the nurse administrator reflects an openness and concern for the values of the nurses practicing in the setting. This openness is demonstrated in a plan for interchange among nurses and administrators about the nursing-care practices in the setting. Concern for the nurses is manifested in a plan that calls for their participation in and responsibility for decision making regarding organizational philosophy, goals, standards of practice, evaluative processes, budget allocations, job descriptions, scheduling, research, educational programs, and mechanisms for change. There are conferences and informal gatherings for interchange, and gentle guidance by the administrator. A sense of freedom to discuss any issue permeates the environment.

The Nurse Administrator

The nurse administrator, as the leader in a nursing-service setting where Parse's theory is practiced, would necessarily be totally committed to that practice. He or she is a role model for other nurses. Thus, a strong knowledge of theory is essential. The nurse administrator teaches the nurses how to live the practice methodology of man-living-health in the setting and guides their progress through continuous dialogue, demonstration, and evaluation. While the milieu within the nursing practice setting is coconstituted by all persons therein, the general direction is set by the administrator. If nurses are expected to live the philosophy of nursing practice by valuing the person and family

being cared for, then the administrator's approach to the nurses must be one of openness, also demonstrating a valuing of each nurse's unique contribution to the quality of care in the setting.

The nurse administrator needs inner strength for the struggle to persist in fostering quality care. This inner strength is called upon as the nurse administrator guides others in the creative venture of practicing nursing from a nontraditional perspective.

Parse's theory is relatively new. It is now being tested in several practice settings. In these settings, nurse administrators have reported that the nurses are excited about their practice and achieve a great deal of personal satisfaction from the care they provide. Improved quality of care, as observed and reported by persons receiving care in these setting is also characteristic.

STRUCTURAL GUIDES IN ADMINISTRATION

The administrative structures, including philosophy, goals, standards of practice, and evaluative processes in a setting where Parse's theory is practiced, reflect the values in that theory. The written and lived philosophy espouse that man is a cocreator of health; thus, the person receiving care in the system is a designer of and expert on personal health patterns. Plans for health-care changes arise from the perspective of the person being cared for, as articulated in the nurse-person dialogue.

The philosophy and goals guiding nursing practice specify beliefs about man, health, and health care consistent with Parse's theory. A few sentences from a philosophy, examples of goals and standards are as follows:

Philosophy of Nursing

The practice of nursing in this health-care system is guided by Parse's beliefs about health and human beings and health-care delivery. Human beings are more than the sum of their parts and are free to choose in life situations. Health is a cocreated process of becoming; it is man's value priorities. The overall nursing practice in this setting is governed by propositions that arise from the theoretical structures of man-living-health. They are:

- Struggling toward dreams discloses the significance of the situation.
- Creating anew uncovers cherished beliefs that lead in a particular direction.
- A different view of the familiar emerges through speaking and moving, while being close to and away from others.

These propositions specify a concern for each person's own dreams, which reflect values and lead in a particular direction. These values are made clear through the person's speaking and moving with others. In this setting, the person is respected as the author of a personal becoming, and nursing practice is guided by the person's own goals for quality of life. Nursing care is delivered through Parse's practice methodology. The focus with the person, then, is on illuminating meaning, synchronizing rhythms, and mobilizing transcendence. A personal health description is written from each person's perspective and emerging patterns of health are identified.

Goals of Nursing Practice

- To enhance the quality of life from the person's perspective.
- To preserve the dignity of the person.

Standards of Practice

Standards of nursing practice and evaluative processes will be consistent with the philosophy and goals. The standards of practice arising from the theory of man-living-health will provide a means for determining the

quality of nursing for persons receiving care in this setting.

Standard I—Personal Health Description

A personal health description will be written from the perspective of each person receiving care. The nurse in dialogue with the person will discuss the meaning of the situation to the person, close relationships of the person, and the person's hopes and dreams.

Evaluation

1. Documentation shows personal health descriptions for all persons receiving care.
2. Health descriptions reflect the meaning of the situation, the close relationships of the person, and the hopes and dreams articulated by the person receiving care.
3. Observations reveal nurse-person dialogue regarding meaning, relationships, and hopes and dreams.

Standard II—Patterns of Health

Emerging patterns of health will be identified with each person as they arise in the nurse-person dialogue.

Evaluation

1. Documentation gives evidence of updated emerging patterns of health. An "emerging pattern of health" is a theme surfacing in discussion. These are paradoxical in nature and reflect both sides of a rhythm. Examples are: "Wants to leave confined setting, yet takes no initiative in planning for the change," "Likes to have multiple connections with people, yet keeps to himself." Activities are planned in relation to the specific emerging patterns of health.
2. Emerging patterns of health and related activities are clearly described.

Standard III—Directional Movement

The directional movement toward changing patterns of health will be formulated by the person receiving care in dialogue with the nurse.

Evaluation

1. Plans for changing certain patterns of health are written specifically from the perspective of the person receiving care.
2. Progress toward change is described by the person and recorded by the nurse.

Evaluative Processes

Evaluative processes flow directly from the philosophy and goals of nursing in a setting. Thus, evaluation would be descriptive in nature. Quality of care is determined by assessment of the emphasis placed on each person's own priorities and how these priorities are lived in practice as viewed by the administrator, the nurse, and the person receiving care. The nature of the documentation and the experience of the person receiving care are also examined as part of the evaluation. The actual living out of the dimensions and processes of the practice methodology are assessed by the nurse and the administrator, and salary increases and promotions are related to this evaluation. Other considerations for promotion are the continuing emergence and change in the nurse as evidenced by initiative for innovation in practice, attending educational programs, and the general way of being with persons receiving nursing care.

In summary, in administering nursing services where Parse's theory is practiced, the leadership strategies, the role of the administrator, the philosophy, goals, standards of practice, and evaluative processes are different from those guided by other theories. What makes this practice of nursing and nursing administration different is its "primary" focus. The primary concern is to enhance the quality of life from the perspective of the person who is receiving care.

The person is the authority on his or her own health and is respected as the author of a personal becoming. The nurse is "there with" the person—illuminating meaning, synchronizing rhythms, and mobilizing transcendence as a primary concern. Administering nursing in this type of setting is a challenging opportunity to test the effectiveness of Parse's theory for enhancing the quality of life of people while further carving out this unique practice methodology.

REFERENCES

1. Parse RR. Nursing science: major paradigms, theories and critiques. Philadelphia: WB. Saunders, 1987.
2. Parse RR. Man-living-health: a theory of nursing. New York, John Wiley & Sons, 1981.
3. Butler MJ. Family transformation: Parse's theory in practice. Nursing Science Quarterly 1988;1(2):68–74.
4. Mitchell G. Utilizing Parse's theory of man-living-health in Mrs M's neighborhood. Perspectives 1986; Winter:5–7.

8

Roy's Adaptation Model: Theories for Nursing Administration

Sister Callista Roy
James Anway

THE PURPOSE of this chapter is to propose a theory of the organization as an adaptive system. Roy's Adaptation Model (RAM) of nursing is used as a framework to identify concepts, theorize, and develop propositions about nursing administration. The model developed rapidly in nursing education in the 1970s. There were a few implementation projects in nursing practice during the 1970s as well, but in the 1980s, the model has been used fairly widely in health-care agencies.

A growing conviction has emerged about the relevance of the adaptation model to nursing service administration. Mastel, Hammond, and Roberts[1] discussed some of the issues involved in administering an implementation project. Roy[2] described the model as applied to several aggregates, including the social organization as an adaptive system. However, neither of these publications, nor any other to date, has realized the potential of systematic theory development and application of the model in nursing service administration. Our chapter aims to fill this gap.

The application of RAM in nursing service administration is a quantum conceptual leap. The strategies lie in identifying the parallel assumptions and principles in nursing science, from Roy's perspective, and in organization science.

Nursing and management are character-ized by continuing evolution, recognition of other scientific advances, and particularly by development and refinement as practice disciplines. Today's organizations, and the beginning of organization theory, have their roots in the Industrial Revolution.[3] Principles from the physical and behavioral sciences have been used to improve the administration of organizations, and numerous conceptual approaches have been implemented to enhance the effectiveness of complex organizations.

Nursing science, and Roy's approach to it, likewise have historical roots and make broad scientific assumptions.[4] The interrelationship of theory, research, and practice is evident in the development of the Roy nursing model over the past 25 years, as it is in the field of administration.

The scientific and philosophical basis of the elements in the Roy model will be discussed and used as the basis for theorizing about nursing administration. The acronym RAM will refer to Roy's Adaptation Model, and RAMA will be used for the Roy Adaptation Model in Administration.

SCIENTIFIC AND PHILOSOPHICAL ASSUMPTIONS

The scientific assumptions of RAM are based on systems and adaptation theories. Von Bertalanffy, the originator of general systems theory, states that "organization runs right through all levels of reality and science."[5] (p. 42) Systems theory is concerned with the interactions of components in a system—system being defined as a complex of interacting elements. von Bertalanffy adds further clarification by stating that general systems are nonmechanistic, that is, regulative behavior is not determined by structural or "machine" conditions, but by the free interplay of organismic forces. Systems theory has been used widely as a theoretical framework from which to understand, analyze, and approach the administration of organizations, for example, in Epstein's approach to planning for change.[6] (p. 47)

Gillies[7] notes that the nurse manager works within, among, and on a variety of systems. She highlights the importance of recognizing that each system has both inputs and outputs. Each can be viewed as a self-contained unit, and at the same time individual systems are integrated with other systems. Holism and integrated functioning are basic premises of systems theory.

The systems framework enables the nurse manager to identify the place and function of subsystems, and to visualize internal and external factors as an integrated whole. The systems within which management operates are complex.

According to Roy, a system is described in its simplest form as a structure and process involving input, internal and external feedback processes, and output. She further emphasizes the system characteristics of holism, interdependence, and interrelationships.[4] In speaking of the community aggregate, Roy[2] indicates that each subsystem has its own goals and objectives. In addition, Roy's view of the aggregate system highlights the interaction of any single system with its suprasystems.

A second set of scientific assumptions for RAM focuses on the concept of adaptation and its relationship to systems theory. Ryan describes three essential elements of a successful system. Systems have (1) goal direction, (2) feedback, and (3) the ability to change or adapt.[8] All normal behavior is purposeful, then, including the effective behavior of organizations: to be effective, a successful management system needs to reflect a unified purpose. Feedback regarding the effect of management actions is the element that enables participants in the system to analyze and evaluate information from the environment. The system that has the ability to recognize the need for change, and be responsive to new input, has the capacity for adaptive change.

Roy has drawn on the work of Helson[9] to describe adaptation as a positive response to the environment. Helson took the concept of adaptation from biology and sensory physiology and developed it in psychophysics. Later research related Helson's notion of Adaptation Level to the social psychology of the person. Quoting Helson, Roy notes that "adaptation is a process of responding positively to environmental changes in such a way as to decrease responses necessary to cope with the stimuli and increase sensitivity to respond to other stimuli."[10] (p. 37)

Roy views the person as an adaptive system, always interacting with other people and with the environment. She focuses on the person's ability to pool the effect of stimuli that have different effects on human behavior. Some environmental factors have a more immediate, almost causal effect, and in Helson's terminology are called "focal stimuli." Other factors affecting behavior are the context of a situation. A person is affected by these factors as he or she takes in and responds to the environment. They are weighed by the person as cognitive processing of the situation takes place and are called the "contextual stimuli." A person's response may also be influenced by factors within oneself, factors that cannot be precisely measured by the investigator of a person's Adaptation Level. Helson refers to these as "residual stimuli."

Roy maintains that the classification of stimuli as focal, contextual, and residual is useful for both nursing practice and research. Identifying the immediate focal stimuli helps the nurse prioritize patient needs and identify critical independent and dependent variables for research. Recognizing contextual stimuli adds meaning to patient behavior and serves to locate important intervening variables in clinical or laboratory studies. Residual stimuli refer to the nurses' hunches about factors that are influencing a situation, but which the nurse has not been able to validate as directly affecting patient behavior. In research, residual stimuli may be the intervening variables that for some reason have not been measured, but need to be recognized in the interpretation of findings. Focal, contextual, and residual stimuli, in systems terms, are the inputs to the person as an adaptive system, whether from inside or outside the person.

Just as the scientific assumptions from systems and adaptation theories are integral to the relationships and propositions in Roy's theory of the person as an adaptive system, so too are the philosophical assumptions of RAM. As described in greater detail elsewhere,[4] the philosophical assumptions about the adapting person in society involve humanistic values and the principle of veritivity. This principle suggests that the individual is rooted in absolute truth as distinct from a position of philosophical relativism.

The humanistic values of creative power, purposeful human behavior, intrinsic holism, and individual and interpersonal integrity are values aligned with those of many nurse managers. In fact, they are mirrored in a number of textbooks on nursing leadership and management[7,11] and in discussions of individual needs, enpowerment, stress, and communication.

Roy's description of the philosophical principle of veritivity affirms a common purposefulness of human existence. This principle states that it is not just the individual that is valued, but the individual in a social context. Roy's[4] explication of this principle is particularly useful for nurse managers. Managers have responsibility beyond the individual level. They are responsible both for the productivity of groups in relation to established goals and for the effectiveness of organizations. In the RAM perspective, this two-fold responsibility expands the social aspects on human activities. Roy[4] discussing veritivity, notes that human activity and creativity are used for the common good and are rooted in the value and meaning of life, and of all human existence.

MAJOR ELEMENTS OF RAM AND RAMA

According to Roy, the focus of nursing is comprised of five major elements: the person, the goal of nursing, health, environment, and nursing activities. These elements circumscribe and direct the practice of nursing. Each can be correlated with analogous elements identified for management. Hodge and Anthony[12] provide a list of such elements and describe them as the "basic building blocks" that help explain the behavior of people in organizations.

The Person and Organization

In clinical nursing, the person is the recipient of nursing care. As noted, the RAM view of person is as an adaptive system with processes for relating to the environment and with observable output. In her early writing, Roy[13] identified the cognator and regulator subsystems as the central coping mechanisms whereby the adaptive person takes in and processes environmental stimuli. Later, Roy[14] described each coping mechanism in detail and developed 36 propositions related to the intact and effective use of the cognator and regulator processes that generate the output of an adaptive system. Based on systematic observations of clinical situations, Roy has described this output in four categories referred to collectively as effector modes. The activity of the cognator and regulator is observable by noting behavior in each of the four adaptative modes: the physiologic, self-concept, role function, and interdependence.

The organization in administration[12] is the parallel system to the person in nursing. An organization is composed of interrelated departments, which function interdependently, to maintain integrity, productivity, and growth of the organization. The central focus of RAMA is the development of the nursing organization as an adaptive system. This system has stabilizer and innovator central mechanisms, and its own system modes.

The Goal of Nursing and Administration

The goal of nursing, according to RAM, is to promote the person's adaptation in four modes, thereby contributing to health, quality of life, or death with dignity.[10] (p. 38) The nurse helps the person manage his or her environment, to effect appropriate adaptive responses.

The goal of nursing service management is to ensure the most effective delivery of services to clients by adapting organizational systems and their resources. Successfully achieving this goal in Roy's terms will be evidenced by adaptive responses, that is, those which promote the survival or change (even discontinuation) of an organization. To become effective, to remain healthy, or to evolve, people in organizations need to remain open to adaptive change in response to environmental influences.

Individual and Organizational Health

One outcome of adaptive responses is health. Roy[10] defines health as both an outcome state

and a process. For the individual person, health involves being and becoming an integrated, whole person. Health defined as integration implies a continuous process of change throughout life: one is being and becoming until, and perhaps after, the time of mortal death.

Adaptation and change are frequently cited as organization phenomena.[12] Adaptation is believed to be directly related to wellness, and therefore ultimately to the survival and growth of an organization. Like people, organizations can be conceived of as suffering from various illnesses and manifesting a variety of symptoms.[15] (p. 40) According to Beer, "healthy organizations sense changes in the environment and make adaptations in the way they function to accommodate new environmental demands."[16,17] Organizations that are not adaptable to relevant stimuli are unlikely to remain viable or healthy over time.

Environment

Environment is the next major element in the nursing model. For the nurse, environment generally refers to the world within and around the person. As noted earlier, RAM describes the person's environment as internal and external stimuli, classified as focal, contextual, and residual. Stated broadly, the environment includes all the conditions, circumstances, and influences surrounding and affecting the development and behavior of persons or groups.[10] (p. 39) Management of the environment is a key to nursing intervention for the individual.

In administration, environment refers to the conditions internal and external to the organization. The conditions, for example, pertain to the physical setting in which goods and services are delivered; the national, regional, and local fiscal conditions and levels of consumer demand; and the availability of nursing and medical resources. The assessment and management of environmental factors are as significant for nursing administration as they are for nursing care.

Nursing and Managerial Activities

Nursing activities in relation to a client include the full range of actions best described by the steps of the nursing process: assessment, planning, (that is, diagnosis and goal setting), intervention, and evaluation. Assessment involves analysis of both behavior and stimuli; diagnosis involves synthesis of data from assessment; goals are set based on the person's adaptive status; interventions are designed to manage the stimuli to enhance adaptive behaviors; and evaluation compares behavior after nursing intervention, with the goal of care.

The managerial process involves planning, organizing, staffing, leading, and controlling.[17] Identification of these functions is based on the classic writings of Fayol, a French entrepreneur of the late nineteenth and early twentieth century. Goal-setting in management, as in nursing, is considered a key aspect of effective managerial activity.

RAMA THEORY OF THE ORGANIZATION

Our theory of an organization as an adaptive system describes internal adaptive mechanisms conceptualized specifically for this system. The observable outputs of organizations are conceptualized as system-specific adaptive modes. Using these conceptualizations, some sample propositions are developed as they relate to the two dynamic internal processors activating the four adaptive modes.

Adaptive Subsystems

The nursing theory of RAM and the parallel theory of RAMA are based on an understanding of the internal dynamism of adaptive systems. For individuals, Roy identifies the regulator and cognator subsystems as sources of adaptation.[13-14] These subsystems function as internal processors to actively promote survival, growth, and reproduction. The regulator in RAM responds automatically through neural-chemical and endocrine channels[14] and includes physiological processes to maintain homeostasis as well as to adapt to environmental stimuli. The cognator, on the other hand, is the person's coping mechanism that responds through four cognitive-emotive channels: perceptual-information processing, learning, judgment, and emotion.[14] This subsystem enables the person to analyze incoming stimuli, formulate an adaptive response, and effect a deliberate response.

The organizational adaptive subsystems in RAMA are called the stabilizer and innovator. Organizational systems, in this perspective, have two overriding goals—one related to stability, the other to change. These two goals of organizational systems are described by many authors using a variety of terms. Leontiades,[18] for example, refers to steady-state and evolutionary management. In nursing administration, McFarland, Leonard, and Morris[11] discuss growth and maturation as well as system maintenance.

In identifying the inner dynamism of the organization as an adaptive system, Roy uses the term "stabilizer" to refer to the structures and processes aimed at system maintenance. Just as the adaptive person has a set of neural-chemical-endocrine mechanisms and engages in processes that act to maintain homeostasis and equilibrium, so the adaptive organizational system has mechanisms and engages in processes that act to stabilize the organization. Stabilizers involve the established structures, values, and daily activities whereby staff accomplish the primary purpose of the organization. For example, in nursing service, the stabilizer subsystem includes the structures and activities designed to meet the needs of clients. When the stabilizer subsystem is intact and operating effectively, the organization is maintained.

The second adaptive subsystem in RAMA is the "innovator." This subsystem involves the structures and processes for change and growth in organizations. Just as the cognator of the person involves cognitive and emotional channels for responding to a changing environment, the organization has parallel information and personnel processes for innovation and change. The innovator dynamism of an organization involves cognitive and emotional strategies for change to higher levels of potential. Both established long-term and short-term strategies are included—for example, strategic planning activities, think tanks, team-building sessions, and social functions. When the innovator subsystem of an organization is intact and operating well, new organizational goals emerge and new growth and mastery are achieved.

Adaptive Modes

Roy defines the adaptive modes as a classification of ways of coping, which manifest cognator and regulator activity.[14] Each adaptive mode provides the clinician with a functional category in which to classify client behaviors and identify the influences of behaviors in one mode acting as stimuli for another. These categories are not intended to be mutually exclusive since they are integral to the person who functions as a whole. The classifying of behavior and stimuli, however, has been useful in organizing nursing assessment and in identifying relevant theory and research for practice. For individuals, Roy identifies the physiologic mode—including, needs for oxygenation, nutrition, elimination, activity-rest, and protection—as well as sensory input, electrolytes, and neurological endocrine function—as the first of four adaptive modes.

The second adaptive mode for the individual is self-concept, which is defined as "the composite of beliefs and feelings that one holds about oneself at a given time, formed from perceptions particularly of others' reactions, and directing one's behavior."[19] (p. 169) An individual's self-concept serves to preserve psychic integrity, balance the individual's perceptions with those of others, and promote and maintain a sense of integrity.

In RAM, the role function mode relates to the individual's behavior in society. It is defined as the functioning unit of society, the set of expectations about how the person occupying one position behaves toward a person occupying another.[20] Role performance is overt, can be evaluated within established norms, and is applicable to all individuals in the society.

Finally, the interdependence mode of RAM is concerned with the close relationships of people.[21] In this mode, adequacy and satisfying relationships with others are emphasized. Given the social nature of people, developing and maintaining significant social relationships during health and illness is an important part of adaptive functioning.[22,23]

To enhance the application of RAM concepts in management, the analogous RAMA perspective, consistent with organization and systems theory has been developed. In the analog, the physiologic mode is physical system; the role function mode is role system, the self-concept mode is interpersonal system, and the interdependence mode is the interdependence system.

ORGANIZATIONAL ADAPTIVE MODES AND THEORETICAL PROPOSITIONS

Physical systems are a critical part of organizations because they include basic, necessary, and often measurable components of organization performance. A physical system, in the context of RAMA, is defined as the basic operating resources and conditions without which an organization cannot maintain even rudimentary functioning. Included in this system are: personnel resources, physical plant and equipment, security and fiscal resources, and occupational and employee health. Problematic fluctuations in the quality and strength of one or more physical system is inevitable over time. However, prolonged ineffectiveness of physical system functions, for example, related to fiscal health to equipment, or information systems have dramatic, negative consequences: Most organizations cease to function without telephones and computers.

The role system relates to job performance. Roles are action components and it is through role performance that work is accomplished. The work done is designed to contribute to the accomplishment of an organization's mission. The mission can be defined as the assigned task or function of an organization. Role subsystems include the functions of administration, as well as information management, decision making, and performance measurement.[17]

Based on the principles of self-concept according to RAM, the interpersonal system of RAMA reflects how people and organizations (individuals and groups in organizations), perceive themselves because of environmental feedback. Interpersonal relationships; personnel management; individual, group and organizational self-image; social milieu; and culture comprise an organization's interpersonal system.

Recognizing the importance of social relationships, the interdependence system is defined as involving both private and public contacts that result in interpersonal relationships, established both intra- and interorganizationally. Intraorganizational contacts serve to facilitate information access by employers, managers, and staff as well as communicating individual needs. Subcomponents of the interdependence system include the governing political system and tax laws; availability of resources, supplies, and equipment; government regulations; ecological concerns; and the general economic climate. Becoming increasingly recognized by managers are activities related to interorganizational relations and organizational exchange. In 1974, Kast and Rosenzweig[3] projected the increasing emphasis on problems that we find in the 1980s related to the interface among organizations.

Table 8.1 summarizes components identified for each RAMA adaptive mode. These adaptive modes, or systems, encompass the relevant phenomenon in the nurse administrator's universe. Identification of these components helps to ensure a focused, conceptually sound, and comprehensive approach, from which to identify management problems and formulate practice interventions.

We think that RAMA paves the way for theory development and research about nursing service organizations as adaptive systems. Four theoretical propositions and their premises have been derived to describe how stabilizer and innovator subsystems may operate in relation to the RAMA modes and to the goals of an organizational adaptive system.

Premise 1: Adaptive systems expend energy toward goals.
Premise 2: Organizational systems have goals designed to promote stability and change.
Proposition: Energy expenditures in an organizational system promote health if directed toward system maintenance and system change goals.

Premise 1: A hierarchy of priority exists among adaptive modes.
Premise 2: Focus on the highest priority occurs in times of change.
Proposition: Changes in physical systems tend to become focal stimuli for energy expenditures in the role, interpersonal, and interdependence systems.

Table 8.1 RAMA Adaptive Mode Components

Physical Systems	Role Systems	Interpersonal Systems	Interdependence Systems
Fiscal health	Management process/role performance	Interpersonal relations	Internal Information access
Occupational health	planning	Personnel management	Organizational policies
Staff physical fitness	organizing	Conflict management	Communications
Environmental safety and security	staffing leading controlling	Self-concept/image	Communications *External* Resources/supplies
Organization design	evaluation	individual group department	
Technological applications	Information management	division company	Political system democratic socialistic
Physical environment		Organizational dress code	communistic
	Decision making		
Physical location/ neighborhood	Networking	Job satisfaction	Judicial/legal
Physical plan/structure and equipment	Corporate performance measurement	Values	Economic climate
Recruitment and retention of staff		Social responsibility Social health/welfare Informal work groups Environmental factors demographics culture social milieu	Governmental regulations Ecology/pollution/conservation Customer needs Market Organizational exchange Interorganizational relations

Premise 1: The interrelationships between and among the adaptive modes change in differing circumstances.

Premise 2: Self- and role systems have been noted to merge in persons as adaptive systems under certain conditions (See Silva[22] and Roy[23]).

Proposition: When organizational systems are stable, role and interpersonal systems operate separately, but in times of change these systems tend to merge.

Premise 1: An adaptive system cannot respond equally to all internal and external stimuli.

Premise 2: A given administrative action will affect each adaptive mode to a different extent.

Proposition: The organizational system develops priorities among internal and external influencing factors, which determine the intensity of the effect of a change on any one mode; these priorities, however, are fluid.

Each of these propositions, and others that can be developed from RAMA, has implications for practice. For example, in terms of the second proposition, agency mergers can be viewed as a change in a physical system that triggers intense activity in all other modes. Given the physical system changes attendant with organizational mergers, nurse managers in these settings revise roles and handle conflicts and related individual issues in the interpersonal systems. Specific research hypotheses can be derived from these and similar propositions. For example, an administrative research nurse may ask questions about the effectiveness of providing anticipatory role-playing before implementing structural changes in the organization.

APPLICATIONS OF RAMA

According to Horton, "the concept of the general management function characterizes the general manager as an analyst of conditions affecting his area of responsibility and therefore, as a diagnostician of the interpersonal and group relationships, values and norms in the organization.[24] (p. 92) RAMA offers administrators a conceptual framework for assessing organizational problems necessitating management attention and intervention. Using RAMA, the nurse administrator has a guide for assessing patients and organizations.

Roy views the behavioral response of the person as being either an adaptive or an ineffective response.[10] Applying RAMA to administration, it is useful to classify the behavior of the organization being assessed as either adaptive or ineffective. Adaptive behavior is defined as that which meets organization goals. High levels of organizational adaptation will result in goal attainment that is acceptable to the society served. Conversely, ineffective organizational behaviors will block goal achievement.

To assess a nursing problem, as noted earlier, Roy addresses (1) focal stimuli, or stimuli immediately confronting the person; (2) contextual stimuli, either within persons or coming from the environment; and (3) residual stimuli, such as attitudes, traits, culture, and beliefs that have an indeterminate yet potentially significant effect on a situation.[10] Like the person, the organization is affected by influencing stimuli. A focal stimulus is the primary input, which precipitates a management focus, and is either positive or negative. For example, nurse administrators are affected by a scarcity of experienced clinical nurses, particularly in acute-care settings. The contextual or contributing stimuli are salary levels, expanded job opportunities, attrition, and the widespread proliferation of staffing agencies.[25]

Residual stimuli include the recent experience of nursing personnel staffing cuts and changing attitudes toward pay equity.

Once influencing stimuli are identified, the nurse administrator is in a position to develop management interventions to maximize the impact of the stimulus input, thus maintaining adaptive function and preparing the way for system growth. The goal of the nurse manager then, is to contain the stimulus within the organization's adaptive zone or in a positive sense, to broaden the range. The concept of an adaptive level is parallel with the notion of an adaptive health level. Adaptation level sets up a zone within which stimulation will lead to a positive or adaptive organizational response.

It appears that in every organization, different degrees of adaptation or levels of organizational health exist from one time to another and at any one time in the several adaptive modes. Further, the specific adaptation health level of an organization, department, or unit, is measurable and can be quantified in terms of RAMA. For example, a corporation's end of year balance sheet can reflect the organization's health-performance level. Measures of job satisfaction, in the interpersonal mode of the same corporation at year's end, can reflect a different health-performance level.

In summary, RAMA enables assessment of organizations through integration of the adaptive modes with stabilizer and innovator functions. Adaptive versus ineffective behaviors related to a specific mode are identified. Additionally, the influencing stimuli are identified. Finally, the nursing process has been used to describe each problem leading to management interventions and evaluation.

Figure 8.1 provides an overview of this assessment process.[26] Initially, the manager (a) identifies an actual or potential management problem requiring RAMA assessment and categorizes the problem under one of the four adaptive modes, and (b) collects behav-

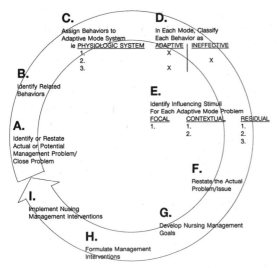

Figure 8.1   RAMA Nursing Process from assessment through Evaluation: A through E are assessment; F and G are planning; H and I are intervention, and A is evaluation.

ioral data pertaining to each problem. In step (c) related behavioral data is listed under the selected adaptive mode header. Then parallel to the system's header (d) the behaviors are categorized as either adaptive or ineffective. Determination of the number of adaptive or ineffective behaviors related to the selected problem gives the practitioner some idea of its significance.

To analyze a problem further, the identified management problem (not each behavior), is evaluated (e) in terms of focal, contextual, and residual stimuli. In step (f) the management problem is then restated for increased specificity. Next, (g) the management goals are identified and (h) interventions are formulated. Finally, (i) implementation is accomplished. To close the system loop, the results of the interventions are evaluated and the problem is either closed or the RAMA nursing process assessment cycle is repeated.

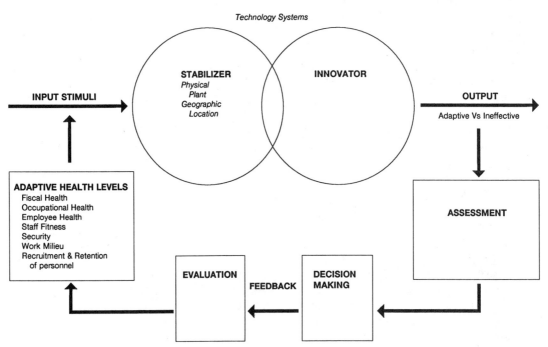

Figure 8.2   Physical Mode of the Organizational Adaptive System

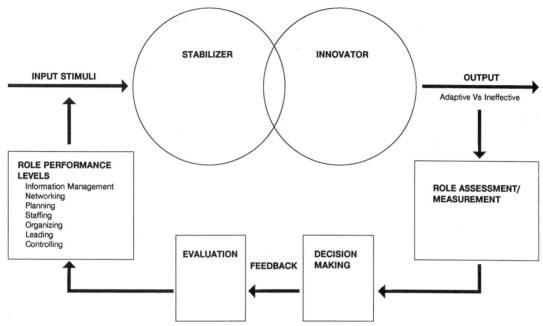

Figure 8.3 Role Mode of the Organizational Adaptive System

Figures 8.2 through 8.5 illustrate how the assessment process works specific to each adaptive mode.

In the physical system mode (Figure 8.2), the input stimuli are processed by the stabilizer and innovator subsystems. The stabilizer focuses specifically on things like the physical plant and the geographic location of the system. Outputs in this mode are assessed as either adaptive or ineffective. The assessment provides the basis for decision making and evaluation to be fed back into the system. Adaptive health levels related to fiscal, occupational and employee status are the result and then are themselves inputs to the system. A similar process follows with each of the modes.

The role system mode (Figure 8.3) specifically generates role performance levels related to factors such as information management, networking, leading, and controlling. The interpersonal system mode (Figure 8.4) receives specific output such as demographics

and culture. The adaptive health levels of this system relate specifically to elements such as self-concept and image, job satisfaction, and interpersonal relations. Finally, particular inputs to the interdependence system mode (Figure 8.5) include customer needs and market factors. Results from this mode of operation pertain specifically to elements such as information access, organizational exchange, and interorganizational function.

Evaluating administrative effectiveness is problematic at best, in fact, it has been said that "no agreed-upon body of objective standards exists by which to judge managerial performance.[27] (p. 26) To facilitate evaluative assessment of nursing organizations, a scale has been developed to numerically rank levels of organization health based on RAMA. Figure 8.6 describes a format that could facilitate identification, presentation, and tracking of an organization's level of health performance. Quantification of adaptation levels can provide the manager with specific, sub-

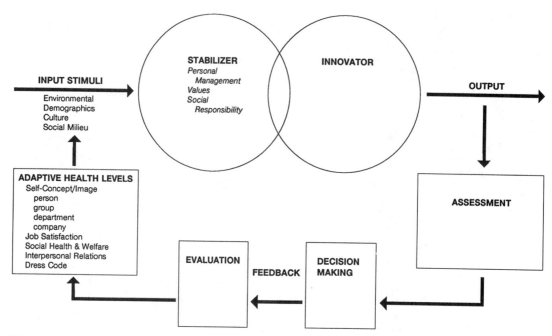

Figure 8.4   Interpersonal Mode of the Administrative Adaptive System

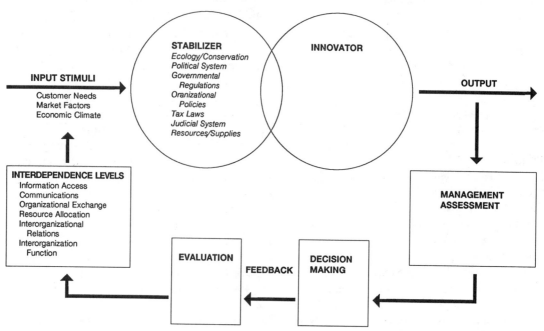

Figure 8.5   Interdependence Mode of the Administrative Adaptive System

ORGANIZATION HEALTH LEVEL

ADAPTATION LEVEL	PHYSICAL SYSTEM	ROLE SYSTEM	INTERPERSONAL SYSTEM	INTERDEPENDENCE SYSTEM
*9				9*
8				8
7				7
6				6
5				5
4				4
3				3
2				2
1				1

SCORE _____   _____   _____   _____

MEAN _____

OVERALL TOTAL _____

Figure 8.6 Organization Health Level. (Used and adapted with permission, courtesy of Mary McFarland.)

stantive information upon which to make decisions. Use of this matrix requires evaluation of each applicable component of the modes; data base programs are readily available and could greatly simplify the process required to develop, store, and update an organizational health evaluation. In conducting the evaluation, the nurse administrator relates the data base to the evaluation criteria to derive a value from 9 to 1 that reflects the level of adaptation. When this process is repeated for each mode, and the profile compared over time, the evaluation can be used as a planning guide.

To conclude, the Roy Adaptation Model of nursing has been used in nursing education, practice, and research the past 25 years. In this chapter a theory of the organization as an adaptive system, based on Roy's scientific and philosophical assumptions, and essential model elements, has been proposed as a further development of the original conceptual model. The development of each component of RAMA, and the education, practice, and research that can derive from it, emphasize organizational goals, stability, and change, as well as environmental impact. The sample propositions generated suggest hypotheses and indicate the potential for further development of theory and research-based nursing management.

Several specific applications have been presented, including an assessment guide, visualizations of subsystems, and a mechanism for administrative planning and evaluation based on level of organizational health. The RAMA approach to nursing administration is a scientifically based conceptual framework relevant to unit managers, department supervisors, and executive administrators. From this framework, problems can be identified, and new plans can be developed and implemented. RAMA applications include problem solving with staff. Aggregate department performance can be assessed, modified, and thus improved. Development of sound guidelines for a peer review program, monitoring quality of patient care, and establishing quality assurance standards are all potential uses of this model.

Nursing service administrators can play a role in further developing and testing RAMA, as well as other nursing models for administration. This growth can be facilitated by personally testing the concepts and theoretical propositions in practice. Additionally, administrators can allow students, researchers, and clinicians access to the organization for the purpose of testing administrative models, and can provide insights and guidance in the interpretation of findings from such projects.

Research opportunities for RAMA, and all other developing nursing management theories, remain relatively untapped. The Roy Model seems well-suited scientifically, philosophically, and developmentally for application to nursing service administration.

REFERENCES

1. Mastal MF, Hammond H, Roberts M. Theory into hospital practice: An implementation project. J Nurs Adm 1982;12(6):9–15.
2. Roy C. The Roy Adaptation Model: Applications in community health nursing. In: Proceedings of the eighth annual community health nursing conference, University of North Carolina, Chapel Hill, NC, 1984.
3. Kast F, Rosenzweig J. Organization management: a systems approach. New York: McGraw-Hill, 1974.
4. Roy C. An explication of the philosophical assumptions of the Roy Adaptation Model, Nursing Science Quarterly 1988;1(1).
5. von Bertalanffy L. Organismic psychology and systems theory. Massachusetts: Clark University Press, 1968.
6. Epstein C. The nurse leader: philosophy and practice. Reston, Virginia: V Reston Publishing Company Inc, 1982.
7. Gillies D. Nursing management: A systems approach. Philadelphia: WB Saunders Co, 1982.
8. Ryan B. Nursing care plans: a systems approach to developing criteria for planned evaluation. J Nurs Adm 1973;3(3):50–58.
9. Helson H. Adaptation level theory. New York: Harper and Row, 1964.
10. Roy C. Introduction to nursing: an adaptation model. 2d edition. New Jersey: Prentice-Hall, 1984.
11. McFarland G, Leonard H, Morris M. Nursing leadership and management: Contemporary strategies. New York: Wiley, 1984.
12. Hodge B, Anthony W. Evolution of organization theory and management. Boston: Allyn and Bacon Inc, 1984.
13. Roy C. Adaptation: A conceptual framework for nursing. Nursing Outlook, 18(3),43–45.
14. Roy C, Roberts S. Theory construction in nursing an adaptation model. New Jersey: Prentice-Hall Inc, 1981.
15. Frost T. The sick organization, part 1: neurotic, psychotic, sociopathic. Personnel 1985;62:40–44.
16. Beer M. A social systems model for organization development. In: Cummings T, ed. Systems theory for organization development. New York: John Wiley and Sons, 1980.
17. Koontz H, O'Donnel C, Weihrich H. Essentials of management. New York: McGraw-Hill, 1982.
18. Leontiades M. Management policy, strategy, and plans. Boston: Little, Brown, 1982.
19. Driever M. Theory of self-concept. In Roy C, ed. Introduction to nursing: An adaptation model. 1st ed. New Jersey: Prentice-Hall Inc, 1976.
20. Malaznik N. Theory of role function. In Roy C, ed. Introduction to nursing: An adaptation model. 1st ed. New Jersey: Prentice-Hall, Inc, 1976.
21. Tedrow M. Interdependence: Theory and development. Introduction to nursing: An adaptation model. 2d ed. New Jersey: Prentice-Hall, 1984.
22. Silva M. Needs of spouses of surgical patients: A conceptualization within the Roy Adaptation Model. Scholarly Inquiry for Nursing Practice 1987;1(1):29–44.
23. Roy C. Response to "Needs of spouses of surgical patients: A conceptualization within the Roy Adaptation Model." Scholarly Inquiry for Nursing Practice 1987;1(1):45–50.
24. Horton F. Reference guide to advanced management methods. United States of America: American Management Association Inc, 1972.
25. Cohen A. Nursing shortages will there be another nursing shortage? An analysis of the factors affecting today's market. Hospital Topics 1986;64(6):23–24.
26. Anway J. An organizational health assessment based on the Roy Adaptation Model. Presented at the 4th Annual Phyllis J. Verhonick Research Course, Washington, DC, 1986.
27. Stoner J. Management. New Jersey: Prentice-Hall Inc, 1982.

9

Application of the Roy Model to Nursing Administration

Colleen K. DiIorio

A MAJOR EMPHASIS of nursing since the 1960s has been the elaboration of a theoretical basis for nursing practice. The need to underscore practice with a body of knowledge propelled Roy and others to develop conceptual models to define and circumscribe that knowledge said to be "nursing." The Roy adaptation model, which gradually evolved from her work and that of her colleagues, is a synthesis of systems and adaptation theories applied to humans. The usefulness of the model for understanding and directing nursing practice has been demonstrated in a variety of clinical settings.

Using the case study approach, authors have described applications of the model to assessment of and intervention for clients who have a variety of dysfunctions.[1-2] Further development of the model has led to its incorporation in practice settings[3] and served as a basis for nursing curricula.[4] In addition, Roy and others have used the model as a framework for the study of families and communities.[5-8]

This chapter builds on previous work of Roy and Marshall, who have applied the model to the study of communities and groups.[6-7,9] The purpose of this chapter is to discuss the key components of Roy's model—adaptation, system theories, and humanistic values—as they relate to the administration of nursing in clinical settings. Theories of management and organizational behavior, to-gether with the writings of contemporary nurses, are interwoven to present a view of administration using a nursing framework.

ROY ADAPTATION MODEL

Since the inception of the Roy adaptation model, its refinement, integration, and utilization have concentrated on the individual. Roy's own work has included an initial application of the framework to aggregates of individuals such as families and communities.[6-7] However, to apply the model to nursing administration, we must sharpen the focus on its central theses and begin to reconceptualize the essential elements as they relate to organizations. This effort requires extrapolating elements in the model that are applicable to groups, and modifying other elements that focus only on the individual.

The first section of this chapter presents an overview of Roy's model and a brief description of the changes necessary to bridge the gap between the application of it to individuals and to nursing administration. The major components of the model—person, health, environment, and nursing—are used to organize the discussion. Nursing administration as an adaptive system is discussed in the second section; the chapter concludes with a discussion of four administrative adaptive modes.

Person

According to Roy, the concept of person is an individual or an aggregate of individuals such as a family, community, or organized group.[5] Within the Roy framework, the person is conceptualized as an adaptive system in constant interaction with a changing environment. Based on systems theory, a person as a living system has inputs, outputs, controls, and feedback. Inputs from the environment and feedback from outcomes serve as stimuli to which the person's adaptive system responds. Adaptive responses are necessary to maintain the integrity of a person's system; ineffective adaptation results in the loss of system integrity.

Nursing administration as an organized group of individuals can be viewed as an adaptive system. Nursing administration is constantly interacting with the environment of the health-care system to achieve the goals of nursing and of the organization. As the environment of health-care systems change, adaptive responses are necessary to maintain the integrity of nursing's administrative systems.

Adaptation to changes in the environment proceeds through the coping mechanisms of regulator and cognator subsystems.[5] In the individual, regulator mechanisms occur automatically as needed and include neural, endocrine, and chemical responses that are activated under stress. Cognator coping mechanisms, on the other hand, are learned reactions to a changing environment and involve cognitive-emotive responses. Roy has identified four cognitive-emotive channels in the individual: perceptual-information processing, judgment, learning, and emotion.[5]

Since the regulator mechanisms have been derived from an understanding of the physiological functioning of the individual, a direct comparison to nursing administration is difficult. Further work is needed to identify automatic coping mechanisms in organizations that parallel the physiological regulators, although the lay-offs, hiring freezes, and wage controls typical of organizational crisis may be examples. A more direct comparison, however, can be made between the cognator mechanisms in individuals and those of nursing administration. We can postulate that the cognative channels for coping at the system level are manifested through information processing and decision making. These processes are learned responses to the changing environment of nursing administration and lead to changed system outputs—to varying levels of quality in patient care, personnel development, and research, for example.

As described by Roy, coping mechanisms are manifest through adaptive responses in four modes.[5] Thus far, only the adaptive modes of individuals have been described. These are the physiological, self-concept, role, and interdependence modes in which the focus is on maintaining biological, psychological, social, and affiliative integrity. Although examined separately in the model, considerable overlap of the four modes is apparent. According to Roy, this attests to the holistic nature of persons as living systems.[8]

The physiological mode focuses on five basic needs of the individual system, for oxygenation, elimination, nutrition, activity-rest, and protection; on the sensory, neurological, and endocrine functions; and on fluid and electrolyte balance. The spiritual and psychological aspects of individuals are inherent in the self-concept mode. The role and interdependence modes emphasize social adaptation focusing on the integration of persons into roles in families, communities, and society and on the reciprocal interactions of love, respect, trust, and caring.[5]

Reconceptualization of modes at the group level is necessary for nursing administration. Reconceptualization must underscore the uniqueness of groups, while at the same time maintaining the essence of the modes. The following administrative adaptive modes are presented for the reader's consideration: managerial function, role function, professional actualization, and interdependence. Each of these modes will be discussed in more detail later in the chapter.

Health

Roy defines health "as a state and process of being and becoming an integrated and whole person"[10] (p. 8). This contemporary view of health emphasizes development of the full potential of human beings and is derived from Helson's theory of adaptation,[11] and from the World Health Organization's definition of health.[12] Central to Roy's definition of health is the concept of integrity. Adaptive responses to environmental stimuli help maintain integrity of the individual and lead to goal achievement. The goals of the person system, as identified by Roy, are survival, growth, reproduction, and mastery.[5] Maximum health is the total functioning of individuals in biological, psychological, social, and affiliative dimensions and leads to goal achievement. Whereas ill health is a temporary or permanent state in which individuals are affected in one or more dimensions, rendering them unable to achieve fulfilling lives.

Health of managerial systems can also be defined in terms of integrity. The overall goals of nursing administration are survival, growth, productivity, and mastery as evidenced by the system outputs of patient care, human resources maintenance, and research. A healthy nursing administration is one in which goals are met, and the system maintains integrity and is able to develop to its full potential. Inability to adapt to the stimuli impinging on the system results in ill health, as evidenced by lack of system integrity. Such a lack of integrity may be displayed through symptoms of disruption among employees, for example, high turnover, absenteeism, or job dissatisfaction and high infection and accident rates among patients.

Environment

Environment is defined as "all conditions, circumstances, and influences surrounding and affecting the development and behavior of persons or groups"[6] (p. 58). The external environment is all that is outside the system, and the internal environment is inside the system. At the individual level, the external environment includes personal space, weather conditions, friends, relatives, and coworkers; and the internal environment includes basic life processes such as neural transmission, oxygenation; and mitosis. At the group level, economic conditions, organizational settings, and level of technology are considered part of the external environment. Whereas individual member characteristics—such as personality and leadership style—and group characteristics—such as shared values and attitudes—are considered part of the internal environment.

Roy's definition of environment is made more manageable by the division of environmental stimuli into focal, contextual, and residual. Focal stimuli are those that immediately confront a system and make it in need of an adaptive response. Contextual stimuli are all other stimuli present in the environment influencing a situation. Both focal and contextual stimuli can be identified and validated. Stimuli that affect behavior, but cannot be validated, are called residual stimuli.[5] Examples of residual stimuli are beliefs, attitudes, and cultural determinants that may have an immeasurable effect on a given situation. Residual stimuli may become contextual or focal if their role in a given situation can be validated.

Nursing

The fourth concept, nursing, is defined by Roy as the practice of promoting adaptation in each of the four effector modes by use of the nursing process.[5] The nurse applies the nursing process by first collecting data about human behavior in the four modes. This initial collection of data about behavior is termed "first-level nursing assessment." The nursing process continues with "second-level assessment," which is the identification of focal, contextual, and residual stimuli that are impinging on an individual system. After data are collected, the nurse can make a diagnosis that involves making a statement about the adaptive condition of an individual in relation to desired outcomes. The nursing process continues with setting goals that lead to adaptation, implementing plans, and evaluating outcomes. Successful application of the nursing process promotes the adaptive function of individuals and the integrity of person systems.

Nursing administration, using Roy's model, can also be defined as promoting adaptation in four modes. Although the focus is different, administrative decision making is similar to decision making in the nursing process. The nurse executive assumes responsibility for collecting data through the assessment of organizational behavior (first-level assessment), identifying stimuli impinging on the system (second-level assessment), developing goals and plans to promote adaptation, implementing plans, and evaluating outcomes. Through these processes the integrity of an organizational system is maintained and moved toward the development of its full potential. The practice of the nurse executive is based on a synthesis of managerial and behavioral theories and an understanding of organizational units as adaptive systems in continuous interaction with their internal and external environments. Figure 9.1 presents a diagrammatic representation of the relationships of key components of Roy's model as adapted for use in administrative systems.

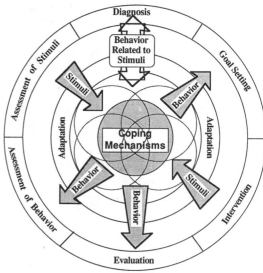

Figure 9.1   A Diagrammatic Representation of the Roy Model as Adapted for Use in Administrative Systems. (Adapted from Andrews HA, and Roy C. Essentials of the Roy Adaptation Model. N.Y.: John Wiley and Sons, Inc., 1983.)

NURSING ADMINISTRATION AS AN ADAPTIVE SYSTEM

The idea that organizations, as well as living beings, function as open systems was introduced into the management literature in the early 1960s.[13] Although a radical change from the traditional thinking of the time, studies have since demonstrated, that in rapidly changing organizations, adaptation to the environment is essential for growth, productivity, and survival.[14] In this respect, the Roy adaptation model is consistent with current managerial thinking and complements the open systems and ecological views of organizations.

Inputs

Within the open-systems framework, administration is viewed as a subsystem of the organization. Figure 9.2 depicts a view of

Inputs

Processes

Outputs

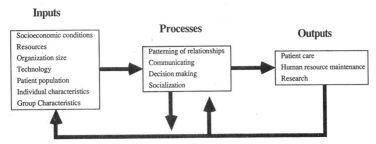

Socioeconomic conditions
Resources
Organization size
Technology
Patient population
Individual characteristics
Group Characteristics

Patterning of relationships
Communicating
Decision making
Socialization

Patient care
Human resource maintenance
Research

Figure 9.2 Nursing Administration as an Open System. The first column of this figure shows the inputs into the system; the second column shows the processes; and the third column shows the outputs. Arrows are drawn from the inputs to the processes and from the processes to the outputs to denote the direction of relationships. The feedback function is also shown. (Adapted from Roy C. The Roy adaptation model: applications in community health nursing. Proceedings of the Eight Annual Community Health Nursing Conference, Department of Public Health Nursing, University of North Carolina. Chapel Hill, NC, May 20–23, 1984.)

nursing administration as an adaptive system. Inputs into the system emanate from the external and internal environments. It is generally agreed that the external environment of an organization is comprised of common stimuli related to cultural, economic, legal, political, and educational conditions.[13] Although conditions are often unique to a given health-care facility in a given geographic area, regional and national policies can precipitate variations in conditions at the local level. Witness, for example, the recent changes incurred by the implementation of prospective payment for medicare patients in most U.S. hospitals. Compare the payment impact on county hospitals located in inner-cities with the impact of the new regulations on well-endowed private hospitals in upper-middle-class localities.

The environment in an institution, but outside the nursing organization, is also considered part of nursing administration's external environment. This environment includes, among other things, material and human resources, size of the facility, level of technology, executive policy making, and relationships with other organizations. An important function of the nurse executive is to determine the status of the environment im-

mediately external to nursing administration. Included in this function are identifying nursing needs, patient needs, and the type and quality of relationships to other departments in an institution.

The internal environment of nursing administration is that which emanates from within the system. This environment consists of the goals and objectives of nurse administrators, characteristics of individual members, and characteristics of administrative groups as a whole. Long- and short-term goals provide direction for the work of administrators. As goals and objectives change, so does the nature of work. For example, extensive recruitment efforts may be necessary to attract nurses to work on new nursing units. As positions are filled, administrators adapt by shifting their focus to developing the skills of nurses and maintaining the stability of work units.

Individuals bring to their jobs certain characteristics such as personalities, abilities, needs, and desires. In an analysis of the corporation, Naisbitt and Aburdene note that the three most important qualities that individuals offer an organization are information, knowledge, and creativity.[15] These qualities affect the processing of information, matter, and energy within a system. Group characteristics that affect administrative systems include the norms and size of groups, the use of power, interpersonal relationships, attitudes, and values. Feedback from group processes, such as information sharing and problem solving, can also serve as stimuli that influence the administrative system.

Processes

The role of administration is to process inputs in such a way as to maximize stated outcomes. Using Roy's model as a guide, administrative processes through which inputs are changed into outputs can be categorized as patterning of relationships, communicating, decision making, and socialization.

Patterning of Relationships

Patterning of relationships, to a large extent, is influenced by the structure of an organization, leadership style, and use of power. An organizational chart depicts the formal patterns of authority and describes legitimate organizational relationships based on hierarchical position. In organizations, there are also informal relationships among members based on interpersonal preference, rather than on formal position. Naisbitt and Aburdene refer to the mixture of formal and informal relationships as a lattice structure that brings together and mixes information from a variety of sources.[15]

Leadership styles influence the types of relationships developed in an organization. For example, an authoritarian leadership style demands more distance between the leader and followers than a democratic leadership style, where an exchange of information between members is encouraged. Contingency theory advocates the use of a flexible leadership style that changes depending on situational conditions. A flexible style allows for varying relationships contingent on interpretations of a situation.

The use of power in organizations also serves as a means of structuring relationships. Legitimate power derived from one's position in an organization can be exercised within the limits of that position. Del Bueno asserts that power is acquired, not given, and is essential for maintaining one's place in an organization.[16] Since power begets influence and control over scarce resources, gaining and retaining power underscores a significant number of organizational relationships. Building coalitions, lobbying, bargaining, and increasing one's visibility are all political strategies used to get and keep power.[16]

Communicating

Communicating is the process through which a system assimilates information and transmits it to other systems. Indeed, it is a process that links an organization together. The transmission of information underlies the basic managerial processes of data gathering, planning, problem solving, supervising, and evaluating. The importance of communication to the task accomplishment of the manager is reflected in the observation that managers spend 80% of their time communicating.[17] Organizational communication can proceed through formal channels consistent with the hierarchic structure of an organization, through informal channels developed through relationships with others, and through nonverbal cues. Regardless of the method of communication, feedback is essential to determine the accuracy of the information conveyed.

Decision Making

Decision making is a vital component of the transfer and conversion of matter and energy into organizational outputs. Decision making is based on both patterns of relationships and communication. Patterns of relationships determine which individuals can make which decisions, and communication skills govern the acquisition of information necessary to make effective decisions. The anatomy of a decision can be dissected into information and perception.[13] Information provides the data for a decision, whereas perception of the situation governs the interpretation of thatinformation. It might be added that previous experience and cognator effectiveness are useful in guiding the decision-making process.

Socialization

Socialization is inherent in the preparation and support of individuals in the performance of their roles in an organization. The focus of socialization is the role development of individuals from novice to expert practitioners. A basic premise here is that the cost of human resources is the most important expense necessary to manage organizational outcomes. The way in which socialization occurs has an effect on the quality of outputs, that is, on patient care and productivity. Nursing administration must effectively process the knowledge, creativity, and information available from nurse managers and staff nurses to yield high job-performance (quality patient care) and high job-satisfaction. Appropriate avenues for socialization are orientation and inservice education. Less formal, but equally effective avenues, are mentoring and networking.

Outputs

The outputs of administrative systems are patient care, human resource maintenance, and research. Although nurse administrators do not provide direct care for patients, they assume responsibility for activities that directly influence patient care. These include hiring and maintaining nursing staff; communicating with other departments that pro

vide support services to nursing; and developing and implementing policies related to nursing care. Assessment data related to the quality of patient care outputs may be collected through reviews of quality assurance reports and management information related to length of hospital stay, medication errors, and accident and mortality rates.

The second output, human resource maintenance, encompasses staff support and development. Information on the effectiveness of nursing administration in meeting the objectives related to staff support and development can be obtained through data about absenteeism, turnover rates, overtime, number and frequency of promotions, ratio of technical to professional nurses, salary scales, and funding for continuing education.

Research, the third output, can be assessed by a review of the number and types of research studies being conducted. Implementation of research findings, research journal clubs, and collaborative ventures with other departments can also provide useful assessment criteria.

ADMINISTRATIVE ADAPTIVE MODES

In the following section Roy's four adaptive modes are discussed in terms of administrative systems. Roy has described four modes of individual systems through which manifestations of the cognator and regulator activity (coping mechanisms) are actualized. As previously stated, these four modes—physiologic, self-concept, role function, and interdependence—can be reconceptualized to understand coping mechanisms at the nursing and organizational levels. Each of the four proposed adaptive modes for nursing administration are presented. The theoretical basis of each mode, as well as the use of the nursing process to assess functioning in each mode, are addressed.

MANAGERIAL FUNCTION MODE

Theoretical Basis

The physiologic mode of individual systems encompasses basic life processes of human beings such as oxygenation, elimination, and circulation. Although there is no direct comparison to bodily functions at the administrative level, basic functions of managers are presented as an analogue for consideration.

The basic functions of managers are vital to the integrity of organizations, just as basic physiologic functions are vital to the health of individual systems. The managerial function mode encompasses those tasks that are traditionally viewed as managerial tasks and are fairly consistent among administrators regardless of setting. Through the basic functions of planning, organizing, staffing, leading, and controlling, managers seek to maintain a high level of job performance and a high level of job satisfaction among members of their work units.[13]

Planning

Considerable amounts of time and energy are invested in determining organizational goals and the means to obtain them. Members of an administrative system must be visionaries who can see beyond the daily demands of the work setting and provide direction for the future. Nurse administrators must be able to assess the impact of the rapidly changing health-care environment on the practice of nursing and plan accordingly to provide quality patient care.

Organizing

When goals are agreed upon, the work of administration focuses on the use of human and material resources to support the stated goals. In developing measures to meet goals, administrators consider both the constraints of an organization as well as its assets.

Staffing

Staffing refers to the advertising, interviewing, selecting, hiring, maintaining, and counseling of personnel working on nursing units. The role of administrators is primarily to ensure a sufficient number of qualified nursing personnel to meet the needs of the patient populations served. In some situations, nurse managers are responsible for scheduling the hours of work for nursing personnel on patient units. The staffing responsibilities of nurse administrators, however, may become obsolete as more professional nurses determine their own schedules and negotiate with other nurses to provide unit coverage.

Leading

The work of administration in regard to the management of personnel, as succinctly stated by Naisbitt and Aburdene, is "to reinforce, refine, and refocus the vision of the organization, while supporting the people aligned to it."[15] The contemporary view of leadership emphasizes support rather than supervision of workers. The philosophy underlying this statement is that, in general, workers themselves know their job best, want to do a good job, and will do so if supported and given a say in their work. This contrasts with the old view that workers must be prodded and continually supervised to do well. Support for employees consists of assisting individuals to achieve maximum work performance, recognizing achievements, providing opportunities for contributions, and listening to concerns and complaints. Nurse administrators face the additional challenge of supporting professional practice in institutional settings.[18]

Controlling

The controlling function of administration is met through continual assessment and evaluation of the outcomes of an organization or service. Nursing administration has the responsibility to determine if patients are receiving quality care and nurses are maintaining competency in their practice. Administrators use a variety of sources to evaluate outcomes. These include infection rates, mortality rates, critical incidences, medication errors, patient complaints, turnover, absenteeism, and interpersonal conflicts.

Nursing Process

Assessment of managerial functioning provides nurse executives with an indication of how a system is coping with environmental change. A first-level assessment is based on the five managerial functions just described, and entails the collection of data regarding behavior in planning, organizing, staffing, leading, and controlling. Consider, for example, a nurse executive who is concerned about an increased number of resignations over the previous two months, leading to shortages of nurses for several shifts. Two head nurses have stated that the staffing crisis on their units is so acute that new admissions cannot be accepted. In this situation, the nurse executive must first gather data about current staffing problems. Information will be obtained to determine the extent and impact of the nursing shortage on patient care.

Collection of data leads to a second-level assessment, which is the identification of factors (stimuli) responsible for the nursing shortage. Using Roy's model, the nurse executive will classify the identified factors as focal, contextual, or residual stimuli. In the situation just described, the administrator may determine that the focal stimulus is the low pay scale in his or her hospital. The contextual stimulus may be the area-wide nursing shortage that has precipitated vacant positions in that hospital. The residual stimulus may be the recent purchase of the hospital by a private corporation.

A statement relating observed behavior

to the responsible stimuli is called a nursing diagnosis.[5] Diagnosis, using Roy's terms, is a judgment about the adaptiveness of an individual's behavior in relation to desired outcomes. In the example I have described, the nurse administrator's diagnosis could read: Ineffective internal mechanisms for handling competition and areawide nursing shortage.

Nurse executives rely on their background in nursing and managerial science to guide them in assessing and diagnosing organizational responses. Knowledge derived from nursing and management provide nurse executives with rationales for judging behaviors as adaptive or ineffective (maladaptive). Adaptive behaviors evident in the managerial mode include development of realistic goals, objectives, and plans for goal achievement. Other manifestations of adaptation might include adequate staffing to meet the needs of patients and of nurses. Maladaptive behaviors are evidenced by confusion about goals or objectives, divisiveness regarding work load, conflict over plans for goal attainment, and staffing problems.

The nurse administrator's next step is to set goals that transform ineffective behaviors into adaptive behaviors. The goal of the managerial function mode is to maintain and enhance effective (adaptive) managerial functions, while transforming ineffective functions to adaptive behavior. Goal statements similar to those Roy recommends for individuals are worth considering. According to Roy, a goal statement consists of three entities: the behavior to be observed, the change expected, and the time frame for achievement of the goal.[5] A goal statement for the case of inadequate staffing might read: Staffing patterns (observable behavior) will meet patients' needs (change) at all times (time frame). Since nursing resignations are also a problem, an additional goal statement may be: Nursing resignations (behavior) will be reduced (change) within two months (time frame).

Promotion of adaptation is contingent on the management of stimuli influencing ineffective behaviors. The intervention methods recommended by Roy include changing the focal stimuli, managing contextual stimuli, and broadening the adaptation zone (level).[5] In choosing interventions, the nurse executive considers previous goals. If the nurse administrator in the above example plans to decrease the acuity of staffing problems, he or she will choose interventions based on the probability of success in resolving the problem. In this case, he or she might appoint a task force comprised of nurse managers, staff nurses, and hospital administrators to examine the issues related to the shortage and to generate recommendations. It also may be imperative to discuss the competitiveness of salaries with hospital directors and financial officers, and to negotiate higher salaries.

Finally, as with any intervention process, evaluation focuses on comparing postintervention to preintervention behavior. If interventions have been effective, a change in behavior will have occurred in the predicted and desired direction. In this case, a decrease in nurses' resignations and stable staffing patterns would be indicative of effective intervention.

ROLE FUNCTION MODE

Theoretical Basis

The role function mode described by Roy can also be applied to the study of nursing administration systems. This mode is concerned with social adaptation—the behavior of one person relating to another.[5] The theoretical background of this mode is based on the research of Parsons and Shils,[19] Erikson,[20] Goffman,[21] and Banton.[22]

Roy classifies roles as primary, secondary, and tertiary. The primary role is related to the developmental stage of an individual; secondary roles are assumed by individuals to carry out tasks associated with their primary role; and roles engaged in for short periods of time and complementing primary and secondary roles are called tertiary. In nursing administration, the primary role of the nurse manager is that of a nurse. The developmental aspect of this role is reflected in the varying degrees of clinical and managerial experience each nurse brings to a given management position. The secondary role is the management position held by the nurse, for example, head nurse, supervisor, director, or vice-president. Membership on committees and task forces constitutes the tertiary roles of nurse managers.

Two behavioral components of role—instrumental and expressive—form the basis of role assessment. Parsons and Shils[19] define instrumental behaviors as those performed by a person as part of his or her role. Instrumental behaviors can be objectively assessed and identified; are characteristically goal oriented; and are used for the transmission of information and skills. Role mastery is the desired outcome of such behaviors. Examples of instrumental behaviors exhibited by nurse managers are decision making, staffing, communicating, and budgeting.

Expressive behaviors involve a display of feelings or attitudes; direct feedback is the intended outcome. Although these types of behaviors do not receive as much attention as instrumental behaviors, they are responsible for the maintenance of interpersonal relationships among coworkers. Examples of expressive behaviors in administrative settings include encouragement, mentoring, and concern for others.

Role partitions or role performance requirements in the Roy model have been identified by Nuwayhid.[23] The four role partitions focus on the individual as a client in a health-care setting. For nursing administration, Mintzberg's action roles of managers provide an analogue for understanding the role performances of nurse managers. Mintzberg[17] describes interpersonal, informational, and decision-making roles and the relationship of each to authority.

In "the interpersonal role," the manager plays the part of a leader, figurehead, and liaison. As the name implies, the major focus in this role is on relationships with others, relations varying from the directiveness of a leader to the graciousness of a host. The instrumental component of this role involves leadership and communication skills, whereas the expressive component involves comforter and mentor skills.

In the "informational role," the manager plays the part of a monitor, disseminator, and spokesperson. The emphasis in this role is on receiving and conveying information. Communicating and information processing are examples of instrumental behaviors, whereas feedback on performance, encouragement, and discussion are expressive behaviors.

In the "decision-making role," the manager plays the part of disturbance handler, resource allocator, negotiator, and entrepreneur. Emphasis is on the use of information to make decisions. Instrumental skills involve problem solving and conflict resolution, whereas expressive skills involve maintaining harmonious relationships, caring, and concern about the effects of decisions on others.

Nursing Process

Assessment of behaviors using the role function mode provides nurse administrators with an indication of how others are coping with environmental change. In assessing the role function mode, the nurse collects data related to the manager's primary role. Assessment includes background information such as age, gender, and number of years in nursing and in management. Information is also collected about instrumental and expressive behaviors in primary and secondary roles using

the role-partition framework; tertiary roles are assessed as needed.

The assessment continues with the identification and labeling of role behaviors as adaptive or ineffective, and the identification of focal, contextual, and residual stimuli affecting behaviors. To assess adaptation, Roy has identified stimuli she believes may be common to the role function mode[10] and applicable to the role of manager, including social norms, physical makeup, chronological age, self-concept, knowledge of expected behaviors, physical and emotional well-being, and performance.

In addition, to assist with the nursing diagnosis and judgments about adaptiveness of behavior in this mode, Nuwayhid and Schofield have identified four common adaptation problems: role transition, distance, conflict, and failure.[23–24] "Role transition" is the process of assuming new and different roles. Effective role transition is exhibited by the display of expressive behaviors, and a few of the instrumental behaviors associated with a role. Ineffective role transition is apparent when there is a display of expressive behaviors but an insufficient manifestation of instrumental behaviors.[23] "Role distance" exists when an individual displays both expressive and instrumental behaviors, but the behaviors differ significantly from those prescribed for the role.[24] "Role conflict" occurs when an individual fails to exhibit the instrumental and expressive behaviors of a role because there are incompatible expectations about role behaviors from one or more persons in the environment, or because he or she occupies two or more roles requiring prescribed behaviors that are incompatible.[24] "Role failure" exists when an individual fails to display both the expressive and instrumental behaviors of a role.[23]

Consider, for example, a 25-year-old nurse who has recently assumed the position of head nurse on a 25-bed neurology unit. Her previous clinical experience consists of two years of primary and associate nursing on the same unit. She has had no managerial experience nor has she taken any courses in management. Her primary role is that of a nurse, and her secondary role is that of head nurse. Instrumental behaviors associated with her role include scheduling, planning, bugeting for the unit, and communicating with supervisors and staff nurses. Expressive behaviors associated with the role include efforts to mentor staff, expressions of concern about work load, and complaints to supervisors about staffing problems.

In the case of this inexperienced head nurse, the nurse administrator may diagnose the problem as ineffective role transition due to lack of managerial knowledge and experience. A goal statement for the new head nurse, focusing on the desired adaptive behavior, might be: The instrumental skills of this first-line manager will improve following a managerial training course.

The selection of interventions to enhance role mastery will be dependent on an accurate assessment of behaviors as well as on knowledge of the specific methods to promote adaptation. A person's ability to adapt depends on the degree of change required and the present adaptation level of the individual.[10] In the case of the head nurse, following the intervention, behavioral outcomes will be compared with the desired outcomes to determine the effectiveness of the chosen interventions.

PROFESSIONAL ACTUALIZATION MODE

Theoretical Basis

Roy describes self-concept as the "composite of beliefs and feelings that one holds about oneself at a given time"[6] (p. 58). The focus of the self-concept mode is psychological and spiritual adaptation requisite for psychic integrity of individuals. Since the focus of this mode has been individual adaptation, recon-

ceptualization is necessary to discuss behaviors at the organization level. Group theory postulates that members of a group develop a perception of the group as a whole. This perception may be analogous to the self-concept of an individual. Although it is meaningful to explore this idea of group self-concept in this mode, I have elected an alternative approach based on the work of contemporary nurses. This approach is the exploration of the ideas of professional actualization and professional development.

The theoretical basis of this mode is derived from Styles and Benner.[25–26] In a careful and thoughtful analysis of the relation of standarized criteria for professions to nursing, Styles suggests that actualization should define practice.[25] Actualization, defined as the achievement of one's fullness, stems from a system of beliefs that provides direction to the profession.[25] Styles asserts that the actualization of individual members of a profession (self-actualization) is requisite to actualization of the profession.[25] Styles[25] has further identified three fundamental attitudes she believes essential for the nurse seeking self-fulfillment: "Social significance," which conveys the nature and importance of nursing, is a sense of mission and social sanction; "Ultimacy of performance" is commitment to doing one's best work; "Collegiality and collectivity" are the conviction that responsibility and authority are shared and that the wholeness of the profession must be preserved.[25]

Basic to the process of actualization, or being the most or best that one can be, is the development into an expert practitioner. The work of Benner sheds light on the progression of the nurse from novice to expert.[26] The Dreyfus Model of Skill Acquisition, which proposes that experience and education together support the development of skilled practitioners, served as the framework for her research. Through participant observations and interviews with nurse clinicians, new graduates, and nursing students Benner identified five levels of clinical nursing practice: novice and advanced beginner, and competent, proficient, and expert practitioner.[26] Based on her findings, she concluded that the development of skilled performance moves from reliance on rules and principles, to reliance on experience. An inherent component of clinical role development is the ability to shift one's focus from the parts of a situation, to the whole of a situation.

The role of nursing administration is to support the development and implementation of models for professionals who practice in institutional settings. The purpose of the models is to support professional actualization and the development of skilled practitioners. Primary nursing was an early and fairly successful attempt to incorporate professional responsibility, accountability, and performance into a model of practice. Westorick[18] has developed a model that emphasizes independent nursing practice by the bedside nurse. The components of the model also address interdependent nursing functions, carrying out physician's orders, for example. Preliminary findings indicate that implementation of the model in selected areas of practice has been associated with greater job satisfaction and autonomy.[18] The philosophical perspective of Styles and the research of Benner can serve as a basis for the development of other models of professional nursing practice in organizational settings.

Nursing Process

Assessment of the professional actualization mode provides nurse executives with an indication of how an organizational system copes with changes that affect professional actualization and professional practice. The three fundamental attitudes of Styles and the five levels of clinical practice identified by Benner form the bases for assessment in this mode. In the first-level assessment, information is gathered about the value of nursing to nurses, patients, and others; about the commitment of nurses to doing their best work; the support of nursing staff by administration; colleagial relationships among nurses and administrators; and about the level of job performance displayed by individual nurses. Information may be gathered through formal and informal discussions, surveys, and performance evaluations. Behaviors indicative of an inability to adapt in this mode include a high rate of turnover, high job-dissatisfaction, and interpersonal problems. Although these behaviors are similar to maladaptation in other modes, the cause of the ineffective behaviors relate to inefficient functioning in the professional actualization mode. Thus, ineffective behaviors can be attributed to feelings of powerlessness, alienation, apathy, low sense of control, fatalism, and helplessness.

Consider, for example, the concerns of staff nurses who complain that their ability to practice professional nursing is severely impaired by the autocratic leadership style of their head nurse. Preliminary information reveals an unusually high turnover rate of nurses on the unit and a high level of job dissatisfaction. More extensive investigation indicates that the skill level of the majority of the staff nurses ranges from proficient to expert, and that authority is not shared with these skilled practitioners. The focal stimulus in this situation is the leadership style of the head nurse, and the contextual stimuli are the skill levels of the staff nurses. The nursing diagnosis could be: Inability of the staff to practice professional nursing because of an incompatible environment.

Goal setting in this mode is highly dependent on the collaboration between management and staff. For effective adaptation, the nursing groups must be reasonably aligned in terms of philosophy and beliefs about nursing. To enhance adaptation, inconsistency about expectations can be identified and reckoned with prior to choosing appropriate goals and interventions. The chosen interventions can focus on changing or managing the stimuli that influence ineffective behaviors, while at the same time reinforcing stimuli that have positive effects. For example, authoritarian head nurses who build barriers to professional practice can be replaced by nurses who are supportive of professional practice. Positive aspects of the situations, such as primary nursing or control over work schedules, can be reinforced.

INTERDEPENDENCE MODE

Theoretical Basis

Interdependence is defined as close relationships among people and involves the exchange of love, respect, and value.[5] Roy contends that it is through social interaction that the need for affectional adequacy is met.[5] The theoretical basis of the mode, as applied to nursing administration, is derived from the work of Tedrow;[27] Randall, Tedrow, and VanLandingham;[28] Naisbitt and Aburdene;[15] and Kotter.[29] Tedrow notes that the mode encompasses the need for nurturance, belonging, approval, and understanding.[27] Significant others and support systems provide channels through which needs are met and assessed in terms of receptive and contributive behaviors. In nursing administration, significant relationships and support systems are those that are vital to the efficient functioning of an organizational system. Nurse administrators' significant others include hospital administrators, nurses, physicians, and patients. Support systems are those in which exchange of information and services is essential for the efficient functioning of the nursing administration system. Examples of other systems include dietary, pharmacy, housekeeping, and laboratory departments. Receptive behaviors in which the system receives respect and value from another are exemplified by the provision of assistance to nursing administration from other departments. Contributive behaviors, those in which the system gives respect and value to others, are exemplified by recognition, service awards, and research awards given to staff nurses.

The epitome of the interdependence mode expressed at the group level is alignment. Naisbitt and Aburdene state: "When people work to their full capacity, when they feel in sync with their coworkers, when everything comes together on cue though completely unplanned, alignment is present."[15] (p. 30). Kotter notes that in organizations, relationships exist among various organizational elements.[29] For example, nursing administration has relationships with staff nurses, other hospital departments, and patients. Kotter asserts that when four structural elements—the individual and his or her agenda, network, and organizational unit—"fit" together, they are aligned.[29] Where alignment exists, the organization is stable and efficiently processes materials, human energy, and information. If, however, the relationships among the elements are not aligned, a state of nonalignment exists, which results in system ineffectiveness.

Although not addressed in detail by Kotter, or Naisbitt and Aburdene, mutual respect and the valuing of elements in an organization underlie alignment. Administration respects individual workers and provides opportunities for individual achievement and creativity. The individual, in turn, works to his or her fullest potential and is self-directed. Mutual respect and the valuing of one another result in high job-performance, effective decision making, and administrative functioning. Productive mentoring and networking are also considered expressions of alignment. Mentoring is assisting less-experienced individuals to "learn the ropes"; and networking is cooperating and exchanging resources.

Nursing Process

Assessment of adaptation in the interdependence mode proceeds from identification of significant relationships and support systems, to identification of receptive and contributive behaviors in each relationship. Second-level assessment involves the identification of related stimuli and the labeling of behaviors as effective or ineffective. Tedrow identified eight stimuli commonly affecting adaptation in this mode.[27] Three of those stimuli are common to nursing administration systems and include the need to give and receive respect and value; the expectations of relationships and awareness of needs; and the nuturing ability of individual members of a system. Two additional stimuli are knowledge of behavior in organizational systems and knowledge of the needs of employees in organizational settings.

Consider, for example, a nurse administrator of a large medical center who approaches the dean of a nursing school about the possibility of collaborating on research projects. The proposed joint venture would consist of faculty presenting minisessions on research methods and working with staff nurses on projects. Staff nurses, as a consequence, would have the opportunity to practice and improve their research skills, and faculty would have access to patients they wish to study. Nurses from both settings will contribute to collaborative projects and both organizations will benefit.

In this example, the receptive behaviors, relative to nursing administration, include staff development in research and public recognition through authorship on articles; whereas the contributive behaviors include assisting faculty with data collection. The nursing administration diagnosis in this example could be: Adequate supportive behaviors related to relationships with nursing education.

Since the behaviors are termed effective in promoting adaptation in the interdependence mode, the goal of nursing administration is to reinforce behaviors leading to collaborative research projects. Reinforcement might include funding of research projects, recognition for completed projects, and development of a research center. Administrative actions like these will generate interest in research and serve to enhance both the quality and quantity of nursing research. Periodic review and evaluation of the joint venture is expected and completes the nursing process in this mode.

In summary, the Roy adaptation model, with its emphasis on systems theory and humanistic values, is congruent with a number of perspectives in management science. The model provides nurse executives with a framework useful for managing nursing services and patient care. This chapter presents an overview of Roy's model and an initial attempt to apply the model to nursing administration. The major components— person, health, environment, and nursing— have been addressed and related to nursing administration using descriptions of four administrative adaptive modes.

REFERENCES

1. Limandri BJ. Research and practice with abused women: use of the Roy adaptation model as an explanatory framework. ANS 1986;8(4):52–61.
2. Janelli LM. Utilizing Roy's adaptation model from a gerontological perspective. J. Gerontol Nurs 1980; 6(3):140–150.
3. Mastal MF, Hammond H, Roberts MP. Theory into hospital practice: a pilot implementation. J Nurs Adm 1982;12(6):9–15.
4. Roy C. Relating nursing theory to education: a new era. Nurse Educ 1979;4(2):16–21.
5. Roy Sister C. Introduction to nursing: an adaptation model. 2nd ed. Englewood Cliffs, NJ: Prentice-Hall Inc, 1984.
6. Roy C. Application of the Roy model. In: Asay MK, Ossler CC, eds. Proceedings of the eight annual community health nursing conference conceptual models of nursing applications in community health nursing.Chapel Hill, NC: Department of Public Health, May, 1984.
7. Roy C. Roy adaptation model. In: Clements IW,

Roberts FB, eds. Family health a theoretical approach to nursing care. New York: John Wiley and Sons, 1983.

8. Hanson J. The family. In: Roy C, ed. Introduction to nursing: an adaptation model. 2nd ed. Englewood Cliffs, NJ: Prentice-Hall Inc, 1984.

9. Marshall LA. The nursing care group. In: Roy C, ed. Introduction to nursing: an adaptation model. 2nd ed. Englewood Cliffs, NJ; Prentice-Hall Inc, 1984.

10. Andrews HA, Roy C. Essentials of the Roy adaptation model. New York: Appleton-Century-Crofts, 1986.

11. Helson H. Adaptation level theory. New York: Harper & Row Publishers, 1964.

12. United Nations. Everyman's United Nations, 8th ed. New York: UN Office of Public Information (UN Publication E.67.I.2 March 1968.

13. Schermerhorn JR Jr, Hunt JG, Osborn RN. Managing organizational behavior. 2nd ed. New York: John Wiley and Sons, 1985.

14. Burns T, Stalker G. The management of innovation. London: Tavistock, 1961.

15. Naisbitt J, Aburdene P. Re-inventing the corporation. New York: Warner Books Inc, 1985.

16. Del Bueno D, Freund C. Power and politics in nursing administration: a case book. Owing Mills, MD: Rynd Communications, 1985.

17. Mintzberg H. The nature of managerial work. New York: Harper & Row, 1973.

18. Westorick B. Clinical practice model: from institutional to professional nursing. Philadelphia: Lippincott, 1988 (in press).

19. Parsons T, Shils E, eds: Toward a general theory of action. Cambridge, Mass: Harvard University Press, 1951.

20. Erikson EH. Childhood and Society, 2nd ed. New York: WW Norton and Company Inc, 1963.

21. Goffman E. Encounters. Indianapolis: The Bobbs-Merrill Company Inc, 1961.

22. Banton M. Roles: an introduction to the study of social relations. New York: Basic Books Inc, 1965.

23. Nuwayhid KA. Role transition, distance and conflict. In: Roy C, ed. Introduction to nursing: an adaptation model. 2nd ed. Englewood Cliffs, NJ: Prentice-Hall Inc, 1984.

24. Schofield A. Problems of role function. In: Roy C, ed. Introduction to nursing: an adaptation model. Englewood Cliffs, NJ: Prentice-Hall Inc, 1976.

25. Styles MM. On nursing toward a new endowment. St. Louis: CV Mosby Company, 1982.

26. Benner P. From novice to expert: excellence and power in clinical practice. Menlo Park California: Addison-Wesley Publishing Company, 1984.

27. Tedrow MP. Interdependence: theory and development. In: Roy C, ed. Introduction to nursing: an adaptation model, 2nd ed. Englewood Cliffs, NJ: Prentice-Hall Inc, 1984.

28. Randall B, Tedrow M, VanLandingham J. Adaptation to nursing: the Roy conceptual model made practical. St. Louis: CV Mosby Company, 1982.

29. Kotter JP. Organizational dynamics: diagnosis and intervention. Reading, MA: Addison-Wesley Publishing Company, 1978.

10

Rogers's Theory and Nursing Administration: A Perspective on Health and Environment

Martha Raile Alligood

NURSING is coming of age as a discipline. Nurse administrators, educators, and practitioners are more united today than they have been in the recent past. One factor contributing to this unity is graduate nursing education. Academe has prepared a sizable body of nurses for service and education. Although prepared to function in different areas, the common values in the core of their advanced nursing education have fostered unity and a recognition of the need for theory in nursing.

Application of nursing theory to the management of nursing care has begun. Conceptual models are being used to guide practice, and theories of nursing are being tested by researchers. An eagerness and willingness to apply nursing theory in nursing administration is also increasingly apparent.

It should come as no surprise that using nursing theory to improve practice is as important for nursing administration as it is for clinical nursing. In the past, nurse administrators have often been educated in programs outside the discipline of nursing. Subsequently, in some cases, they have not played a contributing role in the building of nursing knowledge. They have, however, contributed to the uniqueness of the management perspective in nursing.

Today, nurse administrators are recognizing the importance of contributing to the development of nursing and management knowledge to an equal degree. The nation's nurse executives are applying nursing and organization theory to their nursing administrative practice, and they are using theoretical perspectives to view both clinical and administrative undertakings in new and different ways. One new way of thinking about nursing administration is fostered by Rogers's theory of unitary human beings.

In the discussions that follow, I describe Rogers's unique perspective of people and environment by first reviewing the major building blocks and principles of her theory. My presentation of these ideas is followed by some thoughts about Rogers's theory. Special attention is paid to the idea of environment, and to a lesser extent, to health. Both are reconceptualized, somewhat, to be useful for understanding the delivery of nursing services. In the last section of the chapter, selected research is reviewed apropos of nursing administration.

A SCIENCE OF UNITARY HUMAN BEINGS

Rogers's science of unitary human beings specifies human beings as nursing's phenomena of concern. Dr. Rogers describes the long history of concern among nurses for people and their world, and proposes a conceptual framework specific to that concern. The four building blocks in her theory are energy fields, openness, pattern, and four dimensionality.

Energy Fields, Openness, Pattern, and Four Dimensionality

According to Rogers[1], "energy fields" constitute the fundamental unit of analysis. "Field is a unifying concept. Energy signifies the dynamic nature of the field. Energy fields are infinite." Energy fields exist for human beings and their individual environments.

The human field, called the unitary human being, is "an irreducible, four-dimensional energy field identified by pattern and manifesting characteristics that are different from those of the parts and cannot be predicted from knowledge of the parts."[1] The environmental field, likewise, is defined as "an irreducible, four-dimensional energy field identified by pattern and manifesting characteristics different from those of the parts."[1]

The idea of energy fields is an abstract way of thinking about people and environments. In Rogers's perspective, each person is an energy field embedded in his or her own environmental field. Interaction between the two fields is characterized by invisible waves that form a pattern. Human energy fields operate as integrated wholes at all times and form increasingly diverse field pattern.

The second concept in Rogers's theory is "openness," which describes the infinity of energy fields. Rogers proposes a universe of open systems, stating, "energy fields are open—not a little bit or sometimes, but continuously. The human and environmental fields are integral with one another."[1]

The third concept is "pattern." According to Rogers, "pattern is defined as the distinguishing characteristic of an energy field perceived as a single wave. Pattern gives identity to the field. The nature of the pattern changes continuously. Each human field pattern is unique and is integral with its own unique environmental field pattern."[1] As noted, the energy of the human and environmental fields emanates in waves and interacts in a continuous, ever-changing pattern. Waves of energy from the evolving pattern manifest the characteristics of the field that we routinely see as the characteristics of persons and environments. Although the energy fields are integral, and manifestations of the field are in a pattern, the pattern is always changing. Changes in human growth and development, for example, as we commonly think of them, are pattern phenomena of an energy field.

The fourth concept is "four dimensionality," which, Rogers states, characterizes human and environmental fields, "as a nonlinear domain without spatial or temporal attributes. All reality is postulated to be four dimensional. Four dimensionality is postulated to be a given. It is not something one moves into or becomes. It is a way of perceiving human beings and their world."[1]

Rogers refers to the relative present to describe four dimensionality: for each human energy field there is an environmental field that is relative to it and is, therefore, unique. It is important to understand that the environmental energy field is not just a physical reality, although what we know about physical environment are environmental field manifestations. A person's environment, at any point in time, may also be future wishes, past recollections or present musings. We may be "tuned" to where we are, or, as the saying goes, be "a million miles away."

These are the building blocks of Rogers's

theory. They are four distinct concepts, which, when considered in relation to one another, form a conceptual system and provide a new way of understanding reality.

Principles of Homeodynamics: Resonancy, Helicy, and Integrality

The principles of homeodynamics, as described by Rogers, elucidate the nature and direction of change in energy fields. "Resonancy" is continuous change from lower to higher frequency wave patterns in human and environmental fields.[1] The frequencies of the human and environmental fields vary and manifest changing human characteristics. "Helicy" is the continuous, innovative and diverse human and environmental field patterns characterized by nonrepeating rhythmicities.[1] This simply means that wave patterns are always new, creative, semipredictable, or predictable. The human and environmental fields are constantly changing together. And "integrality" is the continuous, mutual human field and environmental field process.[1] Integrality suggests that energy fields pass through one another; in that they are integral. The two fields continuously interact, and the pattern of interaction changes. Manifestations of this changing pattern are what we commonly refer to as human behavior.

HEALTH AND ENVIRONMENT

The concepts central to nursing science are human beings, nursing, health, and environment. Gueldner, in the next chapter, will address human beings and nursing. In this section, I will discuss Rogers's perspective on health and environment using relevant research to make particular points for nursing administration.

"Health," according to Rogers, is an idea that is value-laden as illustrated by differing cultural health practices. The notion of

health, therefore, is not addressed to any great extent in her recent writing. Earlier, health was dealt with briefly and in the context of the traditional goals of nursing education and practice. According to Rogers, the goal of health has served to provide important evidence of nursing's long history of concern with something other than illness.[2]

Health, in the theory of unitary human beings, may be suggested as a behavioral index of the well-being of people in a particular culture or subculture. Taking as a premise that health is a value, that what is thought of as healthy by a person in one culture may be perceived of as unhealthy in another, it follows that the meaning of health behaviors are culturally determined.

An example of the cultural meaning of health is described by Malinski and derives from her work with the Navajo. Congenitally dislocated hips are common in this cultural group. Surgical repair of a dislocation actually makes sitting crossed-legged and riding horseback, both normal everyday activities among the Navajos, uncomfortable—even impossible. Health, as defined by the Navajo, therefore, is significantly different than the perception of health held by the average middle-class American.[3]

The U.S. health-care system is also characterized by cultural diversity. Some organizations are very small, and are located in outlying communities serving highly homogeneous populations. Other institutions are nearly megalithic, having billions of dollars for services that run the gamut from the highly technological organization-based variety, to outpatient services for heterogeneous populations. The organizational cultures fostered by this array of systems is as varied as the cultural values of the clients who are served. And health is perceived in varying ways depending on the individual and organizational cultures involved. In low-income, rural communities with few resources, good health care may be thought to exist when transportation of any kind is available to pick up an injured field hand from the side of a remote back road—to at least prevent death. In middle-class, urban communities, the idea of health is quite different; here all that modern medicine has to offer, and that insurance carriers will bear, comprises a major industry marketed as health care.

"Environment" is the second basic unit of study. The importance of the environment to the unitary development of people has been a consistent theme in the evolution of Rogers's theory. The importance of environment to nursing can be traced to Nightingale who stated in *Notes on Nursing*:

In watching disease . . . the thing which strikes the experienced observer most forcibly is this, that the symptoms of the sufferings generally considered to be inevitable and incident to the disease are very often not symptoms of the disease at all, but of something quite different—of the want of fresh air, or of light, or of warmth, or of quiet, or of cleanliness, or of punctuality and care in the administration of diet, of each or of all of these.[4]

Although Nightingale's conceptualization of the environment is different than Rogers's, it is important, nonetheless, to note the emphasis on person and environment in the writings of both. It is impossible to think about environment in nursing without immediately associating the idea with Nightingale and Rogers. Both have made their imprint on nursing in more ways than one, but certainly on theoretical nursing, and more specifically, on the meaning of environment and its centrality to health and well-being.[5]

Although there is some recognition of the importance of environment to nursing science, the development of nursing knowledge with respect to environment has progressed slowly. The relatively small emphasis on environment has led some to ask for its reconceptualization.[6] Others have sought to understand the environment in terms that are more than physical. Understanding people and en

vironments in terms of patterns and holism is a challenge at this stage in the development of scientific nursing. The Rogerian conceptual system identifies the phenomenon of concern as people in continuous interaction with their environment.

Conceptualizing human beings and environment as a holistic, unitary, irreducible reality has not been easy. Ference[7] describes the difficulty of the task in her discussion of the development of nursing science. Using Kuhn's[8] three classes of problems in the development of scientific paradigms, she describes the evolution of research that tests and extends Rogers's theory. The three phases are (1) determining the class of facts, (2) matching facts with theory, and (3) articulating theory.

In the 1960s at New York University, studies were conducted that represented the first phase—determining the class of facts. The themes of these early studies were human development, person and environment interaction, human and environmental field relationships, and body-image field boundaries.[7] Many of these studies were cluster studies addressing themes aligned with Rogers's ideas.

By the early 1970s, the following concepts were being empirically examined: time, space-time, field independence, locus of control, and differentiation.[7] During the initial period of determining the class of facts, investigators struggled to conceptualize and study people in unitary interaction with the environment. Those early efforts have provided the basis for later studies classified by Ference as phase two in the evolution of theory—when facts are matched with theory.[7] Ference cites Rawnsley's study as the beginning of the second phase in the science of unitary human beings, which continues to this day.

Examples of empirical investigations that test Rogers's theory, especially those that pertain to environment, are described in the section that follows. The potential usefulness of these studies for nursing administration is also discussed.

EMPIRICAL STUDIES AND THEIR IMPLICATIONS FOR NURSING ADMINISTRATION

Ference[9] completed a study in 1979, that was based on the principle of resonancy. It was from this study that the first instrument for measurement of Rogers's theory was developed. Time experience, creativity traits, differentiation, and human field motion were assessed by Ference in her investigation.

Subsequently, other studies have been designed to test the efficacy of Rogers's principles. The early studies have been basic investigations inasmuch as theory derived deductively has been tested without consideration of the application to practice. These basic studies have tested broad principles. Alligood's[10] investigation, for example, was designed to test helicy, which describes the nature and direction of human development as continuously innovative and increasingly diverse. Empirical linkages were developed to operationalize the human characteristics suggested by Rogers's homeodynamic principles in order to test for the presence of human field pattern manifestations and their proposed relationships. Creativity and actualization were used to operationalize innovativeness and diversity. A measure of empathy was used to assess the principle of integrality. This basic study tested the relationship of two of Rogers's principles, helicy and integrality, and introduced empathy into the science of unitary human beings.

Cowling[11] also examined helicy. This investigator operationalized helicy as mystical experiences and differentiation; creativity was used as an index of the innovative characteristics of helicy. The findings of the Cowling study, and those of Alligood, tended to support the predictive ability of Rogers's principles.

Barrett[12] examined helicy and introduced the idea of power into the science of unitary human beings. Power was conceptualized as a person's knowing participation in developmental change. The idea of knowing participation in change had been suggested earlier by Rogers. But description of the manifestation of participation as power, as described by Barrett, represented a major extension of the Rogerian perspective.

Barrett developed an instrument, using Rogers's theory to structure the content of the items. In the study, human field motion was used as an indicator of the direction of change, and power as an indicator of the nature of change. Power was operationalized as awareness, choice, freedom to act intentionally, and as involvement in change. Barrett hypothesized, correctly, that there would be a positive relationship between human field motion and power.

Creativity, actualization, human development, empathy, and change are all ideas nurse administrators consider important. It is essential that managers find ways of designing organizations where the energy fields of people and environment form pattern in ways that they, and those who work with them, consider healthy. It is equally essential that human development and actualization be understood. A major function of the administrator is identifying ways of patterning fields to assure integrated behaviors for clients and employees.

There are a number of avenues suggested by Rogers that have received little, if any, attention in nursing administration. One is understanding how unconscious energy is transformed into patterns of energy in the environments of higher- and lower-frequency organizations. A second is understanding the actions that generate patterns of meaning in varying organizational cultures for hospitalized people away from the familiar frequency patterns of their everyday environment.

The implications for nursing administration of a nursing theory that addresses power is equally important. Power is fundamental in political theories, many of which have received considerable attention of late in nursing administration. Many political models assume that power determines whose interests prevail where resources are limited; power in organizations is understood in terms of who is dependent on whom for scarce resources. Participation in change as a measure of power is aligned with the idea that power is the inverse of dependence. Understanding patterns of dependence and power by analyzing participation in decisions about how resources are allocated is a promising way to improve understanding of the distribution of resources to individuals and organizations.[12]

The following applied studies, using the Rogers's perspective—which may also prove useful in developing a new way of thinking about nursing management—are those by Rawnsley,[13] McDonald,[14] and Gueldner.[15] To understand helicy, Rawnsley studied the perceptions of the speed of time for the old and young, and the dying and nondying. She found, as expected, that an orientation to the future was more apparent among the young. But she also found that, regardless of age, time passed slowly for the dying. Rawnsley concluded, therefore, that what seems like a lack of patience among the terminally ill may in fact be explained by their change in time estimation. Based on the findings of this study, improved understanding of time estimation and intervention in the management of individual and group care is warranted.

McDonald examined middle-aged women who had arthritis pain and studied the relationship of pain reduction to visible light waves. She found that women exposed to blue light waves of shorter duration experienced a greater reduction in pain than women exposed to other light waves. McDon-

ald also noted that pain was progressively reduced as the duration of exposure to blue light was increased. The idea of environmental management of pain is not new since certain climates have for years been noted to reduce pain and have other health benefits. Likewise, ultraviolet light treatment of infant hyperbilirubinemia may serve as a model for the development of a nursing intervention for blue light treatment of arthritis patients experiencing pain. Recognition of the significance of research findings (such as McDonald's) by nursing administrators will hasten their adoption into nursing practice.

Gueldner[15] studied the relationship of imposed motion, human field motion, and restedness and found a significant relationship between human field motion and feelings of restedness. In nursing administration, the provision of environments that foster rest for clients and employees is important for people of all ages.

Rogers's theory stimulates explorations of the interaction between people and their environment for improved understanding of the well-being of clients and professionals. The knowledge we have about the use of blue light for individuals in pain can be used to expand our understanding of nursing interventions for people with all kinds of pain. Many studies have been done in management relating levels of work and safety to lighting. By combining what is understood about patients' perceptions of pain, and the social and psychic pain experienced by workers under varied environmental conditions, Rogers's theory can be extended to nursing administration.

In conclusion, I have presented the science of unitary human beings as a conceptual system from which principles and theories have been derived and tested. Although an understanding of the applicability of this perspective for nursing practice has evolved slowly, there is increasing widespread support for nursing practice and administration that uses and tests Rogers's theory.

Early findings from basic research tend to support the predictive ability of a number of Rogerian principles. The focus on concepts such as actualization, change, and empathy as well as implications for a nursing administrative theory of power are also important. Barrett's suggestion that conceiving of power as knowing participation in developmental change opens new avenues for research in nursing administration.

Applied research supports the need to examine patterning shifts in energy fields related to the administration of care for different types of clients, and to environmental overload and deprivation.[13] Findings from applied research studies that link dying with time perception, blue light treatment with pain reduction, and increased motion with restedness demonstrate the implications of Rogers' conceptual system for nursing practice and mandate nursing management consideration.

The corps of nurses who are educated in graduate nursing programs provide a unifying force for the discipline of nursing. Their awareness of the need for conceptual systems of nursing from which to develop a basis for research and practice is clearly apparent. It is this group of nurse administrators who will provide managerial and clinical leadership for future nursing research—research that frames long-standing problems using new world views for a unique nursing perspective of administration.

REFERENCES

1. Rogers ME. Science of unitary human beings. In: Malinski VM, ed. Explorations on Martha Rogers' science of unitary human beings. Norwalk, CT: Appleton-Century-Crofts, 1986.
2. ME Rogers. Nursing: A science of unitary man. In: Riehl JP, Roy C, eds. Conceptual models for nursing practice. 2nd ed. New York: Appleton-Century-Crofts, 1980.
3. Malinski VM. Nursing practice within the science of unitary human beings. In: Malinski VM, ed. Explorations on Martha Rogers' science of unitary human beings. Norwalk, CT: Appleton-Century-Crofts, 1986.
4. Nightingale F. Notes on nursing: what it is, and what it is not. Philadelphia: JB Lippincott, 1859/1946.
5. Meleis AI. Theoretical nursing: development and progress. Philadelphia: JB Lippincott, 1985.
6. Chopoorian TJ. Reconceptualizing the environment. In: Moccia P, ed. New approaches to theory development. New York: NLN, 1986.
7. Ference HM. Foundations of a nursing science and its evolution: a perspective. In: Malinski VM, ed. Explorations on Martha Rogers' science of unitary human beings. Norwalk, CT: Appleton-Century-Crofts, 1986.
8. Kuhn T. The structure of scientific revolutions. 2nd ed. Chicago: The University of Chicago Press, 1970.
9. Ference HM. The relationship of time experience, creativity traits, differentiation, and human field motion. In: Malinski VM, ed. Explorations on Martha Rogers' science of unitary human beings. Norwalk, CT: Appleton-Century-Crofts, 1986.
10. Alligood MR. The relationship of creativity, actualization, and empathy in unitary human development. In: Malinski VM, ed. Explorations on Martha Rogers' science of unitary human beings. Norwalk, CT: Appleton-Century-Crofts, 1986.
11. Cowling WR III. The relationship of mystical experience, differentiation, and creativity in college students. In: Malinski VM, ed. Explorations on Martha Rogers' science of unitary human beings. Norwalk, CT: Appleton-Century-Crofts, 1986.
12. Barrett EAM. Investigation of the principle of helicy: the relationship of human field motion and power. In: Malinski VM, ed. Explorations on Martha Rogers' science of unitary human beings. Norwalk, CT: Appleton-Century-Crofts, 1986.
13. Rawnsley MM. The relationship between the perception of the speed of time and the process of dying. In: Malinski VM, ed. Explorations on Martha Rogers' science of unitary human beings. Norwalk, CT: Appleton-Century-Crofts, 1986.
14. McDonald SF. The relationship between visible light-waves and the experience of pain. In: Malinski VM, ed. Explorations on Martha Rogers' science of unitary human beings. Norwalk, CT: Appleton-Century-Crofts, 1986.
15. Gueldner, SH. The relationship between imposed motion and human field motion in elderly individuals living in nursing homes. In: Malinski VM, ed. Explorations on Martha Rogers' science of unitary human beings. Norwalk, CT: Appleton-Century-Crofts, 1986.

11

Applying Rogers's Model to Nursing Administration: Emphasis on Client and Nursing

Sarah Hall Gueldner

CONCEIVING of Rogers's Science of Unitary Human Beings as a basis for administration requires that the nurse, whether a staff nurse or an administrator, understand Rogers's unique ideas of the (a) human energy field, (b) environmental energy field, and (c) human-environmental field interaction. Additionally, it is important that the would-be Rogerian administrator relinquish some traditional views of administration and consider a perspective based on Barrett's[1] unique definition of power as repatterning power. Finally, the process of administration itself needs to be viewed within the broader Rogerian perspective, which purports that both humans and their environmental fields change continuously and innovatively as they evolve together.

Since an overview of the Rogerian system was presented in Chapter 10, in this discussion the focus will be on the administrative features of human-environmental field interactions as defined and described by Rogers[2] and Ference[3], and on the concept of repatterning power, as described and tested by Barrett.[1] Emphasis will be on the relationships between nursing administration, nursing, and clients. Administrative behaviors consistent with the Rogerian perspective will be described.

ESSENTIAL CONCEPTUALIZATIONS WITHIN THE ROGERS SYSTEM

Principle of Helicy

Helicy is the principle of homeodynamics that postulates "the nature and direction of human and environmental change is continuously innovative, probabilistic, and characterized by increasing diversity of human field and environmental field pattern and organization emerging out of the continuous, mutual, simultaneous interaction of the human and environmental fields and manifesting nonrepeating rhythmicities".[4] This principle describes the continuous creative development (evolution) of the human-environmental fields as they evolve together.

Repatterning Power

Barrett has derived a new theory of power (repatterning power) that is consistent with the Rogerian concepts of energy fields, open systems, pattern, and four dimensionality. Barrett defines power as "the capacity to participate knowingly in change as operationalized by awareness, choices, freedom to act intentionally, and involvement in creating change." (p. 18)[5] Thus, repatterning power concerns the process of change and is proposed by Barrett to be an index of helicy.

According to Barrett, people experience

repatterning power as a feeling of enabling strength and as a cognitive recognition of choices interacting with behaviors for desired evolutionary outcomes. Such outcomes are postulated to be innovative, creative, and probabilistic. Choice is inherent in the assumption of repatterning power, and human freedom, responsibility, and courage are manifestations of choice. Power "describes the way people interact with their environment, to actualize some development potentials rather than others, and thereby share in the creation of their human and environmental reality."[5] The potential for repatterning power is assumed to exist in all human fields, and is conceived of as a base for nursing interventions.

Human Energy Field

Another essential feature of the Rogerian perspective is the view that each human energy field has the capacity to participate knowingly and purposefully in the changing of patterns. Each human is viewed as sentient and creative and is held in high regard. It is of utmost importance that nurse administrators view those within their purview—including nurses, clients, and all others who interact in an administrative unit—in this way. Similarly, those in adjacent administrative units, including physicians, must be regarded highly. The Rogers perspective assumes that every individual has the capability to create positive changes in his or her patterns of interaction. Further, Rogerian thinking insists that the human field be considered as a whole, and that an understanding of its characteristics cannot be determined from knowledge of its parts alone.

Environmental Energy Field

Each environmental field is specific to a given human field and includes all that exists outside of that field. Theoretically, each person is a part of every other human's environmental field, which extends to infinity. Environmental fields, like human fields, are purported to be at least four dimensional, acknowledging the probability of attributes outside those readily discernible through the five senses.

Human-Environmental Field Interaction

Both human and environmental fields are integral with one another and each is open, so that they change continuously and creatively as they evolve together. Pattern distinguishes one energy field from all others; each human field pattern is unique and integral with its own unique environmental field. Energy is the dynamic nature of the fields. Causality is impossible according to the Rogerian perspective.

Administrative System

When considered in the Rogerian perspective, an administrative system consists of all human and environmental fields integral to the system, and is potentially so complex as to extend to infinity. Moreover, the Rogerian-based administrator must consider each administrative system in its totality, rather than by individual units or parts. For this discussion, the term "administrative system" will be used to describe a hypothetical aggregate that includes all human-environmental field interactions that fall within the purview of a designated administrator.

To facilitate discussion, the system being highlighted at a particular time will be referred to as the focal system, while peripheral systems under illumination will be referred to as adjacent administrative systems. It is necessary to remember, however, that administrative systems termed "adjacent" remain integral with the overall system. These figurative distinctions are made only to facilitate discussion.

Nurse-Administrator (not defined by Rogers)

The term "nurse administrator" refers to a variety of roles. In its broadest sense, every nurse is a nurse administrator, because each nurse has management responsibilities related to the nursing care of those clients assigned to his or her care. Likewise, nurse educators are administrators. They manage the learning of students—be they nursing students, patients, families, other nurses, or health-care workers.

In the more traditional sense, the nurse administrator is one who plans, directs, and monitors the work of others as they provide health care for a circumscribed group of clients, in inpatient and outpatient health-care institutions including community-based wellness centers and home-care agencies.

Since much of this discussion will relate to both the staff nurse managing care and to the nurse administrator, nurses and administrators will be referred to hereafter as "nurse administrator."

THE COMMON NURSING-ADMINISTRATIVE GOAL

Whatever the practice setting, it is the goal of all nurse administrators to increase the capacity of each individual in a system to participate knowingly in change. All administrative energy, therefore, should be directed to changes in the environment that will enhance harmonious, symphonic human-environmental field interactions. As positive change is achieved, it follows that the unit will progress toward increased symphony, diversity, and complexity, and thus enjoy increased productivity.

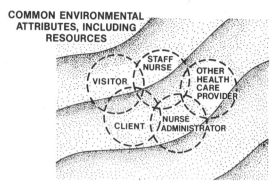

Figure 11.1. An Ordinary Episode in Nursing, Viewed Within the Rogers Framework. This illustration represents a common and relatively simplistic episode within a nursing system. The human energy fields are depicted as circular configurations, with broken lines to denote openness and constant change. In this illustration the nurse energy field is interacting with the energy fields of the nurse administrator, client, visitor, and another health-care worker. As denoted by the broken-line boundaries, the fields of the client, nurse, administrator, visitor, and other health-care worker flow through the same environmental space. The shaded area indicates a hypothetical environmental field within an administrative context, and theoretically extends to infinity. All persons highlighted share the same environment; each human energy field is a part of every other person's environmental field. General environmental attributes such as temperature, humidity, sensory enrichment, available resources, and wave frequencies are common to all in the system.

A HYPOTHETICAL NURSING-ADMINISTRATIVE EPISODE, AS ILLUSTRATED WITHIN THE ROGERIAN CONTEXT

Figures 11.1 and 11.2 depict episodes of nursing administration in the practice setting, as viewed through the Rogerian perspective of human-environmental field interactions.

The illustration in Figure 11.1 represents a common and relatively simplistic episode in a nursing system. The human energy fields are

Figure 11.2. A Representation of the Complexity of a Nursing Situation, as Viewed Within the Rogerian Perspective. This illustration represents the complexity and interrelatedness of a hypothetical nursing situation at a single point in time, when viewed within the Rogerian framework. Each human energy field is a part of every other environmental field, and general environmental attributes, including resources, are shared by all individuals within a system. The environmental field, and therefore the possibilities for human-environmental interactions, extends to infinity.

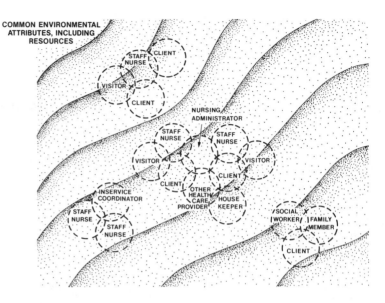

depicted as circular configurations bounded by broken lines to denote openness and constant change. In this illustration, the staff nurse energy field is interacting intimately with the energy fields of the nurse administrator, client, visitor, and another health-care worker. The shaded area indicates the hypothetical environmental field, which extends to infinity. All persons highlighted in this illustration share the same environmental field. It is important to note, too, that each human energy field is part of every other person's environmental field. General environmental attributes (temperature, humidity, sensory enrichment, available resources, and wave frequencies) are therefore common to all individuals in the system.

As denoted by the broken line and overlapping boundaries, fields of the staff nurse, the nurse administrator, the client, visitor, and other workers are open and flow through the same environmental space. Episodes can vary greatly in complexity. Variations will depend on the setting, the number and roles of persons in a unit of supervision, and the functional proximity to other units of administration.

The environmental field of the nurse includes far more than just the persons involved in primary interactions. The system always includes all personnel being supervised by the nurse administrator, all clients receiving care, all visitors in the unit, and all fellow workers. In most instances the environmental field of the nurse administrator at any point in time will also include persons from adjacent administrative units, such as physicians, dieticians, housekeepers, laboratory technicians, and volunteers.

Thus, a more representative human-environmental field, in terms of nurse and client interactions, is depicted in Figure 11.2.

THE NURSING-ADMINISTRATIVE PROCESS WITHIN THE ROGERIAN CONTEXT

From this comprehensive viewpoint, the successful nurse administrator needs to be proficient in assessing the human-environmental interactive patterns operating between each person in his or her administrative unit. It is important to be able to prioritize intentional interactive initiatives.

The well-being of each client is the common and overriding focus of any unit of nursing administration, and all management energy should be directed toward this focus. However, the seasoned nurse administrator knows that interactions involving the client are optimized by synchronized and harmonious interactions in the total system. Persons whose own field interactions are synchronous are in a better position to assist clients to design or modify their field interactions and thereby facilitate maximum health and well-being. The forward-thinking nurse manager, therefore, will be attentive to the interactive patterns of personnel. He or she will design and implement management strategies to enhance positive field interactions between staff members and their respective environments. Ensuring positive interactions will involve the creative use of resource systems and active negotiations; zero-sum interactions will be replaced with situations that foster empowerment in each person in the system.

In a professional community such as nursing, where successful role interaction depends so directly on individual assessment, judgment, creativity, and decision making, it is important to recruit competent individuals who have been socialized to participate intentionally in their own evolutionary development and in the evolution of the profession. The primary responsibility of the Rogerian nurse administrator, in terms of staff development, is to help each nurse use him- or herself as a therapeutic agent and mobilize other resources needed to increase awareness, capacity, and choice. Resources available include colleagues, family, other health-care workers, meaningful orientation programs, creative continuing education opportunities, sufficient supplies and equipment, supportive manpower, and aesthetic, hygienic, and efficient physical facilities.

The Rogerian-based nurse administrator would give high priority to the provision of educational opportunities, since knowing participation in change is based on being informed. Another aspect of Roger's framework is the establishment of open and ample communication systems that reflect a positive view of the contributions of each individual within a system.

Reflecting the positive view of mankind, the Rogerian-based administrative system emphasizes evolution and interaction rather than maintenance and isolation, and encourages creative thinking and problem solving. Where rules and policies are necessary for the smooth operation of a unit, they need to reflect the knowing and intentional participation of the group.

In every way possible, the administrative climate should be open and supportive; the administrative model should be designed to enhance the self-esteem, actualization, confidence, available options, freedom of choice, and opportunities for individual and group development.

From the Rogerian perspective, power is not viewed as strictly within the purview of an administrator, or the physician, or the head nurse, but rather as a process of development participated in by all individuals, including clients. The ideas of "control over," "subordinates," "unilateral change," "coercion," "domination," and even "recipient" are not consistent with Rogers's conceptualization of power. Instead, words such as "informed," "free," "evolving," and "harmonious" describe the characteristics of Rogerian power.

SPECIFIC APPLICATIONS TO PRACTICE AND ADMINISTRATION

While conclusive research findings within the Rogerian system are sparse, they tend to support the findings of environmental studies conducted by industrial researchers.[6–8] These studies show that environmental characteristics are clearly associated with changes in individual well-being and must be taken into account by all nurses, including nurse administrators.

Another characteristic of the Rogerian perspective is consideration of innovative treatment modalities. The findings of investigations using Rogers's framework go beyond traditional environmental concerns such as adequate light, safe noise levels, and efficient layouts, to include more innovative, even futuristic therapeutic modalities. For instance, Ludomerski-Kalamin[9] found that the feeling of well-being was reported to be higher during exposure to blue light (higher frequency, shorter wave lengths) than during exposure to red light (lower frequency, longer wave lengths). Smith[10] demonstrated that a varied auditory environment was more restful to individuals lying in bed than either continuous music or spoken sounds. The findings of investigations of movement[3,11,12] also have important implications for workers and clients. For instance, most health-care institutions have lagged far behind other industrial organizations in providing on-site fitness facilities. Among the more innovative healing modalities under study in the Rogerian system are touch[13] and meditation.[14]

In summary, environments, as defined from Rogers's perspective, should be changed to increase the symphony of human-environmental interactions within each administrative system. Following Rogerian thinking, the nursing environment should be designed to provide each member of the system with ample opportunity for potential development (evolution) through available, free choices and pleasant positive interactions. Creative use of color, space, and light are important considerations for nurse administrators.

Nursing has traditionally been highly structured—medicines and treatments are given with exactness, according to standardized step-by-step procedures, often using equipment and supplies that have been carefully processed and packaged to ensure sterility.

Student nurses are painstakingly taught "the right" way to do each procedure. Aesthetic qualities have too often been neglected by nurse administrators and other health-care workers in favor of sterile, stark, easy-to-clean environments. The Rogerian nurse administrator needs to make sure that creative, less structured practitioners are not forced into rigid routines and procedures that limit their greatest potential contribution—creative problem solving. Environmental fields need to be designed with enough structure so that people feel comfortable and productive, but with enough flexibility to accommodate the more free-wheeling creative patterns of nurses—and clients as well.

Prosthetic or protective interchange may be needed when a persistent negative interaction pattern is observed, or when a recognized potential for problematic patterns exists. For instance, when an inexperienced staff nurse is assigned to the 11 PM to 7 AM shift alone, the nurse administrator should arrange for increased support in the environment. A prominently displayed list of phone numbers to assure quick access to help is one example of such supportive strategies. As the new nurse becomes repatterned, such prosthesics may no longer be necessary. However, in the event that an innovative device or strategy were to emerge to help the repatterning, it should be shared with others.

All nurses are managers of care, because their goal is to maximize the power potential of themselves, their clients, and colleagues in ways that are developmentally beneficial to each individual and to the collective. If nursing-administrative strategies are successful, individuals in a system will become more aware and, therefore, more involved in the process of intentional change as manifested by increased participation. As each individual participates with increasing awareness, systems of a higher order evolve.

REFERENCES

1. Barrett EAM. Investigation of the principle of helicy: the relationship of human field motion and power. In: Malinski VM, ed. Explorations on Martha Rogers' science of unitary human beings. New York: Appleton-Century-Crofts, 1986, pp. 173–184.
2. Rogers ME. Science of unitary human beings. In: Malinski VM, ed. Explorations on Martha Rogers' science of unitary human beings New York: Appleton-Century-Crofts, 1986, pp. 3–8.
3. Ference H. The relationship of time experience, creativity traits, differentiation, and human field motion. In: Malinsky VM, ed. Exploration on Martha Rogers' science of unitary human beings. New York: Appleton-Century-Crofts, 1986.
4. Rogers ME. Nursing: A science of unitary man. In: Riehl JP, Roy C, eds., Conceptual models for nursing practice. New York: Appleton-Century-Crofts, 1980, pp. 333.
5. Barrett EAM. Clinical excellence in nursing international networking. Proceedings of the international nursing research congress Edinburgh, 1987, pp. 17–18.
6. Bartlett F. Psychological criteria of fatigue. In: Floyd W, Welford A, eds. Symposium on fatigue and symposium on human factors in equipment design. New York: Arno Press, 1977.
7. Goldmark J. Fatigue and efficiency. New York: Russell Sage Foundation, 1912.
8. Myers C. Mind and work. London: University of London Press, 1927.
9. Ludomirski-Kalamin B. Relationship between the environmental energy wave frequency pattern manifest in red light and blue light and human field motion in adult individuals with visual sensory perception and those with total blindness. Unpublished doctoral dissertation. New York University, 1986.
10. Smith MJ. ANS 1986;9(1):21–28.
11. Gueldner SH. The relationship between imposed motion and human field motion in elderly individuals living in nursing homes. In: Malinsky VM, ed. Exploration on Martha Rogers' Science of Unitary Human Beings. New York: Appleton-Century-Crofts, 1986.
12. Thomas SD. The experience of intentionality and human field motion: A test of the principle of integrality according to the Rogerian framework. University of Tennessee Center for the health sciences, College of Nursing, in progress.
13. Quinn J. Therapeutic touch as energy exchange: Testing the theory. ANS 1977;6:42–49.
14. Macrae JA. A comparison between meditation subjects and non-meditation subjects on time experience and human field motion. Unpublished doctoral dissertation, New York University, 1982.

12

Nursing Science Theories and Administration

Helen M. Ference

A RESPONSIBLE administration provides direction, gives leadership, and assures that people who are being served are properly positioned to enact their roles and fully engage their knowledge. Nursing theories, which in recent years have guided nursing practice, give direction and distinction to management and nursing administration.

This chapter describes ways of using nursing science to administer nursing services in large and small social systems, such as those found in hospitals, multi-institutional systems, health-care agencies, nursing homes, and corporate practices. The purpose in using a nursing science model is both humanistic and economic. In business vernacular, the bottom line is better care at a lower cost, with greater comfort.

ADMINISTRATION AS DOMAIN DEFINITION

When nurses accept employment in a nursing service, they implicitly agree to conform to the philosophy and objectives of the respective service. Employment acknowledges a certain domain of accountability. This domain is bounded by rules, social norms, and values that are made explicit in the philosophy and objectives of the institution. Further, there is an underlying culture often displayed by the slogans, expectations, rituals and rites of passage.[1] The definition of the philosophical domain of nursing may be subtle, requiring objective signs to describe it. On the other hand, the domain may be explicitly set out in a written form, in which event it is imperative to observe the operation of the philosophy in practice.

In recent years, nursing services have adopted nursing models or conceptual frameworks, one of the strongest advancements for the profession of this decade. The advance of conceptual models derives from thoughtfully developed frameworks. The frameworks logically describe a consistent set of assumptions, constructs, and theories that guide clinical and managerial practice. With established models, such as those described by Rogers, King, Roy, Orem, or Watson, in place, there is structure and coherence in a nursing service. This structure and coherence bring a form of security to the providers of the nursing service.

The definition of a nursing service is found in its philosophy of nursing. From that philosophy, standards of care flow that assure a similar quality of care for similar clients. When the philosophy derives from a set of assumptions of a conceptually complete model, the structure provides a consistency from which standards and quality measures are easily identified. This consistency affords security and a sense of coherence for employees and the people being served. An administration without the substantive knowledge of nursing theory, or with designs of eclectic models used inconsistently in everyday operations cannot function successfully in complex organizations.

TOWARD A NURSING SCIENCE FOR A NURSING SERVICE

It is advantageous from both a philosophic and economic view to adopt a nursing science framework for optimizing a nursing service, as caring is a human process, and the administration of caring likewise is a human process. Ideally, the philosophy of care matches the philosophy of administration in a nursing service. Optimally, staff nurses and administrators practice the art of nursing and nursing administration using the same basic principles in all their interactions.

The "science of unitary human beings" formulated by Rogers[2,3] is a logical construction of nursing theories, principles, and assumptions. Scientific inquiry and research conducted in this framework has resulted in empirical verification of a number of principles.[4,5] The fundamental concepts and assumptions in this framework are:

1. A human being is an *energy field*; the environment is an *energy field*.
2. The *pattern* of human and environmental fields are observable phenomenon.
3. *Openness* of the field is complete, not relatively open, as in general systems theory.
4. The fields are characterized by *four-dimensionality*, which is defined by the synthesis of four coordinates: length, width, depth, and time, called *space-time*.[6]

Based on these assumptions human beings progressively function at high levels of complexity, diversity, and differentiation. While everyday work may seem to be manifested in the form of details and particulate functions, the reality of function lies in the performance of humans as they interface with one another in continuous mutual processes.

> **Resonancy:** The energy field evolves in the direction of higher frequency, shorter wave length from lower frequency, longer wave length.
>
> **Helicy:** The pattern of the field evolves multidirectionally toward greater complexity and diversity.
>
> **Integrality:** The human and environmental field are in continuous mutual process.

Figure 12.1 Principles of Homeodynamics. (From Rogers ME. Science of unitary human beings. In: Malinski VM, ed. Explorations on Martha E. Rogers' science of unitary human beings. East Norwalk, CT: Appleton-Century-Crofts, 1986. Used with permission.)

Each science has a specific language, for its purpose is to bring clarity and new ideas that previously were unknown. The language of a science needs to be understood if it is to be applied in everyday situations. Understanding is facilitated when participants in a social system are engaged in learning the same science.

Rogers has defined three homeodynamic principles, summarized in Figure 12.1, that have been subjected to rigorous empirical testing to demonstrate their predictability.[7,8] The principles of reasonancy, helicy, and integrality are used as the basis for predicting change. The principles have guided research and clinical practice and can also be used creatively to direct nursing services.[9–11]

Assuming that administration exists to support care givers, it is consistent that the philosophy and objectives of nursing service should match those of nursing.[12,13] The principle of "integrality" suggests that the human and environmental fields are in continuous mutual process. This means that every nurse and nurse administrator is reciprocally engaged in mutual processes.

When differing philosophies guide the staff nurse and nurse administrator, the feeling of both is one of disharmony, discomfort and dis*ease*, and occasionally pain. Some nurse administrators have chosen not to be leaders of their nursing service. They have opted instead to be the followers of hospital administrators. When a break between nursing services and nursing administration occurs, it can be said that both fields are in differing relative space-times.

One way of moving into common space-times is by leveling organizational structures to permit continuous movement and open communication between nurses and administrators. Some administrations are top-heavy; excessive hierarchic layers block interactions between executives and staff nurses, resulting in disharmony between the administrators of nursing and the staff. Middle management too, may be on a different wavelength, sharing another time-space that is connected neither to the staff nurses' focus on caring nor to that of the director. Perhaps creating an organizational structure where middle managers are placed in consultative positions would foster the development of a healthy integral nursing service. Staff nurses would share space-times with consultants, serving as evaluators, timekeepers, and standard setters who help pattern their environments toward healthy changes.

Another way of sharing common space-times is through "motion." The theory of motion proposes that as a human field engages in ever-higher levels of human field motion, the pattern evolves toward greater complexity, diversity, and differentiation.[5,10,14] Human field motion expands with increased physical motion,[6] with meditation,[15] with risk-taking,[16] and with higher levels of participation in change.[7]

In the context of the administration of a nursing service, the aforementioned studies suggest that when staff nurses are risk-takers, when they are in motion with their patients, and when they knowingly participate in essential decisions about health care at the patient and institutional levels, they evolve toward greater complexity, diversity, and dif-

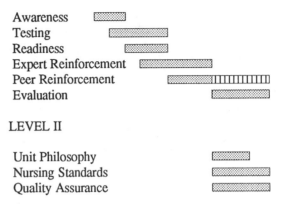

Figure 12.2   Ference Theory Based Practice Time Line

ferentiation. The administrator of the nursing service also experiences a pattern change when there is continuous mutual interaction with staff nurses. The manifestation for the entire nursing service consequently is one of power, feeling of transcendence, lightness, propulsion, and well-being.

INTRODUCING A NURSING FRAMEWORK IN A SERVICE SETTING

Figure 12.2 illustrates a 12-month plan for introducing a nursing science framework. The plan provides time for all participants to learn the framework before advancing to writing the philosophy, standards, and quality assurance programs that maintain the operation of a nursing service in practice.

At level I, the first phase, the nursing framework is introduced through conferences with experts of the science. The awareness phase, a process of learning, generally takes four to six weeks, with a faculty time approximating 10 hours over the period. Planned discussions with the nursing staff can be supplemented with literary resources and annotated references.

In the testing phase, the learner becomes acclimated to the new knowledge. Patient care conferences are conducted focusing on integration of the framework into everyday, real situations. This is the time the learner makes associations for creative changes in practice. The learner might say, "Aha!" or "Now I see." Session leaders guide the images verbalized by learners into the language of the scientific framework. Learners typically move rapidly during this phase, especially when they are participating as a group.

The readiness phase is identifiable when leading students begin using case examples to test the framework. In a group, the more astute learner will be able to identify case problems and diagnose these problems on the basis of nursing science. In this phase, care plans are written and used as examples for other learners. The plans begin to be implemented with much sharing of new modalities of care as the staff integrates the science into their traditional practice.

At the expert reinforcement phase, experts are available at the peak of the learners' change. Feedback is immediate to enable the learner to pattern professional changes into the delivery of care.[17] This phase generally occurs for the serious student after about 30 hours of formal instruction. It is important to anticipate this phase as experts participate in the formal patient care conferences, and are present in the clinical areas, or available for consultation. As the successful learner moves through the various phases, the ability to apply principles and theories to each new situation becomes easier. The frustrated and skeptical learner, however, needs to be placed in a special situation with the expert, or provided with relative space-time that is highly intense. Role modeling with the learner works well for one who has difficulty with imaging and visualization. This phase ends when learners appear comfortable with their new language and conceptions, and rely less on experts.

Experts phase their involvement out by building in peer support processes during the peer reinforcement phase. Since using a nursing framework in practice implies control of one's own practice, it is expected that there be an assignment structure in place that enhances authority and accountability. Primary nursing, for example, must be in place to assure continuity of care and a common relative space-time for patients and nurses. A nursing process audit tool is used by peers to critique adherence of practice to the nursing framework. This reinforces the continuous use of theories, such as motion, evolutionary emergence, and intentionality, to guide nursing prescriptions. Scheduled periodic evaluation of care via conferences, audits of records, and direct observation should be the responsibility of one or two persons, including, the experts, for verification.

Level I is complete after the fifth phase. In a service setting, level I activities generally take up to 6 months. Level II is the administrative and policy level. It involves writing a philosophy from which objectives of care, nursing standards, and quality assurance are derived.

Philosophy of Nursing

The language and concepts of the philosophy of nursing should be consistent with the language and concepts of nursing science. As an example, a philosophical description might be:

Nursing's focus is on the whole person, who grows more complex and diverse with age. Crises are major transformation periods for persons, whereby the nurse engages with the individual to facilitate movement from one pattern to a new pattern. The person functions in continuous mutual process in the environment, as does the nurse. When people are sick, they frequently experience realities that are considered outside of the realm of 'normal.' These altered reality states are explained by a four-dimensional understanding of the human living process. Nurses systematically employ theories of nursing science to skillfully engage with patients experiencing crises and pattern their environments in such a manner as to direct a more complex and diverse evolution of the whole person. Manifestations of this change are experienced as comfort, power, lightness, and a general sense of well-being.[18]

Implicit in this philosophy are the four fundamental concepts of the science of unitary human beings—energy field, pattern, openness, and four dimensionality. The philosophy is articulated in a manner that integrates the concepts with the usual way of perceiving care for people. It is consistent with the language of science. It does not use the language of theories based on different assumptions such as "adaptation", care of the "bio-psycho-social" being, or "compliance."

Nursing Standards

Nursing standards give direction to care deriving from a set of values judged to be appropriate. In the instance of nursing science, the appropriateness of the values has been determined by experienced practitioners.

The assessment tools measure field patterns of the indicators of the whole person. There are two instruments designed specifically within this science, the Ference Human Field Motion Tool,[8,14] and the Barrett Power as Knowing Participation in Change Test.[7] Other indices measured are sleep/wake cycles, near-death experiences, multiple manifestations, and pain/comfort. Assessments are determined as follows:

- *Human Field Motion Tool*, an instrument developed by Ference[5,8,14];
- *Power* as knowing participation in change, an instrument developed by Barrett[7];
- *Sleep/Wake Cycles*, measured by intermittent, continuous dozing;
- *Near-Death Experiences*, exemplified by traumatic encounters, verbal statements

about "dying," "death," or "dead," and descriptions of out-of-body experiences;
- *Multiple Manifestations* as nonverbal and verbal expressions of participation in different and many relative space-times; and
- *Pain/Comfort*, as expressions of agonizing turmoil, or quiet peace.

Assessment of these six characteristics is essential. Secondary assessment of physical movement or immobility, the expression of "time" passing, and creative insights and the presence of significant others are also made.

Diagnoses

Diagnoses are made when the patient identifies a problem; the nurse's focus is on the pattern profile. A pattern that may be "healthy" for one person may be "unhealthy" for another. The problem identified by the nurse and, when possible, mutually with the patient, is generally the manifestation of a pattern profile that is uncomfortable, non-functional, or incongruent with the patient's image of the human environmental field. While nursing diagnoses are being formulated, the goal is to facilitate the patient or client's knowing participation in changing his or her pattern.

Plan and Intervention

Nurses pattern the clients' environmental-energy field in a prescribed manner, in which the nature and direction of change are guided by Rogerian principles of homeodynamics. The nature of change is guided by the principle of helicy. The environmental field is patterned with the understanding that there is continuous mutual process between the human and environmental fields. This is the principle of integrality. The direction of change is predicted by the principle of resonancy.

Modalities of Care

The modalities of care now being used in practice include:

- *Meditation.* Any formalized procedure to place the nurse therapist in a position to move into a selected relative space-time
- *Intentionality.* The nurse therapist strategically patterning the environmental field
- *Innovative Imagery.* Nurse and client participating in the creative patterning of the environmental energy field for the purpose of comfort
- *Field Touch.* Therapeutically using the energy field to propel pattern changes in the shared, relative space-time of a patient, or significant other
- *Imposed Motion.* Rocking or physically moving the environmental energy field[29]
- *Sound Frequency.* Providing any familiar pattern such as singing, vocalizing, story telling, or poetry
- *Light Frequency.* Using blue light or multi-patterned colors of light[19,20]

Evaluation of change is measured empirically by the Ference Human Field Motion Tool. Subjectively, change is evaluated by the patient's professed and demonstrated comfort and sense of well-being.

QUALITY ASSURANCE

Quality is basically an index of intensity or a degree of excellence. There are usually many different grades of quality in services and products. Although grading is not usually done in nursing services, there can be speculations as to what the grades of quality might be. Obviously the more highly educated nurse is a more sophisticated practitioner and can provide a broader range and therefore a higher grade of services to a client, when empowered to do so, than can a technician. Thus, education is a variable of quality. Likewise a clearly structured plan of practice,

which is theoretically based and scientifically sound, provides a higher grade of care than does a mode of practice which is atheoretical, reactionary, and laissez faire.

When practice and administration of a service are organized using a specific set of theoretical constructs, the index, or measure of their functional intensity must match. Therefore, a specific set of quality measures need to be used to judge intensity of function and adherence to standards in accord with nursing science.

Using measures of quality designed for a three-dimensional view of practice to assess practice conducted in accord with nursing science is just as invalid as attempting to use a 12-inch ruler to locate a physical object or event in a system synthesized of temporal and three spatial coordinates. Reality in the nursing science perspective is determinable by a four-dimensional system.

The contrast between three- and four-dimensional measures of safety exemplifies these differences. In a three dimensional framework, the assessment of patient safety may be whether siderails are up, the bed is in a low position, and restraints are secure if a patient is confused. In a four-dimensional framework, constructive mobilization is more important than restrictive immobilization. Thus, safety of the field is assessed by whether there are moving objects in the environment such as people or television sports programs; whether there is a rocking chair, a wheelchair, or a walker available; and whether patients are able to control light color and intensity on demand.

Another standard measured is sleep, often categorized as activity rest. Typically, three-dimensional measurements include whether sedatives are available at bedtime and for repeated dosages for those awakening in the nighttime, and, if patients sleep continuously throughout the night for 7 to 8 hours in one period.

Motion theory in nursing science suggests,

however, that pattern transformations occur with peak human field motion or energy field activity. Fluctuations commonly referred to as activity and rest are varying frequencies of the field where multiple environmental manifestations are experienced. Awakening from sleep is viewed as a natural phenomenon, as an indicator of movement into another relative space-time. This relative space-time is of a different wave frequency. When the frequency is high it appears shorter than the three-dimensional time of a clock. If the interval of clock time were measured it would be short for those in high-frequency space-times and long for those in low-frequency space-times.

Those in crises—the critically ill and the elderly—are people in flux who experience many more sleep/wake cycles in 24 hours than others who are not ill or elderly. Usually their clock-time interval of sleep is much less than 8 hours. Nursing interventions characterized by the intentional imposition of a sleep state when a patient has chosen to be awake may cause confusion—defined as a poorly differentiated experience of many space-times. In the nursing science framework, high-grade assessments are made of whether the patient who awakens in the nighttime is assisted with activity, and whether subsequent nursing activities are planned around the observed sleep intervals.

Outcome criteria too, must match the theoretical model used for practice. Depending on the model in use, the goals differ. Three-dimensional models, such as those developed by Levine[21] and Roy[22] may attend to immobilization when physical safety is the issue. Safe mobilization of the energy field is the concern of the nursing science model when a complex pattern and organization of the field is determined to be coextensive with confusion. An 8-hour norm for sleep intervals is the ideal goal for health according to the traditional theories. The nursing science model, on the other hand, takes as a goal to facilitate the person's pattern transformation by promoting natural sleep/wake cycles that are congruent with manifestations of the energy field wave frequency.

In summary, quality assurance measures are standards that reflect the outcome of the nursing modalities prescribed by the theoretical framework. Quality of care indicators must be valid for the practice standard accepted. Examples of standards derived from nursing science theory have been discussed and compared to those ordinarily considered in three-dimensional practice models.

This section has provided an introduction to nursing science, its assumptions, the Rogerian principles, and a number of theories. Applying the theories of Human Field Motion, power and integrity to the administration of service is a further step. It should be noted, however, that in reality, the application of nursing science both to practice and administration occurs in continuous mutual process.

PATTERNING AN ORGANIZATIONAL ENVIRONMENT FOR NURSING PRACTICE

The application of nursing science theory to administration connotes an organizational and social system comprised of the motion of many people in continuous mutual process. With like thought and practice—that is, similar experiential, multidimensional positions—such a service is organized and harmonious. Little confusion arises because of the commonly held perception of professional practice. The principles that guide human field interactions of patients and nurses, as found in nursing science, also guide the human field interactions of nurses and other nurses.

Barrett's theory of power has special utility for nursing administration.[7] Described as knowing participation in change, levels of power are assessed with an instrument that is found to vary directly with human field motion, as defined by Ference. A group of nurses in a service setting could be evaluated for their level of power. It may be hypothesized that a nurse's freedom to act intentionally and the ability to be creative and use multiple dimensions in care giving capacity can be correlated with quality of care.

In patterning the environmental fields of nurses, using nursing science theory, the insightful nurse administrator applies the principle of integrality. The assumption here is that there is a continuous mutual process between nurses and their environmental energy fields. To find the significant space-time that reflects the appropriate environment, nurses can be asked to select the most influential nurse on their unit. In this way nurses are identifying their source of strength. The product formed by this group selection of all nurses is called a network, specifically "Network of Nurse Influentials."[23] This network is usually highly mobile, with great complexity and diversity of field pattern.

In the classic sense of organization theory and current thought about corporate culture,[24] the network of nurse influentials can be viewed as a mechanism for matching the culture of people in organizations with the strategic vision of administration. By attending to the culture of an organization, Hickman and Silva[24] concur that change is effective, a thought consistent with the nursing science model.

The culture of an organization, composed of intellectual and aesthetic values, shares with similar cultures the same relative space-time. A strategic vision of what the organization can attain in terms of high-quality services can be the creative product of an administration and influential nurses working to achieve new energy field patterns compatible with the practice of nurses, physicians, social service workers, and dieticians in today's service settings. Actualizing this vision can be accomplished through the process of

intentionality, wherein the environmental energy field is patterned toward a higher frequency and greater complexity. The network of nurse influentials is the environmental field of the nurse peer group. The network is also the empowered, who have awareness, see choices, act intentionally, and are creative in change.

Hickman and Silva describe new age skills that must be learned to match culture and strategy and to facilitate effective change.[24] These skills are logically similar to the manifestations that emerge from a complex and diverse energy field. Such skills, or human field manifestations, are creative insight, sensitivity, vision, versatility, focus, and patience.

The process of change in the classic sense is described as thinking, planning, and implementing. In the four-dimensional reality change involves guided imagery to raise insights that pattern a field toward greater complexity and diversity. In a four-dimensional science, planning is the reality of occurrence, in that what is planned well materializes; and implementing is the manifestation experienced once the reality of clear imaging has been achieved. The images created by the cooperative endeavors of nurse administrators and nurse influentials become operationalized by nursing peers integrating the actions of the high frequency group. The change can be both observed and measured with nursing science instruments.

To enhance the network of nurse influentials, each person can be positioned with a mentor "of the same wavelength," that is, one sharing the same relative space-time who can assist with guided imagery—a form of foreseeing directions and strategic planning.

For achieving the transformation envisioned by an administration using the nursing science model, an economic incentive or whatever is of perceived value can be awarded to the nurse influential who achieves an exemplary transformation for a peer group, or to the mentor who best uses guided imagery to facilitate transformations. In the context that the application of nursing science yields probabilistic outcomes, the awards should be predicated on patient-care outcomes: Patients should be more comfortable and feel better prepared to care for themselves.

HYPOTHESES TESTING IN NURSING ADMINISTRATION

The quality of service that nursing administration provides can be addressed through research conducted to determine if, how, and why management makes a difference to the nursing practice for patients. In some circumstances it is merely assumed that any administration is better than no administration at all. The following discussion represents examples of a number of hypotheses that could be tested that derive from a nursing science framework.

Hypothesis 1 *There is a relationship between the guided imagery of nursing administration and the power of the nursing service.* A few highlights are appropriate, in addition to the discussion presented, with regard to the network of nurse influentials. When a group holds a common image, the image serves to direct change that is synchronized and realistic. In the four-dimensional perspective, the image is reality. Performance is the manifestation of the image. The guiding principles here are resonancy, which implies that the change will be toward higher frequency, and the principle of integrality, which implies that there is a continuous mutual process between the environmental and human fields. Power will increase in a group when the direction of environmental change is toward a higher frequency.

Hypothesis 2 *Common intentionality by nursing administration and nursing service is requisite to pattern transformation.* Fundamentally, being sincere and genuinely entering into a space-time with others leads to pattern changes that are comforting and productive. Intentionality is an active process based on the principle of helicy. Where common intentionality exists, change occurs in the direction of greater complexity and diversity for everyone involved. The field pattern becomes more differentiated, more creative, and encompasses a multiplicity of differences.

Hypothesis 3 *The power of nurses to prescribe environmental conditions for clients is related to cost-effective pattern transformations.* In the nineteenth century, Nightingale[25] wrote extensively about the environmental conditions of hospitals, sick rooms, and wards. As a nurse, she saw the need to attend to health and to the hygiene of unsanitary environments. In this century, attention continues to focus on the physical environment of the sick and needy. Intensive care units have had a considerable impact on health and pattern transformation. Were nurses who use nursing science actively involved in hospital environmental control, different colors of light, music patterns, and holograms might well be integrated as normal environmental components to facilitate guided imagery. A truly therapeutic environmental milieu is virtually nonexistent in today's health service organizations. Nursing has the knowledge, capacity, and responsibility to determine whether such environments can make a difference in patient well-being and recovery.

Hypothesis 4 *Assistants to nursing service directed to deliver selective, imposed motion for patients in crises, the immobilized person, and elderly will yield cost-effective service in terms of greater human field motion, creativity, and patient comfort.* Motion is essential to human development.[8,14,26–28] As nurses' work becomes increasingly demanding and fewer nurses are available to deliver total care, human and technological options need to be considered to provide what is scientifically known to influence the comfort and well-being of patients. Given today's knowledge of motion, to not walk or turn a patient, and to restrain a confused person is unacceptable. Hypothesis 4 is based on economic necessity and derived from the principle of resonancy. There are known correlations between imposed motion and human field motion.[14] High human field motion correlates with creativity, differentation, and complexity of the field. A person feels better with imposed motion. A small set of imposed motion tasks could be studied to determine whether earlier discharges from service agencies can occur, particularly for the elderly and when provided by trained assistants to nurses.

THREE-STRAND HELIX: BETTER CARE, IN A SHORTER TIME, WITH MORE COMFORT

In economic terms, the bottom line for health services may be better care at lower costs. In terms of nursing science, we may view our mission as a three-strand helix comprised of better care, shorter time, and increased comfort for clients and nurses alike. Nursing science has grown exponentially in the past two decades. The discipline has identified a body of knowledge that is unique in the Rogerian science of unitary human beings. Nurses have learned that they are professionals and that there are useful models on which to base practice and prescription.

More and more nurse administrators share the new relative space-time of today's dynamic clinical practitioners. There are many environmental patterns modifiable by administrators that encourage practitioners to grow, to be creative, and to engage in the complexities of human field transformations.

Insightful administrators understand health economics. They also understand that scientific nursing models are the domain of professional nurses and therefore provide ample opportunity for consumers to be exposed to professional cost-effective nursing.

Science in practice improves care and assures quality graded as excellent. When nurse administrators are in a continuous mutual process with nurses giving care, a new reality emerges and excellence in nursing service and nursing administration are at hand.

REFERENCES

1. Deal T, Kennedy A. Corporate Cultures. Reading, MA: Addison-Wesley, 1982.
2. Rogers ME. An introduction to the theoretical basis of nursing. Philadelphia: FA Davis, 1970.
3. Rogers, ME, Science of unitary human beings. In: Malinski VM, ed. Explorations on Martha E. Rogers' science of unitary human beings. East Norwalk, CT: Appleton-Century-Crofts, 1986.
4. Ference HM, Foundations of a nursing science and its evolution: A perspective. In: Malinski VM, ed. Explorations on Martha E. Rogers' science of unitary human beings. East Norwalk, CT: Appleton-Century-Crofts, 1986.
5. Ference HM. The relationship of time experience, creativity traits differentiation, and human field motion. In: Malinski VM, ed. Exploration on Martha E. Rogers' Science of Unitary Human Beings. East Norwalk; CT, Appleton-Century-Crofts, 1986.
6. Ference HM. Comforting the dying, nursing practice according to the Rogerian model. In: Riehl J, ed. Conceptual Nursing Models. East Norwalk, CT: Appleton-Century-Crofts (in press).
7. Barrett EA. Relationship of human field motion and power. New York: New York University, 1983. University Microfilms Publication No. 84-06, 278.
8. Ference HM. The relationship of time experience, creativity traits, differentiation, and human field motion: An empirical investigation of Rogers' correlates of synergistic human development. New York: New York University, doctoral dissertation, 1979. University Microfilms Publication No. 80-10, 281.
9. Ference HM. Proceedings: Matching the Rogerian Model of Nursing to Clinical Practice. Spokane, WA: Intercollegiate Center for Nursing, 1981.
10. Ference HM. Synergistic human development and human field motion of adults. In: Proceedings, Research Conference. New York: Upsilon Chapter, Sigma Theta Tau, 1980; New York: Mt. St. Vincent's College, 1980.
11. Ference HM. The structure, security, and coherence of practice through nursing models. In: Proceedings, Nursing Knowledge: Improving practice through theory. Anaheim, CA: Sigma Theta Tau, 1985.
12. Ference HM. Teaching nursing models in diverse clinical settings: the Rogers' model. In: Proceedings, Nursing Knowledge: Improving education through theory. Savannah, GA: Sigma Theta Tau International, 1986.
13. Ference HM. Workshop: Practicing in the Rogerian Framework. New York: Mount Sinai Medical Center, 1986.

14. Ference HM. Digest, The Human Field Motion Tool: Work Form. Carmel, CA: H. M. Ference, 1986.
15. Macrae, JA. A comparison between meditating subjects and non-meditating subjects on time experience and human field motion. New York: New York University, doctoral dissertation, 1982. University Microfilms Publication.
16. Lindley P. Relationship of sensation seeking to human energy field motion. University of Rochester, master's thesis, 1981. University Microfilms Publication.
17. Ference HM, Baker C. The relationship of students' ability to perform psychomotor skills and their experiences during controlled simulation that forces intrinsic reinforcement. Columbus, OH: The Ohio State University Funded Study, 1977–1979.
18. Ference HM. A philosophy of nursing. In: Notes on Nursing Science. Vol. 1 (3). Carmel, CA: Nightingale Society, 1988.
19. Ludomirski-Kalmanson B. Relationship between the environmental energy wave frequency pattern manifest in red and blue light and human field motion in adults with visual sensory perception and total blindness. New York: New York University, doctoral dissertation, 1984. University Microfilms Publication.
20. McDonald SF. A study of the relationship between visible lightwaves and the experience of pain. Detroit, Wayne State University, doctoral dissertation, 1981. University Microfilms Publication No. 81-17, 084.
21. Pieper BA. Levine's nursing model. In: Fitzpatrick J, Whall A. Conceptual Models of Nursing. Maryland: Brady Co., 1983.
22. Tiedeman ME. The Roy adaptation model. In: Fitzpatrick J, Whall A. Conceptual Models of Nursing. Maryland: Brady Co., 1983.
23. Ference HM. Network of nurse influentials: Bringing quality standards to the bedside. New York: Mt. Sinai Medical Center, 1987.
24. Hickman C, Silva M. Creating excellence. New York: New American Library, 1984.
25. Nightingale F. Notes on hospitals with evidence given to the royal commisioners on the state of the army in 1857. 2nd ed. London: Jown W. Parker & Sons, 1859.
26. Neal M. The relationship between a regimen of vestibular stimulation and developmental behavior of the small premature infant. New York: New York University, doctoral dissertation, 1967. University Microfilms Publication.
27. Porter L. Physical-physiological activity and infants' growth and development. New York: New York University, doctoral dissertation, 1967. University Microfilms Publication.
28. Earle A. The effect of supplementary postnatal kinesthetic stimulation on the developmental behavior of the normal female newborn. New York University, doctoral dissertation, 1969. University Microfilms Publication.
29. Gueldner SH. Relationship between imposed motion and human field motion in the elderly. Birmingham: University of Alabama in Birmingham, 1983. University Microfilms Publication No. 83-20, 597.

13

Nursing Theory in the Twenty-first Century

Sydney Pendleton

BASIC to an understanding of nursing theory is an understanding of science and of the contribution of theories and models to scientific knowledge. The nature of science and the role of models and theories in the development of scientific knowledge will be discussed briefly to provide the background for my subsequent discussion of nursing theory.

SCIENCE, THEORIES, AND MODELS

The goal of science is to organize and classify knowledge based on a system of explanation that provides a sense of understanding of relevant phenomena.[1–2] Scientific knowledge consists of statements that describe phenomena. A statement is composed of concepts. A theory, consisting of a set of interrelated statements, describes and explains reality. The concepts in a particular theory are defined, implicitly or explicitly, by the statements of the theory.

Both models and theories are a part of the development of scientific knowledge. Models relate to theory in two basic ways. First, a model may be used to explain or interpret an existing theory. When used to explain an existing theory, a model interprets the theory through simulation, metaphor, or even a physical representation of the theory or of some aspect of the theory. A model makes the theory more understandable by translating the unfamiliar to the familiar.

Second, a model may form the basis for the construction of new theory. For example, a model can be a theory from another discipline used as an analogy. Examples of theories from other disciplines that form the basis for nursing models include both Selye's and Helson's theories of adaptation, Sullivan's work in psychology, and Parsons' action theory. In the development of a body of scientific knowledge for nursing, models based on theories from other disciplines can be used to construct new nursing theory. New nursing theories should describe and explain relevant phenomena and lead to the development of a body of scientific knowledge upon which to base nursing practice.

The theoretical writings in nursing, some called models and others theories, are clearly attempts to develop a scientific basis for nursing practice. The extent to which nurse theorists have succeeded is debatable. Some of the theoretical writings in nursing are theories and others are models. But some are neither theories nor models of the kind that can be used to develop a scientific basis for nursing practice. Many existing models appear to be models of the nursing profession, rather than models from which a theoretical basis for clinical practice can be developed.

NURSING THEORY TODAY

Although nurses beginning with Nightingale have published nursing models, self-conscious development and emphasis on nursing theory has only been evident since the late

1960s. Today there are many nursing models, conceptual systems, and theories, including those of King, Leininger, Orem, Parse, Rogers, and Roy.

These models or theories differ widely in scope and assumptions, but they do have some things in common. All deal in some way with man, nursing, health, and environment. These four concepts were identified by Yura and Torres[3] as common to the conceptual frameworks of 50 accredited baccalaureate nursing programs in the early 1970s. Fawcett refers to these four concepts as the metaparadigm of nursing.[4]

All nursing models or theories purport to view human beings as open systems, however, the extent of openness varies. All espouse holism, but not all to the same extent. The definitions of health vary, as do the goals of nursing. The extent to which the environment and people influence each other, as well as what is included in the environment also vary.

The metaparadigm concepts may be basic to a model of the nursing profession, but I question the assumption that these concepts are really basic to a theory useful for nursing care. Only two of the four concepts—man and environment—are appropriate to a theory that describes and explains the outcomes of nursing interventions. Nursing is a professional discipline, and health is a value judgment. These two concepts are not appropriate to a theory that explains nursing interventions.

Nursing is a profession that is defined legally by the nurse practice acts in each state. It is also defined by the profession itself. An example of the latter is the definition developed by the American Nurses' Association in its Social Policy Statement.[5] Nursing might also be defined as the body of knowledge basic to the profession of nursing.

Nursing, in these senses of the term, is not a concept that is useful in developing a science of nursing.[6] A theoretical definition of nursing could be part of a model of the nursing profession; but to be part of a theory that explains or predicts nursing outcomes, nursing has to be defined in terms of specific interventions.

Health is a concept reflecting a human condition that is deemed acceptable, or good, or desirable in a particular culture at a particular time. What is considered healthy varies over time in different societies, cultures, and environments. What is defined as health is a value judgment, rather than a theoretical concept that is an appropriate part of nursing science. Health, like nursing, might be part of a model of the nursing profession, but it would have to be defined in terms of specific human responses or outcomes to be useful as a concept in a theory that explains or predicts nursing outcomes. Since health is basically a value judgment, any specific outcome might be defined as indicative of good health in one time and place, and as indicative of ill health in another.

A model of the nursing profession is generally an idealized delineation of a nurse's interaction with a patient, or the role of the nursing profession in health-care delivery, and as such can be expected to include the four metaparadigm concepts. Models of the profession describe the role of nursing in society, the role of nurses in the health-care delivery system, or the social or psychological relationships among nurses, patients, and other members of the health-care team. But they do not explain or predict the outcomes of nursing interventions.

Most models of nursing as currently conceived are not theories, nor, in most cases, were they intended to be. In contrast to the models used in the development of scientific knowledge, most nursing models are not models that explain a theory, nor are they models based on theory from another discipline from which new theory for nursing practice can be developed. Theories and models, which will enable us to explain and predict the outcomes of nursing interventions, are needed if we are to develop a scientific basis for nursing interventions.

Describing and explaining what nurses do or should do is a function of the profession, or of the state nurse practice acts, or of a philosophy of nursing; but it is not the proper function of scientific theory. Scientific theory could be developed to describe, explain, or predict the outcome of specific nursing interventions, but not to describe, explain, or predict the activities of nurses. For example, standards of care established by the profession describe and explain what nurses should do. A theory might predict the outcome in terms of human responses to a particular nursing intervention or set of interventions. Neither standards of care nor theories describe, explain, or predict what nurses actually do.

Theories of physics do not describe, explain, or predict what physicists do. However, theories of physics do describe the relationships among various components of the universe. Understanding the nature of the universe allows physicists to predict the outcomes of natural interactions and of interactions resulting from human interventions. Theories of physics predicted that enormous energy would result from nuclear fission. Whether physicists should have used this knowledge to produce weapons is a philosophical question, not a question of scientific theory.

Similarly in nursing: theory may one day be able to predict the outcomes of particular nursing interventions. Whether or not those outcomes are deemed desirable will be a philosophical issue based on the way health is defined by society at that time.

A THEORETICAL BASIS FOR CLINICAL PRACTICE

A theory of how human beings function and interact with their environment is needed to form the theoretical basis for nursing interventions. Knowledge about the nature of environment-human interactions will enable us to predict the outcomes of specific kinds of interactions. A theory that predicts the outcome of specific nurse-patient interactions can be tested and validated. Knowledge of the outcomes of nursing interventions will allow informed decisions to be made about when such interventions are indicated. For example, an intervention might be predicted to lower blood pressure. Knowledge of the interaction of blood pressure with other aspects of human physiology, and of the condition of the specific client, might lead to a decision about the desirability of the intervention based on the current definition of health. In this case, if lower blood pressure were considered healthy, the intervention would be indicated.

Predictive theory, however, would not be prescriptive. No scientific theory can be prescriptive. Prescribing is based on the desirability of a particular outcome. A theory can only predict an outcome. The decision about desirability is a value judgment. The desired outcome of a nursing intervention would probably be described as contributing to or promoting good health. However, as discussed earlier, health is defined by the values of a particular time and culture.

When the outcome of an intervention can be predicted, an individual can make an informed decision about whether he or she should consent to such an intervention. Whether the outcome is defined as healthy or unhealthy, good or bad, is a matter of individual judgment. Even the most cursory historical review of nursing interventions that were deemed desirable in the past amply demonstrates this point. Prolonged bed rest after surgery is a prime example of an intervention that is no longer desirable. Another example is the routine administration of high concentrations of oxygen to premature infants.

NURSING THEORY TOMORROW

In the future, I predict that we will develop one or more models of the nature of interactions between people and their environment. From these models, scholars will derive theories that predict the outcomes of specific nursing interventions. When these theories have been tested and verified, we will be able to predict the outcomes of specific nursing interventions. When we have done this, we will finally have developed a scientific basis for nursing care.

In the process of arriving at this goal, the current array of nursing models will be narrowed to two or three. I predict that the work of Rogers will be among those that survive because it most closely approximates what is needed: a model of the interaction of people and their environment. Rogers' work parallels the development of theory in other fields and is based on historical trends in the evolution of science. Rogers' conceptual system is the basis for a considerable amount of nursing research, and it has influenced other theorists, including Parse and Newman.

Ultimately a comprehensive taxonomy of nursing diagnoses based on a common set of assumptions and on one dominant nursing model will be developed. The complexity of the interactions between people and their environment is impossible to express using the current forms of diagnostic statements. New nursing diagnoses will be completely different, and will be based on a holistic view of human beings rather than on the fragmented human being mirrored in the diagnostic categories formulated by North American Nursing Diagnosis Association. These new nursing diagnoses will identify patterns and relationships rather than causes.

New forms of health-care delivery will evolve, derived from a new nursing model and from changing societal needs. The role of the nurse will change based on new societal expectations, and on new and more sophisticated nursing models. Perhaps in the future, nurses will diagnose patterns of interaction between human beings and the environment and base their interventions on theories that predict how such patterns can be changed. Identification of patterns or relationships as healthy or unhealthy will depend on the the values of society.

Criteria for the evaluation of patient care will be developed based on nursing theories that predict the outcomes of nursing interventions. The problem of evaluating the quality of care will change dramatically when outcomes can be predicted and realistic outcome criteria can be determined with accuracy.

The final decades of the twentieth century are critical for the development of a sound scientific basis for professional nursing practice. Whether nursing develops theories that predict the outcomes of nursing interventions and generates a body of scientific knowledge, or remains based on tradition and common sense will determine whether nursing develops a distinctive role in a changing society or disappears as a profession in the twenty-first century.

REFERENCES

1. Nagel E. The structure of science. New York: Harcourt, Brace and World, Inc, 1961, pp. 1–7.
2. Reynolds PD. A primer in theory construction. Indianapolis: The Bobbs-Merrill Company, Inc, 1971, pp. 3–9.
3. Torres G, Yura H. Today's conceptual framework: Its relationship to the curriculum development process. New York: National League for Nursing, 1974.
4. Fawcett J. The metaparadigm of nursing: present status and future refinements. Image 1984; 16(3):84–87.
5. American Nurses Association. Nursing: a social policy statement. Kansas City: American Nurses Association, 1980.
6. Conway ME. Toward greater specificity in defining nursing's metaparadigm. ANS 1985; 7(4):73–81.

14

Conceptual Model for Theory Development in Nursing Administration

Cynthia C. Scalzi
Ruth A. Anderson

A CONCEPTUAL model of nursing administration is proposed in this chapter that defines its comprehensive sphere of concern and articulates a nursing administration perspective that can be used as a guide for theory development, research, and practice. We introduce terminology and structural concepts as needed to build a new definition of nursing administration that is consistent with the proposed conceptual model.

The model is developed in three stages. In each stage we introduce increasingly complex elements and viewpoints, building toward a system view model. Many of the ideas we discuss during explication of the model have been described in nursing and management. They have not, however, been explicitly described, which is the purpose of this presentation.

STAGE 1: SINGLE-DOMAIN MODEL

The nursing domain is the fundamental element of the single-domain model, illustrated in Figure 14.1 and forms the first level of complexity. In this discussion, "domain" is used to represent an explicit sphere of influence or activity with associated specific goals. At the level of complexity in this single-domain model, nursing administration could be described as the application of administra-

tive knowledge to nursing to provide quality nursing care. The single domain of concern is limited to nursing; the model specifies nursing administration's domain of concern as identical to that of nursing.

Nursing administration's goal in the single-domain model is restricted to assuring quality nursing product. Nursing's goal for the "maintenance, promotion, or facilitation of health"[1] is achieved through a quality nursing product. Any nurse in this model, including a nurse administrator, considers only nursing domain concerns.

Quality nursing is certainly a primary concern of the nurse administrator. However, to view it as the only goal does not capture the comprehensive nature of nursing administration.

STAGE 2: DUAL-DOMAIN MODEL

In the stage two model, the organizational domain with its goal of organizational effectiveness, as illustrated in Figure 14.2, is an additional element of concern and influence for nursing administration. Organizational domain is broadly defined to include various services such as administration, medicine, as well as community institutions. The entire organizational domain is included in nursing administration's sphere of concern to the extent that its components interface with

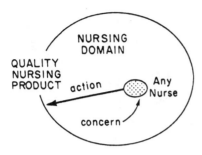

Figure 14.1. Single-Domain Model (one domain, one goal). The nursing domain is represented by the large oval with its goal "quality nursing product" schematically incorporated into the domain structure. A "concern" for the nurse arises from within the domain, shown by the lighter arrow, and in response, some "action," shown by the heavier arrow, is directed from the nurse toward the goal.

nursing. The "interface" between the two domains is the area in which the multiple and diverse concerns of all parties involved interact. Nursing administration, viewed in the context of the dual-domain model, repre-

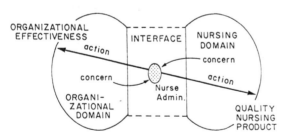

Figure 14.2. Dual-Domain Model (two interfacing domains, dual goals). The nursing and organizational domains are represented by ovals with the nurse administrator positioned at their interface. The dual goals of "organizational effectiveness" and "quality nursing product" are incorporated into their respective domain structures. "Concerns," shown by lighter arrows, can arise for the nurse administrator from either domain, and "actions" in response, shown by heavier arrows, are directed toward one or the other of the dual goals.

sents the point at which clinical knowledge and administrative knowledge interact to define organizational-level nursing actions.

The dual-domain model can be thought of as two dimensional. Conceptually, both domains are on a single level or plane, with goals that may be different, even opposite. The perspective from within either the nursing domain or the organizational domain is that the two domains of concern exist as separate entities with their own distinct sets of goals. We call these viewpoints the "domain perspective" and refer to the distinct sets of goals perceived by individuals using the domain perspective as the "domain-specific" goals.

It is clear that those in separate domains will sometimes cooperate and sometimes compete as they each take actions directed toward reaching their own domain-specific goals. The nurse administrator at the interface is bombarded with conflicting concerns from the two domains but has a responsibility for the goals of both. This viewpoint is called the "interface perspective." The nurse administrator in this perspective strives to weigh concerns arising from both domains and balance actions that may have conflicting implications for the two sets of domain-specific goals.

STAGE 3: SYSTEM VIEW MODEL

The system view model depicted in Figure 14.3 illustrates a perspective of nursing administration expanded beyond the interface perspective. This model portrays a dimension outside or above the plane of the two domains. Structurally, the system view model is a three-dimensional extension of the dual-domain model. In this model, the nursing and organizational domains of concern are interdependent rather than separate and distinct competing elements; they jointly form a "system" of domains with a single set of goals that seeks to maximize the vitality of the

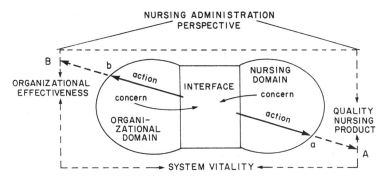

Figure 14.3. System View Model (one system, one set of system goals). The system of concern for nursing administration is represented by the rectangular dashed line encompassing both the nursing and organizational domains and their interface. The single goal of "system vitality" comprising "organizational effectiveness" and "quality nursing products" is incorporated into the system structure. "Concerns" arise from either domain, and "actions" in response are all directed toward the single goal of "system vitality," shown by heavy arrows labeled *A* and *B*. The dashed lines (system view) are visible only from the nursing administration perspective outside the plane of the domains. Without the system view, the actions appear to be directed toward goals in one of the domains, shown by arrows ending at *a* or *b*.

system. The system of domains is depicted in Figure 14.3 by a dotted line to emphasize that it is discernible as a single structure only from the "system plane," a viewpoint acquired by shifting to a higher level of complexity than that of the domain perspectives or the interface perspective. The viewpoint from which the system is visible is the "system perspective."

The system that is nursing administration's sphere of concern has as its elements the nursing domain, the organizational domain, and the interface where the two domains of concern interact. It is the visibility of the system due to a shift in the nurse administrator's perspective that distinguishes the system model from the dual-domain model. An assumption underlying this system view model is that quality nursing care is delivered through viable organizations, and that the effectiveness of such organizations is in turn dependent in part on the quality of nursing. The vitality of the system of concern to nursing administration is thus based on two broad factors that consist of quality nursing and organizational effectiveness.

Within the system view model, the entire

domain of nursing is of concern to the nurse administrator; no part of the nursing domain is omitted. However, the unit of analysis for the concerns arising from the domains expands to reflect the third level of complexity—the system view. Assessment and intervention actions move to the system level rather than the level of direct contact with clients. From nursing's perspective, the nurse administrator operates as the enabler and enhancer of nursing processes and goals. The nurse administrator's tools of nursing action are tools of nursing administration as opposed to those of clinical practice. Similarly, the entire organizational domain is included in nursing administration's sphere of concern to the extent that the components interact and interface with nursing and influence system vitality.

A nurse administrator using the system perspective in this model envisions both quality nursing and organizational effectiveness as jointly constituting the single goal of system vitality. Actions taken in response to concerns arising from either domain are seen as being directed toward the single goal of system vitality (dashed arrows *A* and *B* in

Figure 14.3). Theoretically, the conflict inherent in the second-level model, as a result of trying to accomplish dual and possibly competing sets of goals, is eliminated. However, individuals in either domain have a domain perspective in which the system is invisible, and, therefore, they cannot view the actions as system-oriented; from their perspective, actions seem to be directed to one domain or the other (arrows *a* and *b* in Figure 3).

In the system view model, the nurse administrator uses the system perspective in assessing the multiple concerns that arise, viewing them as system concerns, with the single goal of system vitality. This is in contrast to the second-level interface perspective, where the concerns between the domains with two distinct set of goals conflict.

NEW DEFINITION OF NURSING ADMINISTRATION

A new definition of nursing administration is derived from the system view model. The proposed definition is:

The practice of nursing administration is the use of the system perspective to maximize system vitality through the assessment and management of system concerns. The system of concern to nursing administration is composed of the nursing and organizational domains and their interface. System vitality comprises quality nursing products and organizational effectiveness.

It is thus the use of the system perspective in assessment and intervention that describes and predicts effective administration. A fundamental assumption underlying this definition is the assumption of the system view model: Quality nursing care is delivered through viable organizations, and the effectiveness of such organizations is in turn dependent, in part, on the quality of nursing.

IMPLICATIONS FOR THEORY DEVELOPMENT

The system view model helps to clarify an unrecognized but basic problem in previous attempts to develop nursing administration theory. Generally, theories have been extracted from the nursing domain or the organizational domain and applied to nursing administration practice.[2–4] These extracted theories are essentially domain-oriented or domain-specific theories. As such, the system of concern for nursing administration will not be represented or understood.

For example, theories for nursing have been described as patient-care oriented and as focusing on the nurse-patient relationship.[1,5–6] As such, they reflect what we call the domain perspective for nursing administration; the system is not visible and goals directed toward system vitality are not incorporated. Existing domain-oriented nursing theory cannot properly direct nursing administration action without being expanded to address nursing administration's total concern.

It is clear that nursing theories alone are insufficient to guide nurse administrators in actions pertaining to concerns arising from the organizational domain. Cost containment, productivity, resource allocation, human resources management, and interdepartmental arrangements, for example, are not within the purview of nursing theory. Organizational domain theories have therefore been used to guide nursing administrative action.[2–4] Johnson defines borrowed theory as "that knowledge which is developed in the main by other disciplines and is drawn upon by nursing."[7] Based on the system view model, borrowed theory developed for the organizational domain that does not reflect the nursing perspective will not guide nursing administration action.

In light of the system view model for nursing administration, the concept of borrowed theory needs to be reassessed. The system perspective is not likely to be addressed by any domain-oriented theory, whether the theory is from the nursing domain or is borrowed from the organizational domain. Instead, domain-specific theories need to be expanded or extended from the domain level to the system level of complexity, so that the system view is reflected by the theories. This applies to theory developed in either domain that is encompassed by nursing administration's system of concern.

Research in nursing administration has not focused on developing a body of knowledge.[3–4] The absence of a system view reflecting a higher level of complexity than that suggested by either the domain perspective or the interface perspective may be the cause.

In summary, the system view model has been used to describe the scope of practice in nursing administration. Nursing administration is unique because of the system perspective. Theories for nursing administration have not yet been articulated to describe, explain, and predict actions that will contribute to the attainment of unified system goals.

ACKNOWLEDGMENTS

The authors wish to acknowledge the preliminary work represented by the Nursing Administration Domain of Concern Model in the dissertation of Ruth A. Anderson, R.N., Ph.D.

The authors also wish to acknowledge the assistance of Sondra T. Perdue, Dr. P.H., in helping to clarify and expand our thinking and in adapting the schematic diagrams of the model.

REFERENCES

1. Meleis AI. Theoretical nursing: development and progress. Philadelphia: JB Lippincott Company, 1985.
2. Jacox A. The research component in the nursing service administration master's program. J Nurs Adm 1974;4(2):35–39.
3. Diamond M, Slothower L. Research in nursing administration: a neglected issue. Nurs Adm Q 1978; 2(4):1–8.
4. Trandel-Korenchuk DM. Concept development in nursing research. Nurs Adm Q 1986;1(1):1–9.
5. Chinn P, Jacobs M. Theory and nursing: a systematic approach. St. Louis: The CV Mosby, 1983.
6. Fawcett J. Analysis and evaluation of conceptual models of nursing. Philadelphia: FA Davis, 1984.
7. Johnson DE. Theory in nursing: borrowed and unique. Nurs Res 1969;17(3):206–209.

Conceptual Models of Nursing and Organization Theories

Jacqueline Fawcett
Mary L. Botter
Joan Burritt
John D. Crossley
Barbara Barth Frink

THIS CHAPTER defines and describes conceptual models and theories and explains how conceptual models of nursing can be used in nursing administration. Factors to consider when constructing conceptual-theoretical systems of knowledge are identified, and four knowledge systems for nursing administration are presented.

CONCEPTUAL MODELS OF NURSING

A conceptual model is made up of abstract and general concepts and propositions. The concepts reflect a particular view of the phenomena of interest to a discipline, and the propositions define, describe, and link the concepts in a distinctive manner. Each conceptual model therefore represents a different frame of reference for the phenomena deemed relevant to a discipline. Most disciplines have several conceptual models because relevant phenomena can be viewed in various ways.

Conceptual models of nursing present distinctive frames of reference for the phenomena comprising the domain of the discipline of nursing. Nursing's domain is summarized

in four concepts: person, environment, health, and nursing. "Person" refers to the recipient of nursing actions; "environment," to the surroundings of the recipient of nursing actions, as well as the setting in which the actions occur; "health," to the wellness or illness status of the recipient of nursing actions; and "nursing," to the actions taken by the nurse on behalf of or in conjunction with the recipient.

The many conceptual models of nursing present different perspectives on the concepts of nursing's domain. Brief overviews of Roy's Adaptation Model[1] and Neuman's Systems Model[2] are provided to illustrate two different perspectives.

Roy's Adaptation Model

Roy's adaptation model is concerned with problems of adaptation to the changing environment. Person is defined as an adaptive system, which may be an individual or group that has actual or potential adaptation problems.

Environment is defined as all the constantly changing internal and external stimuli that affect an individual or group. Environmental stimuli include all the conditions, circumstances, and influences surrounding and affecting the development and behavior of an adaptive system. Focal environmental stimuli are those that immediately confront the adaptive system; contextual stimuli are the contributing factors in a given situation; and residual stimuli are other unknown factors that may influence a situation.

Health is defined as a state and a process of being and becoming an integrated, whole person. Wellness is described as adaptive behavior in four modes: physiological, self-concept, role function, and interdependence. The physiological mode is concerned with basic needs requisite to maintaining the physical and physiologic integrity of the human system. The self-concept mode deals with people's conceptions of their physical and personal selves. The role function mode is concerned with people's performance of duties on the basis of their positions within society. The interdependence mode deals with development and maintenance of satisfying affectional relationships with significant others. Illness is described as an ineffective response in one or more of the modes.

Nursing is defined as a theoretical system of knowledge that prescribes a systematic process related to the care of the ill or potentially ill person. The goal of nursing is to promote patient adaptation in all four adaptive modes during wellness and illness. The nursing process component of Roy's conceptual model involves six steps. Step one, assessment of behaviors, involves collecting data regarding a client's physiological, self-concept, role function, and interdependence behaviors. Once the data are collected, the nurse must judge the behavioral responses as adaptive or ineffective. Thus, the primary question is: To what extent is the person adapting to environmental stimuli? Step two, assessment of influencing factors, involves setting priorities for further assessment and identifying the environmental stimuli that

influence a client's behavior and thus contribute to the adaptive or ineffective responses. Step three, nursing diagnosis, involves a behavioral description of the client's adaptive or ineffective responses and identifying the most relevant influencing factors, as well as placing the nursing diagnosis in a hierarchy of importance. Step four, goal setting, involves formulating goals for nursing care. These goals are stated as behaviors expected as the outcome of nursing intervention. Step five, intervention, involves managing environmental stimuli. Management takes the form of an increase, decrease, modification, maintenance, or removal of environmental stimuli. The intervention with the highest probability of reaching the desired goal is selected. Step six, evaluation, requires judging the effectiveness of the nursing intervention. The criterion for effectiveness is whether the desired behavioral goal was attained. The outcome of this step is updating of the nursing care plan.

Neuman's Systems Model

Neuman's systems model presents a different view of nursing's domain. This model is concerned with variances from wellness, the presence of stressors, and the need of the client system to attain and maintain stability. Person is defined as a client system that is a composite of physiological, psychological, sociocultural, developmental, and spiritual variables. The client system may be an individual, group, or community. The system is conceptualized as having a central core of survival factors that is protected by a flexible line of defense, a normal line of defense, and lines of resistance. The flexible line of defense is a protective, accordionlike mechanism that surrounds and protects the normal line of defense from invasion by stressors. The normal line of defense is a state or level of health developed over time and considered normal for the client system. The lines of resistance are internal factors activated to protect and preserve the central core structure.

The environment is viewed as all internal and external factors affecting and affected by the client system. Noxious and beneficial stressors comprise some part of the environment. The stressors may be intrapersonal, interpersonal, or extrapersonal. Intrapersonal stressors are forces that occur within the client system, interpersonal stressors are forces that occur between two client systems, and extrapersonal stressors are forces that occur outside the client system.

Analysis of Neuman's writings suggests that health and wellness are synonymous terms referring to harmony and balance among all aspects of the client system. Wellness may be equated with stability of the client system, which exists when the system's flexible line of defense has prevented penetration of the normal line of defense by stressors. Illness may be interpreted as variances from wellness, which occurs when stressors penetrate the lines of defense. Reconstitution is the movement from a variance from wellness to the desired level of wellness and client system stability.

Nursing is viewed as a unique profession that is concerned with all factors affecting the client system's response to stressors. The primary goal of nursing is to assist the client system to retain, attain, or maintain stability. The nursing process consists of three steps. The first, nursing diagnosis, is based on acquiring an appropriate data base that identifies, assesses, classifies, and evaluates the dynamic interactions among the variables comprising the client system. The primary questions are: To what extent is the client system stable? What is the current level of wellness? Are variances from wellness evident? Actual and potential variances from wellness and available resources are identified by both the client and the caregiver. The second step of the nursing process, formulat-

ing nursing goals, is accomplished through negotiation between client and caregiver. Intervention strategies also are formulated during this step. Nursing interventions encompass primary, secondary, and tertiary prevention. Primary prevention is action taken to retain client system stability and occurs prior to invasion by a stressor. Secondary prevention is action taken to attain client system stability; it occurs in the acute phase just after invasion by a stressor. Tertiary prevention is action taken to maintain the client system stability achieved through secondary prevention. The third and final step of the nursing process involves identifying and evaluating nursing outcomes. The result of evaluation is confirmation of attainment of nursing goals or reformulation of the goals.

CONCEPTUAL MODELS AND NURSING ADMINISTRATION

Most models of nursing have been developed as guides for clinical nursing practice. They may, however, be modified for use in education and administration. Modification requires an adjustment in the four concepts of nursing's domain. When these concepts are particularized for nursing administration, "person" refers to the staff of a clinical agency; "environment," to the surroundings of the staff and the setting in which nursing administration occurs; "health," to the wellness or illness of the staff; and "nursing," to the management strategies used by nurse administrators on behalf of or in conjunction with the staff. When modified more broadly for nursing administration, "person" could refer to the department of nursing as a whole, or to the larger health-care institution. "Environment" would then refer to the relevant surroundings of the department or institution, and "health" to the functional status of the department or institution. "Nursing" would refer to the management strategies and administrative policies used by the nurse administrator on behalf of, or in conjunction with, the department of nursing or the institution.

The utility of any conceptual model de-pends on the degree to which it organizes thinking of, observing, and interpreting the real world. When a conceptual model is used in nursing administration, it provides a sys-tematic structure for addressing administra-tive problems, observing the administrative situations, and interpreting what is seen in organizational settings. A model of nursing management then, represents a particular view of and approach to the administration of nursing services.

Nursing administrative structures and management practices are specified in three rules inherent in a conceptual model. The first rule identifies the distinctive focus of nursing in the clinical agency and the pur-pose to be fulfilled by nursing services. The second rule identifies the characteristics of nursing personnel and the settings in which nursing services are delivered. The third rule identifies the management strategies to be employed.

Roy's adaptation model can be modified for use in nursing administration. In Roy's perspective the distinctive focus and purpose of nursing in a clinical agency is the provision of nursing services designed to promote pa-tient adaptation in the physiological, self-concept, role function, and interdependence modes. The collective nursing staff is viewed as an adaptive system in a constantly chang-ing environment. The department of nursing or the entire health-care institution may also be viewed as an adaptive system. The settings for nursing services are not clearly delineated in Roy's model, although review of the liter-ature indicates that the model has been used successfully in most types of clinical agencies and in most speciality practice areas.[3] Man-agement strategies emphasize facilitating staff, departmental, or institutional adapta-tion to constantly changing environmental stimuli.

Neuman's systems model may also be mod-ified for use in nursing administration by making explicit the rules for administrative structure and management practice that are inherent in this perspective. The distinctive focus of and purpose to be fulfilled by nurs-ing in the clinical agency is the provision of nursing services designed to help client sys-tems retain, attain, or maintain stability by means of primary, secondary, and tertiary prevention. The collective nursing staff can be conceived as a client system that is a composite of physiological, psychological, sociocultural, developmental, and spiritual variables. The department of nursing or the larger health-care institution could also be viewed as the client system. The settings for nursing services are those where primary, secondary, and tertiary prevention are ap-propriate. Thus, this conceptual model could be used in virtually all types of clinical agen-cies, including ambulatory clinics, acute-care medical centers, and rehabilitation units. Management strategies focus on the staff, the department of nursing, or the total institu-tion as the client system of the administrator, who uses management practices that promote system stability.

CONCEPTUAL MODELS AND THEORIES

Conceptual models present global views of certain phenomena. Concepts are not always clearly defined, and propositions are not em-pirically testable. In contrast, theories are more circumscribed. Each theory deals with just one phenomenon. Thus, the concepts and propositions making up a theory are more specific and concrete than those of a conceptual model. The concepts of a theory are usually clearly defined, and the proposi-tions are empirically testable.

Many theories are needed to fully describe, explain, and predict all the phenomena en-compassed by a conceptual model. This is because any one theory deals only with a portion of the domain of inquiry identified by a conceptual model. Each theory, then, more fully specifies selected concepts and propositions of the parent conceptual model.

Theories may be directly derived from a conceptual model, or existing theories may be linked with a model. In either case, the result is a conceptual-theoretical system of knowledge. When an existing theory is linked with a conceptual model, care must be taken to ensure that the model and the theory reflect logically congruent world views about the nature of the phenomenon of interest. One way to determine logical congruence is to determine if both model and theory view the recipient of action as an active participant in the action or a passive recipient of an external action. Another way to determine logical congruence is to determine if both model and theory view the recipient of action as changing constantly or changing only when necessary for survival.

Both Roy and Neuman have derived rudimentary theories from their conceptual models. Roy has developed (1) a general theory of the person as an adaptive system, and (2) theories of the four adaptive modes: physiological, self-concept, role function, and interdependence.[4] Neuman postulated that nursing intervention is structured within primary, secondary, and tertiary modes of prevention, and that these prevention modes facilitate the integrative processes necessary to retain, attain, and maintain client system stability.[2] Recently, Neuman reported that she and her associates are developing a theory of client system stability.[5]

CONCEPTUAL-THEORETICAL SYSTEMS OF NURSING ADMINISTRATION KNOWLEDGE

The theories derived by Roy and Neuman from their conceptual models have not yet been sufficiently developed for use in nursing administration. The search for theories needed to construct conceptual-theoretical systems of knowledge for nursing administration therefore must begin in the organization and management literature. The literature should be reviewed to locate theories that will provide further specification of selected concepts and propositions of a particular conceptual model. No one theory is sufficiently global to deal with all of a model's concepts and propositions. Further, it is unlikely that all theories will be logically congruent with all conceptual models, although some theories may be congruent with more than one model. The remainder of this chapter is devoted to a review of organization theories that can be linked in a logically congruent manner with Roy's adaptation model or Neuman's systems model.

ROY'S ADAPTATION MODEL AND CONTINGENCY THEORY

A logically congruent conceptual-theoretical system of knowledge that can be applied in the area of nursing administration can be constructed by linking Roy's adaptation model and contingency theory. This theory is currently considered the dominant perspective for the study of organizational structure and design in management science.[6]

Contingency theory was developed by Lawrence and Lorsch[7] and Morse and Lorsch.[8] A basic premise of contingency theory is that there must be a "fit" between task, organization, and people. "The appropriate pattern of organization is *contingent* on the nature of the work to be done and on the particular needs of the people involved"[8] (p. 62). The theory thus proposes that organization must be matched to task, task to people, and people to organization.

Contingency theory provides a way of thinking about the complexity of management problems. It addresses the relationship between the structure or design of an organization and each particular situation. A contingency approach to organizational design attempts to match selected environmental factors with selected organizational design characteristics. Lawrence and Lorsch's empirical research revealed that the more complex and diverse the external environment, the more differentiated were the subunits (departments) of an industrial firm, and the greater the need for complex integrating structures such as task forces and coordinators.[7]

A key environmental variable that influences organizational structure is uncertainty, which is defined as the difference between information that an organization has and information that it needs. The amount of information needed depends on the diversity of input and output, as well as the level of goal difficulty. The greater the uncertainty, the more information is needed to make decisions.[9]

Given limited uncertainty, an organization can coordinate activities effectively by relying on a basic hierarchical structure, setting goals, and applying prescribed rules. Organizations operating in highly uncertain environments need flexible, less bureaucratic structures.[9,10] It follows, then, that organizations that exist in relatively simple, stable environments can develop simple, stable structures, whereas those that exist in turbulent, changing, and uncertain environments require more complex, differentiated, and flexible structures.[9]

Proponents of contingency theory have paid considerable attention to the environmental factors that influence performance of tasks. According to contingency theory, the environment in which tasks are carried out influences not only the organizational structure but also organizational performance, including goal setting and daily operations. Three key dimensions of the task environment are clarity of information, understanding of cause and effect relationships, and time span for feedback. When information is unclear, understanding of relationships limited, and feedback slow, an organization has to cope with high levels of uncertainty.[9–11] The amount of uncertainty in the task environment therefore influences task performance.

Other proponents of contingency theory have focused their attention on variables other than task environment. Carlisle has identified two sets of contingency factors in the environment: those that are internal and those that are external to the organization.[12] Internal factors include purpose, tasks, people, technology, and their relationships. External factors include the economy, political pressure, legal issues, sociocultural characteristics, and technology.

When the organizational structure is tailored to fit the situation, achievement of organizational goals is facilitated.[13] Thus, the end result of an appropriate fit between task environment and organizational structure, or between internal and external environmental factors and organizational structure, is an increase in organizational performance. This is not to imply that a particular structure will be suitable for an organization over long periods of time. Rather, to be viable, an organization must be a dynamic, changing entity that functions within a dynamic changing environment. The success of an organization in achieving its goals, then, is a function of its adaptation to the environment.[12]

Roy's adaptation model and contingency theory may be linked to form a conceptual-theoretical system of knowledge that can help nurse administrators more fully understand what structural arrangements will promote the highest organizational performance. The conceptual model concepts of particular interest in this conceptual-theoretical knowledge system are the adaptive system, environmental stimuli, and adaptation. In contingency theory, the organization represents the adaptive system, contingency variables (such as uncertainty of task environment or internal and external contingency factors) represent environmental stimuli, and the organizational structure represents adaptation.

The nurse administrator can use this knowledge system to assess the current situation by preparing a detailed description of the present organizational structure and the characteristics of the task environment. To what extent, for example, is the organization differentiated into various subunits? Furthermore, how clear is the information available to the organization? How much is understood about cause and effect relationships? How much time is required for feedback? How much uncertainty is evident in the task environment? Or, the assessment could be structured according to the internal and external contingency factors identified earlier. The end result of the assessment is determination of the fit between the environment and the organizational structure.

NEUMAN'S SYSTEMS MODEL AND CONTINGENCY THEORY

Contingency theory also can be linked with Neuman's systems model to form a logically congruent conceptual-theoretical system of knowledge for nursing administration. This knowledge system can be used to design the structure of a formal nursing research program, for example, within a clinical practice setting.

The concepts of major interest are the client system and associated variables. Within contingency theory, the department of nursing represents the client system. Client system variables can be represented by organizational structure, people, and tasks. Organizational structure encompasses the structure of the nursing department subunits, practice pattern (primary, team, functional), operating systems (staffing, scheduling, budgeting), and management systems (quality assurance, strategic planning, education). People include all nursing personnel and their creden-

tials and abilities, especially with regard to the conduct of research. Tasks encompass all of the work involved in the conduct of research, as well as the other work that must be done by the members of the nursing department.

Neuman's model directs the nurse administrator to begin the design of the formal nursing research program with a diagnosis of client system variables. Contingency theory specifies the variables as the existing organizational structure and relevant contingency factors. Examples of questions to be asked are: Is the current organizational structure appropriate for the task of research? If not, what organizational structure will accomplish this task? Which members of the nursing department with what credentials are most capable of conducting research? Are additional personnel or credentials needed to accomplish the task? The diagnosis would take the form of a statement regarding the fit of task to organization and to people. The diagnosis will help the nurse administrator match the appropriate personnel resources with the task and organizational structure.

The next step required to establish a formal nursing research program is to set goals. Goals in this situation could refer to the quality and quantity of task performance, that is, ongoing and completed nursing research. Goals could also refer to structural rearrangements or additional personnel needed for continuous research productivity. The goals would be stated as desirable outcomes.

The final step is use and evaluation of interventions designed to achieve identified outcomes. Primary prevention could be used initially to retain client system stability, represented by an appropriate fit of task, organization, and people. Secondary or tertiary prevention might have to be used later if it was determined that the addition of the task of research created an unanticipated stressor and subsequent client system instability.

This conceptual-theoretical system of

knowledge could also be used to investigate the effects of instituting a formal program of nursing research. Examples of research focuses are consideration of the relationship of organizational structure to research program outcomes, the relationship of allocation of human resources to sustaining a viable research program in a clinical agency, and the relationship of the task of structuring research in a practice setting to other forces operating in that setting.

NEUMAN'S SYSTEMS MODEL AND ROLE THEORY

Another logically congruent conceptual-theoretical system of knowledge for nursing administration can be constructed by linking Neuman's systems model and role theory. This theory has been used with increasing frequency by theorists and researchers to describe, explain, and predict the stresses experienced by an employee in the work setting. From an organizational perspective, a "role" is a set of expectations applied to an incumbent of a particular position.[14-16] Roles serve as the boundary between an employee and the organization, tying the employee to the organization and the organization to the employee.[17]

Employees are continually exposed to a variety of expectations in the work environment that may affect their perceptions of their organizational roles.[18-19] At times, an employee may perceive these expectations as incompatible, inconsistent, or unclear. When this occurs, roles can become dysfunctional to both the employee and the organization.

Role conflict, role overload, and role ambiguity have been identified as the three major forms of role-based stress.[20-21] Role conflict is experienced when there are incompatible or incongruent demands placed on a role incumbent.[16,20] Three types of role conflict have been described. Intrasender role conflict refers to a situation in which incompatible expectations of a role incumbent come from a single source. Intersender role conflict arises when the incompatible expectations are generated by several sources. Interrole conflict occurs when role pressures stemming from one position are incompatible with those from a different position.[16,20,22-23]

Role overload is defined as the extent to which the various role expectations communicated to a role incumbent exceed the amount of time and resources available for their accomplishment. This form of role stress is further described as the amount of pressure felt to do more work, the feeling of not being able to finish one's work, the feeling that the amount of work interferes with how well the job gets done, or some combination of these factors. Role overload initially was regarded as the fourth type of role conflict, but later was identified as a distinct and separate form of role-based stress.[21]

Role ambiguity refers to a condition in which the information available to a given organizational position is inadequate or unclear.[20,24] According to Van Sell and associates,[16] role ambiguity may arise when there is ambiguous information regarding (a) the expectations associated with a role, (b) methods for fulfilling known role expectations, and (c) the consequences of role performance.

Although role conflict, role overload, and role ambiguity have been distinguished as different forms of role-based stress, the existence of reciprocal relationships between and among the forms and their dimensions has been noted.[16,24] For example, ambiguity regarding one's role can be associated with intersender role conflict, as when those surrounding the individual attempt to define his or her role; conversely, the experience of incongruous role expectations from different sources can be linked with role ambiguity as information concerning the scope and nature of one's role becomes less clearly defined in light of the conflicting messages and demands.

According to role theory, when the individual perceives role expectations as conflicting, excessive, or ambiguous, a variety of negative health, attitudinal, and behavioral outcomes result. Role conflict, role overload, and role ambiguity represent constraints on an employee's need or desire for achievement, productivity, and predictability; they, in turn, may influence the employee's physical and mental health, attitudes toward the job and life in general, and affect and behaviors while performing the job.[20,24,26]

The Neuman systems model provides a framework from which to view individuals, groups, and communities exposed to stress. Used in conjunction with role theory, the model can assist the nurse administrator to describe, explain, and predict the nature and effects of role conflict, role overload, and role ambiguity experienced by staff in the nursing service setting.

The conceptual model concepts of particular pertinence to a conceptual-theoretical knowledge system linking role theory with Neuman's model are stressors, impact of stressors, and client system stability. The stressors are represented within role theory by role conflict, role overload, and role ambiguity. The impact of stressors and subsequent client system instability are represented by the consequences of role stress, such as illness, negative attitudes toward the job, and inappropriate behavior when performing the job.

Many of the theoretical propositions regarding role-based stress and its outcomes have been supported in studies of both industrial and nursing service employees.[15,17,19,27–28] The conceptual-theoretical system of knowledge formed by linking role theory with Neuman's systems model therefore seems appropriate as a framework for nursing research. Such research could be based on a key postulate of the model that

states that interventions prior to an encounter with a stressor, that is, primary prevention, will help strengthen the client system's lines of defense so that a stressor is avoided or its impact is reduced. In keeping with role theory, primary prevention could be represented by interventions such as opening lines of communication between superior and subordinate, having clearly defined job descriptions and performance evaluation criteria, or establishing reasonable, attainable expectations for employees. Systematic investigation of the effects of such interventions on role conflict, role overload, and role ambiguity, as well as the health, attitudinal, and behavioral outcomes of role-based stress, could provide the empirically valid knowledge needed by nurse administrators to minimize the increasing stress associated with nursing practice. Other investigations could focus on identifying which form of role-based stress is responsible for the greatest client system instability and specifying the differential impact of the stressors, such as health status versus attitudinal outcomes versus behavioral outcomes.

NEUMAN'S SYSTEMS MODEL AND MARKETING THEORY

Another logically congruent conceptual-theoretical system of knowledge of interest to the nurse administrator can be constructed by linking Neuman's systems model and a marketing theory that deals with the process of buying a product or service. Kotler[29] used the notion of stage theories to describe the process of buying, which can be defined as commitment of resources to gain a product or service that meets a perceived need or want. Stage theories assume that the buyer, whether an individual or an organization, does not make an instant, isolated decision to buy a product or service. Rather, the buyer progresses through a series of distinct stages. Kotler proposed a five-stage buying theory, including problem recognition, information search, evaluation of alternatives, purchase decision, and postpurchase behavior.

Problem recognition occurs when the buyer becomes aware of a problem or need. The awareness may be from an internal stimulus, such as an organization's decision to build a new facility, or an external stimulus, such as government mandates for pollution controls at an existing factory.

Information search describes the time and energy expended in an attempt to learn more about the range of options available to resolve the problem or meet the need. The buyer may or may not be aware of all possible options. Initial screening with previously established criteria reduces the set of options of which the buyer is aware to a consideration set. Next, strong choices emerge, and finally, the buyer selects one set of options from the choice set.

Evaluation of alternatives assumes a rational model of decision making on the buyer's part. Alternative evaluation involves consideration of the attributes of each option, weighing the importance of each option, identifying beliefs about the options, specifying utility functions (how the buyer thinks the attributes of the various options will satisfy the want or need), and application of a formal cost-benefit evaluation procedure.

Purchase decision involves purchase intention and the actual purchase decision. Purchase intention can be altered or reversed by the attitudes of others who become aware of the buyer's intent, by unanticipated situational factors, or by changes in the amount of perceived risk attached to the purchase. The actual purchase decision involves the variables of timing and vendor choice.

Postpurchase behavior refers to the level of satisfaction or dissatisfaction that the buyer experiences with the product or service following its purchase. Extremes of satisfaction or dissatisfaction may lead to postpurchase actions such as abandoning the product or service or becoming a vocal advocate for it.

Postpurchase behavior not only influences repeat purchases by the same buyer, but also affects other buyers' purchases.

Kotler's theory was developed primarily from work in consumer purchasing, that is, individuals buying for their own immediate use. The theory is, however, valid for institutional buying when certain formal mechanisms are incorporated into the stages of buying. For example, an organization will have formal written criteria to refer to during the information search, so that the reduction from the total set of options to the choice set is more clearly defined.

Neuman's systems model and Kotler's buying theory can be linked to form a conceptual-theoretical system of knowledge for marketing an existing department of nursing within a larger health-care institution. The use of buying theory by a department of nursing to "sell" itself to the larger institution reflects Neuman's concept of secondary prevention. The goal of application of the conceptual-theoretical knowledge system is an increase in the larger institution's awareness and appreciation of nursing as a unique, efficient, and needed professional service. Achievement of the goal requires penetration of the lines of defense and lines of resistance by a beneficial stressor so that the client system attains a new, improved level of stability.

The concepts of particular interest in the construction of this knowledge system are client system, stressor, flexible line of defense, normal line of defense, lines of resistance, and reconstitution. Within Kotler's theory of buying, the institution represents the client system, and the department of nursing represents the stressor. In this situation, the stressor is regarded as beneficial rather than noxious. The stage of problem recognition represents the flexible line of defense; information search and evaluation of alternatives represent the normal line of defense; the purchase decision represents the lines of resistance; and postpurchase behavior represents reconstitution.

In the model, penetration of the flexible line of defense informs the client system that a stressor is present. At the theoretical level, the problem-recognition stage occurs when the department of nursing increases the institution's awareness of the desire for high quality nursing care among two main consumer groups: patients and physicians. Neuman's model proposes that penetration of the flexible line of defense calls forth a response from the normal line of defense. Theoretically, the response encompasses the stages of information search and evaluation of alternatives. If the institution defines the desire for high-quality nursing care as a high priority, then a purchasing decision will follow. The department of nursing must constantly monitor the institutional response to prevent the lines of resistance from hardening into a no-purchase decision. Perceived risk must therefore be minimized and problems inherent in other options maximized. Reconstitution, in the form of postpurchase behavior, requires the department of nursing that has successfully marketed itself to build on that success by actually providing the promised high-quality nursing care. Documented success will prompt positive postpurchase behavior that should encourage the institution to purchase additional services from the department of nursing, such as an efficiently managed and profitable home health service.

This chapter has illustrated how a conceptual model of nursing provides a framework for viewing phenomena of interest to nurse administrators, and how selected organizational theories provide more detail. The wide utility of conceptual-theoretical systems of knowledge for nursing administration has been exemplified by linking three organization theories with conceptual models of nursing. The resulting knowledge systems have been used to explain assessment of the fit between environmental factors and organizational structure in general, and in the design of a nursing research program in a clinical agency; to develop research questions dealing with effects of role-based stress on nursing staff performance; and to highlight the process of marketing the services of a department of nursing to the larger health-care institution.

The linkage of conceptual models of nursing and organization theories provides a distinctly "nursing" focus for the nurse administrator's work. The resultant conceptual-theoretical knowledge systems help the nurse administrator justify the distinctive perspective and services of nursing within the larger health-care arena. Readers are encouraged to apply the conceptual-theoretical systems of knowledge presented in this chapter and to link other conceptual models of nursing with other organization theories to bring a distinctly nursing frame of reference to the administration of nursing services.

REFERENCES

1. Roy C. Introduction to nursing. An adaptation model. 2nd ed. Englewood Cliffs, NJ: Prentice-Hall Inc, 1984.
2. Neuman B. The Neuman systems model. Application to nursing education and practice. Norwalk, CT: Appleton-Century-Crofts, 1982.
3. Fawcett J. Analysis and evaluation of conceptual models of nursing. Philadelphia: FA Davis Company, Publishers, 1984.
4. Roy C, Roberts SL. Theory construction in nursing. An adaptation model. Englewood Cliffs, NJ: Prentice-Hall Inc, 1981.
5. Neuman B. The Neuman systems model. Keynote address presented at the First International Nursing Symposium on the Neuman Systems Model. Neumann College, Aston, PA. November 10, 1986.
6. Lee S, Luthans F, Olson D. A management science approach to contingency models of organizational structure. Academy of Management J 1982;25:553–566.
7. Lawrence PR, Lorsch J. Organization and environment. Homewood, IL: Richard D Irwin, 1969.
8. Morse JJ, Lorsch JW. Beyond theory Y. Harvard Bus Rev 1970;48:61–68.

9. Bolman L, Deal T. Modern approaches to understanding and managing organizations. San Francisco: Jossey-Bass Publishers, 1985.

10. Kaluzny A, Warner D, Warren D, Zelman W. Management of health services. Englewood Cliffs, NJ: Prentice-Hall Inc, 1982.

11. Gordon J. A diagnostic approach to organizational behavior. Boston: Allyn and Bacon Inc, 1983.

12. Carlisle H. Situational management. New York: AMACOM, 1973.

13. Magnusen K. Organizational design, development, and behavior. Glenview, IL: Scott, Foresman and Co, 1977.

14. Banton MP. Roles: An introduction to the study of social relations. New York: Basic Books Inc, 1965.

15. Brief AP, Van Sell M, Aldag RJ, Melone N. Anticipatory socialization and role stress among registered nurses. J Health Soc Behav 1979;20:161–165.

16. Van Sell M, Brief AP, Schuler RS. Role conflict and role ambiguity: Integration of the literature and directions for future research. Hum Rel 1981; 34:43–71.

17. Schuler RS, Aldag RJ, Brief AP. Role conflict and ambiguity: A scale analysis. Organiz Behav Hum Performance 1977;20:111–128.

18. McGrath JE. Stress and behavior in organizations. In: Dunnette M, ed. Handbook of industrial and organizational psychology. Chicago: Rand McNally and Co, 1976.

19. Szilagyi D. An empirical test of causal inference between role perceptions, satisfaction, performance, and organizational level. Personnel Psych 1977; 30:375–388.

20. Kahn RL, Wolf CM, Quinn BP, Snoek JD. Occupational stress: Studies in role conflict and ambiguity. New York: John Wiley and Sons, 1964.

21. Kahn RL. Conflict, ambiguity, and overload: Three elements in job stress. In: McLean A, ed. Occupational stress. Springfield, IL: Charles C Thomas, 1974.

22. Miles RH, Perreault WD. Organizational role conflict: Its antecedents and consequences. Organiz Behav Hum Performance 1976;17:19–44.

23. Rizzo JR, House RJ, Lirtzman SI. Role conflict and role ambiguity in complex organizations. Adm Sci Q 1970;15:150–163.

24. Abdel-Halim AA. Social support and managerial affective responses to job stress. J Occup Behav 1982;3:281–296.

25. House JS, Rizzo JR. Role conflict and role ambiguity as critical variables in a model of organizational behavior. Organiz Behav Hum Performance 1972; 7:465–505.

26. French JR. Person-role fit. In: McLean A, ed. Occupational stress Springfield, IL: Charles C Thomas, 1974.

27. Jamal M. Job stress and job performance controversy: An empirical assessment. Organiz Behav Hum Performance 1984;33:1–21.

28. Szilagyi D, Sims HP, Keller RT. Role dynamics, locus of control, and employee attitudes and behavior. Academy of Management J 1976;19:259–276.

29. Kotler P. Marketing management. Englewood Cliffs, NJ: Prentice-Hall Inc, 1984.

II

Introduction: Organization Theory for Nursing Administration

Beverly Henry

A FUNDAMENTAL premise on which this book is based is that in a society as technologically complex as ours, and in a profession as complex as nursing, interdisciplinary approaches representing a wide range of worldviews are extremely valuable. While we acknowledge the virtue and power of single-discipline specialization and of acquiring knowledge that is distinctive, we are equally committed in nursing administration to integrating knowledge from at least two fields—from nursing and organization science (the latter term is used interchangeably throughout the volume with management science and administrative science).

Integration of ideas does not, however, occur in a vacuum. The bringing together of ideas from disciplines where perspectives are sometimes similar and sometimes not must be rooted in respect and understanding of what scholars in the disciplines value, perceive as important, and intend to pursue.

For nearly a half century, individuals in and outside of nursing have admonished nurses to integrate knowledge of administration into nursing. Such an integration has been slow in developing—in some cases because of the strong tide of professional conservatism, in others because of arguments that managing is not a legitimate element of the nursing domain, and in a third case because of too little emphasis on the epistemology of interdisciplinary nursing adminis-

tration. Whatever the reasons, the interface between nursing and management science, and between nursing and nursing administration has been a problem.

As editors we are dedicated to what we hope will become a major intellectual endeavor in the future: identifying the cognitive maps of nursing and management for the purpose of theory-finding for nursing administration. Without an understanding of the ideals, basic concepts, and modes of inquiry in the two disciplines, nurses and managers will look at the same things but see something quite different.

Until there is a shared perception of the nature of nursing and the nature of management, nurses and managers will be unable to see the relevance of their coworkers' points of view. Moreover, without an understanding of nursing and management there can be little or no cognitive integration of nursing and organization knowledge and, therefore, no serious theory-building for interdisciplinary nursing administration.

As educators and practitioners in nursing administration, our concern is both with using theory and developing theory. Using good theories casts a bright light on what exists and guides thinking, practice, and research. Theory gives us categories to pigeonhole information and words to understand the events taking place around us. Theories are like stories that help us make sense of important things in new idioms.

Nurses who are administrators and who strive to function effectively need to be knowledgeable about using nursing and organization theory. Nurses also have an intellectual responsibility for theory-finding: for seeing how theories from the natural and social sciences enter and connect with the field of nursing, and how theories from outside the discipline can be altered for nursing administration. Moreover, nearly all academic programs in nursing administration have courses or elements of courses that focus on organization theory. Few in academe would argue with the idea that organization theory has practical value for nursing administration.

One of our premises, however, is that before theories can be used intelligently and before new, refined theories can be found to improve nursing administration, nurses need to be knowledgeable about the theoretical knowledge that already exists.

In Section I, theorists in nursing have told us their stories about nursing administration in their own language, and from a number of different worldviews—some from the perspective of culture; others from the perspective of external control of individual behavior; some from the rational-person, goal-setting perspective; and others from the perspective of social systems. In Section II, six authors describe a number of theories found in management science, some of which have been emphasized in nursing and some of which have not. Although this section is relatively short, we have tried to highlight a number of theoretical perspectives that appear to have special salience for nursing administration, but, for the most part have not been discussed to any great extent in the past.

Dienemann provides the reader with an overview of theoretical perspectives in organization science in Chapter 16. Many of the theories she describes have not been used in nursing administration either to structure thinking in the workplace or for research. She analyzes the theoretical perspectives in organization science, using Astley and Van de Ven's typology, which take either the total organization (macro) or the individual (micro) as the level of analysis.

In Chapter 17, Mark, one of the nurses most knowledgeable about management theory in the country, describes a category of systems theory that is especially appealing to nurses—the structural contingency perspective. She begins her chapter with a description of the historical development of contingency thinking, highlighting the key concepts. Mark cites the researchers and theorists who have made significant contributions to this important paradigm in organization science. Ways of studying the relationships between organizational technology, structure, and effectiveness are discussed, as are the implications for future nursing administration research.

In Chapter 18, Gibbons, chief of nursing service at the Sioux Falls Veterans Administration Medical Center (VAMC), and Krajnak, associate chief at the Dallas VAMC, take one contingency framework—the coalignment model developed by Kotter and Lawrence—and discuss how the model is useful in nursing administration and in-service education. They carefully describe the elements of the coalignment model: four contextual factors—the administrator, his or her agenda, network, and organizational unit; three administrative actions—agenda setting, network building, and task accomplishing; and the relationships among the contextual and action elements. The authors' description of coalignment theory and how it is used to analyze administrative behavior in complex organizations can be extremely beneficial to practicing nurse administrators and to students.

Chapter 19, entitled "The Power of the Nurse Executive," focuses on power and dependence in organizations. The format of this chapter, in two sections, is unique. First, Rotkovitch, former vice president for nursing at Yale-New Haven Hospital, in fascinating, true-to-life vignettes, describes her experiences with power and dependence in complex organizations. Then Nelson, a nurse administrator at the Veterans Administration Medical Center in Tampa demonstrates how a theory of power is useful for analyzing the managerial experiences that Rotkovitch describes.

The theory Nelson uses is one of power and dependence in management. Considerable attention has been paid to power in nursing, especially the last decade. Much less attention has been devoted to understanding the relationship of power to organizational dependence. Nurse administrators function effectively when they understand dependence in management positions, the conflicts for scarce resources that arise where many individuals are highly dependent on one another, and the power dynamics that emerge.

In Chapter 20, White and Green explain how an important perspective in sociology, social exchange theory, can be useful for the field of nursing administration, where the idea of exchange has received little attention. Social exchange theory is based on the premise that individuals and groups function in relationships where there are rewards, costs, and profits. The central idea is that to understand how and why people behave as they do in organizations, one must understand the characteristics of others. More specifically, social exchange theory suggests that social actor *A* is dependent on actor *B*, or groups of actors *BCDE*, to the extent that *B*, or *BCDE*, have and control resources that *A* needs to function effectively.

Throughout this thoughtful, analytic chapter, elements of social exchange are carefully described. Examples are also provided by the authors using the cases of nurses in various settings to improve the reader's understanding of how social exchange theory can be used to understand why people act and interact as they do in the workplace.

In Chapter 21, Frederickson, a nationally recognized scholar in public administration, suggests how knowledge from his field can be used in the development of nursing administration. In the past, nursing has relied heavily on ideas from business administration. The emphasis on efficiency and running health services like private, for-profit businesses is understandable. The high costs of health care, concerns about overly expensive services, and the oftentimes inadequate management that has characterized hospitals warrant the emphasis on productivity and profit.

The fact remains however, that the majority of health-care institutions are public services, and even those that are for-profit, proprietary agencies have public responsibility. And in public organizations, the ideas about administration are somewhat different. Frederickson focuses on three major differences: the conception of public in administration, citizenship, and social equity in organizations as a measure of productivity. He states that honorable administrators of public services oppose unjust policies, genuinely care for the public they serve, act as moral entrepreneurs, and understand that the more one is benefited by society the more one is obligated to benefit society in return.

In this section's final chapter, I argue that to advance nursing administration as an interdisciplinary endeavor, the core knowledge of nursing and management—the epistemology of these fields—must be clarified to a greater extent than in the past before nursing administration can advance intellectually. I suggest that efforts to harmonize nursing and management thus far, have been largely non-intellectual. Rather than focusing on the structure of knowledge in nursing and organization science, the focus has been largely on the characteristics of participants and on problems related to institutional settings. The metaphor and computerized idea spinning are suggested as ways to cognitively connect nursing and management and to generate new knowledge for nursing administration.

16

Theoretical Perspectives in Organization Science for Nursing Administration

Jacqueline Dienemann

NURSES work primarily as employed professionals providing services. They are concerned, as are other professional service providers, about maintaining and increasing autonomy for their practice. In her study, Larson[1] identifies three categories of professionals in organizations. The first are consulting professionals who provide direct services to clients. The second are technocrats, organizational experts employed to manage the effective provision of services. Nurse administrators fit this category. The third are academic professionals, experts in educational technology and the knowledge of a discipline. Nurses in all three categories need knowledge of organization science to understand their work environments and make decisions that enhance performance.

Health-care organizations employ nurses in all three categories. Today's multidisciplinary, multiproduct organizations are diversifying and becoming subunits of larger corporate organizations. Universities, which employ nurses as academic professionals and technocrats, share these characteristics.

Mintzberg[2] refers to service organizations that primarily employ professionals as professional bureaucracies. He notes that power in such organizations is distributed primarily through political interaction. To be effective, professional employees need to understand the distribution of power. Decisions concern-

ing the type and quality of nursing services are often made by individuals at corporate levels who are not nurses. Consequently, it is extremely important for nurses to be knowledgable about how organizations function so as to positively influence executive decisions that affect nursing practice, education, and administration.

SOURCES OF MANAGEMENT KNOWLEDGE

Some nurses rely primarily on tradition and experience to solve administrative problems. They manage largely by using intuition and experience-based decision rules. These informal methods can be effective in stable environments where situations are primarily recurrent and where there is time to learn management skills on the job. But intuitive knowledge and experience, while important, are not sufficient in rapidly changing environments. Contemporary health-care is in a rapid state of organizational change. To capitalize on this change, nurse administrators need to increase their knowledge of organization science.

Disciplinary Knowledge and Theory

Nursing theory defines the events studied in nursing science. Organization theory describes the phenomena relevant to the knowledge of organizations. Nursing administration integrates knowledge from both sciences to design, implement, and monitor productive nursing delivery systems in organizational contexts. To evaluate new ideas and avoid believing that popular, simple solutions will quickly resolve the complex problems related to productivity, employee retention, or strategic planning, nurse administrators need to ensure that changes are based on scientific research and reputable theory.[3] They need to be able to evaluate and use theory and research from nursing and related disciplines.

Nurse administrators may find studies and theories from anthropology, management, sociology, economics, political science, and social psychology relevant to their needs. Moreover, many professional disciplines have administrative subdisciplines with theory that is useful for nursing administration, including education, social work, public health, and hospital administration.

Research and Knowledge

Stetler[4] discusses how research is an important source of knowledge for all nurses. She defines utilization of research as more than the use of research findings and as including the use of research methods, theoretical concepts, and a continuing attitude of critical inquiry.

When evaluating whether to utilize a set of research findings to resolve a problem there are four steps: search, evaluation, comparison, and decision making.[4] First, nurse administrators search the literature for reports of research studies, case descriptions, and reports published on the subject of interest. Second, they evaluate the scientific rigor of the studies. If there are a number of good investigations, they move to step three, otherwise they collect more information from additional sources of knowledge such as published case reports or surveys. Health agencies often have several experts available for consultation such as dieticians, pharmacists, physicians, clinical specialists, and instructors. They then evaluate all sources of information for agreement, conflict, and expertise, and the nurse administrator decides if a recommendation for change is supported by the knowledge acquired.

The third step involves two comparisons. The first is to compare the similarity of the patients and settings used in the various studies under review to the nurse administrator's patient population and setting. The second comparison is of the risks involved with the recommended change, and the risk of no change.

The fourth and last step is decision making based on the comparisons made in step three. There are four choices with respect to the utilization of research findings; rejection, cognitive application, independent application, or interdependent application. Rejection may be necessary where there are no clear recommendations, where there are differences in patient populations or settings, and where the current basis of practice is sound. A cognitive application is deciding that the new information is valuable, but implementing change based on the information is not feasible. Independent application is one involving only single individuals. Interdependent applications involve groups of people, and multidisciplinary teams.

Currently, in nursing, there is considerable argument about the appropriate upper limits of nursing administration roles, about the types of academic programs preparing nurses for administrative functions and what the research and theory in these programs should be.[5] Some suggest that nursing administration encompasses only intraorganizational roles directly responsible for nursing care delivery. Others suggest that nursing administration includes health administrative roles such as product-line management and quality assurance, and interorganizational roles in governments, corporations, and professional associations. Regardless of the outcome of these debates, nurses today perform administrative functions in a wide variety of organizational settings and can benefit from knowledge of the theories and research in organization science.

THEORETICAL PERSPECTIVES IN ORGANIZATION SCIENCE

When first confronted with a problem such as premature employee turnover, there is a tendency for administrators to define the problem as one of "personality conflict."[6] Organization science, however, looks beyond personalities to bureaucratic rules, authority structures, information flow, conflicting goals, corporate cultures, market demands, government regulations, and societal changes.

In organization science, there are many theories that are useful for understanding the problems people face in organizations. Morgan[7] uses the analogy of theories as metaphors to illustrate how various theories illuminate different aspects of organizational life. For example, organizations can be viewed as machines, biological systems, information processing units, cultures, and political systems. Morgan[8] theorizes that it is through metaphors relating previous knowledge to novel experiences that people come to make sense of their world. Each metaphor or image provides a partial, limited, subjective view of objective reality just as different cross-sectional slides of human tissue offer true but partial, limited views of internal organs. Taken together, multiple perspectives offer a richer, multidimensional understanding of what occurs in organizations.

Typology of Organizational Theory

Astley and Van de Ven[9] have developed a typology of organizational theory using four

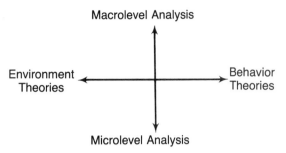

Figure 16.1 The Two Axes of Theories in Organization Science

cells on two axes: (1) micro- and macrolevels of organizational analysis and (2) environment or behavior theories.* The axes are illustrated in Figure 16.1. First, I will focus on the two major axes, and later on each of the four cells.

At the microlevel of analysis, organization theories and research focus on roles, work groups, departments, or divisions in a single organization. At the macrolevel of analysis theories and research address the interactions and comparisons of two or more organizations. Macrolevel analyses focus on organizations in conglomerates, alliances, or geographic areas. Thus, the vertical axis depicts a continuum from individual roles to global comparisons. In health care, microlevel studies oftentimes include those of nursing roles, quality indicators of nursing care on a unit and the life cycle of a hospital. Macrolevel studies include those of regional nursing shortages, restructuring of health-care delivery and comparison of health-care delivery systems in different countries.

The horizontal axis classifies organization theory according to the degree a theory focuses on the environment and structure of organizations, or on the behavior of individ-

---

*Astley and Van de Ven[9] use the terms "deterministic" and "voluntaristic" for the horizontal axis. Scott[12] used "rational" and "social," and Kaylaap[13] uses "economic" and "behavioral" to refer to the same theoretical perspectives. This paper uses the terms "environment" and "behavior."

uals and groups in organizations. Environmental theorists study structures and policies of organizations that support rational decision making and efficient use of human and material resources to effectively achieve organizational goals. Behavior theorists focus on understanding the interactions and subjective perceptions of participants in organizations. Scientists, focusing on organizational behavior often study power, leadership, productivity, cultures, and politics. Examples of studies in nursing administration that use the environmental perspective are those focusing on the functions of head nurses or patient classification systems. Many such studies are cited in the American Organization of Nurse Executive's publication, *Research in Nursing Administration*.[10] The *Magnet Hospitals'* study, which describes the cultures of hospitals able to retain nurses, is an example of a behavioral study.[11]

Each category represents a single paradigm that includes a number of theories at both the macro- and microlevels related because of similar assumptions. Thus, the right and left cells in Astley and Van de Ven's[9] model each represent a single paradigm that includes a number of theories based on similar assumptions about organizational behavior, but originating in different academic disciplines.

Environment Theories

Environment theories are based on the following assumptions:

- people make rational decisions
- organizations are objectively real and can be empirically studied
- research builds knowledge incrementally for prescriptive theory
- behavior in organizations is determined by the missions and structures of organizations
- actions can be evaluated as rational, effective, and efficient in fulfilling organizational missions.

Using the environment perspective, prescriptive guidelines can be generated based on empirical findings. The following is an example of a prescriptive rule: The span of control for a manager should not be more than seven people. A nursing application of this would be: No more than seven head nurses should report to an associate director of nursing.

Environment is the "older" theoretical perspective and is based primarily on studies from economics, sociology, management, and marketing. Three primary lines of theory development in the environment perspective, and the major theorists associated with each, are summarized in Figure 16.2.

Sociology has contributed to two lines of development in environment theory: the systems and bureaucracy perspectives. Systems theory evolved from a closed, single-system approach, to recognition of the importance of the environment in open systems, and later to contingency theory. Simultaneously, Weber was studying management in bureaucracies followed by Taylor, Fayol, and Gulick and Urwick, who studied the functions of management and developed prescriptive guidelines to increase efficiency and effectiveness. Later theorists studied the effect of task and technology on the design of bureaucratic structures. Two macrolevel environment theories are population ecology and organizational ecology.

Economic theory's first contribution to organization science was classical economics, which defined optimal decisions as those based on rationality and self-interest. A truly free economy, in Adam Smith's view, was guided by the "invisible hand" balancing the rational self-interests of all parties. The entire field of management science in economics, business, and engineering devises quantitative models of optimal decision making based on assumptions from classical economics. Public choice theory merges philosophy and economics to emphasize the value of freedom

Systems Theory

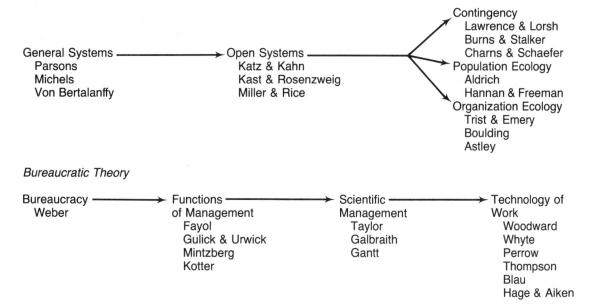

Bureaucratic Theory

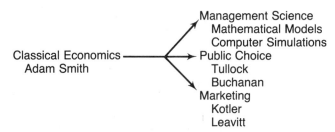

Economic Theory

Figure 16.2 Organizational Environment Theories. Shared assumptions: The purpose of an organization is to economically and effectively fulfill its mission. Reality is external to participants and is objectively studied using empirical methods. Optimal decisions are rational and goal directed. Systems theory is the dominant theoretical perspective in this category of organization theory.

of choice and the factor of self-interest. A third set of theories derived from classical economics and psychology is marketing, which combines analysis of rational self-interest and human motivation to predict which products and associated companies will be most successful.

Environment theorists use Kuhn's[14] rational view of science as building knowledge incrementally through empirical research, using successive dominant paradigms. According to Kuhn, over time, there is a cycle of acceptance by a discipline of one dominant paradigm, recognition of the limits of the paradigm, revolution against the dominant paradigm, competition between alternative paradigms, and the choice of a new dominant paradigm. During the period of a paradigm's dominance, scientists in a discipline accept the same theoretical perspective for directing inquiry and reporting research findings; or, to use Morgan's[7] language, research is directed and interpreted by one metaphor. Research results accumulate to provide an increasingly comprehensive explanation of the field. The theory provides a shared language for rapid dissemination of new knowledge; research results direct priorities for further inquiry. During the periods of competition between dominant paradigms, there is a hiatus in the building of scientific knowledge.

Behavior Theories

Behavior theorists reject the orderliness of Kuhn's[14] theory of the history of science. Knowledge, using their perspective, builds through concurrent multiple studies that incorporate contextual variables using conflicting paradigms, a combination of qualitative and empirical research methods, and a variety of levels of analysis. Knowledge increases through autopoiesis—multiple circular patterns of interaction—rather than by incremental linear additions.[7] Autopoiesis results in a richer understanding of the unique aspects of each phenomenon. Researchers view historical periods in which dominant paradigms direct inquiry, as times of restricted growth of knowledge. By limiting the legitimacy of studies to one theoretical perspective, new knowledge generated through alternative perspectives is ignored. Findings that do not support the dominant theory are rejected rather than pursued as they would be in the process of autopoiesis.[6]

The following are assumptions underlying behavior theories:

- decisions are only subjectively rational
- loosely connected groups of participants provide the actual structure of organizations
- qualitative research methods should be mixed with empirical methods
- organizational mission is a set of conflicting goals

- since the culture of each organization is different, few prescriptive guidelines for action are possible
- effectiveness of an action can only be evaluated retrospectively, and
- effective organizations support the autonomy and accountability of all participants.

Using the behavior perspective, each situation in an organization is unique. Actions should be chosen and evaluated for each specific context. Primary nursing in its ideal form uses this theoretical perspective to support the concept of individualized nursing care coordinated by an autonomous, accountable professional nurse.

The behavior perspective has more recently been applied to organization science and includes studies primarily from management, anthropology, political science, sociology, and psychology. Table 16.1 summarizes the three major theoretical strands and major theorists using the behavior perspective.

Management Theory

The best-known theoretical strand is the merger of management and social psychology that began with Chester Barnard and the studies at Western Electric and identified the importance of shared values and work norms for worker productivity. This led to industrial psychology and the work of Maslow, McGregor, and others who studied human needs and motivation in the workplace. Contemporary research in this area examines worker satisfaction, productivity, job design, and quality of work life.

A parallel line of theoretical development begun in psychiatry was developed in management. Research on small groups, managing change, and organizational development has emphasized the importance of shared governance.

A final overlapping but distinct line of

TABLE 16.1 Behavior Theories of Organizations

MANAGEMENT THEORY

Organizations as Cooperative Endeavors	Motivation/Job Satisfaction/Quality of Work Life	Organization Development/Small Groups/Culture	Leadership/Values/Strategic Management
Barnard	Maslow	Bell Labs	Drucker
Rothlesberger & Dickson	Herzberg	Lewin	Downs
Mayo	McGregor	Likert	Blake & Mouton
	McClelland	Argyris & Schon	Stogdill
	Vroom	Nadler & Tushman	Hersey & Blanchard
	Lawler	Deal & Kennedy	Peters & Waterman
	Oldham & Hackman		Ouchi

ORGANIZATIONAL BEHAVIOR

Decision Making Behavior	Exchange & Pluralism	Power & Negotiation	Symbolic Interaction/Organized Anarchy
Simon	Homans	Gamson	Schutz
Hickson et al.	Thibault & Kelly	Wildavsky	Garfinkel
Allison	Selznick	Pfeffer	March
Cyert & March	Follett	Crozier	Weick
		Dahl	
		Emerson	
		Blau	

CONFLICT THEORY

Role Conflict	Alienation	Radical Theory/Collective Theory
Coser	Durkheim	Marx
Lawrence & Lorsch	Sartre	Marimyama
House, Rizzo & Lirtzman	Jung	Mirow & Maurer
Boulding	Freud	Hegel
Pondy	Fromm	Fox
Sherif & Sherif	Adorno	

Shared assumptions: Each organization has a unique culture and multiple conflicting goals. Reality is an interpretation of each participant's perceptions researched using qualitative methods. Decisions are political and unstable. Management theory is the dominant perspective in this category of organization theory.

inquiry in management focuses on leadership, values, and strategic management. Theorists in this category are Drucker, Hersey and Blanchard, and Ouchi. Strategic management theorists describe how to increase productivity by charging top leadership with the responsibility for the design of strategic plans, which individuals at the lower levels of management then decide how to implement.

Each management level has a different arena of decision making appropriate to its function.

Organizational Behavior

Theorists from sociology, political science, and social psychology have developed theories of organizational behavior. Hickson and others in Britain first described organizations as resource-dependent, open-systems with politically negotiated power structures. This novel view stimulated other theorists to study exchange, power, and perceptions of organizational life. Another related line of theory development led by March and Weick, offered provocative images of organizations as organized anarchies or as mere aggregations of semi-autonomous groups. These two theorists drew attention to situational contexts of action, personal meanings to participants, and the value of loose-coupling for innovation. Peters and Waterman made this perspective widely known among administrators through their best-selling study of outstanding companies, *In Search of Excellence.*[15]

Conflict Theory

The more extreme conflict theories are used primarily in macrolevel studies and include models of alienation, radical theories from political science, psychiatry, philosophy, and sociology. These theories reject bureaucracies as ineffective and describe alternative ways of organizing based on collective action.

In summary, environment and behavior theories each have a body of research based on shared assumptions. And each uses distinctly different methods for collecting and analyzing data. These differences make empirical comparisons between studies problematic. However, many organization scientists are now arguing that theories in both perspectives are valuable and highlight different aspects of organizational life. It is widely recommended that administrators integrate ideas from both categories into their practice.[13]

Environment and behavior theories help nurse administrators become more aware of the relationship of structure to action. Environment theories favor structured, prescribed interactions, which contribute to controlled, effective achievement of organizational missions. Behavior theories favor innovative, spontaneous interaction, which is evaluated for its contribution to organizational success. A nurse administrator can use concepts from both perspectives to create an organizational climate that balances structured coordination and spontaneous creativity to increase the productivity of a nursing department.

MICROLEVEL ORGANIZATION THEORIES

Organizational theories that take the microlevel of analysis are generally well known in nursing administration. Nurses work in organizations and, until the last decade, nurse administrators were primarily concerned with internal operational problems. The largest number of theories and the majority of empirical investigations have been done using microlevel theories. Environment microtheorists have studied work flow, work-group size, professionals in bureaucracies, program evaluation, work measurement, product-line management, and the impact of uncertainty on organizations.[7] Behavior microtheorists have typically studied the power of participants in organizations, motivation, job satisfaction, participation in decision making, and corporate culture. Theories in this latter category direct attention to political and cultural factors in organizations that are not as well addressed by environment theories.[17]

Micro-organizational theories are categorized in two cells on Van de Ven and Astley's model of organization science.[9] The entire model is illustrated in Figure 16.3. Environment microtheories are labeled structural systems theories. In this category, decisions are rational, power is seated in hierarchical structures, and organizational success is measured by appropriate structure and environmental adaptation for effective achievement of organizational missions. Behavior microtheories

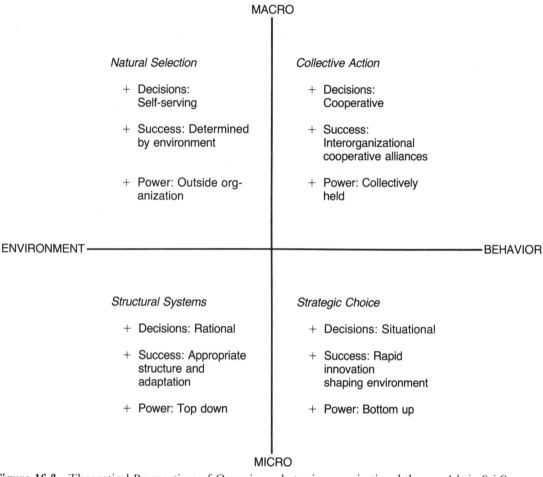

Figure 16.3   Theoretical Perspectives of Organization Science. (Adapted from Astley WG, and Van de Ven AH. Central perspectives and debates in organizational theory. *Admin Sci Quar,* 1983:28;245–273.)

are entitled strategic choice. This perspective views decisions as situationally specific and fluid, power as shared by all levels of employees, and organizational success as a consequence of strategic planning and innovations created to capture fleeting opportunities in turbulent environments.

Structural Systems Theories

Microlevel environment theories of organizations as structured bureaucratic systems are the most widely known.[17] Structural systems

theory was the dominant theoretical perspective in organization science between the 1940s and the 1970s. The work of Parsons and others assessed the functions of organizations for society and identified the ideal characteristics needed to fulfill these functions. Morgan[7] refers to structural systems perspective as the "living organism metaphor." Structural systems theories focus on the qualities of organizational units rather than the people in them. Systems theorists assume individuals share organizational goals and provide feedback for adaptation. The ability of any one person to change an organization is viewed as severely constrained by organizational inertia and environmental constraints.[18] Thus, change according to these theories, is a slow incremental process.

Systems theorists describe organizations as bureaucratic structures in which legitimate power is held by top managers who choose organizational missions, structures, and policies. Middle managers implement the policies to support first-line managers who supervise workers. Workers produce the product or service that achieves the organization's goals. The goals of individual employees and the organization overlap in the ideal structure where shared governance results in higher productivity. Shared governance and interactions between the organization and environment generate feedback to top management which, in turn, is used to plan and adapt organizational goals to fit environmental demands. In other words, research that is done using environmental theories seeks to discover rational, economical, and effective ways to maintain organizations.

Much research has been done in health-care administration using this framework.[19–20] Examples are Alexander's and Randolph's[21] study comparing functional, team, and primary nursing as structures for the delivery of nursing care, and Mark's[22] study of the contribution of task and structure to hospital effectiveness. Charns and Schaefer's[23] book *Health Care Organizations* summarizes many studies using structural systems theories and offers a contingency theory for assessing health-care organizations as structured systems interacting with the environment.

Bureaucratic theories that have developed independently but share the same assumptions are another set of theories in this category. The theories of bureaucracy were briefly described in the earlier overview of environment theories.

Strategic Choice Theories

In strategic choice theories, individual managers in organizations are viewed as actively shaping their environments rather than as adapting to them. This category consists of management theories of cooperation, motivation, organization development, and strategic management; organizational behavior theories of decision making, exchange, power, and symbolic interaction; and conflict theories. Strategic choice theories are less well-developed than structural systems theories. Many are only conceptual frameworks with little or no supportive research. Informal power, culture, and conflict are viewed as important determinants of change and as positive forces for increasing the congruence of organizations with their environments.

The ideal organization, from this theoretical perspective, is a network of loosely coupled self-organizing units that are semi-autonomous. Activity is centralized only to support routine work. Goals are defined by strategic plans but are continuously redefined by rapidly changing situations. Effectiveness, from the strategic choice perspective, is judged by strategic planning and the responsiveness of an organization to innovation and change.[24]

Strategic choice theorists conceive of organizations as aggregations of groups of interacting people with varying motivations and goals. Organizational boundaries, structures, decisions and power bases are viewed as fluid and as continuously redefined through interactions. Rational descriptions of goal-oriented actions are merely retrospective reconstructions based on subjective perceptions of interactions. Reality is shared understandings that guide organizational behavior.

Researchers who are building and testing these theories seek to describe the contextual and process variables that influence the way goals are defined and the way effectiveness is measured in organizations. Some research, primarily about power and politics, has been done in nursing using this view.[25,26] Dienemann's study of the power of nursing schools in universities[27] and Mixon's study of the political processes influencing the passage of the Florida Nurse Practice Act[28] are examples.

VALUE OF MACROORGANIZATION THEORIES FOR NURSING

Until recently, health-care organizations were primarily hospitals, nursing homes, home health agencies, and community health departments. These organizations were generally structured with decision-making power centered in dual hierarchies, one headed by a manager and the others by a physician. Nurse administrators tended to be located in the middle and lower levels of these hierarchies where they were primarily responsible for the daily operation of a nursing department. Consequently, nursing knowledge in administration has focused on individual workers, work groups, and departments—elements addressed at the microlevel of analysis in organization theory.

Today's health-care organizations increasingly are large regional and national corporations that include a wide variety of agencies delivering an array of services. Nurse administrators serve in these organizations as middle managers and executives participating in planning, implementing, and monitoring policy changes, and as first-line managers focusing on daily operations. For the latter group, microlevel theory continues to be the most useful.

Nurse Executives

For executive nurse administrators, however, macrolevel theory provides valuable insights about total organizations. Health care is rapidly reorganizing into fewer, larger, and more comprehensive corporations, a trend

that is creating opportunities for nurses.[29] Macrolevel theory helps administrators identify key stakeholders who are often external to organizations. These theories also describe the importance of interorganizational functions. Serving on advisory boards, government commissions, or in national professional organizations, for example, promotes an organization's image while supplying important information about the environment.

Kreuger,[30] in her review of interorganizational research in nursing-care delivery systems, found little macrolevel research in nursing. Her literature search documented that there is an early awareness of the interdependence of organizations and the importance of mutually beneficial linkages for organizations and their larger communities. Nursing studies of the relative effectiveness of different types of linkages in coping with environmental uncertainty are needed in both the service and educational arenas.

Nurse Educators, Clinical Specialists, and Lower-Level Administrators

Nurse educators need a broad understanding of the interorganizational aspects of health care to effectively design and implement curriculums that prepare nurses to understand aspects of their roles beyond traditional nurse-patient relationships. Students need to be prepared to be sensitive to the importance of viewing the patient as a customer whose satisfaction is essential for an agency's future income. And socializing students to the importance of political action is necessary for improved health-care policy.

Nurses in lower-level administrative and clinical specialist positions need knowledge of organizations beyond their specific work units. Knowledge is needed about ongoing changes in health care if nurses are to participate fully in management decisions. For example, a hospital could be considering a change from providing a service to contracting for it through an external vendor. A head nurse or clinical specialist knowledgeable about organizations could be able to document ways a current hospital service is generating income that is invisible in the existing accounting system. Presenting information about his or her observations in a politically sensitive and convincing manner would assist hospital administrators to make better decisions. It is vital for the welfare of patient services that nurses knowledgeable about organization research and theory exert an influence on corporate-level decisions concerning services added, markets dominated, and resources sought.[17]

Theories of Natural Selection

Macrolevel organization theories address interorganizational relationships and the relationships among large units within corporations. Astley and Van de Ven[9] describe two sets of theories at this level: natural selection and collective action theories.

Natural selection theorists view successful organizations as a manifestation of the survival of the fittest—using a deterministic perspective of interorganizational behavior. In this perspective, organizations thrive that ecologically fit their environment by efficiently meeting society's needs. The environment is the powerful determining agent, defining organizational opportunities and constraints. Natural selection theorists assume that managers have little impact on organizational survival because of their uncertainty about which changes to implement and their imperfect ability to implement decisions. Examples of natural selection theories include: population and organization ecology; classic economic theory; quantified methods of decision making, and public choice.

Theorists taking the natural selection approach assume that managerial decisions are rationally self-serving, although limited by an individual's capability of obtaining and interpreting information. People relate to employers through rational contracts whereby they exchange their labor for desired rewards. They are not motivated to participate in actions that benefit everyone, only those that specifically benefit them. Olson[31] points out that engaging in actions to benefit everyone is illogical. Rational people wait, let others act, and reap the benefits. For instance, if a few nurses gather information about their hospitals' low salaries and petition for a pay raise, all nurses in the hospital will benefit if salaries are increased. It is illogical for everyone in the nursing department to help gather pertinent information. Theoretically, the logical action is to wait and benefit from the raise without expending excessive effort.

Economists view organizations as differentiated by the ecological niches of the markets they serve. Markets, from a natural selection viewpoint, are also studied by population ecologists. For example, Miles and Snow[32] categorize organizations according to the innovativeness of their product lines.

To natural selection theorists, organizations succeed either by completely dominating a market or by creating a market niche outside the interest of dominant corporations. Dominant corporations are vertically integrated—various organizational units in a corporation provide work for other units, thus creating and maintaining their own markets. In health care, an example of vertical integration is hospitals supplying clients to other agencies like home health or skilled nursing homes owned by the parent corporation. Theorists refer to the self-provision of markets by corporations as market-failure because the free, open market is no longer generated by competition among different businesses.

According to natural selection theorists, successful organizations are innovative and able to respond to changing environmental conditions. Organizations that fail to adapt, do not survive. The marketplace changes the distribution patterns of scarce, critical resources through a natural, unpredictable drift, and as conditions change, organizations must adapt or suffer from a lack of essential resources. Consequently, old market niches cease to exist, and innovative organizational forms respond to the newly available, unique market niches that emerge. Thus, a continual process of disappearance of traditional markets, and the emergence of new markets, creates conditions under which organizations must adapt or cease to survive.

Perrow[17] describes the contribution of natural selection theory as offering an explanation of the seemingly paradoxical trend toward the domination of a market by a few, large firms, while simultaneously, small firms continue to thrive in limited, specialized areas of the same market. Perrow urges people to consider the collective action perspective to understand the evolution of organizational forms.

Collective Action Theories

Collective action theories are proposed by scholars who have an alienation or radical theory orientation. Organizations in the collective action perspective are described as densely linked through networks of transactions, dependencies, regulations, and norms that severely constrain action, while demanding constant adaptation. Collective action theories emphasize the importance of political boundary spanning by administrators through memberships in professional organizations, participation on governing boards, contractual agreements between organizations, and other interorganizational arrangements. Using networks and boundary spanning, administrators attempt to create an artificial, vertically integrated, munificent environment that overcomes the inherent alienation and constant flux of the natural environment.

People, according to collective action theories, act within the constraints of customs, laws, and other normative rules of interaction, which limit each person's will. Interactions with others increase a person's freedom by creating new choices and making options available. Individual power increases through decision making, external networking, and boundary spanning.

According to collective action theories, organizations benefit from people interacting cooperatively to make decisions that simultaneously serve an organization's collective interests and a person's individual interests. In effective organizations, there is little or no centralized authority, and decision making by consensus and collective cooperation is highly valued. The power of each participant is increased and the success of the organization is also increased through collective cooperation. Professional group practices, cooperatives, feminist organizations, and profit-sharing agreements are examples of the organizations described by theorists in this school of thought.

Collective action theorists are critical of traditional, rational theory and ask this question: "Bureaucracies are productive for whom?" They posit that natural selection theories blind middle- and lower-level managers to the fact that their labors are exploited to fulfill the goals of owners and executives. They believe that society is structured to inequitably reward owners and the managerial elite through preferential tax systems and favoritism in public works, laws, and governmental regulations.

Collective action theorists argue that the country's wealth could be increased through alternative systems of small-scale organizations that place more value on social equity and quality of life. Ideal organizations would factor in social costs when calculating employee productivity. Every individual would be valued for his or her cooperative contribution to the whole. Theorists who have a collective action view value multiple small organizations with networks to reap the economy of scale, without paying the costs of coordination and impersonality demanded by large organizations. They emphasize that quality of work life should be seriously pursued.

To support the creation and success of a large number of nonbureaucratic organizations, collective action theorists believe more empirical research is needed to find ways of motivating people toward self-regulating cooperative action. Theoretically, where self-regulation and cooperation are the modal forms of interaction the benefits to each person are increased. Collective action theorists view today's governmental policies as mainly destructive—as largely supporting individualistic actions with winners dominating powerless and apathetic losers. They believe the current trend toward large, market dominating organizations is due to manipulation by the power elite, and not to the efficiency of large-scale organizations, a trend contributing to low productivity and slow economic growth.

ORGANIZATION THEORIES FOR NURSING ADMINISTRATION

Between the 1940s and the 1970s, organization science was considered a subdiscipline of sociology with one dominant paradigm—structural systems. Organization science was not recognized as a separate discipline with a unique body of knowledge. Today, organization science is recognized as a discipline with two major theoretical traditions—environmental and behavioral theories at the micro- and macrolevels. Four perspectives have been discussed in this chapter using Van de Ven and Astley's[9] categories of structural systems, strategic choice, natural selection, and collective action. Pinder and Bourgeois[33] argue that an integrated metatheory of organization science is emerging that recognizes and

incorporates the contributions of both the environmental and behavioral views of organizations. Lincoln[34] agrees that a single, dominant paradigm is emerging in organization science but she argues that the strategic choice perspective is central.

Morgan[76] disagrees. He argues that a single metatheory to guide research in organization science is not only impossible, but undesirable. The tension between the four competing major paradigms has expanded knowledge in ways that are beneficial. The pursuit of knowledge about organizations by scientists with different disciplinary perspectives and research methods expands knowledge at a more rapid rate than research that is done by scientists guided by one metaparadigm, using one set of research methods. The multiple disciplinary perspectives of researchers from psychology, economics, sociology, management, anthropology, and marketing offer both a wider breadth of findings and multiple opposing views of the same problems. Moreover, studies by those in subdisciplines, such as nursing administration, discover contextual events and ideas that need to be considered in applying organizational theories to specific types of organizations.

Morgan contends that the contrasting views of reality portrayed by organization theories using alternative metaphors provide a rich understanding of organizations and numerous options for managerial action—far more than any one grand theory. This valuing of rich diversity afforded by tension between theoretical perspectives parallels Carper's[35] conceptualization of the bases of nursing knowledge. Carper categorizes ways of gaining knowledge as empirical, esthetic, kinesthetic, and interpersonal—each is not mutually exclusive, but neither is any one in and of itself, sufficient. Carper argues that both rational knowledge gained from empirical investigations, and behavioral knowledge from aesthetic, kinesthetic, and interpersonal investigations, are valuable.

Nurse administrators in organizations are aware that the objective information rationally gathered and analyzed sometimes conflicts with their intuitive, subjective perceptions. The best managerial decisions incorporate rational and intuitive knowledge. Working in complex organizations involves continuous interaction at both the individual and total organization levels with work groups, departments, and external stakeholders. Comprehending the dynamics of all these interactions simultaneously is impossible. Only through the use of many varied theoretical perspectives can each of the interactions be examined and adequately understood.

Understanding organizations is especially critical today where health care is being viewed less as a public service and more as a private sector, for-profit industry. Health-care organizations are increasingly comprehensive, loosely related, profit-making, and not-for-profit corporations. Organizational expansion has been deregulated and competition has been fostered among health-care organizations, while government health-care subsidies have been drastically reduced. The demand by health-care organizations for nurses with expert knowledge of nursing and management is increasing, while interest in nursing as a career is decreasing. Nursing research is generating increasing evidence that clients need to take a more active role in health care to reduce the leading causes of death and increase their quality of life. Yet health-care organizations have continued to become larger, more impersonal, and only questionably effective in the design of new services for self-responsible adults.

Nurse administrators prepared to effectively deal with social and economic changes and capable of actively participating in decisions concerning health-care service delivery are sorely needed. The multiple theories of organization science can provide valuable insights and assist nurses in their professional practice as care providers, educators, researchers, and administrators.

REFERENCES

1. Larson MS. The rise of professionalism: a sociological analysis. Berkeley, CA: University of California Press, 1977.
2. Mintzberg H. The structuring of organizations. Englewood Cliffs, NJ: Prentice-Hall, 1979.
3. Hitt MA, Ireland RD. Peters and Waterman revisited: the unended quest for excellence. The Academy of Management Executive 1987;1(2):91–98.
4. Stetler C. Research utilization: defining the concept. Image 1985;17(2):40–44.
5. McCloskey JC, Kerfoot K, Molen M, Mathis S. Educating administrators. Nsg & Hlth Care, 1986;7(9):504–509.
6. Gortner H, Mahler J, Nicholson J. Organization theory: a public perspective. Chicago: Dorsey Press, 1987.
7. Morgan G. Images of organizations. Beverly Hills, CA: Sage Publications, 1986.
8. Morgan G. Paradigms, metaphors, and puzzle solving in organization theory. Adm Sci Q 1980;25:605–622.
9. Astley WG, Van de Ven A. Central perspectives and debates in organization theory. Adm Sci Q 1983;28:245–73.
10. AONE. Final Report of the Ad Hoc Committee on Nursing Administration Research. Chicago: American Hospital Association, 1987.
11. McClure M, Poulin M, Sovie M, Wandelt M. Magnet Hospitals. Kansas City, MO: American Nurses Association, 1983.
12. Scott WR. Theoretical perspectives. In: Meyer MW et al eds. Environments and organizations. San Francisco: Jossey Bass, 1978:21–28.
13. Kaalap O. Towards a general theory of managerial decisions: a critical appraisal. SAM Adv Mgmt J 1987:36–42.
14. Kuhn T. The structure of scientific revolutions. 2nd ed. Chicago: The University of Chicago Press, 1970.
15. Lucas R. Political-cultural analysis of organizations. Acad Mgmt Rev 1987;12(1):144–56.
16. Peters TJ, Waterman RH. In search of excellence. New York: Harper & Row, 1982.
17. Perrow C. Complex organizations a critical essay. 3d ed. New York: Random House, 1986.
18. Taylor RN. Behavioral decision making. Glenview, IL: Scott Foresman and Co, 1984.
19. Werley HH, Zuzich A, Zajkowski M, Zagornik A. Health research: the systems approach. New York: Springer Publishing Company, 1976.
20. Calderone GE, Hetherington RW, Williams SR, Lingermann JJ, Hage J. Methods of codification and synthesis of hospital organization research of the

seventies. Annual Meeting American Public Health Association, Medical Care Section, 1983.

21. Alexander JW, Randolph WA. The fit between technology and structure as a predictor of performance in subunits. Acad Mgmt J 1985;28:844–859.

22. Mark B. Task and structural correlates of organizational effectiveness in private psychiatric hospitals. Health Services Research 1985;20(2):199–224.

23. Charns M, Schaefer M. Health Care Organizations. Englewood Cliffs, NJ: Prentice-Hall, 1983.

24. Harmon MM, Mayer RT. Organization theory for public administration. Boston: Little, Brown, 1986.

25. Wieczorek RR, ed: Power, politics and policy in nursing. New York: Springer Publishing Company, 1985.

26. Mason SW, Talbot DJ, eds: Political action handbook for nurses. Menlo Park, CA: Addison-Wesley, 1985.

27. Dienemann J. The power and resources of nursing schools within university settings. Nsg Econ 1987; 5(1):36–41.

28. Mixon PR. Public policy making on a nursing issue. In: Wieczorek RR, ed. Power, politics, and policy in nursing. New York: Springer Publishing, 1985.

29. Coleman JR, Dayani EC, Simms E. Nursing careers in the emerging systems. Nsg Mgmt 1984;15(1):19–27.

30. Kreuger J. Interorganizational relations research in nursing care delivery systems. Annual Rev of Nursing Res 1984;1:155–180.

31. Olson M. The logic of collective action. Cambridge, MA: Harvard University Press, 1965.

32. Miles RE, Snow CC. Organizational strategy, structure, and process. New York: McGraw Hill, 1978.

33. Pinder CC, Bourgeois VW. Controlling tropes in administrative science. Adm Sci Q 1982;27:641–52.

34. Lincoln YS, ed. Organizational theory and inquiry: the paradigm revolution. Beverly Hills, CA: Sage Publications, 1985.

35. Carper BA. Fundamental patterns of knowing in nursing. Adv in Nsg Sci, 1978;1(1):13–23.

17

Structural Contingency Theory

Barbara A. Mark

THIS CHAPTER describes the historical development of structural contingency theory as a major paradigm for knowledge development and theory building in organizational science. Specific concepts incorporated into structural contingency theory are then examined. Finally, a critique of contingency theory is offered, and its utility for knowledge development in nursing administration is addressed.

THE DEVELOPMENT OF STRUCTURAL CONTINGENCY THEORY

Early management theories, the so called "classical" or "scientific management" theories, argued that there was one best way to organize, regardless of the nature of organizational tasks. Over the past 25 years, classical management theory has suffered under increasing criticism and is being supplanted by "structural contingency theory" or more simply "contingency theory." Contingency theory proposed that what constitutes a "good" organizational arrangement will depend on the goals of the organization and the conditions under which the organization is attempting to meet those goals. Implied in such an approach is the idea that organizations, in order to be effective, must develop a structure that is appropriate to organizational tasks and goals and to the environment in which the organization operates.*

Contingency theory originated in the late 1950s when Woodward, a British researcher, attempted to ascertain whether the principles laid down by advocates of scientific management had any relationship to business success.[4,5] One hundred manufacturing firms in southern England were included in the study and were classified in terms of success as below average, average, or above average. Among the factors taken into account in determining the relative success of each firm were profitability, market standing, rate of development and future plans, reputation of the firm in the community, attitudes of management, and rate of supervisory staff turnover.

Woodward first examined the relationship between organizational structure and success, but no consistent pattern emerged. She then classified the firms according to production techniques and complexity of their production systems. "Technical complexity" reflected the degree of control that could be exerted over the production process, as well

*This review will not evaluate the empirical research derived from contingency theory, nor will it address the methodological problems that have lead to inconsistent results. Excellent reviews can be found in Fry[1] and Dalton et al.[2] Neither will this review discuss the conceptual and methodological difficulties inherent in operationalizing the concept of organizational effectiveness. For this, readers are referred to Cameron.[3]

as the predictability of results. The firms were classified according to three types of technology: unit, mass, and process production. An example of a unit production system is the job shop assembling products one at a time; mass production systems include automobile assembly lines; and process production systems include continuous process production such as used in chemical manufacturing.

Woodward found that in each of these classifications, the more successful firms used similar management practices. For example, task fragmentation, role specificity, formality of communication, and use of standard control procedures were all higher in the mass production systems than in either the unit or process production systems. In other words, economic success was associated with the use of management practices that appropriately matched the various techniques of production. Woodward concluded that "different technologies imposed different kinds of demands on individuals and organizations, and these demands had to be met through an appropriate structure." Woodward's study was among the first to question the "one best way to organize" approach of classical management theory. Further, through Woodward's findings, the argument was advanced that technology, defined in terms of the degree of complexity of the production process, was a determinant of organizational structure. In other words, organizational structure was "contingent" upon technology.

In another British study, Burns and Stalker[6] focused on how internal management practices were related to rates of change in the scientific techniques and markets of selected industries. Two polar ideal types of management systems were identified: the mechanistic system and the organic system. The mechanistic system was observed in those firms where conditions were relatively stable and was characterized by the breakdown of tasks into small subtasks, which were often pursued distinctly from the tasks of the

organization as a whole. In addition, these subtasks and the techniques and responsibilities for carrying them out were clearly and precisely spelled out; communication tended to be vertical, that is, between superior and subordinate, and behavior was governed primarily by directives issued by superiors. Loyalty and obedience toward superiors was highly regarded.

In contrast, an organic management system was observed where changing conditions gave rise to fresh problems and unforeseen requirements for action and was characterized by the "contributive nature" of knowledge and experience needed to perform tasks that were understood in the context of the organization's total task. There was continual interaction with others. Communication tended to be lateral, resembling consultation rather than command, and focused on information sharing rather than on issuing directives. Finally, commitment to the "technological ethos" was more valued than loyalty and obedience.

In their conclusion, Burns and Stalker stated that they had

endeavored to stress the appropriateness of each system to its own specific set of conditions. Equally, we desire to avoid the suggestion that either system is superior under all circumstances to the other (Burns and Stalker,[6] p. 125).

Again, the "one best way to organize" approach of classical management theory was called into question. Burns and Stalker, in focusing on the environment, increased the explanatory sophistication of the contingency argument by suggesting that organizational structure was also contingent on the nature of the organizational environment.

In the first U.S. study using contingency theory, Lawrence and Lorsch[7] studied 10 firms and investigated the relationship between effectiveness, environmental characteristics, and states of differentiation and integration. Differentiation arises from the "difference in cognitive and emotional orientation among managers in different functional departments" (Lawrence and Lorsch, [9] p. 11). Differentiation has four dimensions: the degree of investment in particular functional goals (marketing, production, or research); the degree to which managers emphasize "getting the job done" or maintaining peer relationships; the degree to which managers are concerned with short, medium, or long-range issues; and the formality of the organizational structure.

When the state of differentiation exists in an organization, there arises a need for integration; and the states of differentiation and integration in an organization are antagonistic. Integration is the "quality of the state of collaboration that exists among departments that are required to achieve unity of effort" (Lawrence and Lorsch,[7] p. 11). The higher the degree of differentiation between departments, the more difficult it is to achieve integration. If an organization is highly differentiated and not sufficiently integrated, departments tend to develop and highlight their own goals, and these can take precedence over superordinate organizational goals. In addition, if an organization is too highly differentiated, departments can build strong internal boundaries that can lead to an unproductive level of conflict.

Lawrence and Lorsch found that in each industry, (plastics, frozen foods, and containers) highly successful firms had achieved a degree of integration that was appropriate to their level of differentiation. The high-performing plastics organization functioned in the most dynamic and diverse of the three environments, and was the most highly differentiated of the three high-performing organizations. Since turbulent environmental conditions created major problems in maintaining integration, the plastics organization had developed an elaborate set of formal devices—an integrating unit and cross-functional teams—to facilitate conflict resolution and the achievement of integration. In marked contrast, the high-performing container organization operated in a much more stable, less diverse environment. Its functional units were less differentiated and the only formal integrating device required was the managerial hierarchy (Lawrence and Lorsch,[7] pp. 151–158).

To summarize at this point, the research done by Lawrence and Lorsch provided additional confirmation for Burns and Stalker's[6] conclusion that effective organizations operating in environments of high uncertainty require markedly different internal organizational structures than those organizations operating in relatively placid environments. While the studies just reviewed focus on technology and environment as deterministic variables, the rest of this chapter will focus on a further exploration of the concept of technology and its place in contingency theory.

ANALYSIS OF CONCEPTS IN CONTINGENCY THEORY

This section will describe two of the critical concepts in research employing the contingency argument as its theoretical base: organizational technology and structure.

Technology

According to structural contingency theory, one determinant of organizational structure is organizational technology. Technology encompasses several dimensions describing the nature of a given task. In the context of contingency theory, "task" refers not to an individual job, but to the broad range and totality of jobs that contribute to the achievement of organizational goals.

One of the earliest definitions of technology was Perrow's:

The actions that an individual performs upon an object, with or without the aid of tools or mechanical devices, in order to make some change in that object. The object, or "raw material" may be a living being, human or otherwise, a symbol, or an inanimate object (Perrow,[8] p. 195).

Three aspects of technology identified by Perrow are particularly important to an understanding of contingency theory. The first is the number of exceptional cases encountered in the work, or task variability, which is the degree to which "stimuli are perceived as familiar or unfamiliar" (Perrow,[8] pp. 195–196; Van de Ven and Ferry[9]). The second aspect, task difficulty, refers to the analyzability and predictability of the search process undertaken when exceptions (problems) occur. At one extreme is the situation calling for a programmed search that is completed on a logical, analytical basis. At the other extreme, the search arises from a problem that is vague enough to make the task "virtually unanalyzable." In this case, one draws upon the "residue of unanalyzed experience or intuition, or relies upon chance and guesswork" (Perrow,[8] p. 196).

The nature of raw material essential in a task is another important aspect of technology identified by Perrow. If the raw material is well understood, predictability increases and the potential for organizational control also increases. In addition, if the raw material is stable and does not vary, it can be treated in a standardized fashion, whereas if the raw material is highly variable, nonstable, and poorly understood, "continual adjustment" is necessary.

Thompson[10] discussed another critical technological dimension—interdependence. Interdependence refers to the degree to which individuals or organizational subunits are dependent on one another to complete their work. Interdependence is "pooled" when each part of an organization provides a discrete contribution to the achievement of organizational goals. Sequential interdependence results when the outputs of one part of an organization provide inputs to another part of the organization. The most complex type of interdependence, reciprocal interdependence, results when the outputs of each unit become inputs for others. Pooled, sequential, and reciprocal interdependence are increasingly difficult to coordinate because they contain increasing degrees of contingency for organizational units.

Coordination of unit interdependence is accomplished in the hospital setting through mutual adjustments among the diverse professional groups involved in patients' care and often takes the form of intense political activity.[11] In an ongoing series of studies that clearly illustrate the utility of the contingency approach for nursing administration research, a group of Canadian researchers[12–16] has been studying the technology and organization of nursing subunits. In their first study, one of the major purposes was to determine if nursing subunits could be differentiated on the basis of their task characteristics, or their degree of technological indeterminacy. The researchers developed and factor analyzed a questionnaire about the tasks of nursing units. A varimax rotation resulted in a three-factor solution.

The first factor, labeled uncertainty, referred to indeterminacy arising out of the inability to posit specific cause and effect relationships between the work and its outcomes. Items in this scale included the degree to which patients presented multiple and complex problems, the work involved analyzing complex problems, the work required the use of intuition, and techniques quickly became obsolete. The second factor, instability, dealt with the frequency and magnitude of moment-to-moment changes in patients' conditions. Items included the number of emergencies and nursing observations required, and the extent to which work involved technical procedures and equipment; it was directed at patients' physical rather than psychosocial needs. Variability, the last factor, tapped the frequency and magnitude of patient-to-patient differences. Variability included the extent to which patients had dissimilar health problems, nursing care procedures were dissimilar for most patients, patients and their families were included in planning for their care, and day-to-day decisions were repetitive.

Using the Q-technique, the investigators clustered the nursing units into categories based on their degree of technological indeterminacy. Three categories resulted, with pediatric, obstetrical, rehabilitation, and surgical units falling into the first category. In the second category were the auxiliary and psychiatric units, and in the third category were the intensive care units. Category three, containing the intensive care units, was the highest in technological indeterminacy, arising from high levels of uncertainty and instability regarding patients' conditions and uncertainty in nursing techniques. The second category, containing psychiatric and auxiliary units, had moderate levels of technological indeterminacy.

The ability to empirically distinguish one type of nursing unit from another based on a valid categorization of the kind of work done has numerous implications for nurse administrators. Questions might include: What level of decentralization of clinical decision making is most appropriate for a nursing unit with a very high level of task uncertainty, and how does this contrast with the level of decision making on a unit with a low level of uncertainty? Is there a particular skill mix that is more appropriate to one type of nursing unit than another, and does knowledge of unit technology accurately predict these differences? Despite the relevance of these questions, problems related to the technology of nursing units have not yet been addressed.

Organizational Structure

The primary premise underlying contingency theory is that organizational structure must be appropriate to the nature of an organization's task and its environment.[4,5,7–9,17–20] Thompson defined structure as the "internal differentiation and patterning of relationships" by which the organization sets limits and boundaries for efficient performance by "delimiting responsibilities, control over resources, and other matters" (Thompson,[10] pp. 51–54). Structure has also been defined as the "relatively enduring allocation of work roles and administrative mechanisms that allows the organization to conduct, coordinate, and control its work activities" (Jackson and Morgan,[21] p. 87). Organizational structure in general refers to the administrative mechanisms that are developed in an attempt to balance a necessary degree of coordination with specialization of work roles, thus enabling the organization to accomplish its tasks.

In an early empirical study, Pugh and colleagues[20] identified five primary dimensions of organizational structure: specialization, standardization, formalization, centralization, and configuration. The structural dimensions used most frequently in research are centralization, formalization, and standardization.

Centralization is defined as the "locus of authority to make decisions affecting the organization"[20] (p. 76). Later authors[22] have suggested that as tasks become more complex and uncertain and require increased information processing, decision making should occur at lower levels in the organization—near the point where organization members have the requisite information on which to base decisions.

Formalization indicates the extent to which "rules, procedures, instructions, and communications are written"[20] (p. 75) and reflects the degree to which work expectations are clear and explicit. Formalization generally is thought to decrease as technological complexity increases, since as predictability of outcomes decreases, complete specification of the means and ends of work become more ambiguous.

Standardization refers to the extent to which the organization has "standard operating procedures" to be followed in accomplishing organizational tasks. Standardization, as with centralization and formalization, is hypothesized to be inversely related to technological complexity: as the complexity of an organization increases, standardization tends to decrease.

Research focusing on the relationship of technology and organizational structure to organizational effectiveness generally hypothesizes that highly bureaucratic structures—those characterized by high levels of centralization, standardization, and formalization—are most often found in organizations characterized by routine work that is not particularly difficult, and tends not to vary to any great degree, and where individual organization members are not dependent on one another to complete their tasks. When work is less routine, the hypothesis is that one is likely to find an organizational structure that is more flexible, less hierarchical, and less highly formalized. In other words, as technological complexity increases, effectiveness is a function of decreasing levels of centralization, formalization, and standardization.

CRITIQUE OF CONTINGENCY THEORY AND IMPLICATIONS FOR NURSING ADMINISTRATION RESEARCH

Historically, contingency theory grew out of a reaction to the rigid "one best way" approach advocated by the proponents of the scientific management school. The implication of contingency theory, arising out of Woodward's[4,5] research, was that rather than there being "one best way" for all organizations to be designed and structured, the structure of organizations is dependent—that is, contingent—on the nature of its technology, and if

an appropriate "fit" or "match" does not exist between an organization's technology and structure, the organization sacrifices its effectiveness.

Schoonhoven[23] has called attention to a lack of conceptual clarity in contingency arguments, particularly with regard to the failure to define unambiguously such key terms as "appropriate," "consonance," and "fit." The bulk of research based on contingency theory has used either the "environment" or "technology" as the variable posing the contingency. However, even these terms have often been defined imprecisely. Consequently, research has yielded conflicting results.

Problems have also resulted from the failure to identify interaction among the variables. In addition, linearity of the relationships between technology (or environment), structure, and effectiveness has often been assumed but has rarely been tested.[23] Contingency theory, as its label implies, utilizes contingent propositions, in which "a conditional association of two or more independent variables with a dependent outcome" is hypothesized (Van de Ven and Drazin,[24] p. 514). Such contingent propositions imply the existence of an empirical interaction. However, the form of that interaction is rarely specified. Schoonhoven[23] suggests that there are several possible specifications for this interaction. The first, a muliplicative interaction, implying that organizational effectiveness (the dependent variable) is a function of the presence of both technology and structure (the independent variables). A second form of interaction, a maximizing interaction, suggests that for every value of the technological variable ($X1$), there is a unique structural value ($X2$) that maximizes effectiveness (Y). The importance of prior specification of fit becomes critical in the operationalization of the variables, the statement of hypotheses, and the statistical manipulations used in analyzing data.

Schoonhoven[23] also suggests that researchers often do not recognize that the relationships being predicted by contingency theory are symmetrical. In other words, a low value of a structural dimension (decentralization, destandardization), occurring with a low value of a technological (or environmental) variable, should produce effective organizations. Thus, one could argue that an organization in which a low level of decentralization (a high level of centralization) matches its low level of technological or environmental uncertainty will be more effective than the more decentralized organization with a similar level of uncertainty. Schoonhoven derives three specific propositions from this general theoretical proposition:

1. The impact of decentralization on effectiveness is nonmonotonic over the range of uncertainty.

In other words, decentralization should have a different impact on effectiveness depending on the level of technological (or environmental) uncertainty.

Furthermore,

2. In lower uncertainty subunits, increases in decentralization will negatively influence effectiveness.

And

3. In higher uncertainty subunits, increases in decentralization will positively influence effectiveness (Schoonhoven,[23] pp. 353–354).

Some of my own research[25] has examined the relationship of organizational structure and technology to organizational effectiveness in psychiatric hospitals. The structural variables studied were centralization, formalization, and standardization; the technological variables were task difficulty, task variability, and task interdependence.[8,9] Two measures of organizational effectiveness were used: patient care and administrative effectiveness.

The results of that study provided limited support for contingency theory since centralization and standardization were found to exert different impacts on effectiveness depending on the level of task difficulty. Using a multiplicative interaction specification, at higher levels of task difficulty, centralization had a negative impact on patient care effectiveness. In other words, patient care effectiveness was enhanced by the existence of a highly centralized decision-making structure when task difficulty was high, but a high level of centralization decreased effectiveness when task difficulty was low. While this finding is consistent with Schoonhoven's argument of nonmonotonicity, it is not consistent with the assumption of symmetry in contingency theory. The symmetrical property would have been confirmed if, at high levels of task difficulty, a decentralized decision-making structure had enhanced effectiveness.

The findings on standardization, however, supported both the nonmonotonic and the symmetrical assumptions, since at higher levels of task difficulty, standardization was found to have a negative impact on administrative effectiveness, while at the lower range of task difficulty, standardization had a positive impact on effectiveness. Again, inconsistent findings illustrate some of the difficulties encountered when using the contingency approach in research.

In conclusion, this chapter has reviewed the development of structural contingency theory and has examined two of its major concepts: technology and organizational structure. A series of studies using the contingency approach to examine the technology of nursing subunits was described briefly to illustrate the utility of the approach for nursing administration research.

There is little question that managing the provision of clinical patient care in a formal organizational setting is a task that is becoming more and more complex. Not infrequently in the literature for nurse administrators, what is written is prescriptive yet atheoretical. Solutions are offered regarding management strategies, and ways of structuring the organization of nursing units and departments; yet these suggestions are made without systematic and fundamental knowledge of organizational characteristics. Contingency theory certainly has major flaws. Whether it is correctly called a theory can even be questioned. However, it provides researchers in nursing administration with a useful framework to guide the study of relationships between organizational technology, structure, and effectiveness. The information gained from such studies clearly contributes to the development of fundamental knowledge in nursing administration.

REFERENCES

1. Fry L. "Technology-structure research: three critical issues." Academy of Management Journal 1982;25:532–552.
2. Dalton D, Todor W, Spendalini M, Fielding G, Porter L. Organization structure and performance: a critical review. Academy of Management Review 1980;5:49–64.
3. Cameron K. Effectiveness as paradox: consensus and conflict in conceptions of organizational effectiveness. Management Science 1986;32:539–553.
4. Woodward J. Management and technology. London: Her Majesty's Stationary Office, 1958.
5. Woodward J. Industrial organization: theory and practice. London: Oxford Press, 1965.
6. Burns T, Stalker G. The management of innovation. London: Tavistock, 1961.
7. Lawrence P, Lorsch J. Organization and environment. Boston: Harvard University Press, 1967.
8. Perrow C. Hospitals: technology, structure and goals. In: March J, ed. Handbook of Organizations. Rand McNally, 1965, pp. 909–971.
9. Van de Ven A, Ferry D. Measuring and Assessing Organizations. New York: Wiley-Interscience, 1980.
10. Thompson J. Organizations in Action. New York: McGraw-Hill, 1967.
11. Bucher R, Stelling J. Characteristics of professional organizations. Journal of Health and Social Behavior 1969; 10:3–15.
12. Overton P, Schneck R, Hazlett C. An empirical study of the technology of nursing subunits. Adm Sci Q 1977;22:203–219.
13. Leatt P, Schneck R. Nursing subunit technology: a replication. Adm Sci Q 1981;26:225–286.
14. Leatt P, Schneck R. Technology, size, environment, and structure in nursing subunits. Organization Studies 1982a;3:331–342.
15. Leatt P, Schneck R. Work environments of different types of nursing subunits. Adv Nurs 1982b;7:581–594.
16. Leatt P, Schneck R. Sources and management of organizational stress in nursing subunits in Canada. Organization Studies. 1985;6:55–79.
17. Child J. Organization structure and strategies of control: a replication of the Aston study. Adm Sci Q 1972;17:163–176.
18. Child J, Mansfield, R. Technology, size, organizational structure. Sociology 1972;6:369–393.
19. Pugh DC, Hickson D, Hinings C, Turner C. Dimensions of organizational structure. Adm Science Q 1968a;13:62–70.
20. Pugh D. The context of organizational structures. Adm Science Q 1968b;14:110–117.
21. Jackson J, Morgan C. Organization theory. Englewood Cliffs, NJ; Prentice Hall, 1978.
22. Galbraith J. Organization design. Reading MA: Addison-Wesley, 1977.
23. Schoonhoven C. Problems with contingency theory: the assumptions hidden within the language of contingency theory. Adm Sci Q 1981;26:349–377.
24. Drazin R, Van de Ven A. Alternative forms of fit in contingency theory. Adm Sci Q 1985;30:514–539.
25. Mark B. Task and structural correlate of organizational effectiveness in private psychiatric hospitals. Health Services Research 1985;20:199–224.

18

The Coalignment Model and Its Usefulness for Nurse Administrators and Educators

Cecilia Gibbons
Sharon Krajnak

CONCEPTUALIZING policies, objectives, and goals, then developing them into plans of action, and implementing them in programs are essential functions of effective nurse administrators.[1] In the hierarchical structure of today's organizations, the nursing service administrator has the ultimate responsibility for all patient care activities in a nursing division. Ensuring the quality of care provided by nursing staff requires the commitment of nurse administrators to staff development programs that promote and enhance the competence of care providers. As leaders, nurse administrators and directors of staff development need to align their purposes, philosophies, and goals with those of the total organization and the communities served.

The purpose of this chapter is to describe Kotter and Lawrence's[2] coalignment model of administrative behavior and the usefulness of this model for assessing both nurse administrators and educators in their effort to promote quality care. Understanding and using the coalignment model facilitates analysis of behaviors that contribute to effective decisions, actions, and outcomes.

Administrative theory has evolved through at least three phases. During the first, beginning approximately in 1895, Taylor[3] formulated the theory of scientific management that focused on efficiency and productivity. The next phase, beginning about 1927 with Mayo's Hawthorne studies of working conditions, was known as the human relations period. The third phase began in the early 1940s, and subsequently the focus has largely been on systems analysis and contingency theory.[4] Nurses have developed several administrative models using theories that evolved during these three periods.

The coalignment model, grounded in contingency and systems theories, was formulated by Kotter and Lawrence, social scientists at Harvard, in an exploratory investigation of the behavior of elected city officials. In 1979, Henry began adapting the coalignment model for nursing service administration. Using coalignment theory she examined the administrative behaviors of staff nurses in hospitals.[5] Since 1981, many graduate students in the nursing administration program at the University of Alabama in Birmingham have used the coalignment model to analyze nurses' administrative behaviors and the impact of those behaviors on services and organizations.

THE COALIGNMENT MODEL

The coalignment perspective described as a morphogenic systems model, provides a blueprint whereby the context and activities of an administrator can be examined systematically. Focusing on structure, process, and outcome, and the changes in each over time, coalignment theory describes four contextual variables: administrators and their agendas, networks, and organizational units. In brief, coalignment theory suggests that administrative behavior can take on a number of forms in three key processes: agenda setting, network building, and task accomplishing. The four contextual variables and behaviors in three processes are connected in a complex system of interdependencies. These interdependencies can be broken down into relationships between the behaviors in the three processes and among the contextual variables. The actions administrators take in the three processes have a direct impact on the contextual variables; and the context provides resources and constrains behavior.[6] The model also describes dynamics among the contextual variables. In the model, coalignment exists when there is a fit, that is, when there is alignment among all four of the contextual variables. In Table 18.1 the key elements in coalignment theory are outlined.

The three action (process) and four contextual (structure) variables are discussed in the following sections. How we use each variable in analysis of administrative behavior is also described. Our use of coalignment theory is based on the premise that to adequately understand the outcomes of management requires an understanding of managers themselves, their activities, and the context in which their actions take place (the contingencies of their behavior).

ADMINISTRATIVE ACTIVITIES IN THREE PROCESSES

Agenda Setting

Agenda setting is the process by which an individual decides what he or she will do. It encompasses determining short-, medium-, and long-range goals.[7] The manner in which agendas are set varies in each situation and with each individual. In some work situations, there is very little opportunity for creative agenda setting—in situations, for example, that are rigidly governed by numerous regulations. In others, agendas are dictated by supervisors. And in others, managers simply may wish to select agenda items from the continuous flow of requests and ideas they are confronted with on a daily basis.

According to Kotter and Lawrence, agenda setting behaviors can be disjointed and incremental—oriented primarily toward the short run or individual, and sometimes irrationally unconnected.[8] Administrators who set their agendas incrementally have agendas that are generated most often by crisis. Short-run agendas are best where managers are sensitive to immediate problems, are concerned with maintenance rather than with change, and where managers want to have few complications with members in their networks.

TABLE 18.1   Structure, Process, and Outcome Elements in Coalignment Theory

Structure	Process	Outcome
Administrator	Agenda setting	System stability
Agenda	Network building	Administrative effectiveness
Network	Task accomplishing	Administrator survival
Organizational unit		Consumer satisfaction

Short-run agendas, however, create problems because future events are not anticipated and signs of trouble are ignored.[9]

The converse of short-range, reactive, incremental agenda setting is proactive, middle- to long-range agenda setting characterized as holistic and logically interconnected.[10] Functioning as rational planners, administrators develop agendas that are logical and that detail long-term objectives and strategies. Setting long-range agendas requires a high level of technical expertise, and an orientation toward the future. Agendas for the medium- and long-range produce larger changes in the environment, and cause more short-run tensions and complications with network members.[11]

Task Accomplishing

Kotter and Lawrence identify three approaches that are used by managers in their efforts to accomplish the tasks defined in their agendas. The approaches are bureaucratic, entrepreneurial, and individualistic.

When getting a task done "bureaucratically," a manager directs, controls, delegates, and evaluates using all of his or her formal organizational authority. Bureaucratic behavior requires that a manager understand fully the agenda items that need to be addressed; understand the organization and its available resources; possess the administrative skill required to delegate tasks; and know when delegation can be properly exercised.[12]

The manager accomplishing tasks like an "entrepreneur" hustles, creates, and attempts to enlist the aid of others.[13] Formal authority is not used, indeed the manager may not even have much authority. In the entrepreneurial mode, administrators attempt to influence others to assist them in the accomplishment of agenda tasks. To act entrepreneurially, the manager needs to be imaginative and have a wide range of interpersonal skills, as well as

an intimate understanding of the tasks that need to be done.

In the "individualistic" mode, the manager needs only personal time, energy, and resources to accomplish tasks. There is no delegation of responsibilities, nor is there any significant attempt to gain the assistance of others.[14]

According to Kotter and Lawrence, the most effective administrators use all three approaches to accomplish tasks effectively, as circumstance and judgment demand.[15] To mobilize the largest number of resources and have the greatest impact, effective administrators know when to use their official authority, when to act alone, and when to market and sell their ideas.[15]

Network Building

To function effectively and accomplish objectives, administrators and educators must build and maintain networks of positive, cooperative relationships with peers and other organizational members—people who are interdisciplinary health-care providers, workers in ancillary departments, and consumers, or potential consumers in communities.

The nine network-building processes described by Kotter and Lawrence provide a way of understanding how individuals cooperate with one another. Each of the processes is somewhat different and is based on different criteria, established through different behaviors, and has slightly different effects.[16] As depicted in Table 18.2, the network-building processes include: the "utilitarian," in which two parties negotiate an exchange of what each wants for the resources controlled by the other; coercion, where the threat of punishment is used to force the cooperation of others; purposive appeal, where a coalition is formed of people working for or against a common goal; "personal or reference group appeal," where relationships depend on

TABLE 18.2 Network Building Processes

Processes	Prerequisites	Advantages	Disadvantages
Utilitarian	Resources to exchange Network members willing to exchange Negotiation skills	Concrete obligations Low risk	Can be very expensive
Coercion	Network members who allow themselves to be coerced	Quick action Low cost	Risky
Purposive for	Medium- and long-range plans Viable network Communication system	Continuous power generation	Eventual performance production Decreases planning flexibility
Purposive against	Planned continuous effort	Inexpensive Short-range results	Difficult to maintain
Cooptative	Medium- and long-range plans	Inexpensive	Decreases agenda control. May cause conflict and instability
Reference group appeal	Members must feel part of the group. Is effective if you have been a group member.	Inexpensive Safe	None
Friendship	Influential powerful friends. Gregarious personality	Low risk	Time consuming
Charismatic appeal	Charisma	Low risk	None
Formal-Legal Appeal	Rules and regulations Members must perceive legitimate authority	No maintenance	May decrease cooperative effort between members

(Based on Kotter JP, and Lawrence P. Mayors in action. p. 78.)
Adapted from Kotter JP, Lawrence PR. Mayors in action. New York: John Wiley and Sons, 1974, p. 78.

friendship, charismatic appeal, and similar positions; "cooptation," the deliberate addition of people to groups to exact their cooperation; and "formal-legal appeal" where authority is granted by policy or law permitting one person to direct the actions of another.[17–18]

The strongest networks exist where multiple networking processes are employed; and where administrators use each of the processes correctly.

Administrative Contexts

The context in which administrators work affects behavior which in turn is affected by it. The four contextual variables and the major aspects of each, are as outlined:[19]

Individual Administrator
    Cognitive and interpersonal skills
    Needs and drives, values and aspirations
    Personality
Network
    Subcultural traits
    Type and strength of relationships
    Resources available
    Expectations
Agenda
    Short-, medium-, and long-run tasks
Organizational Unit
    Size
    Rate of change
    Location
    Homogeneity
    Administrator's domain
    Nature of interdependent systems

In an adaptation of Kotter and Lawrence's model, Henry examined nurse administrators, their agendas, networks, and organizational units.[20] As noted, the stability of a system and survival of system members are dependent on the degree of alignment or "fit" among the contextual variables.[21]

USING COALIGNMENT THEORY TO ANALYZE ADMINISTRATIVE BEHAVIOR

Using the coalignment model, in the remainder of this chapter an analysis of the administrative behavior of a nurse administrator and staff development director is provided to illustrate the applicability of the model for the evaluation of practice. In the illustrations, the four administrative contexts are described first. Two select administrative behaviors are then described, analyzed, and evaluated in terms of the three key processes and the impact of behaviors in these processes on alignment.

Case 1: Opening a New Unit

The Nurse Administrator

The administrator is master's-prepared in nursing administration with 15 years of progressive managerial experience in a variety of settings. Her clinical background is in medical surgical nursing. She is an energetic, serious individual who has been in her present position for three years. The administrator communicates openly and assertively with others, and values excellence in clinical and administrative practice. Her primary aspiration is to develop a nursing service department that is recognized in the community as progressive and committed to the provision of quality care. Overall, the administrator's total performance is that of a perceptive manager totally aware of what is happening in the nursing department and throughout the medical center.

Agenda

Included in the administrator's agenda are short-, medium-, and long-range plans. Short-range plans are accomplished on a daily or weekly basis. Typical activities include planning the agenda for the weekly nurse executive committee meeting, reviewing weekly nursing budget reports, making daily nursing unit rounds, and meeting with the president of the medical staff. Medium-range plans, which are accomplished within a month to a year, include: recruiting for a vacant clinical nursing specialist position, evaluating a proposed clinical-ladder program, planning the annual nursing administrative retreat, and planning and implementing the reopening of a closed nursing unit following final renovation. Long-range plans require at least one year or longer for completion. Typical of these plans are: ongoing development or revision of standards of nursing practice with appropriate quality assurance monitors; planning and implementing the opening of a new clinical addition to the medical center; evaluating the nursing component in the medical center's marketing program; and ongoing analysis of nursing's cost containment program. Short- and medium-range agendas are primarily based on the annual nursing service goals. Long-range agendas originate from the medical center's five-year plan.

Network

An extensive, strong network provides the nurse administrator with valuable resources to accomplish the tasks in her agenda. Primary network members are people in the medical center and nursing department such as hospital administrators, department heads, nurse managers, and staff. These network members are the key to the administrator's success since they provide her with the essential resources—the information, assistance, and support she needs to accomplish the goals in her agendas. The quality of the resources network members provide has a direct impact on the administrator's agenda.

Generally, the nurse administrator enjoys strong, positive relationships with both her superiors and subordinates. She is well-respected by network members for her diligence and dedication to the nursing department. People in her network expect the nurse administrator to be assertive in matters affecting the nursing department.

Outside the medical center, the nurse administrator has developed strong, cooperative networks with individuals and groups representing other institutions and consumers. This large, heterogeneous network provides a ready supply of valuable resources. A council of citywide nurse administrators comprises her primary, external network. Through members of this network, she is able to compare her nursing department with others in the city in relation to recruitment and retention of nursing personnel, marketing efforts, and nursing practices. She is a member of the National Organization of Nurse Executives, part of the American Hospital Association. Attending national meetings further affords the nurse administrator with an opportunity to expand her network. The primary benefits include valuable information, advice, and friendship.

Other external professional networks include members of the state nurses' association, the state board of nursing, and community nursing-home directors. Members of these networks provide the administrator with essential information about community, state, and national policies and laws that affect the nursing department. Through members of these networks, nurse administrators can have an impact on the formation and implementation of policies affecting nursing.

All members of the nurse administrator's network possess, to some degree, similar traits indicative of the southern American culture. These traits generally affect how the network members interact with one another. An awareness of how this culture affects the relationships between network members aides the administrator in building and maintaining positive, cooperative networks.

Organizational Unit

The nurse administrator, in our case, practices at a 500-bed university-affiliated, regional medical center located in a large metropolitan city with a population of approximately 100,000. Serving a six-county area of two southern states, the medical center's primary service area is comprised of 200,000 individuals living in mostly rural areas. The medical center is a general medical-surgical hospital offering a broad spectrum of specialty services. Twenty thousand patients are treated and cared for annually by 1600 personnel and an active medical staff of 180 physicians. The nonprofit hospital receives funding from both city and county taxation and is governed by a board of trustees. Responsibility for the various hospital departments is divided between four executive vice-presidents who report to a chief executive officer.

One of three hospitals in the city, the medical center, serves as the primary teaching facility for the university's medical and nursing schools. Major employers of the resident population are two large, industrial complexes located on the cities perimeter.

Within the medical center, the decentralized nursing department is the largest employer, with over 700 employees. Administrative staff include, in addition to the nurse administrator, six divisional directors (including the staff development director), and 18 head nurses.

With the administrator as chairperson, a nursing council comprised of clinical nurse specialists, instructors, the infection control nurse, and the quality assurance coordinator, serves as the body from which major nursing-practice decisions emanate. Problem solving and decision making is encumbered somewhat by the large size of the council. The total nursing staff is comprised of registered nurses (40%); licensed practical nurses (28%); and nurse assistants, monitor technicians, and ward clerks (32%).

Administrative Behaviors

In Table 18.3, two administrative behaviors related to the opening of a new patient-care unit are described. The first four columns describe the behavior in each of the three key processes. In the final column, the impact of the behavior on alignment is analyzed and evaluated.

Case 2: Planning a Nurse Internship Program

The Staff Development Director

Many years of educational experience in both academic and service settings, and master's degrees in nursing and education have prepared the director to administer the staff development division. Her clinical background includes experience in critical care and emergency nursing. She has had administrative experience as a head nurse of a surgical intensive care unit. She is a highly motivated, enthusiastic individual who has been in her present position for four years. Under her management, the division's reputation as a provider of quality educational programs has improved significantly in the hospital and in the community. She organizes effectively and demonstrates expertise and skill in the division's varied educational programs.

Development of programs that support the provision of quality patient care is the director's primary aspiration. Programs are designed to reflect the purpose, philosophy, and goals of the nursing department. Overall, the director's performance is that of a highly effective, creative administrator who has the respect of both managerial and clinical staff.

TABLE 18.3   Analysis of the Behavior of a Nurse Administrator

Behavior	Agenda Setting	Network Building	Task Accomplishment	Analysis
Walks to nursing unit undergoing renovation to meet with unit head nurse and vice-president in charge of construction to discuss opening of the unit. Tours the units and finds numerous items needing correction. Calls these to the attention of workers.	*Short:* Identifies aspects of renovation requiring immediate attention and decides on further conversations with the executive council regarding problems. *Medium Range:* Determines staffing needs, time, and sequence to return nurses to the unit. *Long Range:* Determines projected long-term staffing needs, and requirements for capital equipment.	*Utilitarian:* When pressed to open the unit as soon as possible, she agrees that staffing is adequate and the only incomplete renovations are those not essential for patient care. *Purposive:* Enlists the support of the head nurse and vice-president to provide a unit designed and equipped to provide quality care.	*Individualistic:* Uses time and energy to personally monitor the progress of the renovation. Forms her own opinion of the ability of workers to have tasks accomplished by the deadline date. *Bureaucratic:* Understands the needs of the nursing department, and delegates to the unit head nurse the responsibility for assessing staffing needs and determining how quickly previous staff members can be reassigned to the new unit.	These behaviors are effective for strengthening the cooperative relationships among the nurse administrator, and her agenda, network, and organizational unit. But the possibility of some misalignment exists. Although the administrator is responsible for the unit's planning and operation, she is not responsible for the actual construction. A negative response by workers to her criticism and suggestions would indicate a misalignment in her network relationships. If she oversteps her lines of authority, the possibility of a misalignment with her peer network exists.
		Personal Appeal: Fosters a spirit of cooperation by speaking to and encouraging maintenance and construction workers to work as quickly and as efficiently as possible. *Formal-Legal:* Uses her legitimate authority to decide when the nursing unit will be opened.	*Entrepreneurial:* Using interpersonal skills, encourages employees working on completion of the renovation to be as time conscious as possible, and to do a good job in order to avoid complications when the unit opens.	
Meets with chief executive officer and other administrative vice-presidents.	*Short:* Shares information concerning hospitalization and conditions of employees. *Middle:* Gathers data regarding opening of renovated wards. Shares departmental concerns and receives input from others related to their areas of responsibility. *Long Range:* Identifies problems that will affect the future development and functioning of nursing service.	*Purposive:* Used in the finalization of plans to open renovated wards. *Utilitarian:* Used in effecting compromise when negotiating dates for reopening wards. *Personal Appeal:* Used when stressing need to complete all renovations and staff reassignments before reopening.	*Bureaucratic:* Shares in decision-making activities of executive council. *Entrepreneurial:* Effectively solicits help when negotiating the reopening of one ward and the closing of another.	The administrator's behaviors strengthen the relationships between the key members in her context and fosters alignment between herself, her agenda, network, and organizational unit.

Agenda

Short-, medium-, and long-range plans are included in the director's agenda. Her short-range (daily and weekly) plans typically include planning the weekly education staff meeting, conducting evaluation conferences with affiliating nursing students, and providing consultation for members of a workshop planning committee. Medium-range (one to twelve month) plans are based on the annual goals of the nursing department and the education division. They include items such as initiating an annual nursing-school affiliation planning meeting and developing specific standards of nursing education practice with appropriate quality assurance monitors. Long-range (one to five year) plans are derived from the nursing department's five-year plan. Attaining accreditation of the division by the National Accreditation Board of the American Nurses' Association as a coprovider of continuing education, and implementing new major programs such as a nurse internship program, are two items in the director's long-range agenda.

Network

The primary members of the director's network are employed in the medical center and nursing department. These network members include her own education staff (instructors and clinical nurse specialists) and hospital and nurse administrators. Each network member provides the director with essential resources to accomplish the plans in her agenda. For example, divisional directors and the quality assurance coordinator keep her informed about the nursing staff's learning needs on which future education efforts will be based.

Like the administrator, the director has strong, positive relationships with her superiors and subordinates. Mutual respect characterizes these relationships and engenders cooperation between members. She is sought out as a consultant by many hospital employees who expect her to offer assistance willingly.

The director has developed extensive external networks representing organizations and institutions at the local, state, and national levels. She is an active member of a citywide group of hospital educators. This organization provides members with opportunities to share information about educational programs and resources, including workshops, consultants, speakers, and audiovisual materials. The educator group is an arm of the American Society for Healthcare Educators and Trainers of the American Hospital Association.

Other external professional network members include people in the local chapter of Sigma Theta Tau, the state nurses' association, clinical speciality organizations, the American Heart Association, and the American Red Cross. Another primary external network is the dean and faculty at the university and technical schools of nursing affiliated with her hospital. The director's relationship with members of this academic network has a direct impact on the nursing department's recruitment efforts. Since this network provides the director with a forum for sharing with educators, the director is able to have an impact on the skills of nurses who are new graduates.

Organization Unit

As one of five divisions in the nursing department of the medical center, the education division is primarily responsible for the orientation, inservice, and continuing education of all nursing personnel. Responsibility for these functions on a centralized and decentralized basis in each division is divided among four nursing instructors and four clinical nurse specialists. Because the medical center is a multispecialty, university-affiliated hospital, education programs need to meet a variety of complex and diverse learning needs. The diversity of needs requires that the education staff maintain currency in nursing practice, research, and education.

Administrative Behaviors

In Table 18.4, the director's behaviors relative to planning a nurse internship program are described in column one, followed by an analysis of behavior in each of the three key processes. In the right-hand column, the impact of the director's behaviors on alignment is evaluated.

In each case, the representative behaviors of the nurse administrator and educator have been analyzed using the categories of agenda setting, network building, and task accomplishing. For both individuals in our cases, reactive behaviors are absent. Both use foresight to anticipate changing events and plan accordingly. The manager and educator understand that if agenda items are clearly delineated for the parties involved in a change, within achievable time periods, the likelihood of smooth progress toward achieving the internship and opened unit is enhanced.

The administrator and educator in each case use a fairly wide range of network building behaviors. Both have gained the cooperation of others by setting goals, then purposively involving others in the achievement of those goals. In each case, too, they relied on the force of their personal appeal as well as on the legal authority of their positions. In our two cases there was also evidence of the use of negotiation and exchange—of utilitarian network-building.

To accomplish tasks, the administrator and educator used a combination of individualistic, entrepreneurial, and bureaucratic behaviors. By acting like managers, by marketing and selling their ideas in creative and unusual ways, and by being able to act alone when the need arose, both were able to mobilize the

resources that were required to accomplish their goals and enhance organizational effectiveness and stability. In terms of coalignment theory, they were able to move their organizations forward but maintain their stability by keeping the key elements in the organization aligned. In doing so, both enhanced the likelihood of their own survival and the organizations' health.

IMPLICATIONS FOR ADMINISTRATIVE PRACTICE

Analysis of one's own administrative behavior in each unique organizational context is essential for effective performance, self-growth, and personal development. "Self-development of the effective executive is central to the development of the organization."[22] The coalignment model provides a usable, understandable way of analyzing one's actions that is logical and comprehensive.

Following self-analysis, one is able to discern the degree of fit or alignment between oneself and one's agenda, network, and organizational unit. Using the coalignment framework the administrator is also able to identify where nonalignment exists and to estimate the potential factors contributing to the nonalignments and their destabilizing influence.

In summary, the ability to conceptualize organizational policies, concepts and goals and implement plans of action are essential characteristics of the effective nurse executive. Effectiveness is also a result of an individual's ability to analyze use of time and make effective decisions.[23] The coalignment model provides a framework whereby administrative behaviors can be categorized, analyzed, and evaluated for their degree of effectiveness.

According to the model, behavior patterns emerge in particular situations as a function of the four contextual variables; the dynamic relationships among the processes and con-

TABLE 18.4 Analysis of the Behavior of a Staff Development Director

Behavior	Agenda Setting	Network Building	Task Accomplishment	Analysis
Meets with the nurse administrator to present a proposal for a nurse internship program.	*Medium Range:* Plans implementation of the internship program for the next six months. *Long Range:* Plans long-range improvement of the staff development orientation program, and recruitment and retention rates.	*Cooptative Behavior:* Since the nurse administrator has previously expressed some concern about the resources needed to initiate the internship program, the director makes her part of the group, which is supportive of the program, and thereby gains her cooperation. *Purposive Behavior:* Defines a goal others support—the internship program to increase the recruitment and retention of new graduates.	*Entrepreneurial Behavior:* Enlists the nurse administrator's support and cooperation in developing the internship by "selling" her on the idea. *Bureaucratic Behavior:* Plans, directs, and controls future divisional actions that will support the internship program.	These behaviors are aligning the director's network and agenda as she works through her network to accomplish the internship item in her agenda. Her behavior will align the agenda, unit, and network when recruitment and retention rates are improved as a result of the internship.
Attends a meeting with an appointed advisory committee that is planning and developing the nurse internship program.	*Short:* Gives report about a recent discussion with a citywide group of hospital educators about other nurse internship programs in the area. *Medium:* Assesses the progress of the advisory committee and what steps must be initiated and completed during the next several months to ensure the program's success.	*Purposive:* Unites coalition for a successful program and increased recruitment and retention of new graduates. *Formal-Legal:* Provides resources and sets limitations on how the committee plans and develops the program. *Cooptative:* Adds selected people to the committee to gain their cooperation as well as their expertise.	*Bureaucratic:* Delegates but controls the responsiblity for planning and developing the program. *Entrepreneurial:* Seeks the aid of others in planning, developing and later advertising the program.	These behaviors align the director and her network and agenda as a major agenda item becomes a reality through use of internal and external resources. The program has the potential to foster coalignment among all four contexts because the director's actions will align what the organization needs with what is planned and with the contribution of network members.
	Long: Involves representatives from both administration and education, including selected divisional directors, head nurses, instructors, clinical nurse specialists, and unit inservice coordinators, in order to facilitate the change process and increase the long-range success and impact of the program.	*Utilitarian:* Gives committee members recognition for their participation, while gaining their cooperation and expertise.		

textual variables; the nature of the relationships among the four contextual variables; and the proactive elements in an environment that moves a system toward coalignment.[24]

Using the model, five types of administrators can be identified by their patterns of behavior. Each type has a different pattern of behavior as defined by agenda setting, network building, and task accomplishing.

Based on an analysis of the five patterns of administrative behavior, it is readily apparent that use of long-range planning, multiple network-building behaviors, and entrepreneurial and bureaucratic task-accomplishment activities produce the greatest degree of coalignment.

REFERENCES

1. Stevens BJ. The nurse as executive. Wakefield, MA: Nursing Resources Inc, 1980.
2. Kotter JP, Lawrence PR. Mayors in action. New York: John Wiley and Sons, 1974.
3. Taylor FW. The principles of scientific management. New York: WW Norton, 1911.
4. Szilagyi AD, Wallace MJ. Organizational behavior and performance. Santa Monica, CA: Goodyear, 1980.
5. Henry B. Automation and staff nurses' patient management activities. Nurs Adm Q 1982;7(1)64–76.
6. Kotter and Lawrence. Mayors in action, p. 141–142.
7. Ibid., p. 49.
8. Ibid., p. 49.
9. Ibid., pp. 49–64.
10. Ibid., pp. 49–64.
11. Ibid., pp. 49–64.
12. Ibid., pp. 89–93.
13. Ibid., p. 87
14. Ibid.
15. Ibid.
16. Ibid., pp. 65–86.
17. Ibid., pp. 68–78.
18. Henry B. Strengthening our networks. The Florida nurse. Florida Nurses Association, 1986, pp. 9–15.
19. Kotter and Lawrence. Mayors in action, p. 44.
20. Henry. Automation and alignment, p. 29.
21. Ibid., p. 2.
22. Drucker P. The effective executive. New York: Harper and Row, 1985, p. 170.
23. Ibid., p. 29.
24. Kotter and Lawrence. Mayors in action, p. 188.

BIBLIOGRAPHY

Cooper SS. The practice of continuing education in nursing. Rockville, MD: Aspen Systems Corporation, 1983.

Drucker PF. The effective executive. New York: Harper and Row, 1985.

Henry B. Automation and alignment in hospital nursing units. CA: University of Southern California, 1980.

Henry B. Strengthening our networks. Florida Nurse 1985;10:9–15.

Kotter JP, Lawrence PR. Mayors in action. New York: John Wiley and Sons, 1974.

Kotter JP. Organizational dynamics: Diagnosis and intervention. Reading, MA: Addison-Wesley, 1978.

O'Conner AB. Nursing staff development and continuing education. Boston: Little, Brown, 1986.

Porter-O'Grady T. Creative nursing administration. Rockville, MD: Aspen Systems Corporation, 1986.

Puetz BE. Networking for nurses. Rockville, MD: Aspen Systems Corporation, 1983.

Stevens BJ. The nurse as executive. Wakefield, MA: Nursing Resources Inc, 1980.

Szilagyi AD, Wallace MJ. Organizational behavior and performance. Santa Monica, CA: Goodyear Publishing Inc, 1980.

Tobin HM, Wise PSY, Hull PK. The process of staff development. St. Louis: CV Mosby Company, 1979.

The Power of the Nurse Executive

Rachel Rotkovitch

SCAN the *New York Times* or any other major newspaper for the section where hospitals are advertising for top-nursing executives. Most of the ads read alike. They are looking for a nurse with a graduate degree in a health field (not necessarily nursing), with years of proven successful experience in a comparable-size hospital, who will take complete charge of the nursing service and lead it to a most efficient and effective performance. That is the premise on which the applicants for the top-nursing service positions rely as they explore the offer. Unfortunately there is often a discrepancy between the promised authority and freedom to manage the nursing service given during the courting period and the reality of the situation once that period is over and the nurse executive steps into the role.

I know a number of directors of nursing who left their positions after only a short period of time because of such a situation. How many more nursing executives, however, stay on even though their hands are tied and they are, therefore, in no position to fulfill their goals?

In these situations all their hopes and desires are unfullfilled, and the knowledge they possess—which is needed to lead a nursing service to an optimal level of performance—is untapped, as the chief executive officers pursue different agendas and priorities.

It is not my desire to pass judgment on nurse executives who stay in their position even though they are unable to achieve their goals. However, I am on solid ground in stating that in those situations more is involved than the frustration or unhappiness of the incumbent nurse administrator. It is the quality of the nursing care, closely tied with the quality of patient care, that is at stake. Hand in hand with this go the unhappiness and frustration of the nursing staff and the inevitable fallout—turnover of staff, defection from nursing, and something we currently are witnessing—a serious drop in enrollment in schools of nursing. In this context, I would like to share with the readers a theory derived, not by known theoreticians, but by the simple folk living in the small town of Nowagrodek, Poland, where I was raised. It is a story about fish; this is how I remember it:

The only water close to our town was a river, and the only fresh fish came from that river. There were no means of refrigerating food. Therefore, fish brought to the market, which was a large square in the middle of the town where the peasants brought their produce, had to be absolutely fresh and eaten the same day if one wanted to avoid disaster.

I used to watch how the buyers of fish lifted the gills of the fish, then either discarded or bought the fish. The test? The degree of freshness was judged by the color of the gills. When they were red, the fish was deemed fresh; when the gills were grayish, the buyers would bring the fish close to the nose, smell it, and discard it. Hence, the saying that "a fish starts smelling from the head."

It never dawned on me that this test by the simple folk in the small town in Poland where I grew up would become the guiding theory on which, through the years, I based my long professional life as a nurse executive. The truth of this theory has been confirmed and reconfirmed over and over again. That is why I have taken whatever steps were required to make sure, as I was leading a nursing service, to acquire and continually develop the knowledge and skills required to keep this head "fresh." I have urged the same to my colleagues in nursing service and those in the profession of nursing whose responsibility it is to develop and teach the knowledge and skills needed to be competent nurse executives.

If knowledge is the basis of competency, can we assume that the acquisition of it through both education and experience will suffice to be effective in an executive position? I do not think so. The knowledge of the intricacies of one's field of endeavor, in our case, heading a nursing service, is certainly a prerequisite in the pursuit of acquiring the power and developing the clout to achieve one's goals.

However, this represents only one side of the coin. Equally important is the value system we individually cherish, and the sensitivity to the values of our subordinates that we bring to the job, which represents a sine qua non in becoming a successful nurse executive.

For our values are at the core of our personalities. "They influence the choices we make, the people we trust, the appeals we respond to, and the way we invest our time and energy. In turbulent times, they can provide a sense of direction amid conflicting views and demands." In looking back at the many choices I have made during my career, the people I have trusted, and the way I have invested my time and energy I cannot but thank my parents, my teachers, my friends, and all who upheld a value system I have identified with and upheld during the years.

Assuring our patients of the highest possible quality of nursing care is the main responsibility a nurse executive takes on as he or she assumes that role. To fulfill this responsibility, nurse executives depend on the many employees in an organization. Nurse executives achieve their goals through the work of others. These others look to their leader, the nurse executive, for direction, inspiration, and role modeling. To provide this the nurse executive needs to assess whether she or he does, indeed, project a model which will attract and sustain a following. I refer to this assessment undertaking as "taking a look in the mirror of self-criticism." Having done this and having detected the blemishes, which stood in my way of goal achievement, I took appropriate steps to correct those blemishes. Oil of Olay is not the only remedy I use to look well. Indeed, the external appearance and image I project to the hospital co-workers, especially to the management staff and physicians, is important in my being effective as a nurse executive.

The connection between appearance and effectiveness has been confirmed by many studies. And nurses in executive positions have responded appropriately to these findings. About 20 years ago, nurse administrators dressed in white starched uniforms with caps on their heads and had a stern, authoritative demeanor. Moreover, many directors of nursing used to attend conventions and other gatherings dressed the same way. The message this external appearance sent to members of the hospital family was one of distance, unapproachableness, and regimentation.

This has changed. The appearance of most nursing directors and their staff is more reflective of their important positions. One only has to watch the "fashion show" of thousands of nurse executives at any convention and marvel at the transformation. Being dressed as an executive has contributed to the standing of the chief nurse with peer administrative teams and physicians, and has eased relationships with the nursing staff.

Having decided to get out of the traditional attire while at work, and having assisted the rest of the nursing staff to do the same, a nurse executive will, at times, have to respond to objections from physicians and patients alike to this change. I have had to deal with those objections on many occasions and still do. There are complaints from both groups related to their inability to recognize, at a glance, who is a nurse. Before the change in garb, some physicians maintained that they would beckon the first nurse they met on the unit, who was easily identifiable by attire, to assist them in whatever help they needed (retrieving a patient's chart or assisting with a dressing change, and so forth). Now, I reason with these physicians that they should take the time to find out who the nurse responsible for the case of their patients is from the locator board where all the information is recorded, ask the secretary to page her, and find out from that nurse, whose name they now know, the information they seek.

Most physicians recognize the benefits they, the patients, and the nurses get from these new relationships. To convince patients, who for so long have been conditioned to identify nurses as "angels in white," I expressed my rationale in a letter that I mailed to patients. The content of my letter follows.

Dear Ms. K:

In your letter of evaluation of the services provided you by Yale-New Haven Hospital during your recent stay, I read with great interest, your comments on the nursing care. I am pleased to learn that the nursing care you received was good. However, you also referred to the appearance of our nurses which you felt was not professional.

Whether you ascribe your belief about what a nurse whould wear while on duty as stemming from being "old fashioned," or from having been conditioned through the many years of portraying nurses as "angels in white," I respect your opinion.

I will, however, take a few moments to share with you the "other view." To begin with, most nurses in the United States believe that white, being the absence of color, is blah and unstimulating to the eye of the beholder. It has also been established by research, that sensory input plays an important role in helping patients, children, and older people to cope with hospitalization.

Nurses have, for too long, ignored this fact, and in many hospitals and nursing homes they are still not taking advantage of the beautiful colors God created for our pleasure and well-being.

Another reason nurses discarded dressing in white uniforms and caps, is the constraining effect uniformity has on the freedom of the individual to think, make independent judgment, and be innovative. All these faculties are essential to today's nurse if she is to serve the patients and their families at an optimal level.

We recognize that it will take many years of reconditioning of the recipients of nursing services to view each nurse as a person in his or her own right and judge them on the basis of their performance, rather than their appearance.

I want to underscore, that we do have a dress code for nurses, which does provide guidelines as to what is appropriate and what is not to be worn on duty. These guidelines do permit the individual nurse to choose a wardrobe that enhances his or her appearance, self-image, and contribute in creating, in the hospital, an environment that is more like home than the institution it is.

For many patients, this means a lot. Every little bit that relaxes the patients is important to nurses, and we have tangible evidence that when comparing the effect of white starched uniforms worn by nurses for many years to that of pastel colors we encourage them to wear, the colors have an upper hand in creating a relaxed, nonthreatening environment for our patients.

I hope that this little bit of information explains some of the background of the nurses' dress at Yale-New Haven Hospital. I also hope you are well and making good progress toward total recovery.

Sincerely,
Mrs. Rachel Rotkovitch
Vice-President
Nursing

Granted, this kind of a relationship does not develop as a result of a switch in attire only. Many other changes in the nurse executive's environment need to be, and can be, achieved on the way to becoming an effective leader in the hospital setting.

For example, the office from which the

nurse executive operates has to reflect the important role she occupies in the organization. Anyone entering such an office, especially those whose perception of nurses is that they will tolerate any environment or treatment, must wonder, upon seeing the nurse executive's office, at the spaciousness, attractiveness, and comfort. They instantly decide that the person occupying this office is very important and is given recognition by hospital administrators.

It is amazing to watch these reactions from people entering such an office. Moreover, it is gratifying to see the different behavior from some visitors who, under other circumstances, would not be as constrained and on their best behavior. When the office of the nurse executive reflects the standing of that person in the organizational hierarchy, it helps in playing that powerful role.

To summarize, in pursuing the acquisition of power or clout, the nurse executive must not ignore anything, especially the environment and appearance, that paves the way. The records show that the most popular elective course at the Harvard Business School is one entitled Power and Influence. The ultimate goal in any business is to win. Nurse executives are no exception. Very often the question each one of us needs to ask ourself is not so much, what must I do to win? as it is, what must I refuse to do in order to achieve my goal? From the forgoing description of external appearances and office accommodations, it is clear that refusing to occupy a cubbyhole without windows and with electrical outlets on one of the walls (I have been privy to such a set up), or refusing to be straitjacketed in a uniform, are indispensible first conditions in negotiating for a top-nursing position.

The next important prerequisite for success (power) in the top nursing-service position is assuring that the degree of authority as well as the backing of the chief executive will be sufficient to implement programs the

nurse executive has in mind, and to lead an efficient and effective service.

Once the nurse executive has successfully negotiated dress code and a prestigious office, what title and what compensation should he or she be accorded? The latest ANA (American Nurse Association) survey indicates a large percentage of nurse executives are titled vice-president. This title sends a positive message to all concerned; more nursing executives should demand such a designation, especially in hospitals where the head of the organization is titled president and his or her assistants, vice-presidents.

As to salary and other fringe benefits, they are negotiable. Professionals are in a stronger position to negotiate compensation when they are sought after rather than when they are looking for a position. In the latter case, bargaining power is weakened if people so much as signal that they will take the position no matter what. The most appropriate approach, I believe, to achieve a compensation package as a nurse executive is to base the expectation on the parity principle. To be specific, in my current position as vice-president of nursing at Yale-New Haven Hospital, I asked for and obtained a salary equal to that of the other chiefs of health profession services—the chief of medicine, chief of surgery, obstetrics, and so forth.

Receiving such a compensation package represents more than dollars and cents. It represents recognition that the nursing service is a unique and crucial professional service and that the one heading it is equal to the other heads of unique and crucial professional services in terms of compensation. It adds one more building block to the power base a nurse executive needs to be an effective leader.

There are a few more areas a nurse executive has to cover before signing on the dotted line. She must assess who the administrative leaders of the organization are, and what they stand for. This is not a difficult task. Ask those people who should know from personal contact. The best person to ask is the previous nurse executive who worked with the current heads of the organization. I did, and the answer I received was that the chief executive is "God's gift on earth." That was enough for me, coming as it did from a person whose opinion I respected.

Another important item to assess is the salaries of the nurses in the organization. In 1966, when I was sought after and offered the position of director of nursing in a New York hospital, I refused the offer based on what I thought was a significant difference between the nurses' salaries at the hospital and the going rate for nurses in surrounding hospitals. I eventually took the position after I was assured that an across-the-board salary adjustment for all nurses would be implemented. The reason for paying attention to the compensation a hospital accords its nurses is self-evident. Underpaying indicates a disregard by management of the important role nurses play in an organization. The aftermath of low pay is a shortage of competent nurses in the work force, or future union activity. Either of these problems represent a potential deterrent to the nurse executive's effort in bringing a nursing service to the desired operational level. Since, as previously stated, the nurse executive accomplishes his or her mandate through the work of others (nurses), why should she take a job where the work force is not going to be available and, where available, is of questionable quality?

With all the above-mentioned prescriptions for a successful tenure as a nurse executive resolved to one's satisfaction, it is time to say "YES" to the job offer. A written agreement absolutely must be provided to protect the applicant, as well as the hospital. It is done in other industries and businesses, why not in hospitals? Should such a written agreement not be forthcoming, a statement from the nurse—spelling out the main points of employment conditions arrived at by the nurse

administrator and the chief executive—will serve the same purpose.

With these preliminary essentials out of the way, the time to step into the position and assume leadership has arrived. Oftentimes, the nurse executives will need to divide their time between the organization they are leaving and the new organization. It has happened to me several times. Even if enough notification of leaving one's position has been given, there is an obligation, I believe, to assure a smooth transition for the next nurse executive. At the same time, the hospital where the nurse executive is assuming her new position could be in dire need of a signal, particularly to the nursing staff, that the interim period is ending and that the new nurse executive will soon be on board. During the interim, being in the new organization for one or two days a week, will achieve the desired calming influence on a restless and unionization-prone nursing staff.

How many managers would want a union to set foot in their organization? The same is true for the nurse executive. Unionized nurses, no matter under which flag they march, find themselves in an adversary position vis-à-vis their professional leader. Such a situation will invariably create difficulties for a nurse executive. One should prevent unionization from developing, if possible, prior to taking a position and certainly during one's tenure.

Managing without unions can be achieved by filling a leadership vacuum even for one or two days a week before assuming full-time responsibility; and later on, by listening and being responsive to the real and perceived problems that bother the nursing staff. It is almost an axiom that the probability of unions increases not only as a result of a leaderless organization, but because of unresponsive management in an organization or department.

The entry of a union to a nursing service due to default may not be the only undesirable factor that will hinder the nurse executive's ability to fulfill the mandate of his or her position. Other undesirable happenings may develop. I have found that, especially during a leaderless period in a nursing service, a variety of hospital administrators and department heads step in to help "save the nursing service." They do this stepping-in because of a perception that it is their duty, or as an expression of loyalty to the organization.

Confronted with such a situation, the nurse executive must make it clear, beyond doubt, to the well-meaning department heads, that because of the capability of the nurse executive the once-existing vacuum that he or she has filled no longer exists. I still remember vividly when, soon after taking a position as vice-president of nursing, at a meeting of the senior administrative staff, having taken the seat at the head of the conference room table (where you sit conveys a message), I thanked the administrators for filling the void. I also asked them kindly to step out of the role.

Some of my colleagues were visibly shocked. Others smiled and later thanked me for relieving them of a burden they did not really know how to carry. Making the hospital community aware that there is a legitimate nurse executive on board early in one's tenure may shock some. But the benefits of such a strategy far outweigh the drawbacks. The desire of any newcomer on the scene to be all smiles and to be perceived by others as a "nice" person is dangerous.

As a case in point, in 1966 during my first week at a New York hospital, I was invited to participate in a meeting taking place in the board room. I went. There, at the head of the table sat the director of the physical therapy department and the director of medical records. They had called a meeting for all head nurses and clinical nursing directors. What I heard these two department heads say was that they were not pleased with the nursing service. Patients were not arriving for physical therapy on time. The patients' records, still referred to as medical records, were not completed and were not being brought to the department by the nurses at the time of discharge. Controlling my anger, I told all those present that, first, from now on nurses would attend meetings in and out of the hospital only as called for or authorized by nursing administration; and second, that complaints regarding nurses would be directed to nursing administration. I was later told that the shock to everyone present was so great that one could hear a fly. The result? In the future, no one dared call nurses to any meetings without checking with the nursing office. It took time for the nurses to bridge the distance between being intimidated by hospital administrators and being aware of their crucial position and worth. But the first step on that bridge had to be taken, even though I wished it could have been taken a little later in my tenure.

Two months after assuming another vice-president position, a similar event took place at a prestigious university hospital. During my rounds, I stopped at the neuro-intensive care unit. This time I was shocked. There, beside a patient's bed—the patient was flat on his back with a bandaged head—stood a physician holding a coffee cup in his left hand, while pressing the patient's chest with his other hand.

It was clear that he was trying to resuscitate the patient. On the other side of the bed, stood the head nurse and another nurse. When the doctor left the unit I asked the head nurse whether she had noticed that the physician was holding a cup of coffee in one hand and resuscitating the patient with the other? "Yes," she said, "I tell the doctors all the time that it is not acceptable behavior, but they do not pay any attention to me." The head nurse in this particular case did not last long in her position. Anyone in a leadership position, to whom no one pays attention, cannot be effective. The head nurse, as a first-line manager in the nursing service hierarchy, represents the backbone on which the efficiency and the effectiveness of nursing service relies. As to the physician, whom I believed was out of order, after he finished his rounds on the unit, I approached him, introduced myself, and expressed my dismay at his behavior at the patient's bedside. His first reaction? "I object to you telling me how to take care of my patients." "Not so," was my reply, "I object to your bedside manners." More conversation followed. The end result was that we parted friends. But I made sure that news of this incident was widely spread, especially among physicians. The intent was to spread the word that nurses, all nurses in the hospital—whom I was sure shared my values—would not tolerate any behavior, no matter from whom, that would in any way shortchange a patient's welfare.

Having set the stage for nurse-physician relationships, one then needs to nurture patients by using the expertise of both physicians and nurses. Mutual respect and collegiality among nurses and physicians, are at the basis of developing work relationships that benefit everyone involved.

It is my experience that cooperative, productive relationships can be achieved. The great majority of physicians are as dedicated to their patients as the majority of nurses are to theirs. Doctors also work as hard as nurses. And they want to work in an environment of mutual respect and interdependency.

Why then do so many nurses express the desire for better relationships with physicians? I believe this is so because a minority of physicians continue to berate nurses and are not penalized. I have had a number of encounters with such physicians. I invite them to my office (you can see the rationale for having a prestigious place in which to "converse"); occasionally the invitation is for lunch outside of the hospital. In most cases, after our talk, there are no further offenses. On only a few occasions have I found no way

to penetrate the conviction of a physician that nurses are born with placentas but doctors with pedestals.

In attempting to find the reason for such an irrational belief on the part of the medical staff, I have concluded that much of the blame lies with nursing. Nurses in leadership positions have in the years gone by, impressed on student nurses as well as graduates, that physicians are superordinate and nurses are subordinate. Physicians order; nurses obediently carry out orders. Nurses are to stand when a physician arrives on the unit. Nurses carry the patient's chart, open the door, and defer in dozens of ways. Add to all this a plaque I removed from the entrance to a hospital, which merged with the one where I was the nursing executive, that read as follows:

Hold the physician
in honor, for he is essential
to you, and God it was who
established his profession. From
God the doctor has his wisdom.
Thus God's Creative work
continues without cease. He
who is a sinner toward
his Maker will be defiant toward
his Doctor.

Sirach 38, 1–15

Is it any wonder that some physicians—thank God, a small minority—continue to believe in their superiority and therefore relate to nurses as handmaidens? To allow these physicians to get away with unprofessional behavior without penalty deprives the establishment of collegial relationships and thus makes it difficult for nurse executives to achieve their goals.

Nurses who have been conditioned to subservience need to be reconditioned. They must be reminded at every occasion that they are professionals and have the right to expect to be treated as such. They are to be encouraged to report when they are not being treated accordingly. And they must know that no incident of misconduct by anyone will be passed over without appropriate steps being taken.

It has taken decades to condition nurses to be self-effacing. How long will it take to reverse this attitude? In my opinion, as long as it takes to fill the executive nursing positions in our hospitals with nurses who are determined to bring this reversal to fruition. However, determination alone will not suffice. One has to use successful strategies to achieve goals. The nursing staff is the indispensable element with which the nurse executive must strategize.

Therefore, taking stock of the nursing staff is an essential first step in the assessment of who is who on board, and who does what in the nursing organization. I found that the most productive time is time spent in assessing each member of the nursing leadership team by providing the time and privacy for a one-to-one interview. It is good to record the highlights of the information obtained—such as personal background, professional history, length of service in the organization, level of satisfaction with the current status, and desires for the future. Not the least important of the information will be the nurse executive's "gut feeling" about the individual across the table.

One will invariably find a number of staff in nursing leadership positions who are out of place. That being the case, one has to make an effort to find an appropriate alternative place for such a nurse.

Should such a resolution not be feasible, mainly because the incumbent does not agree with the assessment, then there is only one way to resolve the problem. The person has to go. As harsh as it sounds, this is, in my opinion, the best solution for both parties, the nurse and the organization. A case in point comes to mind. One of the clinical directors did not agree with my philosophy and structural model of a nursing service. She shared this with the head nurses in her division, thus creating a serious split in the service. In confronting her with the problem, she admitted having opposing views about how a nursing service should run. With due respect to her views, I told her that the hospital employed me to head the nursing service and therefore she had two choices: to stay on out of loyalty, which is indispensable, and to represent me as expected—which would surely give her ulcers, or seek another position. She resigned.

Filling the nursing director positions with competent and reliable staff is of great importance because it is this group of nurses with which a nurse executive consults, shares, and depends on to carry out the agreed on policies and thrust of the department. The next group essential for the success of a nursing service is the cadre of head nurses. A determination of the need to turn head nurses from a group that believes "nobody listens to us" to one that exclaims "when a head nurse speaks it is like E. F. Hutton speaks" is a tedious undertaking. But it is more than essential. It is tantamount to executive success.

What comes to mind are the first few meetings I once had with a head-nurse group.

The luncheon that preceeded the business agenda was served from brown shopping bags. Wrapped sandwiches, potato chips, and cans of soft drinks were picked up by the head nurses and consumed hurriedly at cafeteria tables. During the discussions that followed, it became clear that staffing patterns were the big problem. Head nurses, they told me, worked Monday through Friday only; their seniority entitled them not to work weekends, evenings, and nights. Part-time nursing staff, they informed me, were not desirable because of the difficulty scheduling these people. In fact, I was told, a letter had been sent to all part-time nurses thanking them for their work, but telling them that unless they worked full time, they were no longer needed.

I saw a close connection between the brown

shopping-bag lunch and the content and quality of the head nurses' discussions. Both were unacceptable. To change the self-image the head nurses had of themselves as minor functionaries, monthly luncheon meetings were instituted where a four-course menu was served at tables with white tablecloths. The head nurses were encouraged to dress in flattering, appropriate business clothes. They were more than encouraged to upgrade their education. They were made aware of what it means to be responsible for the nursing care of patients 24 hours a day, seven days a week. They were taught the principles of financial management and made responsible for the millions of dollars allocated to their cost centers. These and many other changes brought about the reemployment of valuable part-time nurses. And head nurses worked any day, and any shift and time when their presence was needed.

The head nurses reached out for education, and most of them earned master's degrees. They reached a stage where I was comfortable transferring the chairmanship of our monthly meetings to them. They were and are, truly managers, and recognized as intelligent, influential administrators by everyone in the hospital.

The nurse executive, who is looked upon by the rest of the staff as a role model, must set the stage for the desired recognition accorded to the head nurse. If she stumbles in this pursuit, she must get up, straighten out, and hopefully never repeat her faux pas. As a case in point, my husband's secretary, a woman over age 60, was admitted to our hospital for a cholecystectomy. What was found was a diffused cancerous growth that was inoperable. Of course no one told the patient the truth about her condition. I visited this lady daily. One day she said that she

could not understand why she was so weak and that, on top of it, the nurses, when bathing her, asked her to help with the procedure. I promised her that I would speak to the nurses and assured her that she would not have to exert herself anymore.

The head nurse was off duty that day. The assistant head nurse listened to my request in silence. I thought the matter was settled. The next day, when I came to see the patient, the head nurse asked to speak with me. She invited me to her office, asked me to sit down, and proceeded to tell me what she thought of my intervention regarding this particular patient.

The nursing care plan that she, the clinical nurse specialist, and the other nurses devised required that the patient participate in her care, no matter how minimal that participation was to be. Therefore, the nurses did not appreciate my upturning their well thought out care plan. My reaction to this conversation? I was absolutely delighted. Delighted that one of my head nurses had the guts to sit me down and tell me to "butt out." If she did it to me, her "big boss," I was sure she would stand up to anyone else who would interfere, intentionally or unintentionally, in the areas where she is expert.

I made sure that all head nurses knew what happened. I do not remember having repeated this mistake since.

With the right people at the clinical director level and with the strength of head nurses—the group that I refer to as the backbone of the service—a nurse executive is in a powerful position to increase the clout of nursing and advance the quality of patient services.

REFERENCE

Schmidt HW, Posner BZ. Managerial values and expectations. New York: American Management Association, 1982.

Analysis of Power in Nursing Administration: Rotkovitch as a Case in Point

Audrey Nelson

POWER is part of every aspect of organizational life, as Rotkovitch graphically describes. Using power to acquire resources and influence others is an essential function of an administrator.[1] In this section, a theory of power and dependence, developed by Kotter at the Harvard School of Business, is used to analyze Rotkovitch's experiences.

The wave of publications in nursing on organizational power attests to the need for understanding power plays and conflicts among organizational participants. Rotkovitch is one of the five or ten most powerful nurse executives in the country today. To improve understanding of how and why to use power, in the following section I first briefly explain Kotter's theory of power and dependence, then I discuss some methods for managing dependence, and describe strategies for acquiring and using power—referring in each instance to Rotkovitch's experiences.

POWER AND DEPENDENCE THEORY

The degree of dependence in organizations where many people work together is frequently underestimated. Managers get things done through others; everyone realizes this full well. But people often fail to appreciate how getting things done through others involves being dependent on other people to perform in effective, compatible ways. Dependence means being influenced by others and being needful of others for resources—for assistance, information, approval, money, and time.[2] Interdependence exists where two or more parties influence and depend on one another—that is, where two parties have power over one another because each of the parties is, to some degree, dependent on the other for assistance, approval, direction, or any number of advantages.[3]

According to Kotter, power dynamics are inevitable and emerge in organizations because the dependence in managerial jobs is greater than the formal power of control given to people in their positions.[4] Because all relationships involve using power, the ethical and skillful use of power is essential for organizational effectiveness and administrative success.

Kotter also points out that the number and magnitude of dependencies increase as individuals move up in an organization: the higher on the organizational ladder, the greater the number of individuals and groups on whom one must rely, and, hence, the more dependent on others one becomes.[5]

Why is dependency inherent in managerial

jobs? Because labor is divided to accomplish different specialized tasks and because resources are limited.[6] For example, nurses provide nursing care and report to nurse administrators; physicians provide medical care and report to medical chiefs; dietitians provide dietary services and report to the head of dietary. Yet, in each case, nurses depend on doctors, doctors on nurses, and nurses on dietitians for the specialized knowledge and services—the resources that each provides. Thus, there is widespread dependence in organizations.

Moreover, the amount of dependence in an organization, according to Kotter, is directly related to the potential for conflict. Where individuals are competing for the same limited resources, where individuals and groups are needful of others—and therefore dependent, the likelihood of conflict exists. And power is the medium through which conflict is resolved.

Effective administrators are skilled at acquiring and using power. Organizations in which managers use their power appropriately and handle conflict effectively are characterized by original thinking, creative problem solving, and innovative services. Personnel exhibit a healthy competitiveness and respond and adapt quickly to change. Overall, employees are satisfied and enthusiastic about their work and clients are well served.[7]

On the other hand, in organizations where many dependencies exist and conflict is not well managed, there are power struggles, bureaucratic infighting, and self-serving political battles that result in decreased organizational efficiency and increased costs. Where the power to manage dependencies and conflict is only marginal, personnel are alienated and frustrated.[8]

The concepts and relationships described by Kotter's theory of power and dependence are illustrated in Figure 19.1.

MANAGING DEPENDENCE

Dependence is managed best when the power people can develop and use exceeds the number of dependencies they encounter. The authority of one's position is an important source of power. The more formal authority in a position, the greater the likelihood that a person will be able to acquire a large number of resources. But the more formal authority in a position, the greater the job-related dependency.

Positional power used wisely with subordinates and with peers enhances the administrator's ability to accomplish tasks quickly. Recognizing the importance of the nurse executive position in a health service agency is a critical element in managing dependency. One of the ways of assessing the power of a position is by observing the image and status of the department that one will head. Salary, prerequisites, office location and furnishings, and position titles, all provide clues about the status and power of a position. Rotkovitch believes, and rightly so, that the status accorded to nursing services can be assessed by how nurses are treated. And how nurses are treated discloses to the astute observer how the contributions of nursing are valued.

As Rotkovitch noted, however, the power of a position in and of itself is not adequate for the job that needs to be done. Professionals in organizations are not willing to accept mandates without question, particularly if the number of mandates is excessive.[9] Using the power of a position is one way to manage, but it is just that—one alternative. There are others.

Moreover, as Rotkovitch and Kotter point out, there is frequently a discrepancy between the legitimate authority vested in a position by virtue of the organizational hierarchy, and the actual authority needed to manage the large number of dependencies that characterize executive positions. When

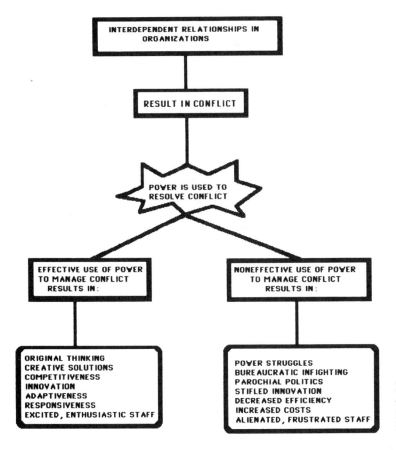

Figure 19.1 Power, dependence, and conflict in organizations. (Adapted from Figure 3-1, Kotter, 1985, p. 36.)

the amount of dependence in a role is greater than the power to cope with dependency, nurse administrators are faced with the dismal choice of leaving their position, or remaining on the job regardless of how ineffective they may be.

A second way of managing dependence is to develop a talent for effectively engaging in what Kotter calls "power dynamics"—those activities in which power is gained or exchanged, and in some cases lost. Rotkovitch exemplifies a nurse executive who is able to accurately assess who has power, what kind of power, how that power is used, and under what circumstances.

Nurses in management positions who use power effectively begin by assessing themselves: Am I able to identify how power is

generated in organizations. Am I able to identify who has power, and what the sources of power are? Am I able to identify and use the power of my position? Do I understand which skills are needed under what circumstances to reduce dependency and to acquire the resources needed by nurses in my department? Do I have the time and energy to engage in power-oriented behaviors?

Successful nurse executives know which questions to ask about their own power-acquiring skills, and which to ask others to accurately estimate the dependence and power in organizations where they work or plan to work. When planning a career and seeking a job, people need to identify their own skills and inclinations for acquiring power and match these with the power-oriented behaviors that will be required in the organization under consideration.

Organizations and jobs require different degrees of power-oriented behavior. In large, complex hospitals, operating in uncertain environments—where resources are scarce, goals are ambitious, formal authority is diffuse, and rewards are granted not for individual but for group performance—job-related dependence is high and the need for power-oriented behaviors is great. Conversely, where an organization is technologically less complex, where the environment is less uncertain and goals are not ambitious, and where individual as opposed to group performance is the measure of successful performance, then there is less job-related dependence and the need for power-oriented behaviors is also lower.

Potential power-dependence problems need to be identified before taking a job. A job should be avoided where the dependencies are greater than one's skill to use power effectively. If the dependencies in a position cannot be eliminated, or additional skill to use power behaviors cannot be developed, then accepting such a position is courting disaster.

A third way of managing dependence is by eliminating unnecessary dependency. When Rotkovitch assumed the position of nurse executive, she quickly sized up and put a stop to the excessive dependence of nurses on individuals in other hospital departments. Recall how she described thanking individuals in various departments for filling the leadership void, then advising them that the control of nursing was in her capable hands, not theirs. Direct and to the point, she gave a clear message that she was in control, that the dependence of the past had ended with her being hired.

Managers also need to be wary of creating needless dependence.[10] Using Rotkovitch's experience as a case in point, while being interviewed for the executive nursing posi-

tion, she recognized that nurses' salaries were not competitive. If she had been unable to negotiate for higher salaries, she might ultimately have found herself highly dependent on a union—a needless and avoidable dependency in her case, and therefore one to be avoided.

A fourth way of managing dependence is by establishing countervailing power over others.[10] Rotkovitch's use of charm and charismatic leadership as power-oriented behavior enabled her to use her personal power to acquire resources from other individuals and groups. This is readily apparent in her negotiation for the director of nursing position. While being interviewed, she successfully marketed her expertise to gain resources such as a better title, pay raises for nurses, and other benefits.

Finally, dependence can be managed by using a wide variety of influencing skills. The skill to influence others is the ability to produce an effect without directly using one's authority and issuing a command. Influencing skills involve the appropriate use of information, relationships, and formal authority. Intuitively and rationally, Rotkovitch understands the various indirect, unobtrusive ways of using power to influence others. For example, she deliberately fostered an image of herself as influential; recall how she described her confrontation with a physician about unprofessional behavior. Following the incident, she noted, "I made sure that news of this incident was widely spread, especially among the physicians."

Rotkovitch also used her influence to enhance the power base of nurses by negotiating higher, more competitive salaries; by revising the channels through which information flowed more speedily to top-level decision makers; and by improving the image of nurses in her jurisdiction. Out went brown-bag lunches, plain everyday dress, and mundane conversations, and in came dining in the board room, dressing for success, and making policy decisions. Rotkovitch clearly understood that her power was linked to the strength of those in her department. All executives are dependent on their subordinates to accomplish personal and organizational goals. Empowering these individuals further enhances nursing's contribution to an organization's overall mission—quality services.

STRATEGIES FOR ACQUIRING AND USING POWER

To stay in a job and to be effective, one must use strategies for getting and keeping power. When first taking the position of chief nurse executive, Rotkovitch strategized. She deliberately designed ways of gaining direct control over the resources she needed to function effectively. She identified the kind of space, staff, authority, equipment, and budget that was needed. Then she took calculated risks, recognizing that all actions affect one's power and that decreasing power should be avoided.

Second, she identified ways of controlling what kind of information was generated and the channels through which data and opinions would flow to have the greatest, most direct impact on decisions. She made it clear to the heads of other departments that communications and meetings with nursing personnel were in her domain and were her prerogative.

Third, Rotkovitch created ways of gaining access to top policymakers so that she could give and take information about patient services to her superiors and subordinates. She refused to accept a position where a strong working relationship with the chief executive officer could not be developed. She bridged whatever communication gaps existed between nurses and physicians to increase nursing's input into decision making, thereby enhancing her own effectiveness and that of the department of nursing as well.

Fourth, power is derived from favorable relationships. An effective executive such as Rotkovitch creates a sense of obligation in a way that is unobtrusive and inoffensive. She markets her professional expertise; her management knowledge is made abundantly clear to administrators and board members, her medical knowledge is made known to physicians, and her knowledge of nursing practice is marketed to nursing staff. She is charming and charismatic and, where necessary, she creates a perception in others that they are dependent on her goodwill and the resources she has at her command.

A final way of acquiring and using power is by paying attention to impression management. A number of examples of how to control the impression that others hold have been cited: how one dresses; one's job title; the size, location, and furnishings of one's office; and where one dines.

A more subtle example is related to those with whom one associates. A method for acquiring power involves associating with powerful individuals inside and outside the organization. In these associations, the nurse executive not only acquires important information and influences the thinking of powerful others, but increases the likelihood that the association will also enlarge the perception coworkers have of the power the nurse administrator holds.

Power influences who gets what, as well as when and how.[11] In today's health service organizations, complex interdependencies increase the likelihood of conflict between key coalitions about how resources are distributed. In administrative positions where there are many responsibilities, where many people report to a single individual, and where teamwork is required for effective overall organizational functioning, there are many interdependent relationships, and the potential for conflict is high. Effective administrators use their personal power and the power of their positions to manage dependencies and the conflicts that necessarily emerge. As Salancik and Pfeffer note, "Power is not a dirty secret, but the secret of success."[12] Rotkovitch has uncovered the secret. She is powerful.

REFERENCES

1. Gorman, S, Clark, N. Power and effective nursing practice. Nurs Outlook 1986;34(3):129–134.
2. Kotter, JP. Power and influence. New York: Free Press, 1985.
3. Ibid., p. 17.
4. Ibid., pp. 16–17.
5. Kotter, JP. Power in management. New York: AMA-COM, 1979.
6. Ibid., p. 11.
7. Kotter, Power and influence.
8. Ibid., p. 36.
9. Kotter, Power in management.
10. Ibid., p. 11.
11. Ibid., p. 16.
11. Morgan, G. Interests, conflicts, and power: organizations as political systems. In: Images of organizations. Beverly Hills: Sage, 1986, pp. 141–198.
12. Kotter, Power and influence, pp. 35–36.
12. Salancik, GR, Pfeffer, J. Who gets power—and how they hold on to it: a strategic-contingency model of power. Organizational Dynamics 1977;5:3–21.

BIBLIOGRAPHY

Archer SE. A study of nurse administrators' political participation. West J Nurs Res 1983;5(1):65–75.
Bacharach SB, Lawler EJ. Power and politics in organizations. San Francisco: Jossey-Bass, 1981.
Baker DC. Persuasion: the power is in the art. Nurs Manage 1986;17(11):59.
Biggart NW, Hamilton GG. The power of obedience. Adm Sci Q 1984;29:540–549.
Bille DA. The emperor's new clothes. Nurs Adm Q 1982;6(4):53–59.
Blackburn RS. Lower participant power: toward a conceptual integration. Academy of Management Review 1981;6(1):127–131.
Booth RZ. Power: a negative or positive force in relationships? Nurs Adm Q 1983;7(4):10–20.
Cavanaugh D. Gamesmanship: the art of strategizing. J Nurs Adm 1985;15(4):38–41.
Clatterbuck SE, Proulix JR. A framework for ethical action in nursing service administration. New York: National League for Nursing, Pub. No. 20-1819.
Clegg S. Power, rule, and domination. Boston: Routledge & Kegan Paul, 1975.
Clegg S. The theory of power and organization. Boston: Routledge & Kegan Paul, 1979.
Cobb AT. Political diagnosis: applications in organizational development. Academy of Management Review 1986;11(3):482–496.

Cochran SJ. The nursing service administrator: a democratic authority figure. Nurs Adm Q 1982;61–65.
Dahl RA. The concept of power. Behav Sci 1957;2:201–215.
Dean DJ. The development of professional and political awareness in nursing. J Adv Nurs 1983;8(6):535–539.
Dennis KE. Nursing's power in the organization: what research has shown. Nurs Adm Q 1983;8(1):47–57.
Donley SR. Nursing and the politics of health. In: Chaska NL, ed. The nursing profession: a time to speak. New York: McGraw-Hill, 1983, pp. 844–857.
Donnelly GF, Mengel A, Sutterley DC. The nursing system: issues, ethics, and politics. New York: John Wiley and Sons, 1980.
Eldridge I, Levi M. Collective bargaining as a power resource for professional goals. Nurs Adm Q 1982;7(2):29–40.
Feldman DC, Arnold HJ. Strategies groups use to gain power. In: Managing individual and group behavior in organizations. New York: McGraw-Hill, 1983, pp. 521–525.
French JR. A formal theory of social power. Psychological Review 1956;63:181–194.
Gillies DA. Obtaining and using power. In: Nursing managment: a systems approach Philadelphia: Saunders, 1982, pp. 301–312.
Gorman S, Clark N. Power and effective nursing practice. Nurs Outlook 1986;34(3):129–134.
Hambrick DC. Environment, strategy, and power within top management teams. Adm Sci Q 1981;26:253–276.
Heinekin J. Power: conflicting views. J Nurs Adm 1985;15(11):36–39.
Henry B, LeClair H. Language, leadership, and power. J Nurs Adm 1987;17(1):19–25.
Hersey P, Blanchard KH. Management of organizational behavior: utilizing human resources. Englewood Cliffs, NJ: Prentice-Hall, 1982.
Hinings CR, Hickson DJ, Pennings, JM, Schneck, RE. Structural conditions of intraorganizational power. Adm Sci Q 1974;19(1):22–44.
Hickson DJ, Hinings CR, Lee CA, Schneck RE, Pennings JM. A strategic contingencies theory of intraorganizational power. Adm Sci Q 1971;16(2):216–229.
Hunter PR, Berger KJ. Nurses and the political arena: lobbying for professional impact. Nurs Adm Q 1986;8(4):66–79.
Kanter RM. Power failure in management circuit. Harvard Business Review 1979;July–Aug;65–75.
Kelly LY. Issues of autonomy and influence. In: Dimensions of professional nursing. New York: Macmillan, 1985, pp. 334–351.
Kotter JP. Power, dependence, and management. Harv Bus R 1977;130–136.
Kotter JP. Power, success, and organizational effectiveness. Organizational Dynamics 1978;27–40.
Kotter JP. Managing external dependence. Academy of Management Review 1979;4(1):87–92.
Kotter, JP. Power in management. New York: AMA-COM, 1979.
Kotter, JP. The general managers. New York: Free Press, 1982.

Kotter, JP. Power and influence. New York: Free Press, 1985.

Kotter, JP, Lawrence, PR. Mayors in action. New York: John Wiley and Sons, 1974.

Kraegel JM, ed: Planned political strategies of organizations. Planning strategies for nurse managers. Rockville, CO: Aspen, 1983, pp. 317–350.

Lamar EK. Communicating personal power through nonverbal behavior. J Nurs Adm 1985;15(1):41–44.

Lapkin D. Leadership: Getting leverage on group power. Nurs Management 1988;17(8):46B–46D, 46F–46H.

Larsen J. Nurse power for the 1980s. Nurs Adm Q 1982;6(4):74–82.

Lind A, Wilburn S, Pate E. Power-from-within: feminism and the ethical decision-making process in nursing. Nurs Adm Q 1986;10(3):50–57.

Lukacs JL. Strategic planning in hospitals: applications for nurse executives. J Nurs Adm 1984;14(10):11–17.

Lukes S. Power: A radical view. New York: Macmillan, 1974.

Mainiero LA. A review and analysis of power dynamics in organizational romances. Academy of Management Review 1986;11(4):750–762.

McCloskey JC, Grace HK. The inherent power of nursing. In: Current issues in nursing. Boston: Blackwell, 1985, pp. 551–552.

McNeil K. Understanding organizational power: building on the Weberian legacy. Adm Sci Q 1978;23(1):65–89.

Mechanic D. Sources of power of lower participants in complex organizations. Adm Sci Q 1962;7:249–264.

Milio N. The realities of policy-making: can nurses have an impact? J Nurs Adm 1984;14(3):18–23.

Mintzberg H. Power in and around organizations. Englewood Cliffs, NJ: Prentice-Hall, 1983.

Mintzberg H. The organization as political arena. J Management Studies 1985;22(2):133–154.

Morgan G. Interests, conflicts, and power: organizations as political systems. In: Images of organizations. Beverly Hills: Sage, 1986, pp. 141–198.

Mouzelis NP. Organization and bureaucracy: an analysis of modern theories. New York: Aldine, 1982.

O'Toole AW, O'Toole R. Negotiating cooperative agreements between health organizations. J Nurs Adm 1983;13(12):33–38.

Peterson GG. Power: A perspective for the nurse administrator. J Nurs Adm 1979;9(7):7–10.

Pettigrew AM. The politics of organizational decision-making. London: Tavistock, 1973.

Pfeffer J. Organizations and organization theory. Boston: Pitman, 1982.

Salancik GR, An index of subgroup influence in dependency networks. Adm Sci Q 1986;31:194–211.

Salancik GR, Pfeffer J. The bases and use of power in organizational decision-making: the case of a university. Adm Sci Q 1974;19(3):453–473.

Salancik GR, Pfeffer J. Who gets power—and how they hold on to it: a strategic-contingency model of power. Organizational Dynamics 1977;5:3–21.

Schein VE. Individual power and political behaviors in organizations: an inadequately explored reality. Academy of Management Review 1977;2(1):64–72.

Shaffer F. Nursing power in the DRG world. Nurs Management 1984;15(6):28–30.

Sweeney SS, Witt KE. Does nursing have the power to change the health care system? In: McCloskey JC, Grace HK, eds. Current issues in nursing. Boston: Blackwell, 1985, pp. 554–572.

Tannenbaum AS. Control in organizations: individual adjustment and organizational performance. Adm Sci Q 1962;7(2):236–257.

Tjosvold D. Power and social context in superior-subordinate interaction. Organiz Behav Hum Decision Processes 1985;35:281–293.

Varricchio CG. The process of influencing decisions. Nurs Adm Q 1982;6(4):8–15.

Weick KE. Laboatory experimentation with organizations. In: March J, ed. Handbook of organizations. Chicago: Rand McNally, 1965, pp. 194–260.

20

Social Exchange Theory for Nursing Administration

Marjorie A. White
Mary Alice Green

NURSING administration as a young subdiscipline of nursing borrows concepts from several bodies of knowledge. The sources include economics, business, political science, sociology, and psychology.

The origin of contemporary, practical thinking related to management in large-scale organizations derives to a large extent from Drucker, known as the "father of management." Drucker[1] describes three aspects of management: (a) work and task, (b) results and performance, and (c) relationships.

The purpose of this chapter is to elaborate on the third category, relationships in organizations. Social exchange theory, in addressing social relationships, provides a theoretical basis for better understanding of health-care settings, nursing administration, and the relationships involved.

Predictions indicate that by the year 2000, more than half of the hospitals in the United States will be part of multihospital systems.[2] These mega-organizational arrangements organize individual institutions under a cooperative agreement or management structure.[3] Nurse administrators are confronted with challenges of such complexity in large organizational systems that it is essential for them to be knowledgeable and skillful in applying relevant concepts from many theory-based disciplines. The challenges nurse administrators face include gaining parity with other administrators in policy-making about quality control, the cost-effective allocation of resources, and the multifaceted dimensions of relationships with clients and staff.

SOCIAL EXCHANGE THEORY

Social exchange theory has been developed during the last two decades by sociologists and psychologists. It provides a framework for numerous middle-range theories that describe events involving everyday face-to-face interactions, as well as relations between and within organized groups.

The basic premise in social exchange is that humans engage in interactions guided by sets of norms. These interactions are based on rewards that are valued by an individual or group. In any given interaction, the goal is to minimize costs as a way of maximizing profits. Reciprocity, social scarcity, and feelings or sentiments are other key concepts.

Several major theorists in sociology, anthropology, psychology, and economics have formulated ideas about social exchange theory: Lévi-Strauss, Homans, Thibaut, Kelley, Blau, Nye, Ekeh, and Mauss are among them. As is often the case, these theorists differ about the proper unit of analysis for social exchange and approach theory development from different points of view.

Social exchange theory derives from two major orientations: the collectivistic and individualistic orientation, in each of which, time and unit of analysis are distinctly different.

The collectivistic orientation was proposed by the French anthropologist, Lévi-Strauss in 1949 (and translated into English in 1969).[4] This orientation supports the idea that relationships between groups in society are important to the extent that they are meaningful to the total society or to special groups within a society. Lévi-Strauss's extensive study of kinship, marriage rules, and clans exemplifies the collectivistic perspective. He defines social exchange as regulated by the rules and norms of society.[5] Time in the collectivistic orientation is viewed as spanning an individual's entire life or career, and a group's duration. The unit of analysis is the group.

The second major orientation, described as individualistic, is associated with Homans[6–7] who focuses on relationships between groups or individuals, and the importance of relationships to the individual rather than to a total group or society. Individual behavior forms the basis for Homans's theory. His conceptual framework consists of three elements: activity, interaction, and sentiment.[6] For Homans, time is regarded as only a short segment in the life of an individual or group. The unit of analysis is the individual.

Definition of Terms in Social Exchange Theory

The ideas and terms used most often in exchange theory are usually defined as follows. "Rewards" are the values an individual holds concerning the enjoyment of pleasures, satisfactions, and gratifications.[8] Rewards also include the status, relationships, interactions, and experiences,[9] which are present both at the beginning of an interaction and, in a specified degree, after an interaction. "Costs" are the uncomfortable feelings an individual has involving status, relationships, or interactions.[9] Nye further defines costs as punishments and rewards that are forfeited.[9] "Profits" are rewards minus costs.[7] Individu-

als strive to maximize profits in any given interaction. Profits are a type of reward that is the residual after costs are subtracted. "Reciprocity" is the act of giving and receiving from others with the obligation to repay.[10] "Norms" are the ideas held by the members of a group about expected behavior under given circumstances.[7] These ideas can be put forth in the form of a statement. "Sentiments" are activities and signs of the attitudes and feelings that individuals exhibit.[7] "Interactions" are situations in which individuals engage in activities and respond to each other.[7] "Activities" are tasks accomplished in relationships with others.[7] "Distributive justice" is the expectation that rewards will be in direct proportion to costs or investments.[7]

Collectivistic and Individualistic Orientations

In further specifying the nature of the collectivistic orientation, Ekeh[5] has extracted from Lévi-Strauss's three selected principles of social exchange: (a) social scarcity, (b) social cost, and (c) reciprocity. Social scarcity is the idea that an individual is limited to certain items or relationships according to social custom. Social cost embodies the idea that the cost of social exchange is assumed by one who gives, but attributed to the larger group outside the direct exchange, rather than to those receiving the benefit inside the exchange.[5]

In nursing administration, an example of a social cost attributed to a larger entity involves the nurse who serves as a speaker at a hospital sponsored workshop, but does not pay the registration fee for the conference. According to custom, the hospital waives the fee by attributing the cost (for the registration fee) to the continuing education department.

Reciprocity incorporates a chain of events in which an individual takes something from others and is expected to return another object of value in kind. As an illustration, the nurse who leaves a unit and asks another nurse to care for his or her patients is expected to reciprocate—to care for the patients of others as the need arises.

Lévi-Strauss[4] further subdivides social exchange into (a) restricted exchange and (b) generalized exchange. Restricted exchange involves two persons, *A* and *B*, who expect reciprocity in a relationship and, as a result, give and take benefits from one another. In a restricted exchange, reciprocity occurs between *A* and *B*: *A* gives to *B*, and *B* gives back to *A*. In an interaction in which the exchange is restricted there is an attempt to maintain equality, to derive mutual benefits, and for each person to be accountable to the other.[4] In generalized exchange, reciprocity occurs in a chain of individuals and events. *A* gives to *B*, who gives to *C*, who gives to *D*, who in turn gives to *A*. An individual never directly receives from anyone to whom he or she has given. Trust is the basis for generalized exchange in that a person expects benefits however indirectly.[5] Figure 20.1 illustrates restricted and generalized exchange.

Ekeh[5] has constructed two types of generalized exchange based on Lévi-Strauss: group-focused exchange and individual-focused exchange. In group-focused exchange, individual *A* at a given time benefits group *BCDE* and the expectation is that the individual as a member of total group *ABCDE* will receive benefits at a later time. In contrast, for individual-focused exchange, group *BCDE* benefits individual *A* and the expectation is that each individual in the group will receive benefits from the group as a whole at a later time. Figure 20.2 depicts the group and individual-focused types of exchange.

In contrast to the collectivistic orientation, Homans's individualistic orientation focuses on exchange in small groups and the important effects of the individual in each group. Homans developed his individualistic perspective as a reaction to collectivism in which the outcome for the group, not the individual, was of greatest importance. Ekeh[5] de-

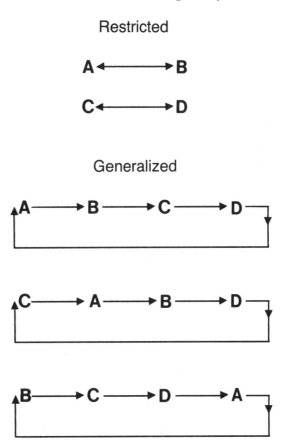

Figure 20.1 Lévi-Strauss's Restricted and Generalized Exchange.

scribed the following four attributes of Homans's social exchange theory:

1. Face-to-face relations
2. Exchange restricted to two individuals
3. Emphasis on psychological and economic needs
4. Utilitarian value of exchange items.[11]

For Homans, it was important to reduce the multiperson group of Lévi-Strauss to dyadic sets as the proper unit of analysis. To improve understanding of face-to-face relations, Homans studied 1500 high-school girls[12] who were asked to select colleagues whom they most admired and who were the most popular. Individual rankings of popu-

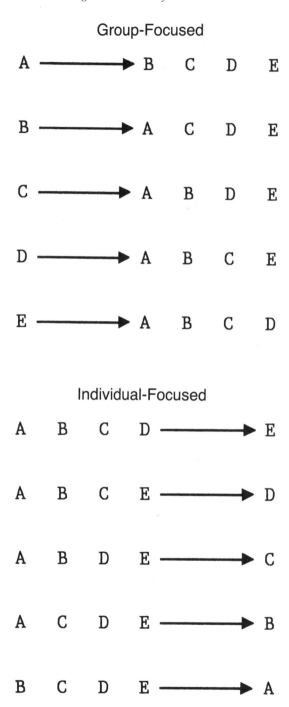

Group-Focused

A ————————▶ B   C   D   E

B ————————▶ A   C   D   E

C ————————▶ A   B   D   E

D ————————▶ A   B   C   E

E ————————▶ A   B   C   D

Individual-Focused

A   B   C   D ————————▶ E

A   B   C   E ————————▶ D

A   B   D   E ————————▶ C

A   C   D   E ————————▶ B

B   C   D   E ————————▶ A

Figure 20.2   Lévi-Strauss's Group-Focused and Individual-Focused Exchange.

larity were assigned by the researchers. The girls also identified their preferences for talking to other girls. Using a sociometric matrix that yielded a status ranking for each girl, Homans's analysis indicated that preferences for interaction were based on the status of the girl who was selected and the girl who was selecting: girls ascribed with higher status preferred talking to girls of higher status; girls of lower status preferred talking to girls of lower status.

The second attribute focusing on dyads was called restricted exchange, although it should be noted that Homans did not use this label himself. Homans analyzed two-person face-to-face contacts and the rewards that each individual received during the interaction. One individual called Person is described as unskillful and needing assistance; the second individual, called Other, provides the assistance Person needs, and receives approval from Person; both Person and Other obtain rewards from this two-person restricted interaction. These everyday face-to-face relations involving restricted exchanges are a significant component of Homans's ideas of social interaction and make up what he calls elementary social behavior.[7]

Third, emphasis on psychological and economic needs also characterizes Homans's perspectives of social exchange theory. From economics, he applies concepts of cost, reward, demand, supply, investment, and profit. He assumes that each individual in an interaction can profit. Profits are rewards minus costs. For example, a reward might include the satisfaction experienced by a group of nurses who have established a home health-care agency and are expanding their services to provide hospice care. The nurses incur costs, however, because of their financial investments, the time spent in developing their business, and because of the uncertainty of their success. The nurses' profit is equal to their feelings of satisfaction minus the cost of resources and the anxiety incurred.

From behavioral psychology Homans applies the concepts of punishment, reward, stimulus, and response to his interpretations of everyday interactions. An example of social interaction involving a stimulus and response is the nurse who works the daytime shift and traditionally arrives at work early. As a response, the night nurse more often than not assembles the bed linen to help the reliable day nurse. However, should the day nurse begin arriving late, the night nurse might not only discontinue helping with the linen, but he or she might discontinue other helping activities as well. And the response might not end there. According to Homans, the response could affect the interactions and attitudes of the single individual—in this case the night nurse—toward another individual—the day nurse; in turn, sentiments are also conveyed to others who are alerted to the possibilities of a similar response.

Utilitarian value of exchange items, as the fourth attribute of Homans's social exchange theory, addresses traditional utilitarian thought from economics, in which material goods and services are the items of exchange. Homans expands the idea of material exchange to include intangible items such as nods, handshakes, smiles, and other affective behaviors. To illustrate the utilitarian value of exchange items in a relationship, consider the case of two health-department nurse supervisors. In their busy schedules, they each give priority to their weekly luncheon meeting. This affords relief from the daily tensions of their jobs. They are close friends and talk about interests in common. Keeping their appointment and talking regularly to continue their friendship serve as examples of utilitarian exchange.

Homans uses a systems approach to analyze small group behavior. "The activities, interactions, and sentiments of the group members, together with mutual relations of these elements with one another during the time the group is active, constitute what we call the *social system*."[13] Relations between activities, interactions, and sentiments each produce a specific outcome. Sentiments—motives, drives, and feelings—provide the initial impetus for activity. An example is the newly graduated nurse who begins work on a unit that has a clinical nurse specialist (CNS). The new nurse admires (sentiment) the knowledge and skill of the CNS and frequently asks (activity) for consultation. If the nurse does not receive the expected response from the CNS, a new sentiment (frustration) arises and the nurse may ask once again (activity).

The structure of activities influences the nature of interactions. Figure 20.3 shows the cycle of relationships in Homans's elementary behavior. To illustrate, multiple shared activities in a job setting yield increased interactions. As interactions increase, the sentiments among members of a group are changed such that their liking for one another is increased.

Interactions, sentiments, and activities that form Homans's elementary behavior function in a social system comprise internal and external subsystems that act and react across a common boundary. In Figure 20.4 the internal system in a work setting is represented by the work group; the external system is represented by the environment, which includes management as well as physical structure.

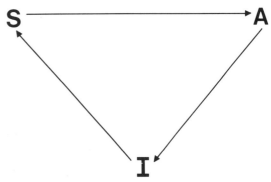

Figure 20.3 Cycle of Relationships in Homans's Elementary Behavior. S = sentiments; A = activities; I = interactions.

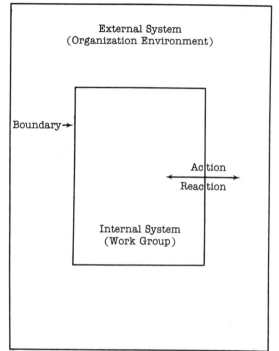

Figure 20.4 Homans's Social System Applied to a Work Setting.

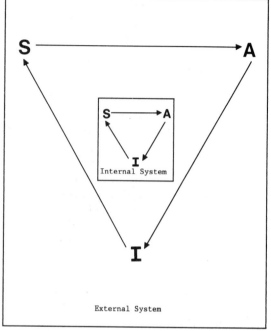

Figure 20.5 Sentiments Activities and Interactions in Homans's Social System. S = sentiments; A = activities; I = interactions.

The relationship between sentiments, activities, and interactions, and the internal and external systems is depicted in Figure 20.5.

Homans's ideas evolved into the five propositions outlined in Table 20.1.

The first four propositions borrow concepts from behavioral psychology in which an individual's past stimulus-response patterns affect present behavior. Major concepts are: similarity, frequency, interval of rewards, and value. The fifth proposition draws from economics and addresses the rule of distributive justice in which the individual expects that rewards will equal costs.

TABLE 20.1   Homans's Five Propositions of Human Exchange.

1. If in the past the occurrence of a particular stimulus-situation has been the occasion on which a man's activity has been rewarded, then the more similar the present stimulus-situation is to the past one, the more likely he is to emit the activity, or some similar activity, now.

2. The more often within a given period of time a man's activity rewards the activity of another, the more often the other will emit the activity.

3. The more valuable to a man a unit of the activity another gives him, the more often he will emit activity rewarded by the activity of the other.

4. The more often a man has in the recent past received a rewarding activity from another, the less valuable any further unit of that activity becomes to him.

5. The more to a man's disadvantage the rule of distributive justice fails of realization, the more likely he is to display the emotional behavior we call anger.[14]

From: Homans G. *Social behavior: its elementary forms.* New York: Harcourt, Brace & World, 1961, pp. 53–55, 75. Used with permission.

To summarize at this point, social exchange theory is based on the proposition that human interaction occurs between two or more individuals. Interaction is based on rewards that are valued: Individuals seek to increase their profits by reducing costs. Interactions take place in settings where a code of norms prevails. French collectivistic thought suggests that the significance of interactions is determined by what is best for a total society or groups. Individualistic thought suggests that the behavior of individuals and small groups is the most significant unit of analysis. In the individualistic perspective, there are internal and external social systems in which activities, interactions, and sentiments form the basic elements.

Social exchange theory offers important ideas for nursing administration. Understanding, structuring, and fostering intricate relationships are the focus of social exchange theory and are essential activities for nurse administrators.

APPLICATION OF SOCIAL EXCHANGE THEORY TO NURSING ADMINISTRATION

Relationships are a key element in the success of organizations—including community health departments, home health agencies, nursing homes, and hospitals. Three organizational components are paramount for the administration of nursing services: the client, staff, and organization. In the remainder of this chapter, social exchange theory is applied to nursing administration using examples to highlight the social exchanges among client, staff, and organization. In the following section, nursing administration refers to the creation and maintenance of an organizational climate for motivating individuals to deliver quality care. Six examples are developed to illustrate how social exchange theory can be used to understand and analyze nursing administration.

Example 1: Exchanges between Specialists and Staff

The first example portrays Lévi-Strauss's idea of generalized exchange defined as group and individual-focused exchange. The concept of generalized exchange is used here to illustrate the relationship between a hypothetical nurse specialist and a group of staff nurses. Our conjecture is based on recent research—used as the starting point, to exemplify generalized exchange. Knaus and associates compared patient outcomes in intensive care units in 13 hospitals.[15] The study demonstrated that the hospital with the lowest mortality ratio employed nurse specialists to assure that standards of care were met. What may exist in these situations is as follows.

To initiate group-focused exchange for *BCDE*, specialist *A* assesses the quality of care during his or her first two months of employment on a pediatric unit. Specialist *A* comes to the situation with personal values about the quality of nursing care and notes that preoperative preparation of children on the morning of surgery is inconsistent and does not meet the established standards of care. In this generalized exchange, the specialist's purpose will be to demonstrate the established standard of care as a model for each nurse to emulate. The specialist therefore arranges to work with all nurses on the mornings they are preparing children for surgery at a cost in time and effort both to his- or herself as well as other nurses in the group. By engaging in this group-focused exchange, the specialist expects that improvement will occur in the preoperative care given by the group of nurses *BCDE*.

After two months, standards of preoperative care are met in a consistent manner. Nurse specialist *A* expects, in this type of exchange and as a member of the total group *ABCDE*, to benefit from the knowledge and expertise that other members of the group might have to offer in the future. For example, *D* has specialized knowledge about long-term hyperalimentation for a child admitted to the hospital, and conducts a conference in which all group members, including *A*, increase their knowledge of parenteral nutrition.

The profits for individuals and the group from this exchange are the satisfactions realized from improved care. The values the specialist holds for high-quality care, minus the costs expended in time and effort with the nurses, represents the profit in the exchange. An additional profit accrues when the specialist can concentrate his or her energy on other problems and units. The same type of profits apply to *D* and to the remaining members of the group because of their newly acquired knowledge.

Example 2: Staffing Needs

The second example portrays the individual-focused type of generalized exchange. An individual-focused exchange can be illustrated by a total group of nursing units *ABCDE* (group), and unit *E* (individual) that needs additional personnel. The nursing supervisor initiates an exchange requesting that *ABCD* each take turns sending a nurse to *E* on four consecutive days. The expectation is that each individual unit, as part of the total group, will in turn receive staffing assistance from *E*, as well as from each other member of the group, as the need arises in the future.

Rewards derive from the staff's belief in the responsibility for helping to maintain adequate care. Costs are the necessary reassignments and the loss of a staff member for a day. Profits are the rewards minus costs: the satisfaction of providing assistance, of carrying out an ethical responsibility, minus the

cost of losing a coworker and the necessary reassignments.

Example 3: Negotiating the Budget

To illustrate exchange between two individuals, the third example portrays reciprocity, restricted exchange, and face-to-face relations. The vice-president for nursing services (Person) in a corporate-owned and -managed nursing home, communicates and negotiates with the vice-president for financial planning (Other) regularly throughout the budgeting process. Other is new to the health-care field and needs assistance from Person if they are to jointly develop a useful, valid budget. Person provides help to Other by scheduling meetings (costs) to inform Other about: (a) the nature of nursing care required by gerontologic patients, (b) clinical specialization in gerontologic nursing, and (c) competitive nursing salaries in nursing homes. Additional meetings are scheduled throughout the fiscal year between the two vice-presidents to discuss unexpected expenditures and to negotiate budgetary modifications. Person receives approval from Other for the time spent focusing on the financial aspects of gerontological services.

In analyzing this situation, the idea of reciprocity suggests the obligation that Other has incurred to repay Person. Repayment becomes a reality when Other allocates funds to ensure that nursing services are adequate and when funds are not channeled into other operations. Both vice-presidents come to the situation possessing knowledge and skill in budgeting. Costs incur to Other when Person schedules the series of meetings to help Other learn about gerontologic care. Profits for both are realized when a budget is formulated in which Person and Other are both invested. Further, Person and Other establish a pattern of reciprocity advantageous for future budget management.

The continued exchange of information by

vice-presidents during and after budgeting is supported by Covalski and Dirsmith.[16] These authors emphasize the need for nurses responsible for budgeting to document reasons for deviating from their budget. They also advocate that nurse administrators describe the unforeseen events outside their control leading to budget modifications, and communicate the extent to which the nursing service is effectively managed within its budget.

Example 4: Relationships in Intensive Care Units

To illustrate Homans's concepts of sentiments, activities, and interactions,[15] the fourth example hypothesizes how patient outcomes in intensive care units can be assessed. In the study described earlier, of intensive care services, by Knaus and associates the purpose of the research was to study mortality rates. Although it was not the main purpose to measure interaction, units with the lowest mortality rates had a greater frequency of nurse-physician verbal exchange.

In analyzing the cycle of relationships, according to Homans and as described in Figure 20.3, the motives and drives (sentiments) of nurses and physicians to maintain high standards of care are the impetus for structuring daily exchanges (activities). These activities result in the exchange of information (interaction) about patient care. Frequent communications are then characterized, according to Homans, by physicians and nurses liking each other to a greater extent. As an outcome, these sentiments and teamwork account for the high-quality care.

Rewards are the satisfactions deriving from the high standards of care that are maintained. Cost for the personnel is incurred by the time and effort spent maintaining daily communications. Profit is the pride of the staff in a hospital with a low-mortality rate.

Example 5: Relationships in Small Communities

To further illustrate the relationship of rewards, costs, and profits in social exchange, the fifth example portrays the nurse administrator in a home health-care agency who is responsible for assigning nurses to care for an 80-year-old woman who has had a stroke. Social relations and the accompanying challenges in community nursing are different than in hospitals. Outside of hospitals, the community is the client. The breadth of relationships requires that the competent nurse administrator respond to the multiple components of a defined community.[17] Administration of nursing services in the community demands knowledge about all related structures from a political, social, and economic perspective.

In this example, a family living in a small, rural community needs assistance in caring for their elderly mother. The needed nursing care is provided by a nurse from a local home health agency. Shortly after care is commenced, members of the family make an angry call to the nurse administrator in charge of the agency because they learn that the nurse also cares for a patient with autoimmune deficiency syndrome (AIDS). The family does not want the nurse to continue caring for their mother because of their concern that she may contract AIDS from the nurse. The family threatens to seek services from another home health agency.

The threat to the community posed by the AIDS patient was discussed heatedly at a recent local community meeting, and several neighbors have been upset about the potential threat of AIDS to other patients receiving care from the agency nurses. Along with the nurse administrator's reassurance to the family that AIDS transmission does not occur indirectly through a second person, the administrator arranges for a presentation at the next community meeting by an epidemiologist and a local physician. Recognition of language as a potent vehicle in this situation serves to facilitate communications between the speakers and community members. Henry and LeClaire stress the importances of messages that avoid mismatches in meanings.[18] In our example, it is essential for the presenters to communicate information about AIDS at the participants' level of understanding. In this potentially charged situation, the meeting serves as a major way of influencing the participants' future actions in which rewards, costs, and profits assume high significance.

A value held by the administrator entails distributing correct information to the community as a basis for trust in agency-client relationships. Protection of an elderly parent represents the rewards (values) held by the family. The administrator's costs involve the threat of failure, which is, in this situation, the potential loss of clients because of the inability to provide acceptable services. Further, the director's time and energy expended in the community presentations represent an additional cost. Uncertainty, fear, and anger aroused in the family constitute costs over and above the worry about a parent's condition. The nurse administrator's profits are the knowledge that the community can be mobilized to solve a problem of relationships between the agency and family.

Economics and politics generate major issues for the nursing director in marketing a type of care that is acceptable to clients and in remaining competitive with other agencies. In a study of 72 public-health nurse administrators, monitoring the sentiments in the community by arranging for the exchange of information is reported as a feasible marketing strategy.[19]

Example 6: The Cost of Enforcing Rules

A final example illustrating how the concepts of reward, cost, and profit in social exchange can be used is provided by a situation where it is necessary to respond to the psychological needs of families as clients. Nurses on a pediatric unit ask the evening supervisor to talk with the parents of a child who want to remain in their child's room throughout the night. Since the child is seriously ill, the parents have been closely involved with care the entire day. In the nurses' opinion, only one parent should stay all night because of the limited space in the child's room. In addition, the staff feel that parents should adhere to the visiting policy, which stipulates that only one parent is permitted in the hospital at night.

For one-half hour, the supervisor calmly listens to the parents' concern, then encourages only one parent to stay overnight in accordance with the visiting policy. At 11 p.m. the supervisor returns to find one parent staying in the room, while the other maintains a vigil in the visitors' lounge. Further discussion results in the parents becoming distressed and adamant about staying close to their sick child. Weighing the situation, the supervisor decides to act as the family's advocate and makes a decision not to persist in enforcing the visiting policy. Complaints from nurses are strongly voiced; the staff feel the supervisor has not supported them.

Rewards for both the staff nurses and evening supervisor embodied the values of parent involvement in implementing the plan for care of the child. Costs in this conflicting situation were related to the time spent by the nurses and supervisor in their interactions with the parents. An additional cost for the supervisor was the sentiments developed by the staff resulting in strained interactions between the staff and the supervisor. For the supervisor, a profit was the knowledge that the parents' expectations were satisfied. For the staff, the costs outweighed the profits— the nurses were hampered in their activities during the night.

In summary, the concepts and relationships described in social exchange theory suggest innovative ways of understanding how nurse administrators manage successful relationships between clients, staff, and other administrators. Whether the nurse administrator is involved in corporate-level decisions, interdepartmental problem-solving, or first-line management in communities, the perspective of the reward-cost-profit framework fosters understanding of the most proficient level of functioning. It is essential for the administrator to assist others to articulate the rewards that each brings to an interaction. Because costs in relationships could lead to dissatisfaction, the astute administrator creates a climate where individuals can express their sentiments. In negotiating relationships among the client, staff, and organization the effective administrator assists individuals to recognize rewards, weigh costs, and come to terms with what are considered reasonable profits. Creating a climate of invigorating relationships in which individuals make use of reward-cost-profit analysis can enhance individuals' pride in their organizational partnership.

REFERENCES

1. Drucker P. Management: Tasks, responsibilities, practices. New York: Colophon, 1974.
2. Harrison JK, Roth PA. Empowering nursing in multihospital systems. Nurs Econ 1987;5:70–76.
3. Freund C, Mitchell J. Multi-institutional systems: the new arrangement. Nurs Econ 1985;3:24–32.
4. Lévi-Strauss C. The elementary structures of kinship. (Trans. unknown). Boston: Beacon Press, 1949/1969.
5. Ekeh P. Social exchange theory: the two traditions. Cambridge: Harvard University Press, 1974.
6. Homans G. The human group. London: Routledge & Kegan Paul, 1951.
7. Homans G. Social behavior: its elementary forms. New York: Harcourt, Brace & World, 1961.
8. Thibaut J, Kelley H. The social psychology of groups. New York: John Wiley & Sons, 1959.
9. Nye F. The basic theory. In: Nye, F, ed. Family relationships: rewards and costs. Beverly Hills: Sage, 1982.
10. Mauss M. The gift. (I. Cunnison, Trans.). Glencoe, IL: The Free Press, 1925/1954.
11. Ekeh P. Social exchange theory: the two traditions. Cambridge: Harvard University Press, 1974, p. 87.
12. Riley MW, Cohn R, Toby J, Riley JW. Interpersonal relations in small groups. Am Soc R 1955;19:715–724.
13. Homans G. The human group. London: Routledge & Kegan Paul, 1951, p. 87.
14. Homans G. Social behavior: its elementary forms. New York: Harcourt, Brace & World, 1961, pp. 53–55, 75.
15. Knaus W, Draper E, Wagner D, Zimmerman J. An evaluation of outcome from intensive care in major medical centers. Ann Intern Med 1986;104(3):410–418.
16. Covalski M, Dirsmith M. Building tents for nursing services through budgeting negotiation skills. Nurs Adm Q 1984;8(2):1–11.
17. Stevens BJ. The nurse as executive. 3rd edition. Rockville, MD: Aspen Publishers, Inc, 1985.
18. Henry B, LeClair H. Language, leadership, and power. JONA 1987;17(1):19–25.
19. Smith A. Public health nurse administrator: coping with competition. Nurs Econ 1985;3:338–340.

21

Nursing Administration as Public Administration: Some Theoretical Perspectives

H. George Frederickson

THE RELATIONSHIP between nursing administration and modern public administration is significant and profound. Both fields are multidisciplinary, which is to say both draw upon many disciplines for their theoretical or conceptual foundations. Both nursing and public administration are practical and applied, the worth of our theories and concepts being daily evaluated by those who practice. Both fields function in the context of large-scale complex organizations. Both fields exist to serve others.

Indeed, the relationship between nursing and public administration makes them the closest of cousins. Over 35 years ago the distinguished public administration theorist, Finer, published the first comprehensive (and still very useful) treatment of *Administration and the Nursing Services*.[1] His focus was the "administration" side of both public and nursing administration.

Many of the essays in this anthology examine the subject of management and organization. Therefore, my focus will be the "public" aspect of public administration, and what I believe should be the public side of nursing administration.

The subject of the public in public and nursing administration is a big one. Therefore, this treatment is of necessity selective and targeted. The targets are three: conceptions of the public for administration; citizenship and administration; and, applications of social equity to administration. The first purpose is to hit these three targets hard enough to demonstrate the closeness of the relationship between nursing and public administration. Because most readers are nurses, the second purpose is to acquaint them with the modern field of public administration.

CONCEPTIONS OF THE PUBLIC FOR ADMINISTRATION

While much of the thinking in modern public administration implies that public means government, in fact, "public" and "government" are two very different words and two very different ideas. The field is not, after all, referred to as government administration. Why? Because the concept of public is not synonymous with the concept of government. "Public" is a prepolitical, pregovernmental, and prebureaucratic word and idea.[3]

The meaning of public traces to two sources, the Greek words *pubes* and *koinen*. *Pubes* was the Greek word for physical, emotional, and intellectual maturity. It means moving from an immature and selfish state to a mature state, moving beyond self-interest to understanding the interests of others. An adult is, therefore, in the public, part of the public, able to understand the relationship between the individual and others, and able to see the consequences of relationships.[2]

The second root word, *koinen*, is the word from which our word "common" derives. Common, of course, means held together, or belonging to everyone. *Koinen* comes from another Greek word, *Kom-ois* meaning "to care with." So, this root of the word public means things in common as well as caring with or concern with.

Taken together, then, public means the mature ability to function in "the common" and to have concern for others. Public describes "things" such as maturity and commonly held goods or items; the "capacity" to comprehend the effects of one's actions on others; and the "idea" of persons working together for the common good.

One way to explicate the meaning of public is to contrast it with the meaning of the word "private." The original Greek word for private has become our word "idiot." Private means being unable to mature and see the significance of relationships between people, and to have a conception of the common good. A second Greek word, *oikos* also means private in the sense of one's family or household. In fact the original meaning of the English word private meant to be deprived of a public life.[3] Palmer reminds us that "the private status that we so value in our day, the life on which we lavish such energy and attention, was once regarded as a state of deprivation."[2]

The public, in contemporary terms, has different meanings. To some, public implies the masses, and ordinary, or vulgar. To others, public means opposition to business or an inclination to collectivism. Public is common parlance in describing schools and universities, parks, libraries, some kinds of radio and television, and so forth. In England, the pub is still, although a business, licensed as a "public house" where anyone can gather.

Much of what we do collectively is public in the sense that it is available to all—theaters, symphonies, parks, the media, and services. This brings us to the critical point: Services are public.

Most services are presented to people in the form of business—as retail shops, utilities, newspapers, dental care, and health care, for example. But these services are also public in the very significant sense that they are available to all. Many services are, of course, provided by cities, counties, states—highways, schools, national defense, international diplomacy—and these obviously are public. Many services are presented to the public by both government and business or nonprofit organizations, as in the cases of public and private hospitals, universities, and utilities. To the ordinary member of the public, the distinctions between public and private utilities are minor, each "taxes" the public as the exclusive provider of services. So, governments, businesses, and nonprofit institutions provide services to the public and are, therefore, public. Indeed, Bozeman boldly states that all organizations are public.[4]

If one is a government employee, then one is obviously in public service. Those who take supervisory or management roles in the public sector are public administrators. School teachers are public servants, as are the police, and, of course, those nurses employed by federal, state, county, and city governments. Nurses with management or supervisory roles in government agencies are public administrators. But what about nurses who are employed by businesses such as doctors' offices or profit-making hospitals, or those employed by nonprofit hospitals and health maintenance organizations? Are they not also public servants?

First, they serve the public in as direct a way as nurses working for government. Second, all nurses are literally licensed by the public, through state governments, to provide effective nursing and health services.

Third, virtually all nongovernmental health service organizations are financed by governmental or insurance funds. If nurses serve the public, if they are licensed by the public, and are paid directly or indirectly by the public, are they not public servants?

In terms of responsibility to the public, should it make a difference to a nurse administrator if he or she is working for a governmental organization, a nonprofit organization, or a profit-making one? In the field of public administration, our answer to that question is no. The nurse administrator's highest obligation is to the public he or she serves. Can an obligation to stockholders or business owners be greater than one's responsibility to the public? No. Can an obligation to legislators or executives be greater than responsibility to the people? No.

While most readers might instinctively agree with this reasoning, it is still too general and vague. What does it mean for both public and nurse administrators to be responsible to the public? Do we understand the public to be a single collective to which we are responsible? Or do we understand the public to be singular, one person distinct from the others? I shall attempt in the next section to set out some ideas about citizenship that provide the administrator with perspectives on the public that are sufficiently concrete to accommodate exercising responsibility to the public.

Neither a nurse administrator nor a public administrator relates to the public from an autonomous position. We, at least most of us, are part of large-scale organizations. To be effective, predictable, and efficient we function in a world of order, organization, hierarchy, procedures, and records. We are bureaucrats, cogs in a bigger machine. Our machines are governmental, business and nonprofit, but still large, complex machines nonetheless. How can we serve the public in a responsible way in the context of our bureaucratic machines? In the third section of this chapter, I shall indicate, through the concept of social equity, how we can serve the public effectively from our organizational homes.

CITIZENSHIP AND ADMINISTRATION

One of the founders of the field of public administration, Woodrow Wilson, pointed out in his seminal essay, "The Study of Administration" in 1887, that in this democracy it is not the monarch that is sovereign but the people.[5] While in Wilson's time, administration was thought of as managerial and technical, he pointed out that in the U.S. context public administration "is, at the same time, raised very far above the . . . level of mere technical detail, by the fact that through its greater principles, it is directly connected with the lasting maxims of political wisdom, the permanent truth of political progress"[5] (p. 10). Wilson also stated, "the principles upon which to base a science of administration for America must be principles which have democratic policy very much at heart"[5] (p. 11). Public administration, then, calls for the active participation of administrators in the policy process and calls on administrators to protect the principles of democratic government.

To Wilson, the administrator had direct responsibilities to citizens, a logic, of course, that traces to the Constitution. In a democratic system, the concept of public refers to the citizens of the political community and assumes that the rights and obligations of citizenship are understood by all. The commitment of administrators in a democratic setting should be to citizens' rights and responsibilities as reflected in the values spelled out in the Constitution.

The public, all of the people in their pregovernmental, prepolitical, and preorganizational state, formed a system of government that did two things. First, it obligated individual members of the public—the citizens—to exercise certain responsibilities to one another. Second, it established a government based on a commitment to values the founding fathers felt should be vouchsafed. These values were taken as true, and included the right to participate in selecting representatives, the protection of private and family rights, the judicial aspects of procedural due process, and perhaps most important, the freedoms and guarantees of the Bill of Rights.[6]

All 50 of the state constitutions are built upon the same model, with virtually the same guarantees. These constitutions have endured the corruption of spoils in the nineteenth century, the great Civil War, several economic depressions, the relentless pursuit of the frontier to the West, and the full inclusion of women and black Americans in the citizenry—what some now regard as the greatest threat of all.

Can effective citizenship survive large-scale, complex bureaucratic organizations? By this I do not mean exclusively or even primarily governmental organizations. General Motors, Proctor & Gamble, the Republican Party, and the American Medical Association are metaphors of contemporary America. The citizen is lost in the sea of huge organizations. Size and professionalization mitigate against direct citizen involvement in policy formulation. A citizen votes, uses services, and chooses between goods offered for sale. He or she is thought of as a client or a customer. But the citizen is seldom thought of as a participant.

Flathman describes participation in "high citizenship" as follows: "Citizens are free, equal, and engaged with one another in pursuing matters of high and distinct human import. Citizenship is the distinctive human activity and the distinctively important feature of the political society"[7] (p. 9). The high-citizenship view is known elsewhere as the "strong democracy" perspective.[8] Flathman argues that only through a commitment on the part of administrators, elected officials, and citizens, to the notion of citizenship,

can there be legitimacy in the exercise of authority in a democratic polity. Legitimacy is critical to the exercise of authority in an effective, yet open, government. Therefore, what should these commitments to citizenship be in administration?

First, that the public administrator has the responsibility for acting directly with citizens. Does this undermine the processes of electoral democracy? Yes, if the public administrator is bent on self-recognition and power. And yes, if the administrator does not understand the point at which his or her prerogatives and responsibilities end, and an elected official's prerogatives begin. Otherwise the answer is no. It is, after all, as critically important for the administrator to enable citizens to participate in policy processes as it is for elected officials. If one assumes that citizens only function to cast votes, then one does not understand U.S. democracy. The administrator who is a public servant has the responsibility to facilitate the routine and regular interaction of citizens with their public organizations.

Would there not, under this approach, be a significant loss in efficiency and economy because of high levels of citizen involvement? And are not such processes inherently slow and cumbersome? Yes, if there is too great an emphasis on process and not sufficient emphasis on closure. As has been said elsewhere, "For the public administrator to be effective, there must be an understanding of the workings of democratic government. Understanding the subtleties of politics and the machinery of government is important. An understanding of the constant process of mediation and adjustment in the policymaking process is important. These arts must be part of the education of public servants"[9] (p. 504).

A second commitment in the citizenship perspective should be to the principles of justice set out in the Constitution. Justice has come generally to mean that which is fair.

While much of what we presently call justice is dealt with through the civil and criminal courts, questions of fairness and equity are dealt with every day by administrators. The next section of this essay will deal further with the subject of social equity.

The third commitment in the citizenship perspective should be to freedom. The constitutional commitments are to many freedoms: of expression, religion, the press, and assembly. In much of the world's history, the biggest single threat to individual freedom has been government. These days, large-scale organizations and the persons who work in these organizations are the perceived threat to individual freedom. It is widely believed that organizations are dehumanizing and threaten the freedom of individuals who work in them and the persons they serve.

However, as I have argued elsewhere, "In fact, it is our large-scale organizations that free us. The U.S. population is better educated than ever before because of large-scale and complex institutions. We are healthier than ever before because of large and intricately-related health service organizations. We may long for the corner grocery store, but in fact, the advantages of the supermarket are compelling. Indeed, the world of large-scale organizations enhances freedom. The trick is to make those organizations changeable and responsive and not allow them to exist primarily for the persons who work in them or profit from them, but for those who are to be served by them"[9] (p. 504). It is evident that we have traded some flexibility, some latitude, even some freedom, for the convenience and security of big organizations.[10]

There can be no better empirical evidence for this than one sees in the field of health care. The infrastructure of U.S. health services has changed dramatically in the past 20 years. In almost all cases, these changes have been in the direction of consolidating smaller units into more efficient, larger units. While cost containment explains some of these changes, the general convenience of size, coupled with creative means of providing alternative services also accounts for the trend toward consolidation.

As significant changes occur in health care and other services, it is a particular challenge to nurse administrators, as well as to other administrators, to be responsive to the public—to facilitate citizen involvement in the conduct of large organizations and to seek opportunities for providing all public services on as equitable a basis as possible.

While this may have the ring of a Sunday school lesson, much of what is being suggested here for the U.S. polity is already underway. Citizens are deeply concerned about the education of their children, but have very serious questions about the effectiveness of public schools. Through a variety of means in recent years, citizens have become involved in the reform of U.S. education. Citizens are deeply concerned about crime and law enforcement; they have serious reservations about the effectiveness of the police, the courts, and the penal system. But they are working together to improve these systems. Effective administrators are working with citizens to sustain and nurture their participation. And the U.S. public is deeply concerned about health care; they have serious reservations about the operation of hospitals, health maintenance organizations, health cooperatives, and the medical professions. We see as a consequence, a significant revolution going on in U.S. health care. Effective administrators, including managers of nursing services, are facilitating that revolution, inventing ways to control costs, promote wellness, and compassionately treat illness.

Through the perspective of citizenship, we are, in the latter half of the twentieth century, learning to respond to the question Cleveland once asked: "How can we get more governance and less government?"[11] Citizens, public administrators and large-scale businesses, are learning how to have broader-based citizen participation in policy processes and in some administrative routines; at the same time they are keeping their organizations effective and responsive. There are myriad reflections of this, including the consumer movement, the environmental protection movement, neighborhood associations, and the sharp increase in U.S. volunteerism.

Finally, and perhaps most importantly, we seem to have learned that our most vexing domestic problems are better solved through a combination of public-private partnerships, through extensive local neighborhood and citizen involvement, and through less social experimentation on the part of the national government. This is not to say that many of the overarching national policy issues such as nuclear disarmament, economic stability, and the social security system are not critical. It is to say, however, that many of our most vexing problems seem now to be closer to solution as a result of local rather than federal action. And it is at the local level that citizens are most effective.

SOCIAL EQUITY, PUBLIC, AND NURSING ADMINISTRATION

If we are responsible to the public through our organizations, and if the public relates to administrators through their role as citizens, how then do we judge organizational effectiveness? What ought to be the calculus of productivity? And how do we calibrate administrative competence? My suggestion is that "social equity" be a standard against which modern public and nursing administration effectiveness be measured.[12]

We begin with *Black's Law Dictionary*, which states that:

In its broadest and most general signification . . . [equity] denotes the spirit and habit of fairness, justice, and right dealing which would regulate the intercourse of men with men: "the rule of doing to all others as we desire them to do us"; or, as is expressed by Justinian, "To live honestly, to harm nobody, render every man his due." . . . it is therefore the synonym of natural right, or justice. But in this sense its obligation is ethical rather than jural, and its discussions belongs to the sphere of morals. It is grounded in the precepts of the conscience, not in any sanction of positive law.[13] (p. 643)

This description of equity is wholly compatible with the values the founding fathers codified in the Constitution. Not only are the protections of the Constitution provided to each citizen individually, it is also made clear that each citizen is entitled to "the equal protection of the law." In the last twenty years, the Supreme Court has interpreted the Constitution to mean that municipal public services, such as the care of roads and the provision of public education must be provided on an equitable basis to the citizenry.[14] Further, the courts have systematically decided that standards of fairness and equity must be included with standards of competence in decisions of initial employment of persons, as well as in promotion and salary decisions.[15] There are many more examples of the applications of principles of social equity in modern jurisprudence.

But the law dictionary indicated that equity is not so much a matter of positive law as a question of morals, a matter of ethics. In the traditions of the field of public administration, the standards by which administrative effectiveness has always been measured have been efficiency, economy, and productivity. In the past 20 years, social equality has been added as a criterion for effectiveness in public administration. This means that the effectiveness of the administrator is judged by others on the basis of standards of social equity. It cannot be that the administrator simply waits for the courts to decide the question of equity. The effective administrator acts in a positive sense to ensure equity, fairness, and justice in the provision of public services, and in the case-by-case application of institutional policy.

The most often used theoretical base for social equity is found in Rawls's, *A Theory of Justice*.[16] The Rawlsean perspective begins with this:

For us the primary subject of justice is the basic structure of society, or more exactly, the way in which the major social institutions distribute fundamental rights and duties and determine the division of advantages from social cooperation. By major institutions I understand the political constitution and the principle economic and social arrangements.[16] (p. 7)

Rawls begins with the conception of each person—regardless of genetic inheritance, historical or social situation—as having a basic citizen's entitlement. Discourse and thinking about each citizen should be conducted behind a "veil of ignorance," or in other words, using a set of rules that do not take into account the specific social or genetic conditions of the citizen. In the abstract, then, no person knows his or her place in society, class or social status. In the abstract, each person does not know whether he or she is more rather than less advantaged. It is obvious, then, that the principles of justice that are chosen must advance the condition of the least advantaged person, since one could easily be that person. Once this intellectual device is accepted, Rawls suggests his two principles of justice, which are:

1. Each person is to have an equal right to the most extensive total system of equal basic liberties compatible with a similar system of liberty for all.
2. Social and economic inequalities are to be arranged so that they are both (a) of the greatest benefit to the least advantaged, consistent with the just savings principle, and (b) attached to offices of positions open to all under conditions of fair equality and opportunity.[16] (p. 302)

The application of Rawls's theory of justice does not mean that all inequalities will disappear and that all goods will be equally distributed. There will always be disparities in income and status. But there is an irreducible minimum of primary goods (such as self-respect, rights and liberties, powers and opportunities, income and wealth) that are due every person. And that minimum must be met.

In application, the conception of social equity obliges the public and nurse administrator to operate within the context of a set of principles that balances concern for efficiency, economy, and productivity with concern for equity. Of course, most of us work in organizations that do not affect, at least in a grand way, the distribution of wealth. But we do distribute services, and we decide, both on a case-by-case basis, and on the basis of social classes or categories, who is entitled to what. Social equity means having a higher quality of law enforcement in areas in which the poor reside than in areas where the rich live. Social equity also means that health-care services will be more extensively provided for those with greater need. This use of the standard of equity in a formal and specific way, as an ethical or moral responsibility, is wholly compatible with the Constitution, with contemporary philosophy, and with many modern administrative or professional codes of ethics.

In conclusion, the intellectual origins of modern public administration included the idea that effective administration in a democracy requires virtuous citizens. Virtue in this case means the voluntary observance of norms of personal behavior in accord with recognized laws and standards of morality. "The founders believed that the ultimate measure of a state was the level of virtue achieved by its citizens. However, they rejected the argument that the government should use its power to produce such virtue."[17]

Virtue implies action. The virtuous citizen is active in public (not just governmental) affairs and engages in moral philosophy. This citizen believes that the United States' founding values are true, not just majoritarian preferences. The virtuous citizen takes moral responsibility for the guarantee of the founders' values and rights. Finally, the virtuous citizen understands civility and engages in tolerances and forbearances toward the views of others[17] (pp. 114–117).

The public administrator, including the nurse administrator, must first strive to understand citizenship and to be a virtuous citizen. In the context of other virtuous citizens, the public and nurse administrator becomes what Hart describes as the honorable bureaucrat.

Public administrators have extensive control over public (not just governmental) bureaucracies. Because they are not elected they have a special moral obligation to never compromise founding values. "Whether through partisan decision, economic considerations, presumed administrative efficiencies, or professional neutrality. They must be active proponents of the regime values"[17] (p. 116).

The honorable public or nurse administrator, therefore, assumes the following four duties. First, fundamentally unjust policies are opposed and if asked to administer dishonorable programs, the administrator will resign. Usually public administrators deal with routine matters. But sometimes they are faced with a policy issue of moral significance. "This calls for a moral heroism not often associated with bureaucracy. However, there are innumerable examples of bureaucrats who have made great sacrifices for their moral convictions. The point is that the U.S. regime values require that kind of heroism, whether from virtuous citizens or from honorable bureaucrats"[17] (p. 117).

Second, it is essential that honorable public administrators genuinely *care* for the public they serve. And the public must believe that bureaucrats truly care for them. In this era of professional narrowness on the one hand, and citizen self-interest on the other, we have an absence of feelings and caring between citizens and those who attempt to administer public organizations. While it is idealistic, there can be no doubt, that one of the keys to administrative effectiveness in public life is the capacity to care for the public, both collectively and individually.

Third, the honorable bureaucrat is a moral entrepreneur. "It is the willingness to take moral risks that is important to honorable bureaucrats. They must always attempt to reduce the number of rules, laws, and compulsions upon citizens, and the only way to do this is through trust. The public must always be treated as virtuous citizens who can be depended upon to honor their commitments"[17] (p. 118).

Fourth, honorable public administrators believe in noblesse oblige. They believe that the more one is benefited in society, the more one is obligated to benefit society.

Taken together, noblesse oblige, caring, risk taking, and understanding moral significance characterize the honorable public and nurse administrator. They nurture a virtuous citizenry, and the people honor them.

REFERENCES

1. Finer H. Administration and the nursing services. New York: Macmillan, 1952.
2. Palmer PJ. The company of strangers. New York, Crossroads Publishing, 1981.
3. Mathews D. The public in practice and theory. Public Administration Review 1984;44:120–126.
4. Bozeman B. All organizations are public. San Francisco: Josey Bass Publishing, 1986.
5. Wilson W. The study of administration. Political Science Quarterly 1887; 2. Reprinted in Shafritz, JM, Hyde, AC, eds. Classics of public administration. Oak Park, IL: Moore Publishing, pp. 8–9.
6. Rohr J. To run a constitution. Lawrence, Kansas: The University of Kansas Press, 1986.
7. Flathman R. Citizenship and authority: a chastened view of citizenship, News for Teachers of Political Science 1981;30:9–19.
8. Barber B. Strong democracy. Berkeley: University of California Press, 1986.
9. Frederickson HG. The recovery of civicism in public administration. Public Administration Review 1982; 42:501–508.

10. Scott WG, Hart DK. Organizational America. Boston: Houghton Mifflin, 1979.
11. Cleveland H. The chronicle of higher education. October 28, 1981, p. 11.
12. Frederickson HG. Symposium on social equity and public administration. Public Administration Review 1974;34:1–51.
13. Black CB. Black's law dictionary. St. Paul, Minn: West Publishers, 1957.
14. Chitwood SR. Social equity and social service productivity. Public Administration Review 1974;34:29–43.
15. McGregor EB. Social equity and the public service. Public Administration Review 1974;34:18–29.
16. Rawls J. A theory of justice. Cambridge, MA: The Belknap Press of the Harvard University Press, 1971.
17. Hart DK. The virtuous citizen, the honorable bureaucrat, and 'public' administration. Public Administration Review 1984;44:111–120.

22

Epistemological Approaches to Interdisciplinary Inquiry for Nursing Administration

Beverly Henry

FOR NURSING administration, an important question is, How should the knowledge of nursing and management* be combined to build theory and improve practice? The purpose of this chapter is to discuss epistemological approaches to interdisciplinary nursing administration where nursing and management knowledge are integrated.

In the first section, the focus is academic disciplines and the considerations involved when ideas about nursing and notions about management are combined for interdisciplinary studies. In the latter sections, metaphor and ideonomy, the science of ideas, are described as mechanisms for facilitating the development of knowledge.

Integrating knowledge from nursing and management has been widely recommended in nursing.[1–5] Less attention has been paid to how integration should develop. It is the *how* of integrating knowledge that is focused on in this chapter.

*The terms "management," "administration," and "organization science" are used interchangeably throughout the chapter.

THE NATURE OF DISCIPLINES AND INTERDISCIPLINARY ENDEAVORS

An academic discipline is characterized by a unique structure of thinking. A discipline is more than a restricted area of facts. Sowell has made the following statements. "Mathematics is not just a subject matter but an intellectual discipline, with its own peculiar structure of reasoning. Chemistry and economics have their own very different intellectual structures, as do other fields."[6]

Sowell continues by noting that there is a tendency to blithely talk about interdisciplinary studies where knowledge from a number of disciplines is "integrated." Importantly for our purposes, he tells readers that mastering any single discipline entails years of work, mastering several disciplines takes decades, and "integrating" knowledge from multiple fields may well be the effort of a lifetime.[6]

Because of the magnitude of the intellectual effort involved in developing truly interdisciplinary programs, many academic undertakings called "interdisciplinary" are far from being even "multidisciplinary". They are "nondisciplinary" instead: each field is treated as a separate subject matter rather than as a structured method of analysis. They are shallow endeavors that degenerate into fashionable crusades and are characterized by "thematic courses that focus on topics (not intellectual structure)."[6]

Observations such as these are worth our serious consideration. The task ahead is to assure that nursing administration inquiry—education and research in the field—contributes to nursing's intellectual enterprise and does not undermine it. In our effort to make nursing administration interdisciplinary, what is created could be "nondisciplinary," comprised merely of a series of courses focusing, for example, on finance, marketing, and policy analysis.

Development of the parent discipline of nursing as a serious, nationwide, intellectual effort is barely underway. Some may argue, therefore, that it is premature to ask questions at this early stage about how nursing administration can become interdisciplinary. Others may disagree with the assumption that interdisciplinary inquiry is preferable to single or multidisciplinary efforts for the advancement of knowledge. Still others may wonder whether or not any of the professions, as applied practice disciplines, do more than borrow knowledge.

These perspectives are important. My belief however, is that nursing administration is a professional practice for which interdisciplinary inquiry is appropriate. This belief derives from practical short-range concerns about how nurses function with respect to organizations, and from less immediate but equally critical concerns about the advancement of nursing knowledge. At work, the interface between nurses, nurse administrators, and nonnurse managers is abrasive. In the profession, the interface between nursing as a discipline and nursing administration as a subdiscipline is equally problematic. Attending to the core knowledge of nursing administration therefore is important lest faculty be ill-equipped to educate practitioners

capable of collaborative work, and lest nursing administration become little more than a "fashionable crusade"—a shallow nondiscipline devoid of a defined cognitive structure.

EPISTEMOLOGICAL APPROACHES TO INTERDISCIPLINARY PROGRAMS

Educators and seasoned practitioners are responsible for preparing future nurses who can effectively manage health care and the environment of care—organizations. In epistemological terms, we are charged with the task of providing students not merely with the latest information and subject matter on topics apropos of nursing and management, but with the facility to see and understand the similarities and differences in the structure of knowledge—the cognitive maps—of the two disciplines.

The map or structure of any single discipline incorporates, among other things, the elements illustrated in Figure 22.1. To understand a discipline, one must be knowledgeable about its general ideals, basic concepts, and observational categories—as well as its modes of inquiry, types of problems, and standards of proof.[7]

A multidisciplinary endeavor is symbolized by the upper half of Figure 22.1, representing the parallel but separate domains of nursing and management. For nursing administration that is multidisciplinary, there is little if any integration of knowledge: the two domains are viewed largely as separate.

In the lower half of the figure, the diagram represents the combining of knowledge for nursing administration. Integration supports development of interdisciplinary practice, education and research which in turn feeds back new, modified knowledge to the nursing and management domains.

Students educated in programs where serious consideration is *not* paid to the knowledge of both nursing and management are less likely to function effectively in the workplace.

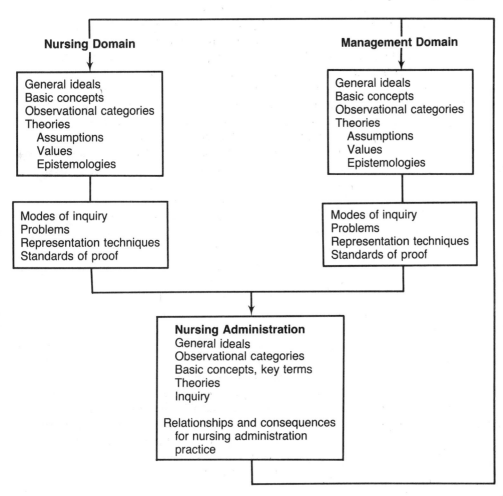

Figure 22.1   Integrating Knowledge from Nursing and Organization Science for Nursing Administration

If nurse administrators are not cognizant of the general ideals, key terms, and observational categories, at least, in the discipline of nursing, how can they understand the clinical nurses with whom they work? Likewise with respect to management science: if nurse administrators are treated to naive education where theoretical frameworks (with their accompanying assumptions and values) are not clear, and where the perceptual apparatus of management is not elucidated, how can they understand what their coworkers see and say? How can they get along in reasonably effective ways with managers rooted in other disciplines? Moreover, if nurses are not grounded in both nursing and management science, how can they be expected to use and generate new knowledge for nursing administration?

Nursing and management are alike in some ways and different in others. With respect to their similarities, in both nursing and public administration, decision making is pluralistic and highly visible. In the two fields, the emphasis is generally on service as opposed to profit and on measuring effective goal attainment.[8]

Nursing and business administration, on the other hand, can be remarkably different. Business administrators march to a drummer that places an exceedingly high value on efficiency, market forces, and profits. Conversely, nurses put a high value on the equitable provision of the finest quality of service for the greatest number. When problems in the workplace arise, a business administrator seeks ways of making an operation more efficient.[9] Nurses focus on quality—on what is equitable—and that is "total patient care" regardless of cost. Each has dissimilar ideals and construes work and how to solve problems differently. Since they are talking different languages (using different basic ideas and terms), oftentimes neither understands the other, goals are at variance, and conflicts result.

Because problems like these are only too familiar, it is important to ask: How can the differences and similarities in the cognitive structures of nurses and managers be best understood? How can we comprehend nursing and management science to produce the finest integrated knowledge for interdisciplinary inquiry that contributes to improved practice?

METAPHOR AND INTERDISCIPLINARY INQUIRY: MANAGEMENT SCIENCE

According to Petrie,[7] for effective interdisciplinary endeavors, at a minimum, participants must learn the "observational categories" and "key terms" in each discipline. One way to understand what others see and what key terms mean is to examine a discipline's metaphors. Metaphor in this context is defined broadly to include the visual pictures created by a discipline as well as its theories or models.

Metaphors do more than merely embellish discourse. They imply the ways of thinking and observing in a discipline that are manifestations of a discipline's unique or shared worldview. The metaphor, as Morgan[10] notes, "exerts a formative influence on science, on our language, and on how we think . . . We use metaphor whenever we attempt to understand one element of experience in terms of another" [p. 12].

Hanson describes the part that languages—key terms used by disciplinarians—play in the development of knowledge. Because knowledge, at a fundamental level, is linguistic, people using alternative metaphors and different languages in those metaphors have difficulty understanding what others apprehend and how education and research should best proceed.[11]

In nursing, the usefulness of the metaphor as a way of understanding is attested to by a number of authors. Fagin and Diers, for example, support delineating the metaphors of nursing.[12] Henry and LeClair have described the usefulness of languages and metaphors for nurses at work in complex organizations.[13] And Marriner, in her synopsis of nursing theory, classifies theories using four metaphors: nursing as humanistic art and science, as interpersonal relationships, as systems, and as energy fields.[14]

Different metaphors produce a variety of insights about the world. In epistemological terms, metaphors provide alternative observational categories and terms, which in turn enable us to comprehend not only the many diverse aspects of individuals, groups, and organizations, but also the different cognitive maps in various disciplines.

Morgan has developed a classification of theory in management science using metaphors that is helpful for identifying the similarities and differences between nursing and management. My premise is this: If we systematically compare the basic ideals, key terms, and concepts in nursing and management, an important first step has been taken in epistemological understanding of how to proceed with the integration of knowledge for nursing administration. By comparing nursing and management metaphorically, the world-views in the two disciplines become clearer and mutual understanding is less problematic. Moreover, as Petrie suggests, by understanding metaphors, "the gap between the differing categories and concepts of different disciplines" can be bridged[7] (p. 42).

According to Morgan, theorists conceive of management and organizations largely as machines, biological organisms, information processing systems, cultures, political systems, psychic prisons, and as systems of transformation, and domination.[10] Each of these metaphorical categories are shown in Table 22.1. The major ideas (epistemology), basic concepts, and a number of representative contributing theorists are also included.

Machine Metaphor

Where organizations are thought of as machines, the following ideas dominate: goal-setting, efficiency, rationality, strict accountability, and the idea that human behavior can be segmented into roles and reduced to the laws of matter in motion. Mechanistic thinking is manifest, for example, in Taylor's scientific management, in Weber's bureaucracy, in the study of motion by Gilbreth, and in the idea of management by objectives (MBO) developed by Drucker and others.[†]

Organismic Metaphor

Where organizations are viewed as living organisms, the cognitive map of biology has

influenced management science. The central epistemology is that organizations, like organisms, have needs, are dependent, and exist in external environments to which they are "open" if they wish to remain "vital." The idea of organizations as living systems is apparent, for example, in the Hawthorne studies by Roethlisberger and Mayo; in the needs studies of Maslow, Argyris, McGregor, and Herzberg; in organizational development theory by Blake and Mouton; and in the contingency theory of Woodward and Lawrence and Lorsch.

Brain Metaphor, Information Processing

Organizations as thinking systems, as brains, is a somewhat newer metaphor. The work of Simon, March, and Cyert on information processing and decision making as "satisficing" is central to this perspective. Cybernetic strategies described by Bateson as learning-to-learn, Schon's idea of double-loop learning, and the idea of holographic thinking as developed by Bohm and Wilber are prominent.

Culture Metaphor

Organizations are also viewed as cultures, and organizational subunits as subcultures. The concept of enactment and organizational reality draw on the work of anthropologists. Among the foremost theorists are Pascale and Athos, Pondy, and Schein. Smircich describes how organizations enact their environment. Pondy and Schein discuss legends, languages, and rituals in organizations. Values and traditions are described by Peters and Waterman.

Flux and Transformation Metaphor

In this metaphor, flux and change are fundamental. The universe at any given moment is

[†]On this and the next few pages, names of individuals are cited but references are not provided. The reader is referred to the useful book by Gareth Morgan, *Images of Organization*, for bibliographic citations.

TABLE 22.1   The Epistemologies, Basic Concepts, and Representative Theorists for Eight Metaphors in Management Science

Metaphor and Epistemology	Basic Concepts	Representative Theorists
Organizations as machines Organizations are rational and operate efficiently.	Bureaucratic Interlocking Roles Precision Efficiency Goal-setting Mechanical interaction Stimulus-response Rationality	Taylor Gilbreth Weber Drucker
Organizations as organisms Organizations are living, dependent, needy systems embedded in environments; effective organizations are "vital," open systems.	Needs Open systems Environmental relations Adaptation Coping Boundary Contingency Organization health Ecology Matrix	Roethlisberger Mayo Maslow Herzberg McGregor Argyris Trist von Bertalanffy Blake, Mouton Katz and Kahn Woodward Lawrence and Lorsch
Organizations as brains Organizations are understood in terms of information processing, intelligence, learning.	Decision making Bounded rationality Information processing Double-loop learning Holographic systems Intuition Cybernetics	Simon March Cyert Bateson Wilber Bohm
Organizations as cultures Organizations are socially constructed realities understood through patterns of shared meanings.	Values Beliefs Norms Rituals Traditions Language Enactment	Pascale and Athos Peters and Waterman Pondy Schein Van Mannen Smircich
Organizations as flux and transformation Organizations are systems of change in which the future is enfolded in the present.	Flowing unbroken wholeness Implicate order Explicate order Autonomy Circularity Self-reference Closure to environment Dialectic	Bohm Maturana, Varela Ulrich Probst Maruyama

TABLE 22.1 (Continued)

Metaphor and Epistemology	Basic Concepts	Representative Theorists
Organizations as political systems Organizations are systems of governance; there is a politics of organizational life.	Interests Conflicts Power Politics	Michels Burns and Stalker Pettigrew Pfeffer Wildavsky Morgan
Organizations as psychic prisons Organizations are unconscious extensions of family relations; ways of organizing are manifestations of individual psychodynamic processes.	Entrapment: conscious, unconscious Groupthink Prison-like qualities of cultures and groups Obsessive control Mentors Regulatory sadism Patriarchal authoritarianism	Laing Marcuse Mitroff Foucault Maccoby
Organizations as instruments of domination Organizations use employees, communities, world to achieve domination.	Exploitation Iron law of oligarchy	Weber Michels Marx Perrow Foucault Braverman

thought of as having an inner logic with all things enfolded within it. Rather than thinking of organizational systems as open to the external environment, in this perspective systems are self-referential. Thus, change and transformation are understood not as adaptive responses to external environmental change, but as internally self-generated.

Political, Psychic Prison, and Domination Metaphors

For the political metaphor, knowledge of organizations is developed in terms of governance, interests, conflicts, and power. Other key terms in this perspective are authority, politics, scarce resources, control, pluralism,

and cooperation. Where organizations are conceived of as psychic prisons, the idea of self-mastery and organizational control are fundamental. And where organizations are thought of as instruments of domination, exploitation, classes in organizations, occupational disease, workaholism, and stress are the main ideas.

METAPHOR AND INTERDISCIPLINARY INQUIRY: NURSING SCIENCE

In Table 22.2, nursing theories and theorists are categorized using the same metaphorical classifications and analogous epistemological

TABLE 22.2 Nurse Theorists and Basic Concepts in Nursing Theory Apropos of Nursing Administration, Classified by Organization Metaphors

Metaphor and Epistemology	Basic Concepts	Representative Theorists
Individuals and groups as machines Individuals and groups are rational and efficient.	21 nursing problems Goals Goal behavior Disciplined response Role	Abdellah Peplau King Orlando Riehl-Sisca Johnson Henderson
Individuals and groups as organisms Individuals and groups are viewed organismically as living, dependent entities with needs, embedded in environments to which they are open.	Nursing systems Needs Environment Adaptation Coping	Orem Adam Watson Peplau Roy Neuman King Barnard Johnson Levine
Individuals and groups as brains Individuals and groups are understood in terms of how they learn, their intelligence, and how they process information.	Judgment Holography	Wiedenbach Newman Benner
Individuals and groups as cultures Individuals and groups are understood through shared patterns of meaning.	Culture, care Humanistic-altruistic values	Leininger Watson Travelbee Orlando Wiedenbach
Individuals and groups as flux and transformation Individuals have an inner logic and engage in circular patterns of interaction that are self-referential: living systems close in on themselves to maintain stability.	Cocreating reality Transcending Resonancy, helicy, integrality	Parse Newman Fitzpatrick Rogers Watson
Individuals and groups as political systems Individuals and groups are viewed as rulers, in terms of governance and politics.	Self-governance	Hall
Individuals and groups as psychic prisoners and as prisons Psychodynamic processes account for actions.	Anxiety Out of awareness	Hall
Individuals and groups as instruments of domination Individuals and groups use others to achieve their ends.		

statements for individuals and groups.‡ What becomes apparent from the categorization is the similarity of basic concepts in nursing and management science. Incidentally, one could just as easily begin with the visual pictures portrayed by nursing metaphors—to identify where the gaps or overlaps of concepts for the two disciplines lie, and classify organization theory accordingly.

Many of the early nursing theories use concepts and describe relationships that suggest a mechanistic, or a combination of the mechanistic and organismic perspectives. The predominant ideas in nursing theory where a mechanistic view prevails are that ideally, individuals set mutual goals, work rationally toward achieving those goals, and people in segmented roles respond and behave in predictable ways that can be maintained or modified.

Just as thinking of organizations as biological systems pervades the worldview of social scientists, systems thinking is every bit as widespread in nursing. The concept of needs, for example, is foundational in many nursing metaphors, as are the concepts of adaptation, coping, environment, open systems, system vitality, and health.

A number of nurse theorists conceive of nursing using the metaphor of culture: Leininger, Watson, and Travelbee for example. And the theoretical perspectives of Rogers, Fitzpatrick, Newman, and Parse, appear to have a cognitive map for nursing very much like that of the transformationist.

The overlap in the cognitive maps of nursing and organization science are not surprising. Nursing theory draws heavily on the same body of science as does organization theory. Moreover, a strong argument can be made that nursing theory, at this stage of its

evolution, is largely theory of nursing care management; nursing theory to a significant degree addresses the management of care by nurses for individuals, small groups, and families.

Note, however, the few nurse theorists using the ideas of intelligence, information processing, judgment, and decision making as central themes. Moreover, there are few, if any, nursing theories that view individuals and groups—their care, environment, and health—as political systems. It is with respect to these perspectives that there is the greatest gap between nursing and management science.

What this metaphorical analysis does, however crudely, is to sort a number of the major concepts in nursing and management into understandable observational categories that identify where ideas in the two disciplines overlap and where they do not.

In the future, useful and important theories of nursing administration may be those that connect knowledge about human responses to health and illness with the ideas of information processing, cybernetics, political systems, transformation, and flux. To increase knowledge of nursing organizations as systems of transformation, inquiry would address the following types of questions: If organizations and environments are one, what patterns of relations define organizations? How does change in one organizational system transform all others? Because system patterns have to be understood as a whole, where do we begin our analysis?[10]

New knowledge for nursing is needed that reflects thinking at the cutting-edge in the natural, physical, and social sciences, and supplements existing theories in nursing that use ideas in the popular machine and organismic perspectives.

Ideonomy and Interdisciplinary Inquiry

Another approach to the development of interdisciplinary knowledge is suggested by

---

‡For both nursing and organization science, contributing theorists have been classified using the metaphor that seems to best represent the predominant ideas in their respective theories.

Terms

	Nursing		Management	
care	caring	organize	organizing
suffer	suffering	cost	costing
comfort	comforting	authority	authorizing
touch	touching	technology	technologizing

Two-Word Descriptions

caring organize | organizing care |

suffering cost   costing suffer

| comforting authority | | authorizing comfort |

| touching technology | | technologizing touch |

Analogies

Caring is to organizing as suffering is to costing.
Comforting is to authorizing as touching is to technologizing.

Questions

Can caring be organized?
Can suffering be costed?
Can comforting be authorized?
Can touching be technologized?

Figure 22.2   Combining Ideas from Nursing and Management

ideonomy and the computerized spinning of ideas. Whereas metaphors might be useful for identifying the gaps and overlap in the cognitive structures of nursing and management, ideonomy may be useful in delineating new conceptual knowledge.

Gunkel defines ideonomy as "the science of the laws of ideas and of the application of such laws to the generation of all possible ideas in connection with any subject, idea, or thing."[15] Lists of ideas—of concepts and notions in varying grammatical formulations—are developed on a subject, computerized, then woven together using all possible combinations. Much of what is generated is senseless. But some connections suggest new insights. Gunkel calls this matchmaking "idea combinatorics" and uses the matchmaking as a warm-up for ideonomy's serious goal of generating new insights for researchers.[15]

In nursing administration, suppose we develop lists of the key ideas in nursing and management, then generate combinations of those ideas, searching as we go for previously unseen connections. Perhaps what will be found will be ideonomical analogs for management that derive from nursing, and for nursing that derive from management.

In Figure 22.2, there is a short list of major concepts in nursing and management. Observe what happens with even these few ideas when they are systematically combined. Note, too, some of the derivable analogies and research questions.

Some combinations are nonsensical. But others are not. The combinations around which lines are drawn may be worth considering further. Perhaps the ideas of "comforting authority" and "touching technology" offer new ways of thinking and new categories important for the cognitive structure of nursing administration.

The analogies which can be developed may also be useful for generating useful models of nursing administration that find their roots in the ideas of nursing, health, and environment. Some educational programs for nursing administration are currently structured using macroanalogical models: the individual is to nursing as an organizational unit is to nursing administration; individual health and well-being is to nursing as organizational health and well-being is to nursing administration; and so on. In the future, the corresponding elemental micro-ideas in the domains of nursing and management can be merged for education and research in ways we have only begun to imagine.

NONEPISTEMOLOGICAL APPROACHES TO INTERDISCIPLINARY EFFORTS

Considerable efforts have been made in the past to understand the interdisciplinary aspects of nursing administration. The majority, however, are largely of the variety Petrie refers to as "nonepistemological." Attempts to develop interdisciplinary inquiry, which are not cognitive or intellectual, focus on the (1) dominant idea or driving force that spurs an interdisciplinary undertaking, (2) the characteristics of participants, and (3) institutional settings. A driving force in an interdisciplinary endeavor is a clear, recognizable notion deriving from some practical, external necessity. Characteristics of participants are the competence and interest of the individuals involved. And institutional setting is the place where time, money, and encouragement for an interdisciplinary effort is provided.[7]

Historically in nursing—except for the decade and a half between 1960 and 1975, when the thrust was clinical specialization—nursing administration has been a recognized, domi-

nant force. The idea that inquiry for nursing administration is legitimate has achieved a measure of acceptance. And this acceptance has resulted largely because of factors external to nursing, the foremost being the economic necessity that nurses remain in control of nursing. Extensive discussion exists in the literature about the characteristics of programs and faculty and the managerial skills that characterize effective nurse administrators. Courses, subject matter, and the rationale for the various topics that should be in nursing administration curriculums are also described as deriving, for the most part, from problems in the workplace. Considerable attention is paid, too, to whether nursing administration should be a major or minor area of study, at the master's or postmaster's levels, and whether programs are best placed in schools of nursing, or in schools of business or health administration.

Nonepistemological considerations like these are highly important to interdisciplinary endeavors. Alone, however, they are not sufficient if nursing is to develop as a discipline, and if interdisciplinary education and research in nursing administration are to become a reality. The task at this stage is to delineate more clearly than in the past, knowledge of nursing administration that represents an integration of knowledge from nursing and management science.

REFLECTIONS AND PROJECTIONS

Knowledge in our field is needed for practice that is intelligent, education that is credible, and for good research. Nursing administration is a sizeable component of today's master's and doctoral programs. Knowledge generated and disseminated in schools of nursing characterizes some of these programs. In others, students acquire knowledge in multiple disciplines: most often in nursing and business or health administration.

Regardless of the institutional setting, inquiry for nursing administration by definition is at least multidisciplinary, comprised of information from nursing and management. A goal in nursing, which is fairly widely valued, is that nursing administration should be interdisciplinary: it should represent an integration, even a modification of nursing and management knowledge.

The time when nurses were unable to identify nursing models by name,[20] one hopes, is behind us. And more and more nurses are broadening their understanding of the theoretical perspectives in organization science. The basic concepts, observational categories, and theories in the two disciplines are clearer to us in 1988 than they have been in the past.

Using metaphors can help clarify the multiple realities and connections between key terms and observational categories in nursing and management. Ideonomy as well may be useful in generating new ways of thinking about how concepts in the two fields can be combined to generate interdisciplinary knowledge, first for nursing administration, and ultimately for nursing and management.

REFERENCES

1. Arndt C, Huckabay LM. Nursing administration: theory for practice with a systems approach. St. Louis, MO: CV Mosby, 1980.
2. Brown B. Clinical nursing: a Basis for administrative excellence. In: Brown BJ, Chinn PL, eds. Nursing education: practical methods and models Rockville, MD: Aspen, 1982, pp. 109–115.
3. Jacox A. The research component in the nursing service administration master's program. J Nurs Adm 1974;4:35–39.
4. Leininger ML. This I believe . . . about interdisciplinary health education for the future. Nurs Outlook 1971;19:787–791.
5. Stevens BJ. Education in nursing administration: where are we and where should we be? In: Slater CH, ed. The education and roles of nursing service administrators. Battle Creek, MI: WK Kellogg, 1978b, pp. 21–38.
6. Sowell T. Recipe for change on campus. The Wall Street Journal, June, 1987.
7. Petrie HG. Do you see what I see? The epistemology of interdisciplinary inquiry. Journal of Aesthetic Education 1976;10(1):29–43.
8. Harmon MM, Mayer RT. Organization theory for public administration. Boston, MA: Little, Brown, 1986.
9. Dunlop JT. Business and Public Policy. Cambridge, MA: Harvard University Press, 1980.
10. Morgan G. Images of organization. Beverly Hills, CA: Sage, 1986.
11. Hanson NR. Patterns of discovery. Cambridge, Great Britain: The University Press, 1958.
12. Fagin C, Diers D. Occasional notes, nursing as metaphor. New England Journal of Medicine 1983; 309(2):116–117.
13. Henry B, LeClair H. Language, leadership and power 1987;17(1):19–25.
14. Marriner A. Nursing theorists and their work. St. Louis: CV Mosby, 1986.
15. Stipp D. An idea man who thinks in lists. The Wall Street Journal 1987;109(105):28.
16. Jacobson SF. Studying and using conceptual models of nursing. Image: Journal of Nursing Scholarship 1987;19(2):82.

III

Introduction: Research Themes and Methods for Nursing Administration

Beverly Henry

THE PURPOSE of Section III is to provide readers with discussions of themes and methodologies that appear to be especially useful for future research in nursing administration. Our premise for including these is that research—not just theory—is needed to advance nursing knowledge and practice.

A second and more important premise is that as practitioners and educators, it is paramount that we understand (1) the research questions being asked, (2) the investigative techniques being developed and introduced into nursing administration, and (3) the implications of the methodologic techniques in use, and those that need to be used.

Even a cursory review of research in nursing administration suggests that relatively few methods have been used—largely simple statistical measures of variance and correlation. Moreover, little attention has been paid in our inquiry to the epistemological overlap of the concepts, modes of inquiry and standards of proof in nursing and management. The questions being asked in nursing administration, the standards of proof, and the specific methodologies we adopt all need scrutinizing to elucidate what should be studied, which methods should be developed by nurses that are unique to nursing, and which should be incorporated into the field.

The momentum for research in nursing administration is building. The *National Nurs-*

ing Administration Research Priorities study,[1] the emphasis on the research function of the nurse executive as outlined in the *Guidelines on the Role and Functions of the Hospital Nurse Executive*,[2] and the definition and priorities developed by the American Organization of Nurse Executives[3] have provided an impetus. But there is a long way to go.

To enlarge our understanding of research for nursing administration, Section III opens with chapters by Hinshaw and Alexander. We selected these authors for the following reasons. Hinshaw, perhaps more than any other nurse scientist in the country, is in a position to assess how contemporary trends in nursing and government affect present and future research in nursing administration. Alexander, one of the nation's finest young nurse researchers, is well informed about methods and themes in management science. Hinshaw analyzes programs of nursing research and the implications of these for advancing the science of nursing administration. Alexander examines research methodologies and themes in two of the fields adjacent to nursing administration—business and public administration. She describes the implications of advances in both fields for inquiry in nursing administration. The chapters by these authors, taken together, provide the reader with a perspective of the values, ideas, and research methods in nursing and management science. Both perspectives are integral to the development of empirically testable knowledge for nursing administration.

The chapters that comprise the body of this section are clustered in two groups. The first six describe methodological approaches for basic academic research where the primary goal is to advance knowledge about nursing administration science. The last six describe methodologies for applied administrative research where the goal is more apt to be generating information to solve a problem in a particular organization.

All research in nursing administration should both meet the test of scientific validity and be useful to practitioners. The methodologies are categorized as basic (context-free) or applied (context-specific), depending on whether a methodology is more oriented toward theory-building or toward problem-solving, simply to structure Section III in a way that is useful.

As with the volume as a whole, chapters in this section are not intended to provide a complete collection of research themes and methodologies apropos of nursing administration. Our goal has been simply to provide readers with a sense of the broad sweep of methods which appear useful for nursing administration—from the more qualitative to complementary quantitative methodologies, and from the more basic to a number of highly practical approaches.

Contributing authors have something to tell us, in various ways, about the study and practice of nursing administration. The authors represent a wide range of backgrounds, but by and large they are nurses with experience in both education and practice. Consequently, we think that their views will be of interest and of use to investigators in the university and in health service agencies.

Hinshaw introduces the section in Chapter 23 with a discussion of research programs in nursing. She categorizes major streams of scientific inquiry for the field as nursing productivity; nursing care requirements; re-

source allocation; nursing care costs; quality of care outcomes; nursing staff stress, satisfaction, and turnover; and new nursing roles. Concerned that future research builds and tests theory, she suggests that investigators use knowledge from a number of basic and professional disciplines to build a coherent body of theoretical yet practical and useful knowledge.

In Chapter 24, Alexander takes a close look at recent scientific developments in business and public administration. Having reviewed the major research journals in both fields, she carefully describes the concepts and methodologies pertaining to organizational behavior, personnel management, and organizational theory.

In Chapter 25, entitled "Philosophic Inquiry for Nursing Administration," Giovinco increases our sensitivity to the importance of inquiry that is not only empirical, but also philosophical and epistemological. She suggests that before any investigation of phenomena begins, the wise researcher engages in the careful questioning characteristic of philosophic inquiry: about what a problem or issue actually is, and what it means. Philosophical questioning is examination of general, yet persistent and pervasive characteristics of basic problems. The author describes the dimensions and stages of philosophic inquiry and compares formal inquiry to common sense as a way of building knowledge. She continues with a brief discussion of epistemology. Epistemology as a theory of knowledge encompasses finding resolutions to nagging questions, beginning with analysis of concepts and proceeding to the development of propositions and the making of intelligent statements about reality.

Parse, in Chapter 26, describes the value of the phenomenological research method for nursing administration. The author begins her discussion by helping the reader understand the importance of qualitative approaches in science. Next, she describes the phenomenological movement highlighting the contributions of Bretano, Husserl, Heidegger, Merleau-Ponty, and Sartre. The essentials of the phenomenological method are described in careful, lucid language. In the final portion of the chapter, Parse formulates a number of useful research questions and provides the reader with directions for applying the phenomenological method in nursing administration.

Keddy, at Dalhousie University in Halifax, Nova Scotia, adds a unique international flavor with Chapter 27. Her style of writing is delightful. Drawing on her knowledge of historical analyses of directors of nursing in Canadian hospitals, and on studies of nurses in Newfoundland, Keddy supplies us with graphic, readable portrayals of times past. She then relates past events to contemporary choices by way of emphasizing the usefulness of history in science and everyday management.

In Chapter 28, Smyth describes case study methodology: the varying types of cases, myths about case studies, and some of the issues related to reliability and validity. She points out that the case study is one of the earliest and most valuable methods used in nursing. A number of important nursing studies using the case approach are described. Based on her review of articles in a leading journal for nursing administration, she concludes that while many single example cases are described in the literature, few investigators use the case study as a scientific method. Examples are provided of the kinds of problems that can be addressed using the case method to provide a well-documented foundation for nursing administration science.

Pendergast, a biostatistician, is the author of Chapter 29, entitled "Some Approaches to the Analysis of Repeated Measurement Data." Pendergast is one of the country's leading young scientists focusing on analysis of repeated measurement data for health care. Although we know of no studies in nursing administration that have used the advanced analytic techniques she describes, some may be underway: a number of important investigations in health services and management science have been done using these techniques. Repeated measurement models—including one- and two-factor ANOVA and MANOVA as well as nonparametric and categorical models to assess how changes in time and in other predictor (independent) variables affect response (outcome) variables—hold special promise for improved longitudinal testing of the effects of interventions that are designed to improve quality care.

The next six chapters describe research methodologies for quality assurance, productivity measurement, patient satisfaction, inservice education, and individual decision making. Jones leads with an overview of quality assurance. She begins by defining the meaning of quality health care. The components of quality assurance programs are analyzed, starting with establishing standards and criteria, proceeding to data collection, comparing current practices to set standards, and feeding back results for improved courses of action. In this carefully written chapter, Jones provides the reader with a total systems view of how to assure quality care for patients. She introduces the reader to the problems of defining outcome criteria where the outcomes may or may not be attributable solely to nurses. Accessibility to care, continuity of care, cost containment, and the requirements of quality assurance systems are also addressed.

Brett's chapter is next. A researcher at Robert Wood Johnson University Hospital in New Jersey, Brett focuses on the measurement of outcomes of nursing care. She describes a systems model of quality care comprised of three levels of analysis—the patient, nursing, and nursing organization—and four elements of analysis relative to the specificity and size of targeted populations. Brett points out that instruments to measure patient care outcomes are fewer in number and relatively newer than measures of structure and process. Two of the outcome measures discussed are the Patient Indicators of Nursing Care (PINC) and the Criterion Measure of Nursing Care Quality based on Orem's self-care model. In her concluding comments, Brett provides the reader with useful suggestions for future efforts designed to assess the results of nursing.

An expert on productivity measurement in nursing, Edwardson provides us with workable definitions of health care and nursing productivity in Chapter 32. She points out that increased productivity does not necessarily mean that quality will be lessened. To assess labor productivity, she describes the personnel, technological, and managerial elements that appear to hold the most promise for improved understanding of how best to increase productivity.

In Chapter 33, LaRochelle discusses one of the outcome measures touched on by previous authors, patient surveys. She provides an historical overview of survey research and describes the strengths and weaknesses of the methodology. Her discussions are especially useful for nurse administrators who need to evaluate data that has been collected by the survey method, or who are faced with the complex task of designing surveys.

Hefferin, associate chief for research at the Wadsworth Division of the Veterans Administration Medical Center in Los Angeles, addresses the many aspects of evaluating the effectiveness of in-service education pro-

grams in Chapter 34. She emphasizes that directors of in-service who are attuned to cost effectiveness first assess which programs are priority; second, oversee the provision of educational activities; and third, use the best possible evaluation mechanisms to assess how educational interventions have improved the quality of care.

In the closing chapter, Freund discusses individual decision-making styles using type theory. She reviews Jung's and Myers-Briggs's theory, describing four cognitive processes—extraversion and intraversion preferences, perceptive and judging orientations—and how these are validly and reliably measured by the Myers-Briggs Type Indicator (MBTI). Applications are described that are useful in education and administration for assessing patterns and preferences in the way people take in information and make decisions. Freund's discussion provides the reader with the information necessary to improve understanding of various cognitive structures and develop profiles in ways that are useful for administrators and educators.

REFERENCES

1. Henry B, Moody L, Pendergast J, O'Donnell J, Hutchinson S, Scully G. Delineating nursing administration research priorities using three futures methods. Nursing Research 1987;36(5):309–314.
2. American Hospital Association. Role and function of the hospital nurse executive. In: Guideline document. Chicago, IL: American Hospital Association, 1985, pp. 1–3.
3. American Organization of Nurse Executives. Blue Ribbon Committee for Nursing Administration Research. Final report. Chicago, IL: American Hospital Association, AONE, September 1986.

23

Programs of Nursing Research for Nursing Administration

Ada Sue Hinshaw

UNDERSTANDING the knowledge base for administrative decisions and long-term policies is extremely important to the profession's ability to utilize and manipulate such information for improvement of the delivery of nursing care. The American Organization of Nurse Executives (AONE) recently reinforced this importance in their official statement on nursing administration research: "A driving factor in the organization's appointment of a Blue Ribbon Committee on Nursing Administration Research is today's emphasis on precise measurement of health-care quality and cost. (Thus), the Board determined that for AONE to be effective in influencing health-care policy, legislation, and reimbursement, a substantive data base in nursing administration research is essential."[1]

Nursing administration research was defined by the Blue Ribbon Committee of AONE as "the scientific inquiry of factors which influence the effective and efficient organization and delivery of high quality nursing service."[2] As such, research in nursing administration focuses on the systematic examination of the relationships among nursing services, the quality of the outcomes of care, and the organizational and environmental elements that influence the delivery of services.[3] The major purposes of nursing administration research, from the AONE association's perspective, are to enhance the processes and outcomes of health care, and to influence the analysis and development of health policy.

Nurse scientists functioning in the arena of nursing administration research have the responsibility for generating and testing theoretical models for the concepts, factors, and relationships involved in the delivery of nursing services. In addition, they must assume responsibility for monitoring their own and their colleagues research programs to provide a continuous evaluation of the "state of the science." It is important for nurse executives to have immediate access to research results that are scientifically credible and can be judged useable by certain standard criteria.[4] As the AONE report suggests, "As sound nursing administration research based on valid and reliable methodologies continues, nurse executives will have available a professional data base that can be used to insure effective, high quality nursing care in a cost-conscious health-care environment.[5]

The purpose of this chapter is to systematically evaluate the major areas of nursing administration research. The evaluation will focus on:

- The primary dimensions and areas of study that have been conducted,
- The strengths and weaknesses of these bodies of information, and

251

- The concerns raised within each area of research.

In addition, the issues regarding the broader perspective of nursing research will be raised from both a substantive and methodological stance. Finally, the research priorities, as delineated by the profession, will be outlined.

AREAS OF NURSING ADMINISTRATION RESEARCH

Nursing administration research represents a broad base of information and knowledge for study. As the earlier definition suggests, the avenues of study are multiple and complex. A number of the major areas of research for this field will be considered:

- Relationships among nursing care requirements, nursing resource allocation, nursing costs, diagnostic related groups (DRGs), and quality client outcomes (nursing productivity),
- Relationship of quality of care and cost outcomes for clients,
- Nursing staff stress, satisfaction, and turnover,
- Development and testing of new roles for professional nurses.

Nursing Productivity

Describing and testing models for explaining productivity for nursing care has been the focus of discussion and controversy since the 1930s, with the early discussions focusing on the predictions for staffing and scheduling. Curtin and Zerlich[6] define productivity as the relationship between inputs and outputs when considered from the perspective of the general systems model. This definition is refined by Davis and Levine in the Proceedings of the Georgetown University Conference on Nursing Productivity as "a measure of work accomplished per level of resources applied."[7] Thus productivity indicates how effi-

ciently resources are being used to accomplish certain defined and desired outcomes. Participants in the Georgetown Conference identified and discussed three major models for nursing productivity: the Medicus Model, the Johns Hopkins Model, and a model developed at Georgetown University Hospital. These models have in common a general systems orientation to the understanding of antecedent or input conditions, which are manipulated in order to result in certain defined client and service outcomes.

Because of several recurring problems, which are identified with the orientation of nursing productivity as a conceptual model for nursing administration research, this discussion will not center specifically on nursing productivity, but rather on the broader category of nursing administration, acknowledging that other factors than those that are traditionally considered productivity concepts are involved in that particular arena of content.

The major concern with using the nursing productivity model is that it is an industrial approach to a professional process. The model assumes that nursing administration and the delivery of care results in an output that is highly standardized as well as precisely predictable in terms of "units" of goods produced, and labor or hours of workers performing routinized and repetitive tasks. The process of delivering nursing care, however, involves a high level of professional judgment, specifically, because such care is not completely routinized, nor does it consist of only repetitive tasks. Thus, while the conceptual model defined for nursing productivity has been extremely helpful as an analytical approach, it brings a perspective that by its very nature makes certain assumptions. First, it assumes that the characteristics of the input factors to be dealt with are highly standardized and understandable. Second, it assumes that the care process will be routinized and repetitive. Third, it assumes that outcomes will be well defined and precisely predicted. These three assumptions are *not* always consistent with the actual delivery of nursing care.

To consider the state of the science of nursing administration research, the concepts and relationships that generally make up the nursing productivity model will be discussed, rather than the grand theory perspective of the nursing productivity model itself. My analysis will focus on the nursing research that has been conducted examining relationships among nursing care requirements, nursing resource allocation, and nursing care costs, as well as on diagnostic related groups and severity of illness measures. Each of these major construct areas needs to be considered separately.

Nursing Care Requirements

Traditionally nursing care requirements have been measured by various types of patient classification systems. The nursing administration literature is replete with patient classification systems that have been developed to assess current and predict future nursing care requirements of patients primarily in acute care agencies.[8] Usually such classification systems are developed in terms of the amount of nursing care required by a patient based on a specifically defined conceptual factor such as complexity of care,[9] dependency of the patient, or the time required to provide care.[10] If the classification systems are not directly attached to time allocations and resources needed, then they are generally related to resource indices as a second step in the classification process. Such classification systems have also been developed for specialty units—such as emergency rooms and intensive care units—and are currently being produced for ambulatory care settings as well.[11]

The major purpose for the development of such factor or profile classification systems

has been to provide the information needed for guiding the staffing and scheduling of nursing personnel, both in terms of the number and type of personnel required. In addition, the classifications provide basic information about a patient's level of care, over a period of time, on which to base long-term budgeting and justification of nursing resource allocations.[12]

Several recurring issues have haunted this particular program of research in nursing. A major problem has been the consistent difficulty in developing within such classification systems, not only the interdependent functions—that is, the activities and nursing actions required or conducted with other health care professionals—but also the independent actions that are initiated by nurses.[13] Independent nursing actions include family intervention, planning and referral, support and consultation, as well as teaching, assessment, and observation.[14] Categories that include these actions are very difficult to establish in a classification system: the actions are less precise, it is more difficult to obtain reliability among staff as they classify patients in terms of these actions, and it is difficult to define the activities as having been conducted or not conducted by nursing personnel. Such categories also tend to be overused and to become a constant in a classification system, which then making it difficult to discriminate among patients on the basis of independent actions.

A second major concern in terms of patient classification research has been the need to relate nursing care requirements of patients, not only to nursing work load, but also to other entities, such as diagnostic related groups, and to nursing diagnoses. Halloran considered nursing time, as estimated from the Medicus patient classification instrument, in relationship to patient condition (defined in terms of nursing diagnoses) and in terms of diagnostic related groups.[15] His findings suggested that nursing conditions or nursing diagnoses explained twice the variation in nursing care time as predicted from the patient classification systems (52%) as did the medical diagnostic related groups classifications (26%). Halloran suggested that nursing care time is predicted better by a patient's nursing diagnosis, than by either medical diagnostic or demographic characteristics, indicating that nursing care is not physician prescribed. This then underscores the need to have incorporated in patient classification systems the independent actions, as well as the interdependent functions characterizing nursing care.

Another major concern in the development and use of patient classification systems over the years has been developing systems that are both reliable and valid. Validity is the issue described earlier—that classification systems contain all of the major types of nursing care requirements, actions, and functions involved in the delivery of care, both independent and interdependent. In addition, reliability has been of concern. A number of studies are reported that outline the need to ensure both the reliability of instruments and the reliability of personnel who use the instruments—two totally separate issues and both basic to obtaining accurate information from classification systems.[16]

Nursing Resource Allocation

A major area of research, in terms of nursing resource allocation, is the staffing and scheduling of nursing care personnel. In addition to research focusing on the amount of time required for nursing personnel to care for defined or classified levels of patient needs, other types of research programs have been conducted. A number of studies have investigated the value and cost of scheduling an all registered nurse (R.N.) staff. For example, Minyard, Wald, and Turner concluded after conducting a work sampling study and examining over 175 activity samples, that nursing

personnel used far less personal or nonproductive time than did either the licensed practical nurses (L.P.N.s) or nurses' aides.[17] The differences were not only statistically significant, but clinically impressive as well. R.N.s spent 11% of their work time engaged in nonproductive activities, while L.P.N.s and nurses' aides spent 17% and 24% respectively. Hinshaw and Atwood reported in a study of all R.N. staffing versus variable staffing on one highly acute medical unit, that "All R.N. staffing" consistently resulted in more positive staff and patient outcomes combined with a trend toward less cost for such outcomes.[18] The outcomes studied were group cohesion, job satisfaction, and perspectives of the quality of care among the nursing staff; patient outcomes included patient satisfaction and individualization of patient care; cost factors included sick time, compensation time, and turnover.

Other studies have reported investigations of the efficiency and effectiveness of 12-hour staffing patterns compared to 8-hour and 10-hour staffing patterns. The attempt in these studies has been to define the most desirable type of scheduling for either R.N. or variable types of employees.

The literature is rich with studies describing the differences in various types of delivery patterns—for example, between primary nursing and team nursing. The major thrust of this program of research has been evaluating and testing a philosophical approach to a particular type of assignment pattern for nurses—primary nursing. The intent of the conceptual thrust in primary nursing is to increase the autonomy and control over information and care decisions of professional nurses. The intent of this orientation is to ensure the professional role of nurses in a basically bureaucratic organization, to lessen role conflict, and to increase professional input about the care of patients. The assumption in primary nursing is that with increased professional control and opportunity for input, the quality of care is higher. The impact of this conceptual orientation on the delivery of care is manifest largely by staffing and scheduling in a way that allows for the implementation of the primary nurse concept. Thus much research in nursing administration has focused on staffing and scheduling mechanisms as well as on the ability to integrate the philosophy of autonomous professional action in complex organizations.

Giovanetti, in her summary article on the "Evaluation of Primary Nursing" in the fourth volume of the *Annual Review of Nursing Research,* suggests that the research on primary nursing and the desired outcomes are "equivocal."[19] If one looks at the outcomes of the approximately 12 studies reported in the literature, the findings in terms of patient satisfaction and other similar factors are ambivalent.[20–22] The findings are similarly inconsistent when quality of care is the outcome variable under investigation. However, when multiple outcomes are considered in relationship to primary nursing, the findings, including quality, care plans, and job satisfaction are generally supportive of primary nursing. In Giovanetti's investigations of primary nursing, her results conflicted with the majority of studies in this area; that is, team nursing was preferred to primary nursing with respect to a number of factors.[23–24] Thus, the data from the research programs focusing on assignment patterns and the organizing structures on nursing units remain inconclusive.

The research conducted in the arena of staffing and scheduling of nursing care personnel has been varied. Many diverse topics have been investigated. Moreover, there has been minimal replication for the various research programs except with respect to primary nursing.

In addition to the lack of replication, one other major concern in this area of research needs to be articulated: Many of the studies on staffing and scheduling have been done in a single acute care agency, or on only one particular patient care unit. Thus, much of the existing data are difficult to generalize to conditions on other patient care units, or in other types of acute care hospitals.

Since these studies are usually not generalizable in terms of the unit or sample, an alternative is to attempt to generalize through a particular conceptual or theoretical framework. However, most of the reported projects tend to be empirical or operational in nature. Few develop a definitive conceptual or theoretical framework and systematically test it. Thus, generalizability through a theoretical system is usually limited as well.

Nursing Care Costs

Identifying the costs of giving nursing care has been a major area of nursing administration research over the past several years with the advent of the prospective payment system for hospital care. The driving forces for such research programs are related to the following needs: (1) to identify not only the cost of nursing service but also its revenue generating component, (2) to charge patients for nursing services on an equitable basis (those receiving less complex nursing care would pay less and vice versa) and (3) to identify the ratio of nursing care in relationship to other services provided to patients in terms of the budget or allocation base negotiated with hospital administration. The need in the profession to view nursing as a professional, autonomous provider of service in a bureaucratic organization has heightened interest in identifying revenue that can be generated through the delivery of nursing care to various types of patients. Such a change in costing and in allocating income projects a different image of professional nurses.

The research approaches to costing out nursing care are varied. Riley and Schaeffers, identifying two categories of nursing costs—direct and total—suggested that it is possible to relate nursing costs definitely to patient classification instruments, thus discriminating among high and low complexity, or more or less time that is given to clients.[25] Reitz developed and tested a Nursing Intensity index, which is comparable to a Diagnostic Related Groups index, but based on the concepts of nursing intensity and various types of patient functional health parameters.[26] The Reitz instrument is used at the point of discharge or at postdischarge for determining the degree of nursing care provided to patients. Reschak, Biordi, Holm, and Santucci investigated the Relative Intensity Measures (RIMs) in contrast to patient classification system methodology for identifying the cost of nursing.[27] In essence, they concluded that it is possible to accurately, objectively, and inexpensively account for the cost of nursing services by DRGs using a patient classification system.

The inclination toward linking nursing costs to patient classification systems has been to take advantage of a major data collection system already present in many acute care agencies. Sovie, Tarsinale, Van Putts, and Stunden concluded in their investigation "A Correlational Study of Nursing Patient Classification, DRGs, Other Significant Patient Variables and Costs of Patient Care," that a four-category system of nursing acuity adequately accounts for the variation in nursing care requirements, and unbundling the nursing costs from the room costs enhances nursing's accountability in patient care.[28] They suggested that the average direct nursing costs in the mean room costs vary from 18% to 24% and that nursing needs of individual patients in any one DRG category are extremely variable. In the Sovie and associates investigation, coupling DRGs with nursing patient classification data enabled a budget prediction that reflected 87% of the actual adjusted expenditures. Walker's study at Stanford, analyzing two methods for identifying the relative costs of nursing care, suggested that approximately 12% to 20% of total hospital charges are for nursing care provided in general care units.[29] However, Walker's research suggested that the level increased dramatically in the critical care arena: in these units, 55% of the daily room charge was for direct nursing care. This would substantiate the need to cost-out nursing care based on a variable that conceptualizes the complexity and intensity of patient care.

Research programs focusing on costing out nursing care are proliferating because of the economic pressures for such information. A number of different approaches and conceptual models are being developed and tested which, in terms of the "state of the science," bodes well for results that can be trusted. The various approaches and models begin to provide a consensus on the major issues—such as actual cost per type of patient and percentage of nursing care involved, either in the direct total hospital cost or in the room cost by service. The current difficulty with research in this area is the lack of replicated information from which to develop nursing administration policy.

Relationship of DRGs to Other Major Nursing Productivity Factors

The major thrust of nursing productivity research programs has been to understand and explain the relationships between diagnostic related groups, patient classification systems, nursing resource allocation, and costs for the delivery of care. There has been a scramble to understand such relationships in almost every other professional group delivering health care as well as in nursing. Caterinicchio[30–31] and Joel[32–33] have written extensively of the multiple sets of studies investigating the development and use of a Relative Intensive Measure using a case mix nursing performance approach, better known as RIMs. This method essentially yields an empirically derived, patient specific, case-mix adjusted length of stay statistic that can be used to appropriate nursing costs by case. However, Grimaldi and Micheletti[34] criticized this particular methodology, suggesting that the per diem method, or the by-case-by-day method makes no allowance for variation in patient's specific diagnosis or the related nursing care requirements. Other authors, as noted earlier, have attempted to relate the diagnostic related category classifications to the traditional patient classifications used in hospital agencies to allocate nursing resources.[35–37] These studies suggest that classification according to a nursing complexity type of index varies highly within each DRG, particularly for general medical-surgical units. The variation is less for intensive care units where the nursing care complexity tends to be high.

A study conducted by the American Nurses' Association entitled "DRGs and Nursing Care"[38] suggested several principal findings: (1) that the DRGs relative cost weights generally appear to reflect differences in nursing resource requirements, (2) some DRGs were interpretable groupings of patients, both in terms of total hours of nursing care and the daily pattern of nursing resource consumption, (3) nursing costs accounted for between 20% and 28% of hospital costs for two-thirds of the DRGs in the study (21 DRGs studied in total), and (4) sufficient variations in nursing resource utilization patterns and nursing costs were found to suggest that further study of nursing care, length of stay, and DRGs is warranted as a potential mechanism for refining prospective pricing. This study differed from others in the sense that most other projects suggest that DRGs' relative weights do not appear to adequately reflect the specific differences in nursing resource allocations.[39–40]

Most of the research in this arena acknowledges the complexity of the relationships involved with DRGs and nursing care requirements, nursing resource allocation, and cost. The studies suggest that rather than the more simplistic direct relationship between any two nursing productivity factors, it is a combination of the various types of classification systems that will ultimately provide the best explanation for nursing care costs and requirements. For example, Sovie[41] suggests that when DRGs are coupled with nursing patient classification data, the two together are an excellent predictor of nursing resource consumption. She accounted for 87% of the actual adjusted expenditures for nursing care, given the consideration of both classifications simultaneously. Thus, we need to consider both a severity of illness index (a medical assessment) and a nursing intensity index together in attempting to explain nursing care costs. Thompson[42] as well as Thompson and Diers[43] suggest that further study needs to be targeted to the extension of existing staff models (patient classification systems) to create nursing time estimates for the total length of hospitalization for each patient. Thompson points out that the DRG payment system is based on the premise that to contain total case cost, all of the subsets of that cost must be included. If an important component of case cost, such as nursing, cannot be measured, it weakens the structure of the entire total program. Thompson and Diers suggest that two major criticisms of the DRG prospective pricing approach are, first, whether DRGs measure severity of illness more generally, and second, how they measure the different kinds of nursing resources consumed in the treatment of patients.

Thus, numerous research programs have been conducted to consider the relationships among the various nursing productivity factors—nursing care requirements, resource allocation, and costs as influenced and understood through the diagnostic related prospective pricing system. There is a strong need for replication in terms of these various investigations. The study of such relationships, as well as the development and testing of systems for costing out nursing care in other types of health care systems—home health care and nursing homes—is important.

Quality of Care Outcomes and Cost of Care

Objective and systematic evaluation of nursing care has long been a priority in the profession. Numerous research programs have targeted the identification of major patient care outcomes and their relationship to the delivery of nursing care. Early in these research programs the major focus was on the development of outcome criterion measures to assess the quality or effect of nursing practice on patient progress.[44-47] In 1975, Lindemann[48] suggested that the determination of reliable and valid indicators of quality nursing care was a high priority for investigating nursing's influence on patient welfare, and that essentially this field of research could not move any further until, (1) major patient outcomes could be identified in terms of nursing impact, and (2) that measurement systems to index such outcomes had been developed. Over the years, particularly in response to this priority, a number of various types of quality of care instruments have been tested and published: the Nursing Audit by Phaneuf,[49] the Slater Nursing Competency Rating Scale,[50] the Quality Patient Care Scale,[51] and the Rush-Medicus system.[52] The need to develop such reliable and valid indices of quality and of outcome remains a priority concern in the profession.

In addition, numerous descriptive studies have been conducted describing the relationships among major structure, process, and outcome factors, which explain the quality of care for patients. The Donabedian model[53] stimulated the use of structure-process-outcome—a general systems perspective. Outcome studies have focused primarily on identifying patient indices that are thought to be amenable to nursing influence. The major focus of these studies has been patient health knowledge, preventive behaviors, and self-care skills. The types of studies vary from Horne and Swain's[54] early work in 1978, in which they developed 539 outcome criterion measures reflecting 18 self-care demand categories describing patient outcomes for adult medical-surgical hospitalized patients, to patient outcomes that could be expected as a result of nurse-influenced iatrogenic conditions.[55] Again, in most of these outcome studies, the emphasis of the research has been on the development of patient outcome indicators rather than on the relationship of these indicators to other major influencing factors in nursing care.

Lang and Clinton[56] suggested in their *Annual Review* chapter of the "Assessment of Quality of Nursing Care" that the majority of the structure and outcome studies have examined the relationship between patient responses and human resource requirements which occur when changes are made in the delivery of nursing care or the organization of health personnel. Included have been studies of nursing assignment patterns as they affect patient outcomes and the impact of nurses in various roles such as that of the nurse practitioner. Studies in which research has examined the relationship between process and outcome elements have been primarily concerned with evaluating the effect of patient education programs and the use of clinical judgment on particular patient outcomes.

Studies which included variables that were structure, process, and outcome oriented in nature focused on the implementation and evaluation of standards for nursing practice as they affected quality of care. It is in this area of research that Lang and Clinton[57] recommend that the greatest emphasis be placed in future nursing administration research. Why? First, because data are still relatively sparse in terms of the interactional effects of structure and process variables as they affect outcomes for clients. Second, because there is a need for comparative studies since many current research programs have focused on a single-patient care unit of an agency, rather than on broader theoretical and generalizability factors. Third, because problems that have plagued this area of research continue to be of concern—the ability to identify major patient outcomes that are primarily the result of nursing care, and once identified, the ability to measure the outcomes reliably and validly. Fourth, Lang and Clinton suggest that regardless of the design issues and the methodologic problems, there is a need in this field of research for more rigor in submitting "data to inferential testing." Essentially this means there is a need to construct various nursing care intervention systems that can be deliberately manipulated in relationship to known and desired quality of care outcomes.

Since about 1974, there has been an additional emphasis on balancing the outcomes of quality care with the cost of such outcomes. This trend is clearly evident in Lang and Clinton's[58] text when they discuss the structural factors studied in relationship to the assessment of quality care. The types of cost factors measured vary from salaries, absenteeism, turnover, and patient day-cost, to investigating health-service utilization costs such as length of stay and hospitalization rate. Fagin and Jacobson[59] in their *Annual Review* chapter on "Cost Effectiveness and Analysis in Nursing Research" outline a number of areas in which cost effectiveness analysis has been conducted. However, little nursing research is available on the conduct of cost-benefit analysis. Cost-effectiveness analysis is defined as identifying the effectiveness of particular interventions using explicit quantitative methods to measure net cost. Cost-benefit analysis suggests that both costs and benefits must be placed in quantitative monetary terms and considered in ratio. In their review, Fagin and Jacobson identified only 10 studies of interventions dealing with the quality of care outcomes, which had systematically considered the cost effectiveness of such interventions, and a more limited number of studies using cost-benefit analysis. Thus, there is a dearth of studies investigating the balance between what can be delivered in terms of quality, and the costs that are incurred.

Nursing Staff Stress, Satisfaction, and Turnover

The setting for major research programs investigating nursing staff stress, satisfaction, and turnover has been primarily acute care agencies. However, a few studies have also been conducted in hospice and nursing home settings. The thrust of this area of study is to understand the effect of an organization on professional nurses who are employees in a bureaucracy. The basic assumption is that nurses who are more satisfied and less stressed deliver a higher quality of care for patients, and insure less cost in terms of attrition. The reported cost of turnover among registered nurses varies depending on the general or speciality unit to which the registered nurse needs to be oriented.

There are a number of studies reported in the literature investigating the effect of different organizational and interpersonal factors as they influence nurse satisfaction and job stress. Pincus[60] in a study of 327 professional nurses investigated the effects of nurses' perceptions of different organizational factors on their job satisfaction and job performance. The study results indicated that certain aspects of communication (such as with a supervisor) and the climate in which communication occurs, are influential contributions to job satisfaction and to a lesser extent, to job performance. Blalack[61] suggested that maturity, self-actualization, the opportunity to help people, a feeling of accomplishment, opportunities for growth and development, and a feeling of self-ful-fillment were among the most important needs of registered nurses if they are to consider themselves satisfied with their profession. Other scientists, such as Prescott and Dennis,[62] studied staff nurses' perceptions of the formation of hospital policy and their role in policy formation as affecting their authority, influence, and autonomy.

A number of investigators have pursued a causal modeling approach to the study of termination or turnover among nurses—Price and Mueller,[63] Curry, Wakefield, Price, Mueller, and McClosky;[64] Weisman, Alexander, and Chase;[65] and Hinshaw and Atwood.[66] Price and Mueller's work has consistently used sociologically based variables such as opportunity, routinization, centralization, instrumental communication, integration, and pay as they affect job satisfaction of the potential employee, which in turn influences commitment and intent to stay, which in turn influences actual turnover. Weisman and Alexander, in their work, also considered the variable of professional autonomy, while Hinshaw and Atwood focused more on professional factors. The Anticipated Turnover Model proposed by Hinshaw and Atwood[67] suggested that certain individual factors, including mobility opportunities and initial intent to stay in an agency, influenced staff's response to factors such as group cohesion (integration), job stress, control over nursing practice, and individual autonomy in decision making. In turn, individual response to these organizational factors influenced two different types of satisfaction: organizational job satisfaction and professional job satisfaction, which were predicted to be the major factors influencing anticipated turnover and in turn, actual termination from an agency.

Basic findings from the studies conducted by these three different groups of investigators are quite similar: anticipated turnover, or intent to leave or stay, is a major predictor of actual turnover; job satisfaction is a major predictor of anticipated turnover or intent to leave or stay; as are variables such as kinship responsibility, and organizational commitment, in Price and Mueller's[68] and Weisman and Alexander's[69] research. In addition, Weisman and Alexander, and Hinshaw and Atwood found that autonomy was a significant predictor of satisfaction.

For Price and Mueller,[70] task repetitiveness, autonomy, promotional opportunities, and fairness of rewards were important determinants of job satisfaction, while for Hinshaw and Atwood,[71] important determinants were group cohesion and job stress in conjunction with control over nursing practice and professional autonomy. In Hinshaw and Atwood's work, two additional findings were evident: job stress did not have a direct effect on anticipated turnover, but instead affected anticipated turnover only through the variable of organizational and professional job satisfaction. This is an important finding since it means that job satisfiers can be manipulated as retention strategies for combatting job stress, in order to decrease anticipated turnover and increase actual retention. Second, there were two types of job satisfaction that were important to professional nurses: organizational job satisfaction which included factors such as pay (rewards) and administrative style; and professional job satisfaction which included factors such as the ability to deliver quality care, time to deliver quality care, and a general enjoyment of the job.

A number of studies focusing on stress, satisfaction, and turnover have investigated the effect of job stress on critical care or other speciality groups. Norbeck's research[72] supported the hypothesis that higher levels of perceived job stress are related to lower levels of job satisfaction and to higher levels of psychological symptoms of illness among critical care nurses. These results essentially substantiated the findings of Bailey and Claus[73] reported in the early 1980s. Kosmoski and Calkin[74] studied the factors that influenced critical care nurses' intent to stay in their position, indicating that the best predictor was satisfaction with work activities. Similarly Gordon and Goeble[75] found in studying satisfaction among psychiatric staff nurses, that limitations inherent in team nursing were a major source of professional goal dissatisfaction. Being able to use creative strategies, such as leading inpatient educational groups and participating in leading assertiveness groups, improved job satisfaction, increased assertiveness, and enhanced professional self-image.

With each of these studies, the descriptive data for the speciality subgroup is important information, but often does not provide for a comparison of the amount or types of job stress, which may differ among staff nurses working in a variety of clinical settings. Hinshaw and Atwood,[76] in their research, considered the variables cited earlier and compared the job stress and job satisfaction experienced by staff nurses in various clinical units. Their research suggested that medical-surgical nurses are the most stressed group, while nurses functioning in the specialty areas such as critical care, pediatrics, and psychiatry, are both less stressed and more highly satisfied. In addition, the types of stress varied among the groups. For example medical-surgical nurses were highly stressed by concerns with feeling competent in the care that they were delivering, while critical care nurses were more concerned with stress which resulted from a lack of respect from other health care professionals.

Given the number of studies that have been conducted in the area of nursing staff stress, satisfaction, and turnover, there are still several major areas of concern when the state of the science is considered. First, there is a need

for replication of the specific differences in stress, satisfaction, and turnover across nursing staff functioning in diverse clinical conditions. There is only a minimal amount of data outlining a complex situation, suggesting that retention strategies need to be specifically targeted to various clinical conditions.

Second, there is a need for investigators to adopt similar instrumentation, or at least instrumentation that has been carefully tested in terms of reliability and validity. This issue is critical in order to understand which of the variables have the strongest influence in the causal models predicting the relationship among stress, satisfaction, and turnover.

Third, there is a need to move from descriptive work, in which there is a substantial amount of replication of findings at this point, to the investigation of retention strategies and stress reducing and satisfying interventions. In addition, the outcomes of such intervention systems on the attitudes and actual behaviors of staff nurses in clinical settings need to be studied.

Finally, there is a need to focus on major organizational factors as they influence performance behavior and as these in turn affect patient care outcomes. For example, do dissatisfied nurses who have less integration with their colleagues and feelings of less control over their practice deliver a different quality of care to clients in contrast to nurses who feel strongly a part of their group, less stressed in terms of everyday functions, and in control of their practice? Weisman and Nathanson's[77] early work in the area of nursing staff satisfaction as it influences client outcomes suggests that lower staff satisfaction leads to less compliance in the clinical arena for clients, and to significantly less patient satisfaction with the care received. A number of challenges lie ahead for scholars who are conducting research programs in this area.

Development and Testing of New Professional Roles

There have been a series of studies devoted to investigating new and different professional roles for nurses. These studies vary from examining the orientation provided for nurse executives[78] to a descriptive content analysis of what first-line nursing managers do,[79] to the documentation of clinical nurse specialty activities.[80]

Valuable descriptive information has been compiled on the multiple dimensions of staff-nurse role conception. Role expectations among staff nurses have been linked to turnover and attrition and associated with such phenomena as absenteeism and burnout. A role that has been studied in the last several years by a research team at the University of Illinois is that of the clinical nurse researcher. Hagel and associates[81] surveyed 34 clinical researchers and their respective nurse executives using telephone interviews to identify role conceptions and functions. Similarities between the executives and researchers were that they agreed a doctorate is a necessity for nurse researchers and that clinical investigators should be personable and approachable. Some disagreement existed between the two regarding clinical experience and the need for a solid background in research and statistics. The investigation identified the major characteristics of the roles of clinical nurse researchers, and reported the suggestions from both the nurse researchers and executives, which may help to increase the productivity of nurses in research positions in clinical settings.

To summarize at this point, the research investigating new and varying roles has been primarily descriptive in nature rather than providing a systematic manipulation of such roles to determine more clearly their influence either on colleagues or clients. In addition to intervention studies, it will be valuable to investigate relationships among roles, and factors influencing the adoption of new roles, or the productivity and effectiveness of professionals in new roles.

ISSUES IN NURSING ADMINISTRATION RESEARCH

In considering the "state of the science" in nursing administration research, several general substantive and methodological issues are apparent. A number of these issues have been identified in the prior discussions specific to each area of investigation.

Complexity of Nursing Administration Phenomena

An obvious similarity among the areas of nursing administration research programs is the complexity of the phenomena. Usually, the questions raised are multivariate in nature and oftentimes involve several levels and sections of a health-care organization as they affect the delivery of nursing care. The structure, process, and outcome model for understanding quality of care outcomes is an example of such complexity. As Lang and Clinton[82] note, only a few studies have been conducted which account for each aspect of the model. Instead, the majority of studies concentrate on only one stage of the model.

The complexity issue is also evident with the research on nursing staff stress, satisfaction, and turnover. This area of research illustrates how complexity flows from the interface across disciplines and bodies of knowledge. The problems under study require considering individual factors in relationship to organizational concerns expressed by scientists in several disciplines—in sociology, psychology, management, and economics, for example.

Macro- Versus Microlevel of Analysis

Most nursing administrative research has been conducted with the individual person or patient as the focus. This is a microlevel of analysis and study. Only a few of the research programs use either hospital units or total health care agencies as the unit of analysis. Prescott[83] in her study used the patient care unit. Considering health care agencies as the unit of analysis is rare in nursing administrative literature.[84] Yet, important questions, such as the influence of different types of organizational management structures on the delivery of nursing care need to be studied from this perspective.

In addition, studies that take both the macro- as well as the microlevel as the units of analysis will facilitate the generalizability of research results to multiple types of settings. Often, research questions studied in only one agency cannot be replicated or the results cannot be assumed to be stable in agencies with very different characteristics. Generalizability is often attempted in nursing administrative research through the testing of the theoretical frameworks guiding the studies. By testing and subtantiating the theoretical relationships, the framework can be assumed to also explain the same factors and relationships in other agencies. This assumption can be empirically tested by studying the relationships under various organizational structures and conditions. Thus, while design generalizability of research findings is often difficult due to methodologic constraints, there are other strategies for enhancing generalizability.

One of the major methodologic issues in nursing administration is the ability to use designs that allow for causal inference. As the descriptive studies in the field lead to the development of various interventions for implementation and study, this problem will become critical. There are several methodologic options: the experimental or quasi-experimental designs, or the causal modeling approach. The latter is a strategy for making causal inferences from nonexperimental correlational data.[85–86] This strategy provides an alternative to the experimental design when the conditions of causality cannot be met, such as time ordering or randomization to account for extraneous variables. Nurse scientists need to creatively use these various designs to handle the complexity of the problems studied, the contingencies of field settings, and the need to derive causal inferences from results. Moreover, the more quantitative designs needs to be coupled with grounded theory and ethnographic approaches to provide the rich data base needed for valid interpretations of results, and understanding less well defined phenomena in nursing administration research.

A continuing problem in nursing administration research is the lack of useful instruments—measures which have known psychometric properties—for indexing the numerous concepts of interest. The need for accurate information on which to base administrative decisions and long-term policies dictates that reliable and valid instruments be used. This issue was one of the early concerns cited as a priority in the Delphi Study conducted by WICHE in the middle 1970s. The issue is a continuing one that nurse researchers need to be aware of and account for in their scientific programs. As tested instruments become available, and a repertoire is accumulated, the criticalness of this problem will dissipate although sensitivity to the problem of accurate data will remain.

RESEARCH PRIORITIES IN NURSING ADMINISTRATION

The American Organization of Nurse Executives Ad Hoc Committee on Nursing Administration Research identified 18 research questions organized in 4 general categories which were judged high priority; practice and administrative systems, support services, documentation, and education. These areas and questions were based on two assumptions: (1) cost and quality measures must be inherent in all nursing administration research activities, and (2) the priorities should be revised annually in order to remain current and responsive to the needs of society and the profession.

The first category "practice and administrative systems" contained questions such as, What is the cost-quality impact of differing systems *on* nursing care delivery (primary, team, function, nursing-diagnosis-based)? Category two, "support services," included questions such as, What is the impact of the level of support services in an agency on the requirements for and the effectiveness of the professional nursing staff? The "documentation" category contained questions such as, How can reliable and valid information systems be designed to produce standardized nursing information sets related to the cost and quality of the nursing care system? Category four, "education" included, What is the difference in the quality of decision making of nurses prepared at differing educational levels? and How do we attract and retain the "best and brightest" for the nursing profession?

The questions to be considered when setting research priorities are:

- How do the discipline priorities fit with the major health-care needs of society?
- How can research priorities be identified and operationalized professionally and organizationally while allowing for scientific creativity and guidance of the discipline's body of knowledge?
- Because of the number of high priority areas of study, how can the major questions in each arena be identified still allowing for the addition of new priorities as societal and professional needs change?

In summary, a number of research areas in nursing administration have been discussed and analyzed in light of the "state of the science." Several overall issues and research priorities for this aspect of nursing's professional domain of knowledge have been considered. The need to provide accurate information from which to guide administrative decisions and long-term policies motivates the continual development and testing of theoretical and research programs for nursing administration. Bringing a nursing perspective to research questions—which requires interfacing the knowledge generated from a number of basic and health care disciplines—results in a body of information that is uniquely applicable to the profession's delivery of nursing care, while also contributing to the knowledge base for other disciplines.

REFERENCES

1. American Organization of Nurse Executives. Final report of the Ad Hoc Committee on Nursing Administration Research. Chicago: American Hospital Association AONE, 1986, p. v.
2. AONE, p. 1.
3. Henry BM, Moody LE. Nursing administration in small rural hospitals. JONA 1986;16(7/8):37–44.
4. Horsley JA, Crane J, Crabtree MK, Wood DJ. Using research to improve nursing practice: a guide. Orlando: Grune & Stratton, 1983 (Conduct and Utilization of Research in Nursing Project)
5. AONE, p. vi.
6. Curtin L, Zurlage C. DRGs: The reorganization of health. S-N Publication, Inc, 1984.
7. Davis AR, Levine E. Proceedings of the National Invitational Conference of Nursing Productivity. Washington, DC: Georgetown University School of Nursing, 1986.
8. Giovanetti P. Understanding patient classification systems. JONA 1979;9:4–9.
9. Hinshaw AS, Verran JA, Chance HC. A description of nursing care requirements in six hospitals. Communicating Nursing Research 1977;9:261–283.
10. Giovanetti P. 1979.
11. Verran JA. Patient classification in ambulatory care. Nursing Economics 1986;4(5):247–251.
12. Giovanetti P. 1979.
13. Curtin L. Determining costs of nursing service per DRG. Nursing Management 1983;14(4):16–20.
14. Hinshaw AS, Atwood JR. Independent nursing actions: an integral part of patient classification. Presented at Western Society for Research in Nursing Communicating Nursing Research Conference, Portland, OR: May 1983.
15. Halloran EJ. Nursing workload, medical diagnosis

related groups, and nursing diagnoses. Research in Nursing and Health 1985;8:421–433.

16. Giovanetti P. 1979.
17. Minyard K, Wall J, Turner R. RNs may cost less than you think. JONA 1986;16(5):28–35.
18. Hinshaw AS, Chance HC, Atwood JR. Staff, patient and cost outcomes of all-registered nurse staffing. Journal of Nursing Administration 1981;11(11-12):30–36.
19. Giovanetti P. Evaluation of primary nursing. In: Werley HH, Fitzpatrick JJ, Taunton RL, eds. Annual review of nursing research Vol 4. New York: Springer, 1986.
20. Daeffler RJ. Outcomes of primary nursing for the patient. Military Medicine 1977; 142:204–208.
21. Daeffler RJ. Patients' perceptions of care under team and primary nursing. JONA 1975;5(3):20–26.
22. Ventura MR, Fox RN, Corley MC, Mercurio SM. A patient satisfaction measure as a criterion to evaluate primary nursing. Nursing Research 1982;31:226–230.
23. Giovanetti P. A comparison of team and primary nursing care systems. Nursing Dimensions 1980;7(4):96–100.
24. Giovanetti P. 1986.
25. Riley W, Schaeffers V. Costing nursing services . . . nursing costs per DRG actually represent a small proportion of total hospital charges. Nursing Management 1983;14(12):40–43.
26. Reitz JA. Toward a comprehensive nursing intensity index. Parts I and II. Nursing Management 1985;8, 9.
27. Reschak GLC, Biordi D, Holm K, Santucci N. Accounting for nursing costs by DRG. JONA 1985;15(9):15–20.
28. Sovie MD, Tarcinale MA, Van Putte A, Stunden A. Amalgram of nursing acuity, DRGs, and costs. Nursing Management 1985,16(3):22–42.
29. Walker DD. The cost of nursing care in hospitals. JONA 1983;13(3):13–18.
30. Caterinicchio RP. A debate: RIMs and the cost of nursing care: a defense of the RIMs study . . . relative intensity measures. Nursing Management 1983;14(5):36–39.
31. Caterinicchio RP. Relative intensity measures: pricing of inpatient nursing services under diagnosis related group perspective hospital payment. Health Care Finance Rev 1984;6(1):61–78.
32. Joel LA. DRGs: The state of the art of reimbursement for nursing services. Nursing and Health Care 1983;560–563.
33. Joel LA. DRGs and RIMs: Implications for nursing. Nurs Outlook 1984;32(1):42–49.
34. Grimaldi PL, Micheletti JA. DRG reimbursement: RIMs and the cost of nursing care. Nursing Management 1982;13(12):12–22.
35. Riley W, Schaeffers V. 1983.
36. Reschak GLC et al. 1985.
37. Atwood JR, Hinshaw AS, Chance HC. Relationships among nursing care requirements, nursing resources and charges. In: Patients and purse strings.

New York: National League for Nursing, 1986, p. 99–119.
38. American Nurses Association. DRGs and nursing care. Kansas City: Author, 1985.
39. Sovie et al. 1985.
40. Atwood JR, Hinshaw AS, Chance HC. 1986.
41. Sovie, et al. 1985.
42. Thompson J. The measurement of nursing intensity. Health Care Financing Review 1984;Annual supplement:47–56.
43. Thompson D, Diers D. DRGs and nursing intensity Nursing and Health Care 1985;6(8):434–439.
44. Abdellah FG. Criterion measures in nursing. Nursing Research 1961;10:21–25.
45. Brodt DE, Anderson EH. Validation of a patient welfare evaluation instrument. Nursing Research 1967;16:167–169.
46. Hagen E. Appraisal of quality in nursing care. In: American Nurses' Association Eighth Nursing Research Conference. Kansas City, MO: ANA, 1972.
47. Zimmer M (ed): Symposium on quality assurance. Nursing Clinics of North America 1974;9:303–380.
48. Lindemann C. Delphi survey of priorities in clinical nursing research. Nursing Research 1975;24:434–444.
49. Phaneuf MC. The nursing audit and self-regulation in nursing practice. New York: Appleton-Century-Crofts, 1976.
50. Wandelt MA, Stewart DS. Slater. Nursing competencies rating scale. New York: Appleton-Century-Crofts, 1975.
51. Wandelt MA, Ager JW. Quality patient care scale. New York. Appleton-Century-Crofts, 1974.
52. Haussmann RD, Hegyvary ST, Newman JF, Bishop AC. Monitoring quality of nursing care. Health Sciences Research 1974;9:135–148.
53. Donabedian A. The criteria and standards of quality: explorations in quality assessment of monitoring, Vol. 2. Ann Arbor, MI: Health Administration Press, 1982.
54. Horne BJ, Swain MA. Criterion measures of nursing care quality. Final Report. Hyattsville, MD: NCHSR, US DHEW, 1978 (NTIS No. PB-287 449/36A).
55. Gilson BS, Gilson JS, Bergner M, Bobbitt RA, Kressel S, Pollard WE, Vesselago M. The sickness impact profile: development of an outcome measure of health care. American J of Public Health 1975;65:1304–1310.
56. Lang NM, Clinton JF. Assessment of quality of nursing care. In: Werley HH, Fitzpatrick JJ, eds. Annual Review of Nursing Research, Vol. 3. New York: Springer, 1984.
57. Ibid.
58. Ibid.
59. Fagin CM, Jacobson BS. Cost-effectiveness analysis in nursing research. In: Werley HH, Fitzpatrick JJ, eds. Annual review of nursing research, Vol 3. New York: Springer, 1983.
60. Pincus JD. Communication: key contributor to effectiveness—the research. JONA 1986;16(9):19–25.

61. Blalack RO. How satisfied are hospital staff nurses with their jobs? Hospital Topics 1986;64(3):14–18.
62. Prescott PA, Dennis DI. Power and powerlessness in hospital nursing departments. J of Professional Nursing 1985;1:348–355.
63. Price JL, Mueller CW. Professional turnover: the case of nurses. New York: Spectrum, 1981.
64. Curry JP, Wakefield DS, Price JL, Mueller CW, McClosky JC. Determinants of turnover among nursing department employees. Research in Nursing and Health Care 1985;8:397–411.
65. Weisman CS, Alexander CS, Chase GA. Determinants of hospital staff nurse turnover. Medical Care 1981;19:431–443.
66. Hinshaw AS, Atwood JR. Anticipated turnover among nursing staff study. Final Report. Bethesda, MD: DHHS, National Center for Nursing Research, Grant No. NU00908, 1987.
67. Ibid.
68. Price JL, Mueller CW. 1981.
69. Weisman CS et al. 1981.
70. Price JL, Mueller CW. 1981.
71. Hinshaw AS, Atwood JR. 1987.
72. Norbeck JS. Perceived job stress, job satisfaction, and psychological symptoms in critical care nursing. Research in Nursing and Health 1985;8:253–259.
73. Bailey J, Claus K. Summary of a study of stress in intensive care nursing in northern California. San Francisco: UCSF School of Nursing, 1977–78.
74. Kosmoski KA, Calkin JD. Critical care nurses' intent to stay in their positions. Research in Nursing and Health 1986;9:3–10.
75. Gordon VB, Goble LK. Creative accommodation: Role satisfaction for psychiatric staff nurses. Issues in Mental Health Nursing 1986;8:25–35.
76. Hinshaw AS, Atwood JR. 1987.
77. Weisman CS, Nathanson CA. Professional satisfaction and client outcomes: a comparative organizational analysis. Medical Care 1985;23(10):1179–1192.
78. Schofield VM. Orientation of nurse executives. JONA 1986;16(11):13–17.
79. Beaman AL. What do first-line nursing managers do? JONA 1986;16(5):6–9.
80. Robichaud AM, Hamric AB. Time documentation of clinical nurse specialist activities. JONA 1986;16(1):31–36.
81. Hagle ME, Kirchhoff KT, Knafl KA, Bevis ME. The clinical nurse researcher: New perspectives. J of Professional Nursing 1986;282–288.
82. Lang NM, Clinton JF. 1984.
83. Prescott PA, Dennis DI. 1985.
84. Hinshaw AS, Verran J, Chance HC. 1977.
85. Blalock HM. Causal inferences in nonexperimental research. New York: WW Norton, 1964.
86. Duncan OD. Introduction to structural equation models. New York: Academic Press, 1975.

24

Programs of Administrative Research for Nursing Administration

Judith W. Alexander

NURSING administration is a unique blend of the sciences of nursing and administration. The principles of general administration theory, as practiced in business and government, can be applied to nursing organizations.[1-2] The purpose of this chapter is to review the research programs and methodologies currently employed in business and public administration and to draw implications for practitioners, educators, and researchers in nursing service administration.

To accomplish this in a parsimonious fashion, a review was done of the 1985 and 1986 content of business and public administration journals to discover the nature of current programs of research underway and the methodologies in these fields. Journals included in the review were the *Academy of Management Journal, Academy of Management Review, Administrative Science Quarterly, Journal of Applied Psychology, Journal of Management, Organizational Behavior and Human Decision Processes, Psychological Bulletin, Public Administration Review, Public Personnel Management,* and *Review of Public Personnel Management.* From my review, three dominant categories of research programs emerged along with several issues related to research methodologies. This chapter focuses on the content of research programs and on issues related to research methodology.

RESEARCH PROGRAMS IN BUSINESS AND PUBLIC ADMINISTRATION

In the fields of administration the focus has generally been on organizational behavior, personnel management, and organizational theory. Review of recent journals suggests that these areas of research continue to be the most prominent. As nurse administrators encounter problems similar to those in related fields, application of the results from previous studies to nursing practice and research designs should prove useful.

Organizational Behavior

There are four research topics in the organizational behavior category with important implications for nursing administration: leadership, employee stability, job satisfaction, and commitment. Studies focusing on each of these topics are particularly important for nursing as the 1990s approach and the need to retain nurses increases in part because of the predicted shortage of nurses entering the profession. Organizational behavior research has traditionally emphasized the importance of leadership, stability, satisfaction, and commitment for building a productive work force. Authors publishing in the administration literature continue to support research focusing on these topics. They suggest however, that some dramatic changes should be made in future research programs. The development of meta-analytic procedures has improved the sophistication of critical reviews of research addressing behaviors related to worker productivity and has made possible statements of specific directions for future research.

Leadership

Contingency theory of leadership has been popular since its introduction by Fiedler in the 1960s.[3] The contingency perspective suggests that leadership effectiveness is a function of the interaction between a leader and his or her leadership situation. More specifically, a leader can be either task oriented or person oriented; the situation is defined by three factors—leader-member relations, task structure, and position power. Combining the five factors, what results is eight specific leadership situations (octants) that differ in overall favorability. Peters, Hartke, and Pohlman[4] applied meta-analytical techniques to 33 studies using Fiedler's model and found that the empirical support for Fiedler's theory is based largely on laboratory studies, whereas field studies provide support for only four of the octants. These authors concluded that additional theory construction was needed to make Fiedler's theory useful in practice.

Another leadership theory that has been developed since the 1970s is the leader-member exchange model (LMXM).[5–6] The LMXM is based on the concept of developed or negotiated roles between organizational members: Role making takes place through a series of role episodes in which a focal person interacts with relevant other individuals to define the role that will be played within a particular organization. Dienesch and Linder[7] critiqued the LMXM. Based on the fact that empirically the LMXM explained more variance than other leadership aproaches and that conceptually it gave a more complete picture of leadership processes, Dienesch and

Linder recommended that the LMXM receive more attention from future investigators. They also suggested that the exchange between a leader and member should be defined as a multidimensional construct and measured using the concept of mutuality from social exchange theory.[7] Mutuality implies exchange along the three dimensions of perceived contributions to an exchange, loyalty between members in an exchange, and mutual affection that members in an exchange have for one another based on interpersonal attraction. Attention should also be paid to the interactions between these three dimensions to develop a more complete understanding of leader-member exchange as a developmental process.

Similar critiques were not found in the literature for other leadership theories—those for example that have been popular in nursing such as Vroom and Yetton's[8] model of subordinate acceptance of leader decisions and information availability, and Hersey and Blanchard's[9] theory of subordinate job and psychological maturity. I suspect, however, that if reviews of these theories have been conducted, similar recommendations have probably been made: it seems safe to say that additional theoretical construction and refinement is needed for all leadership theories.

Another important aspect of leadership research since the early 1970s has been the identification and specification of moderator variables. A moderator variable is a factor that "affects the nature of the relationship between two other variables, without necessarily being correlated with either of them."[10] Unfortunately most research on moderators has been unsystematic. Howell, Dorfman, Kerr[10] have developed a typology to identify and classify three categories of leadership moderators according to their impact on leadership outcomes. The first of these variables are leadership neutralizers and enhancers. Neutralizer moderators are factors that create a situation such that no leadership style makes a difference: the situation of highly authoritarian subordinates or lack of leadership expertise, for example. On the other hand, enhancer moderators are those that augment relationships between leader behaviors and outcomes, such as the experience of a subordinate.

The second category of moderators in the typology is leadership substitutes. Substitute moderators are those that make leadership unnecessary. To be a substitute, a moderator needs to provide a logical reason why a potential substitute should provide guidance. A substitute moderator also needs to be a neutralizer and it should have an important impact on outcomes differentiating substitutes from neutralizers. An example of a substitute would be intrinsically satisfying work tasks or employees' professional orientations.

Howell, Dorfman, and Kerr's final category of moderators, is leadership mediators. A mediator is an intermediate factor between the independent and dependent variables. This type of moderator implies a causal process, which, with the mediation of behavioral uncertainty, could be as follows: a task-oriented leader reduces a subordinate's uncertainty concerning job tasks, which in turn leads to a higher level of performance.

One final discovery from my examination of recent administrative research on leadership was a meta-analysis of 17 studies of gender-related differences in leadership.[11] No significant differences were found among men and women: both exhibited equal initiating structure and consideration and had equally satisfied subordinates. This surprising finding is particularly important for nursing, a predominately female profession. Nurses need to realize that making a place for themselves as leaders in health care may not be as highly influenced by gender as commonly thought.

My review of administrative research on leadership suggests several things for nursing

administration. Research is indicated in the areas of: leadership models and the applicability of these to nursing organizations; the impact of gender on leaders in nursing; and identification and specification of moderator variables for nursing leadership. Howell's typology of moderator variables in leadership behavior, perhaps most importantly, provides structure for our future leadership research. Nurse administrators need to be aware of moderating factors affecting leadership and address these variables in research designs.

Employee Stability

Turnover, absenteeism, and attendance have been grouped together in the category of employee stability. The line of research addressing worker stability and factors that are identified as precursors to employee stability are extremely important for effective nursing administration, but they have gone largely unstudied in nursing. Inattention has been more pronounced with respect to nurses' absenteeism than with turnover.

Investigations by Mobley,[12–14] Muchinsky,[15–16] and Price[17–18] are the landmark studies of employee turnover, while the Steers and Rhodes's[19] model of employee attendance has become the cornerstone model for attendance and absenteeism research. Judging from research reports, researchers of organizational behavior generally think that employee absenteeism and turnover are not causally related. Consequently I will discuss each of these phenomena and their implications for nursing administration separately.

Cotton and Tuttle[20] conducted a meta-analytical review of 131 studies on employee turnover and were able to elucidate factors that related directly to turnover: age, tenure, pay, overall job satisfaction, employee perceptions, and the presence of a union were all found to be reliable correlates of turnover, while task repetitiveness, accession rates, and intelligence were found to be weakly, if at all, related to turnover. Additional variables that were not included in previous reviews of turnover research, such as met expectations, behavioral intentions, and organizational commitment, hold promise for future new models of turnover. Cotton and Tuttle[20] concluded that future research is needed that tests models using the factors suggested above rather than simply correlating traditional factors with turnover. Research focusing on turnover seems to be particularly critical for nursing administration since attrition rates among nurses have traditionally been high.

With respect to absenteeism, Brooke[21] pointed out that Steers and Rhodes's[19] model of attendance has considerable utility as a starting point for research, but that the model contains several limitations, which make empirical testing difficult. The Steers and Rhodes model proposes that the nature of a job and the surrounding work environment interact with employee values and expectations to determine employee satisfaction with a job situation. A job situation is made up of the scope and level of a job, role stress, promotion opportunities, and relations with coworkers. The model of attendance differentiates between voluntary and involuntary absenteeism by considering the motivation, pressure, and ability to attend.

Brooke[21] contends, however, that the Steers and Rhodes model of attendance does not clearly specify the content of motivation, pressure, and ability to attend; consequently these factors are neither measured nor included in causal models. Brooke also points out that many of the variables—such as job scope—are not single concepts and have diverse dimensions with conflicting effects on attendance. Moreover, the important variables of job involvement, distributive justice, and employment involvement are omitted. Thus, Brooke presents a model that corrects for the deficiencies in Steers and Rhodes's

model and urges that future researchers take an interdisciplinary approach to this area of inquiry.

In a meta-analysis linking absenteeism and job satisfaction, Scott and Taylor[22] found in 23 studies that a significant negative relationship existed between certain facets of job satisfaction and absenteeism. The meta-analysis also suggested, however, that inconsistent findings concerning the complex relationships between satisfaction and absenteeism could be accounted for by sampling error and instrument problems. They concluded that investigators must correct for statistical artifacts before looking at the impact of potential moderator variables. In an analysis published at approximately the same time as Scott and Taylor's, the three authors Watson, Driver, and Watson[23] suggested techniques that could correct for statistical and instrument problems in absence research, including four methods for inducing or testing for multivariate normality when using multiple measures of absenteeism. However, Watson[23] also noted that another valid alternative would be using nonparametric statistics, a suggestion that could be more appealing for nursing.

Nurse administrators may find it useful to take the research on employee stability and test its generalizability to nursing situations. If the results of previous and future studies are indeed generalizable, then nursing administration will have substantial understanding of the elements on which to develop programs to retain a consistent, dependable nursing staff, one which can contribute to the continuity of patient care.

Job Satisfaction

Job satisfaction has been a well-studied phenomenon in nursing as well as in management. Two meta-analytical reviews of satisfaction have suggested that some of the long-held views about the precursors and results of job satisfaction might not be supportable. Loher, Noe, Moeller, and Fitzgerald,[24] for example, conducted a meta-analysis of 27 studies investigating the relationship of Hackman and Oldham's[25] job characteristics model and job satisfaction. Job characteristics in the model are skill variety, task identity, task significance, automony, and feedback. Changing the characteristics of jobs has been widely undertaken in job enrichment programs. The model postulates that job characteristics affect an individual's psychological state and in turn can be linked to outcomes— to work motivation, job satisfaction, employee stability, and quality of work. In the model, too, the individual characteristics of the need for growth is seen as a moderator of the relationship characteristics of jobs and outcomes. Loher, however, found few empirical studies of actual job enrichment interventions; what was found were correlational studies that weaken the conclusions. For the future, Loher and colleagues advocate the use of multiple methods to assess the factors that appear related to job satisfaction since the results in many previous studies have been confounded by common method variance.

On the outcome side of job satisfaction, Iaffaldano and Muchinsky[26] conducted a meta-analysis of 74 studies on the relationship between job satisfaction and job performance. Their analysis indicated that the true correlation between job satisfaction and performance is low, and much of the variability in results is due to small sample size rather than unreliable measurement of job satisfaction and performance. These results led Iaffaldano and Muchinsky to question the assumption implicit in many organizational programs and policies that espouse improving job satisfaction to achieve higher performance. The assumption that satisfied workers are more productive might be true under some conditions, but the interventions that make the relationship hold constant appear

to be different for each situation and thus cannot be generalized.

Continued study of job satisfaction may *not* be helpful if the intent is to improve worker productivity. Perhaps organizational research, specifically nursing administration research, should begin to address other research programs—such as organizational commitment, mentoring, and organizational structure—to improve employee productivity and quality of patient care.

Organizational Commitment

Commitment has been widely studied in the field of organizational behavior since the 1970s when Porter, Steers, Mowday, and Boulain[27] introduced the Organizational Commitment Questionnaire (OCQ). The idea of organizational commitment has intuitive appeal because of the relationship of commitment to behaviors—such as turnover, absenteeism, and performance—behaviors that are important to nurse administrators as they attempt to stabilize the pool of nursing personnel.

Reichers[28] conducted a review of organizational commitment research to include the multiple commitments individuals have to various groups that comprise an organization. Measuring multiple commitments is a change from the traditional global approach of total organizational commitment that the OCQ measures. Multiple measures could account for two employees being equally committed to an organization, but for entirely different reasons. For example, in a single organization one employee might be highly committed, believing that the organization espouses humanistic values toward employees, while another employee might be equally committed believing that the organization is devoted to quality products at reasonable costs.

Several of the recent studies on organizational commitment[29–30] have used nurses as subjects, which should make the transition from management to nursing science easier for nurses continuing this line of research. It should be noted, however, that unfortunately, the causal modeling done by Curry, Wakefield, Price, and Mueller[30] does not support a causal relationship between organizational commitment and job satisfaction. Perhaps the change to examining multiple aspects of commitment as suggested by Reichers[28] will assist nurse administrators in delineating the multiple precursors and implications of organizational commitment among professionals.

To summarize at this point, my review of organizational behavior studies reveals that investigations from the fields of business and public adminstration hold considerable promise for future nursing administration research. Programs of research that are of particular importance to the advancement of nursing administrative theory specifically, and administrative theory generally, have been presented for the topics of leadership, employee stability, job satisfaction, and organizational commitment.

Personnel Management

Four additional research topics that are apparent based on review of the personnel literature, and worth considering in nursing administration are: pay equity, labor relations, mentoring, and employee assistance programs. These topics have been addressed fairly frequently in nursing administration especially since the early 1980s. Reviewing the current state-of-the-art relative to personnel management, in business and public administration, has yielded useful information for nurse administrators, the high points of which are shared in the following four sections.

Pay Equity

The issues of pay equity and comparable worth have become major social and eco-

nomic concerns in our society. Since nursing has traditionally been one of the women's professions with lower earnings, and the American Nurses' Association has taken the case of pay equity to the courts, research focusing on equitable pay has important practical as well as theoretical implications for nursing administration.

Some of the research on pay equity describes the nature of inequities rather than the antecedents and outcomes. Reichenburg[31] has developed an overview of pay equity theory as well as an update on recent scientific developments in the field. Johansen[32] reviewed reports of inequitable pay studies generated by the U.S. General Accounting Office, U.S. Commission on Civil Rights, and the State of Virginia. These reviews demonstrated that nurses, either in practice or when developing research designs, should be aware that the legal environments differ from state to state, and that strategies for implementing pay equity should be planned and tested accordingly.

Traditionally, job evaluation has been used to determine the relative worth and equitable compensation for jobs in an organization. Research on job evaluation, as a consequence, has a considerable number of implications for comparable worth. Madigan and Hoover[33] conducted a study of six job evaluation methods using 206 state classified jobs. The purpose of their study was to investigate the effects of job classification decisions on the equity of job hierarchies. Additionally, the study investigated to what extent pay structures varied by job classification and if studies of pay equity were sensitive to differences in job evaluation methods: six methods of job evaluation were based on two job rating procedures; on two approaches to compensable factor weighting, that is, the characteristics on which organizations base compensation; and on different criterion structures in statistical weighting procedures. Madigan and Hoover's results indicated that if relative job worth is solely based on job evaluation procedures, then the choice of evaluation method will influence job hierarchies and pay equity.

The implication of these findings is that job evaluation methods are biased by the values of jobs, and if evaluation techniques in health-care institutions are biased, for or against nursing, nursing administrators should be aware of this. Replication of Madigan and Hoover's research in health-care institutions is warranted.

Campbell and Lewis[34] conducted a survey of 558 citizens in the State of Georgia to ascertain what the public thinks of policies on comparable worth for public employees. Comparable worth is pay equity among comparable jobs in a work setting. The results demonstrated that three-quarters of the subjects were in favor of comparable worth, but that overall, the public may not have strong and stable opinions about the direction pay equity policy should take. These findings indicate that the "battle for the hearts and minds of Americans on the matter of comparable worth is only in a very early stage."[34] Nurse administrators need to realize how people feel about comparable worth and to replicate studies among the immediate constituencies with whom nurses work—physicians, hospital administrators, and consumers of nursing care.

Fiorito, Greer, and Dauffenbach[35] examined earnings across different occupational groups by using 1970 census data to determine whether compensable factors are treated uniformly. Results indicated that compensable factors were rewarded differently among occupational groups; however these was little difference in the specific compensable factors considered important across all occupational groups. Fiorito suggested that the variation in rewards could be a source of racial- or gender-related earning difference and that additional research is needed to determine the potential importance of these findings.

A review of the literature on pay equity demonstrates that research on the topic is not well developed and that several avenues for future nursing research are worth considering. The avenues for research include job evaluation, compensable factors in health-care institutions, and how nursing constituencies perceive pay equity.

Labor Relations

Labor relations is an aspect of personnel management that is broadly defined as the relationship between employees and employers. Changes in the Fair Labor Standards Act, since 1966, concerning the maximum number of hours that can be worked before overtime must be paid, and the changing of the law in 1974 to allow for collective bargaining in nonprofit health-care institutions, continue to alter the character of labor relations in the health-service industry.

Johnston and Kurtz[36] examined the response of local governments to changes in the 1985 Fair Labor Standards Act as a consequence of the *Garcia v. San Antonio Metropolitan Transit Authority* decision relating to overtime and compensatory time. The model of pre-existing networks and internal coping that local governments used during this period can be especially useful for nurse administrators who are encountering unexpected changes in labor relations laws and regulations.

The Johnston and Kurtz model proposes a four-step sequence of activities for dealing with unexpected change related to labor relations. The first step is mitigation, or deciding what the likelihood of change is, and what to do where a risk to health, safety, and welfare exist: this step implies the need for risk reduction programs. The second step is preparedness, and involves developing a response plan—training responders, identifying critical resources, and making necessary agreements with responding agencies so that critical services can be maintained; a management awareness program is an example of an activity at this step. The third step is response: this step involves implementing a plan once a crisis occurs to minimize problems. The final step is recovery: this is providing immediate support during the early recovery period immediately following a change, and continuing support as a situation returns to normal. The implication for nursing administration research, of the Johnston and Kurtz model, is to test to what extent nurse administrators scan the political, economic, and sociological environments and follow the steps when responding to changes. If nurse administrators are using this or a similar model, a useful research question would address how effective the model is in handling changing labor relations in nursing.

In a related study, Plovnick and Chaison[37] examined the relationship of economic adversity and impending financial crises in an organization, and the incidence of union concessions and cooperative plans. Although this study examined 69 New England manufacturing firms, nurse administrators should be interested in the results since economic adversity and financial crises characterize contemporary health care. The findings of the New England survey, in which presidents of local unions who had negotiated collective agreements with the firms between 1981 and 1982, indicated that economic adversity alone neither improved the quality of labor-management relationships nor brought about union or management concessions, or cooperative programs. However, the incidence of concessions and cooperative programs was associated with improved quality of labor-management relationships.

Plovnick and Chaison did not propose causal relationships; further research is needed to substantiate their results. An interesting study would determine if similar findings exist in collective bargaining agreements developed for nurses. Additionally, a useful

investigation would determine which type of concessions and cooperative programs are best negotiated in collective bargaining situations and which are best discussed in specially created committees outside the collective bargaining framework.

Angle and Perry[38] studied the importance of organizational commitment, in the context of a labor-management climate, for 22 municipal bus companies. Self-reports of four types of commitment were measured: dual commitment to the employing organization and the union or employees' association; commitment to the organization using the Organizational Commitment Questionnaire;[39] commitment to the union and amount of union participation; and labor-management climate using a scale adapted from the University of Michigan Organizational Assessment Package.[40] The results indicated that dual commitment to the union and the employing organization was significantly higher in cooperative climates and that the relationship between commitment and cooperative climate was moderated by the extent of a member's participation in the union. Organization and union commitments taken separately also covaried with the labor-management climate, but in a less dramatic fashion. If similar relationships hold true in nursing organizations, the intuitively appealing idea that nurse administrators should work to improve cooperative relationships with employees would be upheld.

A final research report on labor relations I reviewed addressed the development of a model of voting behavior in union representation elections. The Summer, Betton, DeCotiis[41] model explained voting behavior in both certification and decertification elections. These investigators postulated that the major factor in a voter's decision was his or her general beliefs about unions and perceptions of the combined union-organization potential to achieve valued outcomes compared to the organization's ability to achieve the same outcomes alone. The model characterizes voters as to whether they are likely to vote for a union, against a union, or to abstain. The authors suggested future longitudinal analysis using the model to discover causal linkages among the suggested relationships, a useful avenue for future nursing administration research.

Studies as diverse as the ones I have reviewed on labor relations, illustrate the widespread possibilities for nursing administration research focusing on this topic. Studies are needed of nursing organizations that are unionized as well as of those that are not. Research is needed that tests and builds models to deal with unexpected changes in labor relations environments, the impact of economic and financial adversity on labor-management relations, the organizational commitment of employees to labor and management, and determinants of voting behavior in collective bargaining situations.

Mentoring

Mentoring is a training and development mechanism that has been espoused since the middle 1970s as having a positive impact on the professional progression of individuals in organizations. In 1983, Hunt and Michael[42] reviewed research on the topic and classified the issues related to research on mentorship into five categories: issues addressing the context, mentor, protégé, career stage, and outcome of mentoring. The many problems adhering to any of these factors suggest a wealth of potentially useful studies for nursing administration.

Verta[43] studied mentoring relationships among women in a district office of the Internal Revenue Service. Her study, using both survey and case study methodology to examine 169 male and female employees, indicated that for mentoring relationships to be successful among women, the obstacles to mentoring must first be assessed. For exam-

ple, attitudes and personality characteristics; domestic constraints; and organizational constraints such as veteran's preference, external constraints, and job qualifications need to be evaluated. Moreover, assessment of these factors should be done in the setting of each organization to determine if differences in obstacles exist for women in advanced positions and for other women in these same organizations. From an analysis of potential obstacles to mentoring, deductions can then be made and applied to the specific career needs of individuals being mentored. Verta characterized this process as a proactive approach and as a comprehensive aid to the career development of women.

Henderson[44] studied the character of mentored relationships in the public sector by interviewing 100 public managers who had both mentors and protégés. He described the mentor as one who is expected to teach, guide, sponsor, validate, protect, and communicate, yet be invisible. The protégé on the other hand was upwardly mobile, competent, dependable, and interested, as well as visible or invisible depending on the circumstances. Henderson's findings indicated that both mentors and protégés could be adverse to organizational programs that impose either mentor or protégé relationships on employees. But both groups typically supported the idea of an organizational philosophy that strongly encouraged and expected executive mentoring to occur.

Formal mentoring relationships have not been common in nursing. Thus the Kram and Isabella[45] research on peer relationships in career development is of interest. Their exploratory study of 25 mentor-protégé pairs in a manufacturing company indicated that peer relationships are important alternatives to conventionally defined mentor relationships. The study findings demonstrate that both mentoring and peer relationships have the potential for providing support during successive career stages, as well as career enhancing, psychosocial, and mutuality functions. For individuals who do not have or want mentors, peer relationships offers unique development opportunities.

More research is needed to explain how individual differences in developmental tasks, self-concept, attitudes toward authority, and intimacy among both partners in mentor or peer relationships shape those relationships. Replication as well as extension of the existing studies on mentoring and peer relationships will make an important addition to nursing's body of knowledge.

Employee Assistance Programs

Employee assistance programs (EAPs) are programs designed to assist employees with personal problems when these adversely affect job performance. Interest in EAPs in private and governmental agencies has grown since the middle 1970s. Kemp[46] surveyed state government EAPs, and Johnson[47-48] examined three municipal EAPs in one study, then in another compared the municipal EAPs with those in 10 private sector organizations. All these investigations were descriptive, providing directions for future studies of factors that need to be considered in the establishment of assistance programs. Moreover each of the investigations pointed out that issues are similar irrespective of settings. Programs are based on humanitarian concerns of assisting employees as well as on pragmatic concerns about the economic and social desirability of rehabilitating previously proven and trained employees, rather than terminating workers because of poor work performance secondary to personal problems.[46]

The success of an assistance program depends on a climate of concern for employees and a commitment from management including: the allocation of resources, careful performance appraisals to spot problem employees, referrals to a program, and support of treatment programs. Decisions that need to be made in establishing an employee assistance program are related to: who will have the authority for establishing the program, whether the program will be in-house or contracted, what services will be provided, and the location of a program—in the department of employee relations, personnel, or the medical department, for example.[46-48]

In nursing, the body of literature addressing problem employees and impaired nurses has grown, largely since 1980. The issue of problem workers is of importance to nurse administrators who can now begin to examine the productivity implications of assistance programs.

In summary, as with the review of research focusing on organizational behavior, this review of personnel management studies has demonstrated that there are many areas ripe for research in nursing administration. A beginning point has been suggested for research programs addressing a variety of topics for nursing related to pay equity and labor relations, as well as to mentoring and employee assistance programs.

Organizational Theory

The four topics that emerged from my review of the organizational theory literature were organizational structure, power in organizations, stakeholder management, and organizational models. Little is available in the nursing literature on these topics. Each provides rich opportunities for future nursing administration research.

Organizational Structure

Organizational structure is the allocation of work roles and administrative mechanisms among individuals to control and integrate work activities. Study of organizational structure has been prominent in the administrative literature since the 1960s. The initial focus of research was on defining the concept of structure and its relationship to technology. More recently, the focus has been on the relationship of organizational structure to strategic decision making and organizational performance. Health-care and nursing organizations have frequently been the subjects of these studies; the results, however, have not generally been used in nursing organizations to improve performance. Current studies indicate that changes in approaches to this topic are evolving that have important implications for how organization structure is studied.

Descriptions of matrix organizational structures and their successes and failures have had a major place in the organizational literature since the 1970s. Matrix structures are oftentimes found in health-care institutions. Thus changes in methods for implementing these structures are particularly important for nursing administration. Joyce[49] conducted a social experiment prior to and following the reorganization of an engineering division of an aircraft manufacturing firm.

The reorganization involved structural changes that implemented a matrix structure. To examine the change in structure, Joyce developed a quasi-experimental design using treatment-effect correlations between design, drafting, and testing groups. The implementation of the matrix structure resulted in predicted increases in the quantity of communication, but decreases in the quality of communication with corresponding decreases in coordination. Overall, Joyce's study supported the view that implementing complex structural changes requires multiple interventions; and that lateral communication channels, necessitated by matrix organizations, should supplement rather than replace traditional hierarchical channels to assure such desirable outcomes as improved coordination. Joyce thought that the observations in his study, relative to communication and coordination, had been overlooked to a significant extent in earlier research on matrix

structures. He recommended, therefore, that future research be more than surveys and laboratory experiments and that social field experiments be used as well. Nurse administrators are in ideal situations to conduct social experiments in the field during the reorganization of many of today's health-care institutions.

Generally, research on structure has begun to focus on such organizational variables as job design. Brass,[50] for example, investigated the interrelationship between organizational technology, structure and job design, and the effects of these interrelationships on employee satisfaction, performance, and influence. His study of a newspaper publishing company assessed these variables using multiple measures and data from at least two different sources. The results indicated that there was a need to integrate individual and organizational perspectives when thinking about the design of jobs. Job design should not be derived solely from an individual-level needs theory approach but rather from the organizational perspective of requisite variety[51] and the appropriate matching of environmental uncertainty and organizational flexibility. Researchers examining organizational structure have always stated that organizations must remain flexible to adapt to uncertain environments. Brass[50] suggested that individuals who successfully adapt to uncertain technologies operate best in organizational structures that allow for autonomy and variety.

Another aspect of organizational structure research has involved examining the relationship of structure and strategic decision making. In the past, the proposition that structure follows strategy has been widely espoused. Fredrickson,[52] however, discusses a growing body of literature that suggests that once a structure is established, the structure influences an organization's strategy formation. Fredrickson[52] described the influence that organizational structure—centralization, formalization, and complexity—can have on strategic decision making, and how this impact can be used to produce a pattern describing different types of organizations' decision-making strategies. He used Mintzberg's[53] forms of organization—simple structure, machine bureaucracy, and professional bureaucracy—for his description. Since the professional bureaucracy is closest to the form found in most nursing organizations, I too use that form for further elaboration.

The professional bureaucracy has complexity as its dominant characteristic, but it also has less formalization and more decentralization than other organizational forms. Because of the parochial views that oftentime characterize members of a professional bureaucracy, strategic problems and opportunities go unnoticed. Moreover, due to the high level of specialization, strategic actions usually only take place after extensive political bargaining. Consequently, the only way executive level management can develop overall strategies is by "patching" together the diverse preferences of professionals into a program strategy, or by allocating resources to individual professionals in hopes that they will work synergistically.[52] Further research is needed that will add empirical evidence supporting and testing this model and specifying how strategic decision making is enhanced, constrained, or molded by professional structures. Very little research in nursing administration has been undertaken on this topic.

Research on the technology-structure relationship has changed in character, as has the structure-strategy relationship described above. Barley[54] proposed, through an examination of two hospital radiology departments in which computer tomography (CT) scanners were introduced, that technology can be treated as a social rather than a physical phenomenon, and that structure is a process rather than an entity. A conceptualization of this sort suggests that identical technologies in similar situations could have different structural outcomes and that these different structural outcomes could be due to differences in the history of organizational members and the degree to which decision makers understand technology.

Barley's[54] approach is complementary to the growing body of knowledge positing that the proper fit between technology and structure has better performance as an outcome. Methodological discussions have been prominent in the 1980s as to the best form for operationally defining contingency relationships. Most authors[55-56] have posited that interaction approaches, whether involving the use of multiplicative models or deviation scores, are inadequate. Thus, Drazin and Van de Ven[56] proposed using a systems approach and "incorporated the concept of equifinality of interpreting fit as a feasible set of equally effective alternative designs, with each design internally consistent in its structural pattern and with each set matched to the contingencies facing the organization."[56] Their systems approach of alternative designs was tested on 629 employment security units. They discovered that with multiple forms of fit, including both selection forms—only the best performing organizations survive—and contingency forms are needed to obtain a comprehensive description of context-structure-performance relationships in organizations. Perhaps Barley's[54] approach to technology and structure discussed above is an example of where the context dimension is an organization's technology and its history using the technology.

Alexander and Randolph[55] used an alternative form of fit to predict performance defined as quality of care for 27 nursing units. They used a measure of fit that assumed for each value of a technology variable there was a best value of a structure variable that resulted in high performance. Fit was the absolute difference between the values of technology and structure. Technology was measured by the instrument developed for nursing units by Overton, Hazlett, and Schneck.[57] The structure instrument was developed by Alexander and Randolph.

This study has important implications for nurse administrators in that a proper fit for technology and structure of nursing units was suggested. The fit between variability of technology and horizontal participation, and the fit between uncertainty of technology and formalization are the important findings. More specifically, Alexander and Randolph[55] suggested that in nursing units where tasks and patient diagnoses vary widely, personnel should be highly involved in decision making and defining tasks. On the other hand, where there is little variability among patients, less horizontal participation enhances the quality of nursing care. To improve the fit between uncertainty and formalization, units with more complex nursing problems should require relatively more rules and procedures to provide quality care, while for units with little uncertainty there should be relatively little formalization.

Further research is needed focusing on the relationship of organizational structure, performance, technology, and strategy on varying types of nursing units.

Power in Organizations

Power is often conceptualized as an interpersonal variable; however, conclusions drawn from studies using the individual level of analysis can be generalized to the organizational level.[58] The most popular and widely discussed individual approach to power is the typology, advanced by French and Raven[59], of reward, coercive, legitimate, referent, and expert power. French and Raven also included a sixth type of power—informational influence, but not as a primary base of power.

Podsakoff and Schriesheim[60] reanalyzed the research studies that used French and Raven's conceptualization and concluded that many of the studies have methodological shortcomings. Most notably, the studies suffer from narrow operationalization of concepts, response bias, and aggregation of individual data to unit responses. Suggestions for future research addressing these problems included the development of multi-item measures of the bases of power; the use of Likert-type scales rather than ipsative ranking procedures that force negative correlations; and efforts to assess the independent contributions of each power base to subordinate criterion variables such as withdrawal behavior, job satisfaction, and performance. Nurse scientists are needed who will take these suggestions and conduct further research so that nurse administrators can find ways to increase their power in health-care institutions as well as in the greater health care and societal environments.

Stakeholder Management

Since the 1970s, stakeholder management has become increasingly important. Stakeholders are individuals, groups, or organizations that have a stake in what an organization does. Some stakeholders are internal to an organization—employees for example. Others are at an organization's interface with its environment—the board of directors is an illustration. And still other stakeholders are external—such as the federal government. Some stakeholders are powerful. Others are not.

Using the ideas developed about stakeholder management[61-63] Blair, Korukanda, and their coinvestigators[64-65] have presented a series of papers at national and regional meetings describing typologies of stakeholder management for health-care institutions. The typologies and accompanying management strategies are based on the potential for threat or cooperation of stakeholders with an organization, organizational resources that stakeholders control, and the bargaining positions of stakeholders.

The strategies developed by these researchers have implications for nurse administrators as they attempt to maximize their power. For example, in a county hospital, clients in the community who have private insurance pose a threat to the nursing department inasmuch as they have the prerogative to choose a private hospital, rather than a county hospital, thereby reducing the revenue to the county hospital. A nursing department could maximize its power through collaborative strategies with consumers to improve the delivery of quality care that increases the department's bargaining power with insured clients. Research needs to be conducted to test whether or not the strategy of increasing bargaining power can be supported empirically.

Organizational Models

Hall[58] described two primary reasons for studying organizations: one is to understand how and why organizations are effective, and the other is to develop organizational theory (p. 261). Both of these reasons are germaine to the understanding and development of nursing administration theory. Organizational models that have been popular since the 1960s are the systems-resource model explicated by Yuchtman and Seashore[66], and the goal-oriented models proposed by Barnard[67] and Etzioni.[68] Since the late 1970s, the new models of population ecology[69-70] and resource dependence[71-72] have been advanced.

The population ecology model uses biological ecology to describe the variety and evolution of organizations. Organizations are distinguished as either specialized or generalized. They survive based on creating a niche in the environment. The resource dependence model suggests that organizations play a role in their fate through political decision making and internal action.

Tolbert[73] studied the pattern of administrative differentiation in colleges and universities, integrating perspectives from the resource dependence and institutional models. In the institutional model, "organizations experience pressure to adapt their structure and behavior to be consistent with their institutional environment in order to ensure their legitimacy . . . and chances of survival."[73] The institutional approach suggests that organizations take various forms because of the institutionalized values and beliefs in society. Tolbert concluded that the use of a single theoretical perspective—either resource dependence or the institutional—is inadequate for explaining organizational processes, and that these perspectives are complementary, not competitive, and should be used together.

Hrebiniak and Joyce[74] integrated theoretical perspectives in a typology of how organizations adapt to their environments: the typology is based on the interaction of strategic choices made by organizations and the determinants in an environment. In a two-by-two matrix, population ecology is the quadrant of low-strategic choice and high-environmental determinism, and resource dependence is in the quadrant of high-strategic choice and low-environmental determinism. Low-strategic choice and low-environmental determinism are characteristic of organizations that adapt by chance or "muddle through,"[75] while organizations categorized as high-strategic choice and high-environmental determinism are typically large firms in highly regulated industries. Hrebiniak and Joyce concluded that this synthesis of perspectives produces a more complete approach to the understanding of organizations.

Hall[58], using the eclectic approach to integrating theoretical perspectives suggested by Tolbert[73], Hrebiniak and Joyce[74] and others, proposed a "contradiction" model intended to be applicable across all organizations. In Hall's view, organizations face multiple and conflicting environmental constraints; second, organizations have multiple and conflicting goals; third, organizations have multiple and conflicting external and internal constituencies; and last, organizations have multiple and conflicting time frames. Future empirical research is needed to test the explanatory power of Hall's model. But this perspective, which synthesizes ideas from a variety of models, has promise for nursing as nurses search for ways to determine which nursing organizations are effective and as nursing administration theory is developed.

In summary, my review of research that is building organizational theory indicates improved research is evolving, but that much empirical testing remains to be done. Nursing administration research is needed that addresses organizational structures—especially matrix designs, the impact of these designs on strategic decision making, and the fit of organizations structured in a variety of ways with technology. Additional avenues for research include bases of power at the organizational level, the impact of stakeholders, and integrated models of nursing organizations.

RESEARCH ISSUES FROM BUSINESS AND PUBLIC ADMINISTRATION

Survey and descriptive research are still widely reported in the administration literature, particularly for problems related to personnel management. New methodologies using meta-analysis, improved qualitative techniques, and advanced quantitative measures—such as causal modeling—are growing in importance.[76] The development of these methodologies will not be elaborated on further in this chapter as they are discussed by others in the book. I will close, however, with a discussion of contexts of studies, research utilization, and units of analysis.

Research Contexts

Of potential interest to nursing administration is the discussion by Blair and Hunt[77] of context-free and context-specific research.

Context-free research involves investigations that are conducted by researchers interested in basic phenomena—such as leadership, mentoring, or organizational structure. Context specific research on the other hand, is more applied, focusing on the unique characteristics of a particular kind of organization—health care, education, or manufacturing.

The context-free approach tends to support basic research that focuses on a restricted range of variables: it is also more microanalytic, generally speaking, too generic to be relevant to administrators, and usually not interdisciplinary. The context-specific approach usually is applied research examining many variables in a single organization, more macroanalytic, relevant to administrators, and interdisciplinary.[77]

Much of the research reviewed in this chapter that was described as organizational behavior and organizational theory research is context-free, while the personnel management research is largely context-specific. Nursing administration can glean ideas from both approaches.

In an attempt to facilitate the development of knowledge from both the basic and applied approaches, Blair and Hunt[77] have proposed a model that provides a research road map for integrating the two. The model depicts a series of reality checks interspersed with research studies. An initial reality check, for example, is conducted with basic and applied researchers to set the stage for systematic research and application. Programmatic research efforts can be undertaken to look at substantive (context-free) as well as problem solving (context-specific) research. Follow-up reality checks can then be used to determine what has been learned, where gaps exist, and how useful the research is for application.[77] This approach to research may initially appear to be time consuming and costly. But it is one that is needed if research useful for both theory building and practice is to be conducted. Blair and Hunt's model can also be useful in developing programs for research utilization in nursing.

Research Utilization

As in nursing, writers in the administrative literature discuss the problem of making research understandable and usable for practitioners. McGuire[78] examined how administrators and researchers vary in their way of understanding and interpreting organizational phenomena. Administrators look for guidelines to action, while researchers value more abstract and conceptual information. McGuire suggested that qualitative research designs could be helpful for examining these differences and moving practicing managers and theoreticians closer together.

An administrative conference, sponsored by the Center for Effective Organizations at the University of Southern California, was held in 1983 to address research that contributed to both theory and practice. The series of papers that resulted from the conference[79] provide some useful insights about how to bring practitioners and scientists together. In nursing we face the same challenge—to bridge service and education—to find ways of combining the talents and energies of researchers and practitioners.

Unit of Analysis

Whether to conduct organizational investigations at the individual, departmental, divisional, or corporate level has always been an issue in administrative science. Why a researcher should choose one unit of analysis over another is not well understood. But history shows that the level of analysis selected makes a difference in the results.[80]

Selecting the appropriate level and unit of analysis is complicated by the likely magnification of the cost of obtaining individual-level data. Additionally, the aggregation of individual-level data to generate departmental and organizational scores has been criticized methodologically except where variance in departments is less than variance between departments.

At this time, the administrative literature does not provide clear answers to the problems related to unit and level of analysis. Researchers in nursing administration therefore must carefully justify the unit of analysis they select, and be scrupulously explicit and rigorous in the interpretation of results.

In summary, new methodological techniques reported in administrative science are beginning to be explored in nursing. The current state of the art in business and public administration, with respect to the issues of context, research utilization, and unit of analysis, provide direction for nurse researchers as they develop increasingly complex, innovative, yet useful research designs.

This chapter has provided a review of research programs and methodologies from the fields of business and public administration in an attempt to connect management and nursing science by providing background information and direction for future nursing administration research. Interspersed throughout the discussion I have tried to portray how the bridge between research and practice is being built in other administrative fields. Investigators in nursing administration need to understand the practice of nursing, nursing administration, and management if their research is to have an impact on the management of nursing services.

REFERENCES

1. Arndt CL, Huckabay LMD. Nursing administration: theory for practice with a systems approach. St. Louis: CV Mosby, 1980, p. 9.
2. Chaska NL. Theories of nursing and organizations: integrated models for administrative practice. In: Chaska NL, ed. The nursing profession: a time to speak. New York: McGraw-Hill, 1983, p. 724.

3. Fiedler F. A theory of leadership effectiveness. New York: McGraw-Hill, 1967.

4. Peters LH, Hartke DD, Pohlmann JT. Fiedler's contingency theory of leadership: an application of the meta-analysis procedures of Schmidt and Hunter. Psych Bull 1985;97:274–285.

5. Dansereau F, Cashman J, Graen G. Instrumentality theory and equity theory as complementary approaches in predicting the relationship of leadership and turnover among managers. Org Beh and Human Perf 1973;10:184–200.

6. Graen G, Novak M, Sommerkamp P. The effects of leader-member exchange and job design on productivity and satisfaction: Testing a dual attachment model. Org Beh and Human Perf 1982;30:109–131.

7. Dienesch RM, Linden RC. Leader-member exchange model of leadership: a critique and further development. Acad of Manag Rev 1986;11:618–634.

8. Vroom VH, Yetton PW. Leadership and decision making. Pittsburgh: University of Pittsburgh Press, 1973.

9. Hersey P, Blanchard K. Management of organizational behavior. 4th ed. Englewood Cliffs, NJ: Prentice-Hall, 1982.

10. Howell JP, Dorfman PW, Kerr S. Moderator variables in leadership research. Acad of Manag Rev 1986;11:88–102.

11. Dobbins GH, Platz SJ. Sex differences in leadership? How real are they? Acad of Manag Rev 1986;11:118–127.

12. Mobley WH, Horner SO, Hollingsworth, AT. An evaluation of precursors of hospital employee turnover. J of App Psych 1978;63:408–414.

13. Mobley WH, Griffeth RW, Hand HH, Meglino BM. Review and conceptual analysis of the employee turnover process. Psych Bull 1979;36:493–522.

14. Mobley WH, Hand HH, Baker RL, Meglino BM. Conceptual and empirical analysis of military recruit training attrition. J of App Psych 1979;64:10–18.

15. Muchinsky PM, Tuttle ML. Employee turnover: an empirical and methodological assessment. J. of Voc Beh 1979;14:43–47.

16. Muchinsky PM, Morrow PC. A multidisciplinary model of voluntary turnover. J of Voc Beh 1980;17:263–290.

17. Price JL. The study of turnover. Ames, IA: Iowa State University Press, 1977.

18. Price JL, Mueller CW. A causal model of turnover for nurses. Acad of Manag J 1981;24:543–545.

19. Steers RM, Rhodes SR. Major influences on employee attendance: a process model. J of App Psych 1978;63:391–407.

20. Cotton JL, Tuttle JM. Employee turnover: a meta-analysis and review with research implications. Acad of Manag Rev 1986;11:55–70.

21. Brooke PP. Beyond Steers and Rhodes model of employee attendance. Acad of Manag Rev 1986;11:345–361.

22. Scott KD, Taylor GS. An examination of conflicting findings on the relationship between job satisfaction and absenteeism: a meta-analysis. Acad of Manag J 1985;28:599–612.

23. Watson CJ, Driver RW, Watson KD. Methodological issues in absenteeism research: multiple absence measures and multivariate normality. Acad of Manag Rev 1985;10:577–586.

24. Loher BT, Noe RA, Moeller NL, Fitzgerald MP. A meta-analysis of the relationship of job characteristics to job satisfaction. J of App Psych 1985;70:280–289.

25. Hackman JR, Oldham GR. Motivation through the design of work: test of a theory. Org Beh and Human Perf 1976;16:250–279.

26. Iaffaldano MT, Muchinsky PM. Job satisfaction and job performance: a meta-analysis. Psych Bull 1985;97:251–273.

27. Porter LW, Steers RM, Mowday RT, Boulian PV. Organizational commitment, job satisfaction, and turnover among psychiatric technicians. J of App Psych 1974;59:603–609.

28. Reichers AE. A review and reconceptualization of organizational commitment. Acad of Manag Rev 1985;10:465–476.

29. Bateman TS, Strasser S. A longitudinal analysis of the antecedents of organizational commitment. Acad of Manag J 1984;27:95–112.

30. Curry JP, Wakefield DS, Price JL, Mueller CW. On the causal ordering of job satisfaction and organizational commitment. Acad of Manag J 1986;29:847–858.

31. Reichenburg NE. Pay equity in review. Pub Pers Manag 1986;15:211–231.

32. Johnansen E. Comparable worth: the character of a controversy. Pub Admin Rev 1985;45:631–635.

33. Madigan RM, Hoover DJ. Effect of alternative job evaluation methods involving pay equity. Acad of Manag J 1986;29:84–100.

34. Campbell JE, Lewis GB. Public support for comparable worth in Georgia. Pub Admin Rev 1986;46:432–437.

35. Fiorito J, Greer CR, Dauffenbach RC. Uniformity and variation in occupational earnings determination: potential sources of incomparable worth. J of Manag 1986;12:61–74.

36. Johnston VR, Kurtz M. Handling a public policy emergency: the Fair Labor Standards Act in the public sector. Pub Admin Rev 1986;46:414–422.

37. Plovinick MS, Chaison GN. Relationship between concession bargaining and labor-management cooperation. Acad of Manag J 1985;28:697–704.

38. Angle HL, Perry JL. Dual commitment and labor-management relationship climates. Acad of Manag J 1986;29:31–50.

39. Mowday RT, Steers RM, Porter LW. The measurement of organizational commitment. J of Voc Beh 1979;14:224–247.

40. Institute of Social Research. Michigan organizational assessment package: Progress report II. Ann Arbor MI: Survey Research Center, ISR, 1975.

41. Summers TP, Betton JH. Decotiis TA. Voting for

and against unions: a decision model. Acad of Manag Rev 1986;11:643–655.

42. Hunt PM, Michael C. Mentorship: a career development tool. Acad of Manag Rev 1983;8:475–485.

43. Verta LL. Women, occupational advancement, and mentoring: an analysis of one public organization. Pub Admin Rev 1985;45:415–423.

44. Henderson DW. Enlightened mentoring: a character of public management professionalism. Public Admin Rev 1985;45:857–863.

45. Kram KE, Isabella LA. Mentoring alternatives: the role of peer relationships in career development. Acad of Manag J 1985;28:110–132.

46. Kemp DR. State employees assistance programs: organization and services. Pub Admin Rev 1985;45:378–382.

47. Johnson AT. Municipal employees assistance programs: managing troubled employees. Pub Admin Rev 1985;45:383–390.

48. Johnson AT. A comparison of employee assistance in corporate and governmental organizational contexts. Rev of Pub Pers Admin 1986;6:28–42.

49. Joyce WF. Matrix organization: a social experiment. Acad of Manag J 1986;29:536–561.

50. Brass DJ. Technology and the structuring of jobs: employee satisfaction, performance, and influence. Org Beh and Human Dec Proc 1985;35:216–240.

51. Ashby WR. Variety, constraint and the law of requisite variety. In: Buckley W, ed. Modern systems research for the behavioral scientist: a sourcebook. Chicago: Adline, 1968.

52. Frederickson JW. The strategic decision process and organizational structure. Acad of Manag Rev 1986;11:280–297.

53. Mintzberg H. The structuring of organizations. Englewood Cliffs, NJ:Prentice-Hall, 1979.

54. Barley SR. Technology as a occasion for structuring: evidence from observations of CT scanners and the social order of radiology departments. Admin Sci Qtrly 1986;31:78–108.

55. Alexander JW, Randolph WA. The fit between technology and structure as a predictor of performance in nursing subunits. Acad of Manag J 1985;28:844–859.

56. Drazin R, Van de Ven AH. Alternative forms of fit in contingency theory. Admin Sci Qtrly 1985;30:514–539.

57. Overton P, Schneck R, Hazlett CB. An empirical study of technology of nursing subunits. Admin Sci Qtrly 1977;22:203–219.

58. Hall RH. Organizations: structure, processes, and outcomes. Englewood Cliffs: Prentice-Hall, 1987, p. 129.

59. French J, Raven BH. The bases of social power. In: Cartwright D, ed. Studies in social power. Ann Arbor, MI: Institute for Social Science Research, 1959.

60. Podsakoff PM, Schriesheim CA. Field studies of French and Raven's bases of power: critique, reanalysis, and suggestions for future research. Psych Bull 1985;97:387–411.

61. Freeman RE. Strategic management: a stakeholder approach. Marshfield, MA: Pitman Publishing, 1984.

62. Mason RO, Mitroff II. Challenging strategic planning assumptions. New York: Wiley, 1981.

63. Mitrof I. Stakeholders and the organizational mind. San Francisco: Jossey-Bass, 1983.

64. Blair JD, Baliga BR, Whitehead CJ, Korukanda AR. Stakeholder management strategies for health care organizations. Paper presented at Academy of Management meeting. Chicago, IL; August, 1986.

65. Korukanda AR, Blair JD. Resource dependence and stakeholder management: strategies for managers of today's health care organizations. In: Proceedings of the Southern Management Association Annual Meeting, November, 1986.

66. Yuchtman E, Seashore S. A system resource approach to organizational effectiveness. Amer Soc Rev 1967;32:891–903.

67. Barnard CI. The functions of the executive. Cambridge MA: Harvard University Press, 1938.

68. Etzioni A. Two approaches to organizational analysis: a critique and suggestion. Admin Sci Qtrly 1960;5:257–278.

69. Hannan MT, Freeman JH. The population ecology of organizations. Amer J of Soc 1977;82:929–964.

70. Aldrich HE. Organizations and environments. Englewood Cliffs, NJ: Prentice-Hall, 1979.

71. Aldrich HE, Pfeffer J. Environments of organizations. In: Inkeles K, Coleman J, Snelser N. eds. Annual review of sociology, Vol. 2. Palo Alto, CA: 1976.

72. Pfeffer J, Salanick GR. The external control of organizations: a resource dependence perspective. New York: Harper and Row, 1978.

73. Tolbert PS. Institutional environments and resource dependence: sources of administrative structure in institutions of higher education. Admin Sci Qtrly 1985;30:1–13.

74. Hrebiniak LG, Joyce WF. Organizational adaption: strategic choice and environmental determinism. Admin Sci Qtrly 1985;30:336–349.

75. Lindblom CE. The science of muddling through. Pub Admin Rev 1959;19:79–89.

76. Perry JL, Kraemer KL. Research methodology in the Public Administrative Review 1975–1984. Pub Admin Rev 1986;46:215–226.

77. Blair JD, Hunt JG. Getting inside the head of the management researcher one more time: context-free and context-specific orientations in research. J of Manag 1986;12:147–166.

78. McGuire JB. Management and research methodology. J of Manag 1986;12:5–17.

79. Lawler E, Mohrman A, Mohrman S, Ledford G, Cummings T, eds. Doing research that is useful for theory and practice. San Francisco, CA: Jossey-Bass, 1985.

80. Freeman J. Data quality and development of organizational social science: an editorial assay. Admin Sci Qtrly 1986;31:298–303.

25

Philosophic Inquiry for Nursing Administration

Gina Giovinco

IN PHILOSOPHIC inquiry, arguments, theories, and even seemingly esoteric issues can be traced to the basic problems in a particular field. All issues have philosophic beginnings and are traceable to two main philosophic questions: What is the real issue versus what we think it is? and What does it mean in terms of explaining, describing, and defining the issue?

The first question asks about the nature or essence of a phenomenon. The second asks about meaning. Raising questions about the nature or essence of phenomena in a particular field builds knowledge in that field. Philosophical questioning, as in metaphysics, is examination of general, persistent, and pervasive characteristics. In nursing administration, philosophical questioning can help account for such phenomena as change, cause and effect relationships, identity, uniqueness, and sameness. What it means to make a change in the organizational structure and function of a health-care facility is a philosophical concern that raises many issues requiring critical thinking.

METAPHYSICS

Metaphysics, as a branch of philosophy, is a system of fundamental principles and involves critically examining the underlying assumptions of a system of knowledge. Metaphysics addresses the claims about what is real and what is imagined. Questions about what is real give rise to epistemology. Epistemology is the study of methods and grounds of knowledge with reference to the limits and validity of knowledge in a particular field. Although the utility of epistemology as a way of knowing continues to be debated, it is generally held that through epistemological processes—critical thinking—one can arrive at fundamental truths about reality.

Fundamental truths help us address questions of meaning and theory development in nursing and nursing administration. Meaning is that which is designated by a phenomenon or is intended to express why experience and reality is as it is. What is nursing administration? What does it mean to be a nurse administrator? Questions like these, about the essence of nursing administration and its meaning, are part of the process of critical thinking and lead to a science of fundamental principles and categories that build knowledge in the discipline.

Knowledge building occurs from meanings derived from words and how they are assembled in sentences that are considered logical by a discipline. Meanings derive from the forms of statements and from the logical relationships of components in statements. Words have meaning only in terms of the something to which they refer; that something constitutes their meaning. For example, when statements are made about staffing, budgeting, cost containment, or efficiency, these terms in statements must have objectively existing referents in order to be logical, coherent, and meaningful. Meaning is crucial to communication because it has to do with how people use words and sentences and how the terms that are used relate to the expectations of others.

Verification of meaning in philosophic inquiry is different from other kinds of inquiry. In clinical science, variables are isolated and studied individually and empirically. Scientific inquiry in the logical positivistic tradition as we know it, provides conflicting recommendations as to the most useful procedures to be used to clarify and advance understanding of phenomenon in a field of study. Philosophy is sometimes referred to as the art and science of argument. It is by its methods rather than by its subject matter that philosophical inquiry is distinguished from other kinds of inquiry.

DIMENSIONS AND STAGES OF PHILOSOPHIC INQUIRY

The following paragraphs illustrate the fundamental steps and elements of philosophic inquiry[1]. The methods suggested by these steps have been derived from a plethora of literature on how to proceed with inquiry.

First, the inquirer becomes aware of a problem or situation that calls for an account or explication. Questions like these are asked: What is the meaning of an efficiently and effectively managed nursing unit? What are the elements in the aforementioned question that are open to debate? At this step, skillful, astute observation is crucial.

Second, various aspects and phases of a situation at hand, differentiating some changes from others, are measured and a tentative, partial description of what is happening is begun. The question asked at this stage is, What is the basis for rational thinking? To respond to this question one must be able to justify that claims are being made and verify the knowledge that comprises the reality related to the issue as it is understood.

Third, these questions are asked: What are the connections among the things that are observed, and how are they measured? What connections are imagined and unexplained? Philosophical inquiry at this stage focuses on what seem to be the most pertinent conjectures as to what could happen with respect to the phenomena of interest under particular circumstances.

Fourth, conjectures might elucidate other facts that should be verified. Some of these additional facts may not have been originally thought to be pertinent, but as inquiry proceeds, a situation could be viewed far differently than it was originally. For example, consider how differently we think of our past views and legislation relative to the deinstitutionalization of the mentally ill. Asking even deeper questions enables us to be farsighted and make decisions where long-range implications are more clearly thought through.

Fifth, transformations using verbal and mathematical logic may be used to clarify and advance understanding and meaning of a situation. What was taken as fact at an earlier stage, might be revised or rejected at this point. Tentative understandings and descriptions of what is, and of its meaning, are revised as necessitated by the demands of society and as knowledge expands.

Sixth, empirical observation might occur. As new conjectures are formulated, they require further observation—for fuller more adequate descriptions—to clarify and advance understanding of the phenomenon of interest. This process of observation, reconsideration, renewed observation, and the raising of philosophical questions is oftentimes referred to as empirical observation, which in turn leads to the formulation of hypotheses about the relationships between elements of a phenomenon.

Seventh, the success of a philosophic inquiry is apparent when there is evidence of extensive critical thinking and generation of a description and explanation of the elements, relationships, and procedures for resolution of a problem. Subsequent inquiries may be used to supplement an original description and explanation of a phenomenon. In some situations new, additional inquiries can reveal aspects and phases of a problem, which demand that there be important amendments to earlier descriptions of thinking about how best to address and resolve a problem.

In philosophic inquiry, there is no end point; consequently philosophers speak of "resolution" to a problem rather than a "solution." A complete, comprehensive description and explanation of even seemingly simple problem situations has never been achieved and never can be because mankind and its problems are dynamic—always in a state of flux. Nevertheless, descriptions and explanations that are as fully developed as possible, given the resources brought to bear, are the objects of philosophic inquiry.

It should be noted, however, that a description of a single element of a complex process of events might be seen as a full description and explanation of an entire event, particularly where single hypotheses relative to small circumscribed elements are tested mathematically. These explanations, then, are falsely assumed to provide evidence of scientific inquiry and scientific proof for larger populations and phenomenon. Relying on incomplete explanations is problematic and defies common sense.

Some extant technological advances are impressive, particularly to those who are not philosophically and mathematically skilled. Others would argue, however, that scientific inquiry is not as advanced as many in society seem to think. For example, in medicine many common health problems remain unsolved, while more and more resources are expended on exotic problems that occur for relatively few.

PHILOSOPHY AND COMMON SENSE

What is common sense, and how does it relate to philosophic inquiry? The term "common sense" is not precise, and the object to which it refers is somewhat ambiguous; for exam-

ple, when we call a viewpoint commonsensical, do we mean that many people hold that view in common, or do we mean that some people hold a particular view in common? Or do we mean that the view is common to people in general? In a fourth instance, when we use the term we could refer to what people who are not specialized in a discipline believe about the phenomena of interest.

Generally speaking, common sense is good, ordinary sense as understood by most people. It is the intuitions of all mankind that are not dependent on special or technical knowledge. Common sense forms a layman's philosophical framework. While essential for human functioning, common sense alone is not adequate for critical decisions: for important decisions both common sense and knowledgeable inquiry are needed.

If one insists on common sense as the final court of appeal when making decisions, confusion often results and experimentation and knowledge development are impeded. Philosophy, it should be noted, does not set out to deny or affirm common sense. In fact, common sense can be the beginning of philosophical inquiry. It is because of common sense that one begins to wonder, question, and try to make sense of the meaning of one's existence. Common sense is an appropriate beginning—an ideal springboard for an epistemological journey—as long as we remain aware of the limitations of managing affairs using only the unreflective opinion of ordinary persons.

EPISTEMOLOGY AND A SENSE OF KNOWING

It should not be thought that philosophic inquiry is appropriate only for those phenomena that are complicated. Philosophic inquiry is also important for the seemingly simple and close at hand. When we say we cannot see the forest for the trees, what we mean metaphorically is that it is easy to miss the obvious—easy to see the elements of a phenomenon and miss seeing the whole, the entirety. It is the obvious or close at hand, oftentimes, that is unfathomable and in which the greatest philosophical questions dwell.

For nurse administrators confronted with myriad problems and situations, all of which often seem equally critical, it is easy to lose sight of the whole. Where the number of problems, especially new problems requiring new kinds of strategic decisions exist, it is easy to address each individual problem for the short term, without getting to the root of the problems, and without seeing the totality of issues and their interrelationships. What results is management by crisis rather than intentional rational administration based on knowledge, theory, and pragmatics.

One of the most frequently quoted maxims by Socrates is, "Know thyself." The philosophical questions, Who am I?—What does it mean to be just this unique self?—are perfect examples of how we can be directed to that which is closest and most obviously at hand, yet in many ways, quite distant.

Mankind's world and attitudes are manifold. What is manifold or multifaceted is often frightening because it is not neat and simple: most persons are threatened to some degree by complexity, and consequently prefer to forget how many possibilities are open to them.[2] The great Viennese philosopher Martin Buber, says, "those who tell of two ways and praise one are recognized as prophets or great teachers because they save men from great confusion and hard choices. They offer a single choice that is easy to make because those who do not take the path that is commended to them live a wretched life." But all simplicity is not wise. What Buber is saying is that to know the world, you must know yourself and take responsibility for the choices you make regarding your reality.

Knowing and the Known

When it comes to philosophic inquiry, it is not enough to identify symptoms; one must identify the root of a problem. But how does one get to know what lies at the root?

To locate something, we must first have some idea about what it is that we are searching for. In other words, to find the answer to a question, we need to be able to recognize the best answers among potential answers. In a sense, we must know the nature of answers in advance; this, of course, is a paradox, and a crucial one that directs our inquiry to a different meaning of knowing.

Common sense, as has been noted, is knowledge of many things. As administrators we might say of our workplace, this institution exists, it has existed for many years, it has many departments offering a variety of services, all of the characteristics of the institution have been recorded and are history. History can be called forth through memories. History brings together the past and present as a way of questioning the future, which helps one to understand the purpose and meaning of the institution.

On reflection, however, we realize that using common sense and historic information alone, while improving our understanding of the meaning of the institution, leaves us with relatively little information about what goes on in the institution. For these reasons administrators cannot be completely satisfied with the information that common sense affords. It is not until one learns how all departments fit together to form the whole of the agency, it is not until one understands the meanings people give to their lives and work that he or she can understand and know an institution.

The Epistemological Journey

If getting to know about a thing involves aspiring to see it—an institution, a profession, and so forth—how does one know when he or she has identified phenomena as they actually are? Thinking about this question is the beginning of epistemology. Once our questions have reached this stage of thought and inquiry, common sense knowledge no longer suffices: epistemology—a theory of knowledge for finding resolutions to nagging questions—is needed. At best, epistemology addresses this question: What do I need to know to be able to claim that a phenomenon is what I say it is?

Epistemology is characterized, first, as seeking to give an account of the nature of knowing in general by analyzing the concept of knowing in all the various contexts in which it is applied. Second, it is characterized as seeking to account for important concepts such as belief, certainty, and truth.[3]

When approaching a problem epistemologically, one of the fundamental tasks is to set out the conditions under which propositions are argued. The object of propositional statements is to establish truths. The truths, or untruths, are then used to support the claims that are made about a phenomenon.

Epistemology also addresses the source of knowledge. One of the sources of knowing is through perception, along with intellectual authority and reason. Perceiving a problem from a single perspective, it should be noted, means the problem is understood in terms of the limitations of a single individual's ability to understand its multiple dimensions. Single-person perceptions, therefore, limit the claims one makes about knowing what a problem is, what it means, and how best to address it. A single individual's experience is neither true nor false, it simply is limited in its meaning. A single individual's knowing is usually not at as high a plane as collective knowing. Collective knowing helps to validate and evaluate what we think we know about a particular problem or phenomenon.

To move to a higher plane of knowing, one has to transcend individual beliefs, assertions, and opinions. A claim based solely on opinion is not useful knowledge unless defended with great care and precision. When a claim is not defended, it is simply a proposal of one way to view a situation—be it a problem or some other phenomenon of interest.

Opinions are usually held less firmly than beliefs, and one soon learns that an opinion is not sufficient evidence to understand and resolve problems, especially not the problems nurse administrators encounter in complex organizations. For example, when a question in a university hospital arises about an increase in wound infections on a particular patient-care unit, and nurses express the opinion that medical students and physicians are not adhering to the prescribed hand-washing routines, knowledge in addition to that derived from opinion will have to be generated to resolve the problem.

Where statements of opinion are given, there needs to be further inquiry, well-founded beliefs, and eventually knowing. What is commonly meant by knowing is that a belief is true and that there are good, even conclusive reasons for believing as one does.[4] The use of knowledge is a distinctly human approach to coping with reality, and knowledge—especially complex theoretical understanding—is something that only human beings appear to be able to acquire and to require for their existence.

Since opinions are a clue to the existence of objective knowledge, as administrators we may claim to know about an issue based on an opinion that is thought to be valid. But until the claim to truth can be justified, we cannot reasonably claim "to know" what is true. Justification of an opinion is needed. Justification refers to the reasonableness of the evidence that supports a claim.

Knowledge, it is clear, is intimately linked with the expression of claims, and expression normally finds its utterance in judgment. But epistemology is really concerned with the question of the grounds of judgment as these relate to knowledge. The central preoccupation of epistemology is with the question of evidence.[5] To use epistemological methods, therefore, questions in metaphysical terms need to be raised prior to any other questions because it is in metaphysical inquiry that one attempts to answer the questions of existence and meaning. Epistemology is a form of philosophical inquiry that investigates the origins, structures, methods, and validity of knowledge.

Let us suppose that a nurse executive claims the problem of a nursing shortage has been resolved for his or her institution. For this statement to have meaning, it would have to be demonstrated that in fact a shortage existed—that the statement was not merely someone's opinion, with no supporting evidence and justification. To supply evidence of this kind of knowledge is to think rationally and reasonably. To ask, for example, shortage in terms of what?—numbers of nurses and hospitals? numbers of occupied beds? numbers in terms of population and morbidity?—is epistemological rationality.

In summary, epistemology is the philosophical science of the nature of knowledge and truth—although the decision as to whether or not a given kind of reasoning is valid or not is a question of logic. Understanding the scope of epistemology will be helpful for considering the relationship of nursing to adjacent disciplines like psychology, management science, and economics, for developing a science of nursing administration. Moreover, an understanding of epistemological processes is useful for the nurse administrator who is responsible for identifying the means and methods for making statements intelligible; expressing knowledge intelligibly; and identifying the meaning in intelligible resolutions.[6]

REFERENCES

1. Handy R, Harwood EC. Useful procedures of inquiry. Great Barrington, MA: Behavioral Research Council, 1973.
2. Buber M. I and thou. New York: Charles Scribner, 1970.
3. O'Connor DJ, Carr B. Introduction to the theory of knowledge. Minneapolis, MN: University of Minnesota Press, 1982.
4. Machan TR. Introduction to philosophical inquires. Boston, MA: Allyn and Bacon, 1977.
5. Gallagher KT. The philosophy of knowledge. New York: Fordham University Press, 1982.
6. Runes DD. Dictionary of philosophy. NJ: Rowman and Allanheld, 1984.

26

The Phenomenological Research Method: Its Value for Management Science

Rosemarie Rizzo Parse

VARIOUS research methods are being explored as ways to expand management science in general and nursing administration in particular. Quantitative methods are no longer the only accepted methods to investigate organizational questions. Qualitative methods offer enticing opportunities to uncover meaning and expand knowledge of human experiences and interpersonal processes.

Traditionally research methods used in management and administration have been borrowed from the natural sciences. It is common to find published studies utilizing quasi-experimental, descriptive correlational, ex post facto, and survey methods to investigate research questions within the domain of management. These quantitative methods are appropriate to answer research questions that seek to understand cause and effect, and associative relationships. They are not appropriate, however, to answer questions related to the meaning and structure of human experience.

As management science, and organizations with high-level technology expand, an understanding of complex interpersonal relationships becomes more important. These interpersonal processes and the meanings of human experiences cannot be adequately or accurately investigated using quantitative methods of inquiry.

To address research questions arising in management science related to human experiences, it is useful to draw on all the social science research traditions. There are a number of methods available for use to investigate meanings and evolve structures of experiences as humanly lived. Three major methods, descriptive (exploratory and case); ethnographic; and phenomenological, all borrowed from the social sciences—are qualitative in nature and appropriate for use when the phenomena to be studied are lived experiences, and the expected outcomes are descriptions and hypothetical propositions.[1]

THE METHOD OF CHOICE

The method used for investigation of a research question is chosen on the basis of the ontology from which the phenomenon to be studied arises. If it emerges from a belief system grounded in the notion of cause and effect, the method of choice is quantitative. For example, if the investigator seeks to know which of two methods of nursing care more effectively produces client adaptation, then a quasi-experimental design may be developed for testing specific hypotheses using instruments to measure client adaptation. If the phenomenon arises from a belief system grounded in the notion that man[*] and environment evolve simultaneously, thus positing the view that human experiences are coconstituted, that is, created in the man-environment interrelationship, not governed by cause and effect, then the method of choice is qualitative. For example, if the investigation seeks an understanding of a feeling of satisfaction, then a phenomenological study may be designed to arrive at a description of that lived experience. In both situations, the findings may be used to enhance the theoretical perspective guiding the study and thus guide development of management practices and stimulate further research.

THE PHENOMENOLOGICAL MOVEMENT

The phenomenological tradition began early in the nineteenth century and perhaps before then. But phenomenology as a method of inquiry first appeared in the last half of the nineteenth century in the writings of Brentano.[2] Brentano's student Edmund Husserl[3] developed the method in some detail, which was later refined by the German philosopher Martin Heidegger[4]. While other German philosophers like Jaspers and Scheler were important in the movement, it was Heidegger[4] who synthesized Husserl's phenomenology with Kierkegaard's existentialism to form existential phenomenology. French philosophers of the early twentieth century, Gabriel Marcel,[5] Maurice Merleau-Ponty[6], and Jean-Paul Sartre[7] expanded the phenomenological movement and formulated phenomenology as a method of inquiry and an alternative to traditional research methods.

[*]The term "man" in this chapter refers to mankind in the generic sense, homo sapiens.

ESSENTIALS OF THE METHOD

It is important at this juncture to explain the term "phenomenology." The term "phenomena," derived from a Greek verb, means to show or appear. The term "phenomenology" means the study of something as it appears.

It also has a more specific meaning in the world of research. Phenomenology is the qualitative research method emerging from the philosophical science of existential phenomenology. The purpose of this method is to uncover meanings and structures of lived experiences by following particular processes of inquiry; it does not seek to show causal relationships.

Foundational to phenomenology is the notion that experiences are coconstituted; the phenomenological methodology takes into account man's participation in life situations.[1,8] Man's participation with an experience is related to the choices inherent in cocreating it, so that an experience is given personal meaning through the way it unfolds. What is experienced is a personal event.[9]

Phenomenology, as a method of inquiry, is the rigorous adherence to the phenomenon as it appears and unfolds in the descriptions of subjects who have lived the experience under study. Analysis of subjects' descriptions reveals the nature of the phenomenon by uncovering the essences and meaning of the experience. The method offers researchers the opportunity to appropriately study human experiences without prescriptive presuppositions that only measure characteristics in discrete categories, eliminating the richness of subjects' personal perspectives of lived experiences. The researcher using phenomenology as a method seeks to find the meaning of the experience in the context of the subjects' lived world, rather than in the theoretical beliefs about the phenomenon.[10–12] To implement the method requires great skill. Novice researchers using the phenomenological method require guidance from a mentor who knows and has used the method.[1,2]

RESEARCH-RESEARCHER DIALECTIC

A critical feature of the phenomenological method is the nature of the researcher's participation in data collection and analysis. The researcher explicitly participates in uncovering the meaning of the experience; this participation is called the research-researcher dialectic.[13] Phenomenological research is often criticized for involving personal participation. Critics say the method produces biased findings; but qualitative researchers merely take into account the researcher's frame of reference and explicitly make it a part of the research report.[13] The subjective interrelationship between researcher and researched is acknowledged in the phenomenological method. While it is a factor in utilizing quantitative research methods, it is neither acknowledged nor made explicit. Before engaging in a phenomenological study, researchers make explicit their personal beliefs about the phenomenon being examined. These beliefs are set forth in a section of the report called the researcher's perspective, which also contains the investigator's theoretical grounding and personal experience with the phenomenon. These beliefs are bracketed by the researcher as he or she proceeds through data collection and analysis. Bracketing is the researcher's temporary suspension of personal beliefs and assumptions about the phenomenon under investigation in an effort to forge directly to the essences of the thing itself as it is appearing.[3]

Data collection and analysis require that the researcher abstract the essences from descriptions made by subjects and translate data from the concrete statements provided by study participants to the language of science.[14] This process of shifting levels of abstraction happens within the researcher's personal frame of reference. These transformational shifts by the researcher expand the body of knowledge in a discipline. These shifts are made through the processes involved in phenomenal analysis. The engagement between researcher and researched phenomenon happens through "contemplative dwelling," which is the profound thinking inherent in the processes of intuiting, analyzing, and describing.[1] Through contemplative dwelling, the researcher's privileged position is joined with the view of the lived experience described by the subject, to create the structure of the experience. The researcher's interpretations are intersubjective; that is, given the researcher's frame of reference, another person could design similar interpretations following the rigorous processes of the phenomenological method.[1]

PROCESSES OF PHENOMENOLOGY

The three major processes involved in phenomenological analysis are intuiting, analyzing, and describing.[1,2] These processes occur simultaneously as the researcher dwells with the subject's descriptions. They require the researcher to adhere to the surfacing meaning of the phenomenon through the strict intentional tracing of its elements and the setting forth of the characteristics of its essences.[2] These processes are consistent with the fundamental presuppositions of phenomenological research articulated by Giorgi.[10,15] The presuppositions are (1) the researcher is required to remain faithful to the phenomenon as described by the subject in the context of the situation as it emerges in everyday life; (2) description is the mode used for data collection and reporting of findings; and (3) the researcher searches for the meaning through rigorous adherence to the rules of phenomenal analysis.

Various Modifications of the Method

There are a number of modifications of the phenomenological method. The two most widely accepted are those designed by van Kaam[16] and Giorgi[10]. Van Kaam's modification has six operations of scientific explication. They are

1. eliciting descriptive expressions;
2. identifying common elements;
3. eliminating nonrelated expressions;
4. formulating a hypothetical definition;
5. applying the definition to the original description; and
6. identifying the structural definition.[1]

The researcher engages in the process of contemplative dwelling with the subjects' descriptions, then identifies the descriptive expressions—statements expressing a complete idea. A common element is an abstract phrase, naming a major theme that arises from a cluster of descriptive expressions and is explicitly or implicitly contained in each subject's description. The common elements are synthesized to form a hypothetical definition. Through further verification, a structural definition is identified. Judges are used to verify the researcher's interpretations of the descriptive expressions, common elements, and the structural definition. A more detailed explanation and example of expressions, elements, and definitions in nursing science can be found in Parse.[1]

The Giorgi[10,15] modification is somewhat different. It includes the following six operations:

1. returning to the subject for elaboration on the description;
2. identifying natural meaning units;
3. identifying themes;
4. identifying focal meanings;
5. synthesizing situated structural descriptions; and
6. synthesizing a general structural description.[1]

The researcher dwells with the subjects' descriptions, identifies areas where further explanation is desired, and then returns to the subject and asks for elaboration on these specific areas of the description. The researcher, in dialogue with each subject's descriptions, identifies meaning units. Themes are then identified for each meaning unit. A theme is the central idea of the unit written in the language of the subject. Focal meanings are identified from each theme. The focal meanings written in the language of the researcher shift the level of abstraction to the language of science. The focal meanings are synthesized to form a situated structural description for each subject; then a general description is written, which synthesizes the situated structural descriptions from all of the subjects.

Scientific Rigor in Phenomenology

Rigor in phenomenological research cannot be judged by use of the quantitative criteria of reliability and validity. These criteria are peculiar to methodologies that measure characteristics. For qualitative research, the criteria of creditability, auditability, and fittingness have been set forth as appropriate for judging scientific rigor.[17] "Creditability" is justified when other researchers recognize the structural description arising from the data as the lived experience being studied. Creditability is enhanced by the explicit articulation of the researcher's perspective of the phenomenon prior to engaging in data collection and analysis. "Auditability" is the criterion of scientific rigor related to intersubjectivity. It is satisfied if other researchers can follow the path from the raw data, through the levels of abstraction to the structural description of the lived experience, and in so doing arrive at a comparable conclusion. "Fittingness," as a criterion of scientific rigor, is satisfied if the findings of the study fit into contexts outside the study situation and if others appreciate the findings as meaningful. The findings must also be congruent with the raw data from which they were derived.

PHENOMENOLOGY AND MANAGEMENT SCIENCE

Phenomenology, as described above, is a research method that can be selected for use in the investigation of lived experiences related to any aspect of management science. Management is intricately involved with interhuman processes. The study of lived experiences, therefore, is important for the expansion of its science. It is important, however, to consider the ontology of the management theory from which the phenomenon for investigation and the research question arise. The assumptions and propositions about the interhuman processes in any theory circumscribe the choice of methodology. If the philosophical beliefs underpinning the theory are cause and effect in nature, a quantitative method should be chosen; if the beliefs relate to coconstitution of experience, and meaning of interhuman relationships is sought, then a qualitative method should be used.

It is important when considering these options to have identified the theoretical perspective of the managers governing the organization. In regard to the administration and management of nursing services, too, it is imperative to know the theoretical framework grounding nursing practice. If the nursing theory governing practice is Roy's model of adaptation, quantitative methods are suitable in that adaptation is rooted in cause and effect relationships. If the nursing theory is Parse's Man-Living-Health, then qualitative methods would be utilized because the theory is grounded in acausal interrela-

tionships and focuses on lived experiences. Management and nursing theories must be congruent to assure harmonious interrelationships in an organization that provides nursing and health care services.

For the phenomenological approach to be the method of choice, the focus of an investigation should be on human experiences in the interpersonal processes relevant to management in general or management of nursing services in particular. Examples of lived experiences appropriate for study when Parse's theory guides the nursing practice in a setting where there is a congruent management theory are: the lived experience of leading others; the experience of living with ambiguity and paradox; the experience of feeling responsible for others; the experience of being frustrated; the experience of having accomplished something; and the experience of persisting.

If any of these phenomena are chosen, the researcher would design the study by first setting forth the research question, for example, "What is the meaning and structure of the experience of living with ambiguity?" The researcher would write a researcher's perspective expressing theoretical beliefs and personal experiences with the phenomenon. Two or more subjects for the Giorgi method and 20 or more for the van Kaam method would be recruited from persons holding nursing management positions. "Adequacy of the sample is achieved when the researcher experiences redundancy in the descriptions. Redundancy is repetition of statements regarding the phenomenon under study."[1] (pp. 17–18)

Potential subjects would be informed that they may withdraw from the study at any time, that their anonymity will be preserved, and that there are no known risks or benefits to participating. Those who agree to participate are invited to respond to the statement, "Describe a situation in which you experience living with ambiguity. Please share all your thoughts and feelings related to the situation." The descriptions would then be analyzed using either the van Kaam[16] or the Giorgi[10,15] modification of the phenomenological method. Each of these proceed in a slightly different manner, but both require contemplative dwelling with the data through intuiting, analyzing, and describing. This leads to the transformational shifts in levels of abstraction to a general structural definition of the lived experience. The findings of the study would be woven into the management and nursing theories related to the interhuman processes guiding the development of administrative strategies in the setting where man-living-health was the theoretical framework of practice.

In summary, phenomenology, a rigorous method of inquiry, uncovers meaning of lived experiences. It is particularly appropriate for use in management science, where phenomena and research questions about interhuman processes are central. It may be the method of choice in a nursing service setting where nursing practice is based on the theory of man-living-health, the central focus of which is man's lived experiences. The findings of phenomenological studies are not merely preliminary or exploratory work for initiating quantitative research studies. Such findings stand on their own and enhance theory that guides the evolution of practice.

REFERENCES

1. Parse RR, Coyne AB, Smith MJ. Nursing research: qualitative methods. Bowie, MD: Brady Communications Company, 1985.
2. Spiegelberg H. The phenomenological movement. Vols. I and II. The Hague: Martinus Nijhoff, 1976.
3. Husserl E. Ideas: general introduction to pure phenomenology. (WRB Gibson, trans.) New York: MacMillan, 1931.
4. Heidegger M. Being and time. New York: Harper and Row; 1962.
5. Marcel G. The philosophy of existentialism. New Jersey: Citadel Press, 1956.
6. Merleau-Ponty M. Phenomenology of perception. (Colin Smith, trans.) New York: Humanitas Press, 1974.
7. Sartre JP. Being and nothingness. New York: Washington Square Press, 1966.
8. Parse RR. Man-living-health: a theory of nursing. New York: John Wiley & Sons, 1981.
9. Ihde D. Experimental phenomenology: An introduction. New York: Putnam & Sons, 1977.
10. Giorgi A. Psychology as a human science. New York: Harper and Row, 1970.
11. Oiler C. The phenomenological approach in nursing research. Nursing Research 1982; 31:178.
12. Parse RR. Nursing science: major paradigms, theories, and critiques. Philadelphia: W.B. Saunders, 1987.
13. Bodgan R., Taylor S. Introduction to qualitative research methods. New York: John Wiley & Sons, 1975.
14. Pelto PJ, Pelto GH. Anthropological research: the structure of inquiry. Cambridge: Cambridge University Press, 1981.
15. Giorgi A, Fischer CT, Murray EL, eds. Convergence and divergence of qualitative and quantitative methods of psychology. In Phenomenological psychology, Vol. 2, Pittsburgh: Duquesne University Press, 1975.
16. van Kaam A. Existential foundations of psychology. New York: Doubleday, 1969.
17. Guba EG, Lincoln YS. Effective evaluation. San Francisco: Jossey-Bass, 1981.

27
Historical Research Methods

Barbara A. Keddy

THE PAST is the future. It is also the present, and so one must search for social and cultural factors in each epoch of history to understand how values, practices, and traits are sustained, altered, or removed from our present everyday world. Journeys into the past can provide fruitful clues that can better help us to not spin our wheels through endless repetitive cycles. How can the nursing profession's past be used to study its present, and more specifically, how can nurse administrators expand their research horizons by adopting a transhistorical perspective to gain more knowledge about nursing administration theory? This paper grapples with these and other issues related to nursing history and its relationship to the management of nursing practice, which until the 1970s, was rarely discussed by nurse administrators, educators, practitioners, or researchers.

Any discussion of historical research must necessarily include a definition of the concept of "history." To gain some perspective, it is important to point out that while there are various positions regarding what constitutes history, generally the positions represent some basic stands. Broadly defined, history is either direct or indirect evidence about trends, issues, practices, or phenomena occuring over time.

Historiography is the writing of history. The historian Carr[1] discusses issues related to historiography in great detail. He says that facts do not make history, "they provide no

ready-made answer to the question 'What is history'?" It is generally agreed by all who either do historiography or discuss the method philosophically that despite efforts to write within a "scientific" tradition of objectivity, historical facts are filtered through the historian's own ideology, values, and approaches. There are, therefore, complex relationships between historians and their historiography. "Just as scientific theories change, then, so does the past in the hands of different historians."[2] However, to take an overly critical view of the real or potential bias of historiography is to risk the presumption that all other types of scientific research or theory are totally unbiased. No writers of philosophical, theoretical, or empirical research can claim to have a tabula rasa.

My argument is not intended as an apologia of historical research, but rather as an attempt to discuss the joining together in a marriage of sorts, historiography and nursing management, while at the same time recognizing that there is no pure form of objective history. To achieve the aim of this paper, however, it is necessary at this stage to point out that there has been considerable struggle in the nursing research tradition to even achieve some small degree of status for historical research. Davies[3] has written, "Although there are encouraging signs that this is now changing, the idea of 'nursing research' is still all too likely to conjure up a picture of the questionnaire and the survey, the researcher in the field rather than the researcher in the library and archive room."

Having set the scene about the difficulties involved in defining history, reporting and interpreting facts objectively, and the relatively low status of historical research in general, let us proceed to discuss aspects of the more positive and potentially fruitful field of untapped information, which could entice nurse managers to try innovative approaches to gathering data in their search for better paths to the management of nursing practice. To that end, it is essential to examine various types of history, which the historian can use as data, and which can assist nurse managers in selecting appropriate methods for their purposes.

ORAL HISTORIES

The amount of oral history being done in North America is voluminous. While generally oral historians are themselves the interviewers, it is also possible to analyze the data of other oral historians who have simply presented verbatim reports without analysis. The term "oral history" is often used synonymously with "telling one's life story," "life review," "reminiscing," "personal interview," or "narrative history." If the method is used in the informative sense when the focus is on factual material,[5] then the oral historian needs to be skilled in aspects other than interviewing, such as in uncovering forms of data—like written records, letters, or literature—that can assure historical integrity. Far too often, oral historians such as the American, Studs Terkel and the Canadian, Barry Broadfoot have been accused of writing collections of stories, presented as narrative without evaluative criteria or analysis. It is difficult to achieve any degree of credibility of this type of documentation particularly if the results are called research findings, although unanalyzed data standing alone can serve as the basis for validating other forms of histor-

ical information. There is a vast amount of oral history to be collected for the purpose of understanding nursing management. Oral histories, however, should not be mere collections of personal interviews without synthesis.

The Process of Oral Histories

How then does a researcher-historian prepare for gaining practical knowledge of an institution, such as a hospital? Olson[6] has written "If you are concentrating on a particular agency, you need to read its annual report, which will explain its structure, the extent of departmental jurisdiction, the budgetary situations, and its accomplishments over the year." If the nurse manager has as his or her aim the intent to review change in, for example, departmental jurisdictions or accomplishments over a 20-, 30-, or even 40-year timespan, a review of the records suggested will provide a beginning stage for developing interview questions and deciding whom to interview. It is, of course, not always possible to interview older head nurses, staff nurses, and administrators who might have died, are incapacitated, or unavailable, but who could provide valuable data about the nature of change in a ward or an entire hospital. It is surprising, however, to find many who are still accessible and willing to provide extensive histories that help to present a clearer picture of why certain values seem inherent in an agency, or why specific practices are difficult to change, or how informal coalitions influence the nature of an institution.

Within the last 25 years the role of nurse managers has changed tremendously. (There are, however, frustrations that, although inherent in most aspects of nursing, changes often are more complex in administration. We generally think that change is too slow, that we have not made advances in the manner we desired, and that more substantial innovations should have occurred in spite of broad historical barriers.) Lest we think nursing hasn't changed, let me use the following example of how things were in nursing administration in 1960. In an interview for an oral history project with an older nurse who became a director of nursing in 1960, in a rather large hospital in Nova Scotia, I asked her to recall her experiences. This anecdote, taken from the data now preserved in the Nova Scotia Archives, gives the reader the opportunity to compare and assess the changes that have occurred in nursing administration over the past several decades.

Keddy: What was it like on your first day as director? Were you frightened?

Mrs. Allan: No. Strangely enough, I wasn't frightened. But I came to a meeting with the board, I met with the administrator and then I came to a meeting with the head nurses, and I started talking about head nurses' responsibilities and I got nothing but a blank. I drew an absolute blank. Because at that time head nurses were doing their share of bedside nursing care. They were acting very much as the senior student back in my training days. They were still doing nursing care, giving medications. When you spoke of head nurses' meetings, principles of nursing, different responsibilities, they were wholly unaware of any of this.

This same nurse had taken a one-year diploma course in nursing management at a university, and she was seen as the most educated nurse in the vicinity—with new and progressive, albeit strange, ideas. She was responsible for having head nurses take a six-week course in management. The hospital at that time did not have medical or hospital bylaws. She and the administrator developed them. It would be interesting at this point to have interviewed the administrator and head nurses to compare their experiences during that era. However, the point of this anecdote is to suggest that it would be even more interesting to take an oral history of that same hospital's nurse administrator today and develop a profile of the changes in values, practices, and areas of jurisdiction that have occurred over a span of each five years—then to relate those facts to such phenomena as the women's movement and women at work.

History can be viewed from any particular era or time span, or from the perspective of any number of individuals involved with an experience, and it can be used not only for comparative purposes but to discern whether certain trends have changed and how new ones evolved. When history is used in ways like these, we are better able to appreciate progress, or conversely point out that, in fact, we have regressed or, as is often the case, only to find that 20 or 30 years later the same problems still exist. As a process, therefore, it is necessary for researchers to understand the nursing administration of a period in time either by reviews of journals or, more specifically, of records and documents generated by individual institutions, than to verify the data with first-hand accounts. In the case of the director of nursing, her entire oral history was validated through journals and records in the hospital archives.

The reader should now be convinced that there are stories available that are worth preserving by obtaining systematic work-life reviews that are culturally and generationally distinct, as well as gender, status, and social-class specific. It then behooves the nurse historian to collect and transcribe the data appropriately. In addition, analysis of historical information enables others to decide whether or not a data set is reliable and valid. How does one proceed, then, to do an oral history accurately and systematically?

As I suggested earlier it is imperative to read relevant documents from earlier times that provide insights necessary to decide on the next stage of the research process. Among the important documents are nurses' notes, financial reports, medical records, correspondence, and other secondary sources such as newspapers and periodicals. Statements of philosophies, goals, and objectives of committees too, provide valuable information often leading younger readers to either gasp in disbelief that times were so different or, that, in fact, little has changed.

It is true that a historian's work could end with a review, summation, and analysis of the oral data. In many cases, this may be all that is needed to provide a good historical overview. For the careful oral historian, however, the job has just begun.

The next stage in the oral history process is deciding whom else to interview in order to generate information from a wide spectrum of individuals who can provide varying perspectives that either complement or contradict existing perceptions of the historical experience being investigated.

Verification of Data

It is obvious at this point that a particular work or life history is by definition unique. For that reason asking one director of nursing or one head nurse, or supervisor about his or her experience confines the research to a single person. However, the stories told by single individuals can be tested by the collection of a number of oral histories that can then be used to identify patterns of regularities. Take these two examples and discover for yourself the similarities in their stories. Each is an anecdotal segment from an oral history of a director of nursing in the 1920s and 1930s in two Canadian provinces.

Keddy: What was your job like as superintendent?
Mrs. Caine: Well, you had to be on call practically all the time because you had the key to all the drugs and anything they wanted, why, you had to go even to the intravenous supplies. There was just the one person. You didn't trust to leave the keys to the night supervisor or where any of the graduates could get it because they would help themselves to stuff whether they needed it or not or more than they were supposed to and the first thing you would know, you'd be out and that would be it. So, we developed a system for when something like that happened. Around that time, they had several bad accidents at night, you know, and I just put my clothes on and went up, me there. I remem-

ber one night, I pulled my slacks right on over my pyjamas and went up and I had a bed gown on and we put men out on Ward D sunporch. We had to put them wherever we had beds. There was a bad accident down Wedgeport way and I was getting this man's arm ready for starting intravenous in and he [the doctor], of course, had no idea that it was me when he got in there. "Well, Mrs. Caine!" he said. What we used to do is we'd stay right there, the operating room girls were right there and we stayed right there until everything had quieted down. Maybe go in the doctor's room and have a cup of coffee and sit and chat there for awhile before we left.

Keddy: What sorts of jobs did you have to do as a superintendent?
Mrs. MacDonald: We went on and got night report from the night supervisor and, of course, saw our sick patients first, and it just depended, if it was a quiet day, there was just a little extra visiting the staff as well as the patients. And if it was a busy day—now I remember one Sunday, now I'm not saying I'm the only one who could do this, anyone could do it, we knew how to run the portable X ray, so when a minor accident came in or some emergency we went down and admitted the patient, and we could do urine (for sugar and albumin), we could do a microscopic, and we had run the portable X ray, and probably had to go up there, the same supervisor—it was 125 beds, and run the operating room. And I remember not thinking a thing about it, and the doctor that day said, "Well, I've never seen the likes of it in this hospital!"

It can be readily seen that the jobs of administration and nursing, nurse administrators, and other health professionals, overlapped considerably. Often, in fact, the director of nursing was the hospital administrator as well.

What were the social implications of these practices? When did the nurses give up these positions to others? What was the reason for changes in jurisdictional responsibilities? In what ways are there still overlapping responsibilities?

A journey through time with nurses over the past several decades provides partial answers to these and other questions: reading the nursing journals of those eras helps to both verify stories and fill in gaps. It is, however, the regularities that provide a clear idea of the trends. With an understanding of how trends change, nurse managers can plan and not fall into old established patterns by seeing the broader long-term picture more clearly.

The idea of oral history is best summed up by the British nurse historian Davies:[7]

A striking development in social history of late has been oral history—the growing concern with what is called "history from below," the views and experiences of the rank and file. These views can sometimes only be captured through the reminiscences of participants, and are subject to all the difficulties and distortions which the retrospective interview method brings. But sometimes letters, local records, journal articles, biographies, etc. can help build up a picture . . .

OTHER TYPES OF HISTORICAL DATA

For the nurse manager, collecting oral histories may seem like an overwhelming task, one that requires time, typists, transcribers, and searching for other forms of documentation. For those who do not have the resources, there are of course other sources of primary data such as personal letters, handwritten notes, autobiographies, reports, minutes, and more recently, audio and visual recordings. A basic problem for many hospital nurses is that until the days of Florence Nightingale few records were kept. At the turn of the century, however, official documents became more plentiful. It is unfortunate though that in most cases very old records stored in hospitals have been unlisted and stored under poor conditions. In the last few decades, historians, librarians, and archivists have made great strides in preserving records from the more well-known hospitals. It is experts in these hospitals that nurse managers can turn to for assistance in uncovering data that can answer research questions.

Secondary data—such as published research, biographies, statistics, edited transcripts, and textbooks—are all examples of additional data that can clearly help the researcher become more familiar with a topic under investigation. Davies[8] writes: "Whether a researcher uses primary sources, secondary sources, or, as is usual, a mixture of both is dictated by the state of knowledge in the area, the way the problem has been formulated, time available, and so on."

However, as with oral histories, it is imperative that all archival data be critically evaluated. As Christy[9] has pointed out, "The goal of the historiographer is to establish truth." Continuing, Christy discusses two processes for establishing the validity and reliability of data, external and internal criticism. In the former, the researcher attempts to determine whether or not the documents themselves are valid. In the latter, internal criticism focuses on establishing that the information in a document is reliable.

It is often difficult to understand the literal meaning of documents written in another era by persons living in another culture, a crucial issue especially when reading biographies or histories of nursing in various localities or parts of the world. Consider the following example regarding cultural meanings from a book written about nursing in Newfoundland in 1934.[10]

On one occasion when the doctor was visiting, he was confronted by a man with a severe toothache who pleaded:

> Doctor, I got a won'erful bad 'ead. I finds he scattering toimes, the last month, but, you know, not so bad altogether. Last night he took me won'erful, Doctor, I wants me tooth hauled.

Nouns are often assigned personalities by the use of "he" and "she" instead of the article "a" and "it," and "won'erful" is literally to mean "full of wonder."

Nevitt, the narrator and interpreter of this quotation, herself a British nurse writing about nursing in Newfoundland, referred to the book entitled, *Among the Deep Fishers* as her secondary source of data. She showed that it was the use of secondary sources that enhanced her understanding of the point she was trying to make in her own historical analysis, that is, that nurses need to develop a sensitivity to the language and customs of the culture they are studying.

But of what interest is this to the nurse administrator you may well ask? Has nursing jargon changed that much in recent years? Do past practices resemble the present and have only the words changed? The answer to these questions seem immediately obvious. What were "blood letting," "stirring blood with citrate," "mustard poultices," "pneumonia jackets" if not nursing interventions?[11] The word "interventions" was not used but that is exactly what these procedures were. Nursing practices have changed, however, from rustic interventions to sophisticated techniques.

What was the first indication of the development of nursing processes? Was it not the nurses' notes? Who was a matron or superintendent if not a director of nursing? What were rule books if not objectives or philosophies? How then can nurses in management continue to avoid using historical research methods? History is the soul of present-day nurse managers; it is their own story.

HISTORY AND THE NURSE MANAGER

There are various theoretical approaches for analyzing the development of hospitals as institutions employing large numbers of nurses. For the most part, there are two main perspectives: the first and most common is the liberal democratic perspective and the second is the political economy view, which although gaining popularity does not have a wide following among nurses. Generally, however, in historical research, a narrative is presented without any explicit mention of the theoretical position of the historiographer.

In the first and more common perspective—the liberal democratic one, data are generally presented as though nursing has

made great strides, many difficulties have been overcome, and we continue to sail forward, taking our place in the world as "true professionals." Histories of nursing in this view reflect primarily the work of great nursing leaders, often presented as biographies of heroines. Historical studies in this tradition are often intended to bring out our sense of pride at what has been achieved without ever addressing and comparing the frustrations of nurses in the past with those of the present. There is a quote in Davies[12] book that says,

We hear a great deal about systems; it seems there was or is an old system, and that there is or will be a new system. Under the former, it is said, all was bad; under the latter, we shall behold perfection.

This quote is taken from the Edinburgh Medical Journal, May 1880, under the heading "A Nurse, Systems of Nursing." In the 1980s we can ask, have we beheld perfection?

In the second perspective, the political economy view, nursing and its historical connectedness to sociopolitical issues is described. Nurses and their relationships to labor unions, feminism, other occupations, and the social class backgrounds of nurses, are generally believed to be the reasons why there are difficulties in the profession today. Let us examine some of the issues using this perspective and explore their usefulness for nurse administrators, and equally significant, for rank-and-file nurses who are care providers and whose stories are often unsung.[13]

Women as Nurses: The Underpaid, Exploited Perspective versus the Great Strides View

While there are some male nurses the numbers are extraordinarily small. For that reason, nursing has traditionally been viewed as a woman's occupation. Any history of women's work in the past century must of necessity study the "short step from idealization of the womanly role in education or nursing, to propaganda which would persuade women to accept jobs as assistants to men, at low salaries, in return for the opportunity to serve."[14] This point of view, the political economy perspective, suggests that history must take into account the following factors in order to provide a more complete understanding of women's work of which nursing is an integral component. There is first of all, the type of women's history that has only just arisen, that is, revealing ordinary rank-and-file lives as part of history, since initially women's history focused primarily on great women.[15] Second, there is the need for women to create a culture of their own born from reading and assimilating history, not fearing it.[16] Third, to avoid tackling history as though it is just a series of advances, it is important to take shorter periods of time and to concentrate on what has been happening outside of nursing as well as in the profession.[17] Fourth, we need to look into the unwritten history of nursing, oftentimes obscured by the early century elite who suppressed revolts against the conditions of hospital work, until the American Nurses' Association was converted to an organization to avoid massive unionization.[18]

There is also the view that Sidel and Sidel[19] forcibly describe when they discuss the Flexner report of 1910, and the issue of hierarchies in medicine. These authors encourage the view that we should not repeat history but study it to understand who has come to dominate health policy. There are, of course, other factors that deal specifically with social class disparities, the division of labor, and historical materialism.

Contrast the political perspective with the popular liberal view held by many nurse-historians. Melosh[20] argues that their "narratives dramatize a history of progress, from the 'Twilight and the darkness' before Nightingale to the triumphs of reform, reorganization, and upgrading education." While Melosh says the liberal view is useful, she also notes that it has prevented nurse-historians from moving beyond the issue of professionalism. She writes:

Nurses are working in an occupation that has consistently employed large numbers of women; in the medical division of labor, nursing occupies a key position that has been largely overlooked in medical history and sociology; it provides a significant example of a major service industry over a century when such work has come to dominate the economy and the labor force. As we bring the questions of medical history, women's history, and labor history to the data of nurses' experience, we shall revise and challenge these formulations even as we forge a stronger and more comprehensive nursing history.

WHAT IS HISTORICAL RESEARCH TO THE NURSE ADMINISTRATOR?

To summarize the issues discussed, I shall focus on three main points: how to do historical research, how to convince others of its viability, and how historical investigations should be processed.

How to Do Historical Research

The researcher or research unit of a hospital or agency planning to do historical research should first know whether or not historical material has been retained and preserved. Moreover, before writing a research proposal, the researcher must know that the information collected, if it is to be primary data collected firsthand, will be kept in a place formally designated for archival material. Other primary and secondary data, which are generally scattered about in various places such as board members' homes, museums, nursing associations, basements of alumni buildings, and so on, can be problematic for inexperienced researchers.

A variety of paths need to be taken as preliminary work before a plan of action can be developed. It is important for the historian to recognize that the ease of access and the location of data will be influencing factors as to whether or not it is feasible to do a study. The idea of hunting through unsorted, scattered about records or collections of papers may be exciting but it is also time consuming. For the academic, it can be rewarding and challenging; for the researcher working under severe budgetary constraints, the unpredictability of this method can pose serious problems. The point to be emphasized is to limit research projects to a size that is reasonable given the amount of time and money available. Nurse administrators are often in a good position to calculate what resources are available and to provide access to institutional archives.

After the hours of search have been assessed it is appropriate for the proposal to be written. As in all research designs, time and money budgets assume great significance. It is, therefore, important for the investigator to establish a time schedule in a strictly adhered to research plan. If the proposal is not written in a polished sophisticated fashion, the existing, oftentimes erroneous perceptions of nursing history will not change. It will be assumed that historical research is a second-rate activity, folksy and rather interesting, but not true research. It is imperative, therefore, that a careful and extensive literature search, research purpose, population to be studied, methods of collecting data, and plan for analysis become integral parts of the proposals that are developed.

There are various strategies for analyzing historical data, such as the more common ones used in qualitative studies like content analysis, a grounded theory approach, or case analysis. Whatever method is chosen, the researcher should strive to present a careful and creative synthesis of the data.

How to Convince Others of the Method's Viability

In writing a history of the nursing service director over the last 100 years, Erickson[21] wrote

Knowledge of earlier practices, values, and orientations of hospital nursing directors and their influence on the role as it is today can contribute to a better understanding of the present situation

and a clearer picture of the future of nursing administration.

Yet review of nursing research by Brown, Tanner, and Padrick[22] verifies the widespread usage primarily of questionnaires and interviews. These authors point out that nurse researchers should use a wider variety of data sources including records and archives, and a broader array of methods. How then do we convince investigators, administrators, and others who control the purse strings in complex health-care organization of the relevance and usefulness of nursing history?

There are several steps that can be taken to plant the seed for the need to preserve our profession's history. It is important, first of all, to create a broad sense of awareness of the history of an agency, an association, a school of nursing, a nursing technique or program, and then to select groups in organizations who will be open minded and eager to encourage greater activity among others whose vision it is possible to broaden.

Consider, for example, approaching a head nurse and asking her to locate the records and minutes relating to the evolution of the unit—then presenting her analysis of the content of those records to the staff in a comprehensive fashion, with help from a nurse researcher, to improve understanding of practices in advanced technological societies.

Or, consider asking a group of nurse administrators to recall past management fads and trends that they have experienced such as management by objectives, motivational dynamics, or Japanese management[23] and present them in a systematic fashion outlining their successes and failures based on minutes from staff meetings.

Other activities worth considering would be to review historically various nursing practices as they have evolved over a number of decades.[24] The list of potential topics is endless. The most significant point is to sell the idea to a group who can see the value of learning from the past and who are willing to accept the responsibility for the preservation of information about their own world of work.

In these difficult economic times, it is obvious that management practice is often of a crisis nature. But has that always been the case? A historical review of past approaches could bring to light the management strategies and personnel development models of 10, 20, or even 50 years ago. Analyzing past management models as evolutionary processes, can give us a perspective of current problems by using comparative techniques. For example, we can examine the kinds of nursing units of today that did not exist years ago and ask ourselves what new technologies, or diseases, or socioeconomic conditions brought about the changes in contemporary institutional systems. How were the problems of yesteryear dealt with? Are the present methods of solving personnel problems, changing current practices, or deciding on management jurisdictions the result of planned objectives or happenstance, and are we underutilizing staff and monetary resources? Why were systems or models of the past changed? Were these changes reactive or planned and pro-active? Only historical analyses of past trends, values, and practices can provide us with the insight necessary to meet the considerable demands of the present.

How to Process Historic Research

Historical data must be processed in a fashion that follows the rigors of scientific research. Models of management can now be looked on as scientific, but past nursing management was no doubt developed intuitively and as the need arose. Professional issues and how they were dealt with in various epochs can be analyzed in a factual systematic manner and can solve problems, which to this point simply exist as raw, unanalyzed phenomena.

Hospitals and principles of practice, variability from one geographical area to another, and women willing to work for low pay and little recognition are all factors that must be taken into consideration while processing data for nursing administration. The end product of historical research is one that will be available for generations to come, and much to the interest of future nurses, historians, and archivists. Lynaugh and Reverby[25] have reiterated that "the historian has to make sense of the available evidence and relate it to larger generalities." As the authors speak of "the renaissance of historical scholarship in nursing," they also ask:

What do we really learn if we read about an organization's development unless we can relate it to larger human events and concerns? How can we understand nursing's difficulties if we don't also consider the cultural imperatives about womanhood and work, and how women either accommodated or changed them?

The ideas of younger nurses will be built on what is preserved from the past and how it is integrated into nursing's present body of knowledge. "As such, it is certain to attract the historical attention of a generation anxious to draw closer to the texture of human experience and to an understanding of the structures that help shape such experience."[26]

REFERENCES

1. Carr EH. What is history? Harmondsworth: Penguin Books, 1970, p. 19.
2. Kruman M. Historical method: implications for nursing research. In: Leininger M, ed. Qualitative research methods in nursing. Orlando: Grune & Stratton, Inc., 1985.
3. Davies C. ed: Rewriting nursing history. NJ: Barnes & Nobel Books, 1980, p. 14.
4. Friedricks R. A sociology of sociology. New York: Free Press, 1970, p. 177.
5. Lo Gerfo M. Three ways of reminiscence in theory and practice. International Journal of Aging and Human Development 1980–81;21(1):39–48.
6. Olson G. Campus cap talk: the oral historian, the law enforcement officer, and the "war in Isla Vista." In: The oral history review. Oral History Association, 10, 1982, p. 4–5.

7. Davies C. Rewriting nursing history, NJ: Barnes & Nobel Books.
8. Ibid., p. 200
9. Christy T. The methodology of historical research. Nurs Res 1975;24(3):189–192.
10. Nevitt J. White caps and black bands. Newfoundland: St. John's, 1978.
11. Keddy B, Acker K, Hemeon D, MacDonald D, MacIntyre A, Smith T, Vokey B. Nurses work world. Scientific or womanly ministering. Resources for Feminist Research 1987;16(4).
12. Davies C. Rewriting nursing history. NJ: Barnes & Nobel Books, p. 41.
13. Keddy B. Private duty nursing days of the 1920s and 1930s in Canada. Canadian Women Studies 1986;7(3):99–102.
14. Prentice A. Writing women into history: the history of women's work in Canada. Atlantis A Women's Studies Journal 1978;3(2):79.
15. The London feminist history group. The sexual dynamics of history. London: Pluto Press, 1983, p. 3.
16. Siverman E. Writing Canadian women's history, 1970–82: an historiographical analysis. Canadian Historical Review 1982;LXIII(4):533.
17. Davies C. Rewriting Nursing History, NJ: Barnes & Nobel Books, p. 13.
18. Wagner D. The proletarianization of nursing in the United States, 1932–1946. International Journal of Health Services 1980;10(2):271–291.
19. Sidel V, Sidel R. Reforming medicine lessons of the last quarter century. New York: Pantheon Books, 1984, p. 219.
20. Melesh B. Doctors, patients and "big nurse": work and gender in the postwar hospital. In: Lagemann E, (ed.) Nursing History New Perspectives New Possibility. New York: Teacher's College Press, 1983, p. 158–159.
21. Erickson, E. The nursing service director 1880–1980. The J of Nurs Adm 1980;X(4):6.
22. Brown J, Tanner C, Padrick K. Nursing's search for scientific knowledge. Nurs Res 1984;33(1):26–32.
23. Smith H, Reinow F, Ried R. Japanese Management Implications for Nursing Administration Journal of Nursing Administration 1984;14(9):33–39.
24. Keddy B, Lukan E. The nursing apprentice: an historical perspective. Nursing Papers 1985;17(1):35–46.
25. Lynaugh J, Reverby S. Thoughts on the nature of history. Nurs Res 1987;36(1):69.
26. Rosenberg C. Clio and caring: an agenda for American historians and nursing. Nurs Res 1987;36(1):68.

28

Case Study Methodology

Kathleen Smyth

MANY leaders in the field of nursing administration are talking about the need to develop a knowlege base unique to this specialty of nursing. Nursing is a practice discipline, hence, the dual mandate of knowledge development and utilization of knowledge in practice must be addressed.[1] Since the early 1970s, we have witnessed how nurse researchers have focused on the development of knowledge using a variety of modes of inquiry: the empirical scientific, philosophic, historic, and aesthetic, most predominantly. In their efforts to address the myriad questions needing investigation, nurse scientists have used multiple approaches and strategies. The focus of this chapter is one of the earliest methods used by nurses—the case study.

My purposes in this chapter are to define the case study as a method of research, to discuss its advantages and disadvantages, describe its use in other fields, and trace its use in nursing. An attempt is made to dispel some common myths regarding case study methodology, and suggestions are offered for future research.

DEFINITIONS

What Is the Case Study Method?

Isaac and Michael[2] have defined case method as an investigation of a social unit that emphasizes a complete organized picture. In using this method, the researcher undertakes a systematic investigation of the background, current status, environmental characteristics, and interactions of an individual, organization, or group.[3]

In nursing, case studies have been written about the life events of a single subject, a specific clinical problem, or selected experiences as they are lived in organizations and as they change over time.[4] The focus of case studies is in-depth determination of *why* a subject thinks, behaves, and develops in a particular manner, rather than *what* his or her status, progress, or actions actually are. Using the type of probing characteristic of case methodology requires collecting data over a period of time. It often involves not only the subject's present state but also past experiences, situational and environmental factors, and interactions of an individual or group within an organization or community. The intensive probing characteristic of case study methodology often leads to insights concerning previously unsuspected relationships, stimulates insights, and suggests hypotheses and directions for future research. Case studies serve to clarify concepts.

Distinguishing case studies from other research strategies, Yin offers the following comprehensive definition. According to Yin, a case study is an empirical inquiry which investigates (a) a contemporary phenomenon within its real-life context, (b) phenomena when the boundaries between phenomenon and context are not clearly evident, and (c) by using multiple sources of evidence.[4]

What the Case Study Method Is Not

Case study research has long been stereo-typed as a weak sibling among research methods because of its alleged lack of precision. However, the method continues to be used in traditional disciplines—in anthropology, psychology, political science, sociology, history, and economics. It has been adopted in many practice fields including medicine, education, and public administration. It is imperative that the case study, as a research method, be understood as distinct from case history, the case study as a teaching strategy, and ethnography.

How the Case Study Method Differs from Case History

Glaser and Strauss[5] distinguish between case history and case study. Case study method focuses on describing, verifying, and generating theory by using comparative analysis of multiple cases. Psychoanalytic theory, for example, is based for the most part on Freud's carefully documented case studies of psychiatric patients. A case history, by contrast, provides readable imagery, showing how a theory can be used to comprehend human experiences. The case study entitled *Anguish: A Case History of a Dying Trajectory* by Glaser and Strauss, is an example.[6]

The Case Study as a Teaching Strategy

Case studies, as teaching strategies, popularized in the fields of law, business, and public policy now are widely used in virtually every academic field. The main purpose of using a case in the classroom is to establish a framework for discussion and debate among students. Stevens in the text, *Educating the Nurse Manager*, describes the usefulness of the case study format for nursing education.[7] When using case studies for educational purposes, it is important to realize that not every teacher employs the actual case study nor reflects a complete or accurate account of actual events. In a "real case study," the uniqueness and variations presented by the central figure in the case are important factors. Many nurse instructors, however, use nursing cases to teach students about the care of a typical patient. The use of a case study in this way is a normative content lecture in disguise.[7] Hypothetical cases can be created, however, that do test important critical thinking skills essential for clinical and managerial situations.

How the Case Study Differs From Ethnography and Other Qualitative Research Methods

Although the case study method is commonly associated with ethnography, it is not a method of naturalistic inquiry exclusively using techniques of participant observation. The case study method, although descriptive by definition, may or may not require a qualitative format for data collection: case studies can employ experimental designs.[8–9] The case study is an approach that can be applied to a variety of problems and questions and, more importantly, it is one, as noted, that is not rigidly restricted by procedural considerations.

The case study method when selected does not imply the generation exclusively of one type of data[10–12] as is oftentimes the case when qualitative methods are used. Triangulation, use of more than one method or instrument to observe or measure the same phenomenon, can be used when doing a case study.[12–13] A combination of qualitative and quantitative data may be collected for an intensive case study.

The Unique Advantages of the Case Study

The case study methodology has several advantages. First, it permits the researcher to decide on the sources from which data will be acquired to a greater degree than do other methods. Second, using the case method the investigator specifies the amount and type of data that will be collected throughout much of the course of the study. And third, it permits flexibility to begin or terminate an investigation depending on the investigator's purposes.

"Case study," and "single case design," are terms used interchangeably. Single-case research is frequently reported in practice-based disciplines, for example, in medicine,[14–16] psychiatry and psychology,[17–21] social work,[22–23] education,[24–26] and administration.[27–28] Increasingly, researchers are recognizing the importance of single-case investigations for the development and expansion of knowledge. It should also be noted that important methodological and conceptual advances have occurred with respect to this method over the past few years, in part because of The Case Study Institute, Inc. (now COSMOS), established in Washington, D.C., under the leadership of Robert Yin.

Additional advantages of the case study methodology include the following. First, case study research provides an important knowledge base that is unattainable through large between-group experimental designs. Second, case study research as a methodology is not limited to the study of a single client. It is uniquely suited to the evaluation of organizational processes involving large numbers of people. Third, case study research provides an important alternative to traditional large sample experimental designs particularly where objections of withholding treatment from clients in the "no treatment" control groups is problematic.[29] In case study research, treatment can be implemented, and data can be collected and analyzed immediately. Fourth, case study and single-case research designs promote the development of measurement technologies that can be used repeatedly over the period of study. For example, direct observation, rating scales, and self-monitoring reports can be used as repeated measures throughout a case study. Repeated measurements, when obtained by a single case or multiple cases, allow for in-depth analysis of variability and covariation over time.[4]

TYPES OF CASE STUDY INVESTIGATIONS

Kratochwill[30] described several different types of case study investigations that have been used in psychology and can be applied to nursing research. The typology of cases is depicted in Table 28.1 and the three types and characteristics of case studies are described in the following sections.

Nontherapeutic Case Study

Nontherapeutic case studies generate descriptive or biographical information. Dougherty's study entitled *Becoming a Woman in a Rural Black Community*, is an example of a nontherapeutic descriptive case study.[31] Through observations and interviews, Dougherty, a nurse anthropologist, describes the

TABLE 28.1   Types and Characteristics of Case Study Investigations

Type	Characteristics

Nontherapeutic case study
  descriptive-uncontrolled
  biography-autobiography
	Researcher is interested in nonclinical investigation. Such areas as anthropology, education, and psychology are examples, (including traditional biographies).

Assessment-diagnosis case study descriptive case	Researcher employs various theories, psychometric instruments for diagnosis or description of cognitive or social behavior.

Therapeutic-intervention case study
  uncontrolled
  pre-experimental
  clinical replication
	Researcher is primarily interested in a clinical disorder-treatment and can either describe the natural course of case disorder or design an intervention to treat client's problem.

social organization and cultural forces in a rural community. As a nontherapeutic case, this study provides in-depth knowledge of the rites of passage of a black female adolescent during pregnancy, childbirth, and motherhood.

Assessment-Diagnosis Case Study

Sociologists, psychologists, and educators often use assessment case studies to deepen understanding of learning problems. Case studies of this type have important implications for diagnosis and intervention. By employing various psychometric techniques and procedures, an assessment profile is developed of various areas of functioning.

Assessment case studies are also intended to provide an example of the application of theory. Parse, a nurse educator, explored the question of how retirement changed the way couples talked to each other. In this assessment case study, the meaning of retirement to participants was analyzed using a phenomenological theory developed by the researcher.[3]

Therapeutic-Intervention Case Study

A number of case studies have been done in nursing to develop a comprehensive picture of the variables directly related to clients' history, care, or treatment. Nurses in the clinical setting are confronted daily with unique client situations that warrant in-depth analysis of the experiences of patients. Case studies in nursing that are therapeutic intervention studies include, first, the investigation entitled *Open Heart Surgery on Children: A Study in Nursing Care* by Blake.[32] In this study, the researcher describes in detail the nursing care of a four-year-old child before and after open heart surgery. The case portrays the ways in which the child and her parents react and deal with hospitalization, nursing care, and medical treatment. Using

Erickson's theoretical framework, Blake selects themes from her observational recordings to describe preoperative and postoperative nursing care. She describes ways her hypotheses might be tested with other sick children. Throughout the case study, Blake shows how to systematically develop and test the validity of hypotheses generated in descriptive cases.

White, a nurse sociologist, in an intervention case study of an Appalachian family, describes family conflict.[33] After collecting observational data for eighteen months, White reported on how a family managed their conflict. Using Dahrendorf's conflict theory, she describes the pattern of change in family relationships and her nursing interventions to assist the family.

Baltes and Zerbe's study titled *Reestablishing Self-Feeding in a Nursing Home Resident*, is an example of a therapeutic case study.[34] These researchers hypothesized that a change in environmental conditions would result in a change in the subject's self-feeding behaviors. They designed their study to include a base-line assessment and treatment plan using continuous reinforcement to initiate and maintain self-feeding behaviors. The protocol included a treatment package employing skills based on a Skinner's operant behavior model. When an intervention is being demonstrated or assessed, it is useful to collect data over an extended time period and, when possible, to subdivide the time frame into base-line, treatment, reversal, and reinstitution phases.[4]

Another example of an intervention case study is one done by Martinson[35], who studied 66 families, case by case, over a period of six years, to investigate the feasibility and desirability of home care for dying children. Resio and Verhonick[36] used the case study design to analyze the characteristics of patients who had developed decubitus ulcers. Durand[37] described the impact of an intensive care program on a five-year-old boy with

Down syndrome. Other investigators have used the case study design to examine health from a cross-cultural perspective.[38]

By far the most common type of case studies are those developed in the clinical fields of medicine, psychology, and psychiatry to evaluate the effectiveness of various treatment modalities. In case studies, classical experimental and statistical controls are often absent. Consequently, the data that are generated must be interpreted with considerable rigor. Single-case studies are generally pre-experimental. Threats to validity are a problem for investigators using intervention case-study methodology.[4] To reduce the threats to validity, well-controlled experimental time-series designs are recommended.

NURSING ADMINISTRATION RESEARCH

Case studies, because they examine many factors related to a single organization, or to a number of groups, are useful in nursing administration research. The case method is appropriate when the goal is: to provide insight into organizational problems that deserve extensive analysis, to gain background information, to design a major subsequent experiment, and to illustrate, by specific in-depth examples, more generalizable statistical findings.[30]

The case study design uses a full range of data sources, including interviews, observation, records, and documents. Information about an organization can be collected both retrospectively from historical documents, and concurrently, for example, by studying the activities of administrators in an organization over a period of weeks, months, or years. Poulin's study of nurse executives is an example of this.[39]

Case studies are potentially appropriate for two types of problems: the study of emergent unique organizations, and the study of organizational processes. Kaluzny's and Veney's study is an example of the latter.[40] These investigators assessed informal social control in a medical group practice setting and studied the way control influenced physician performance. Through analysis of taped interviews with primary care physicians, categories of control behavior were devised and behaviors were analyzed to identify patterns of control.

Wilson's study,[41] entitled "Deinstitutionalized residential care for the mentally disabled: the Soteria House approach," is an example of a therapeutic case study. It illustrates how a researcher can use this type of design to study a community based residential care facility for diagnosed schizophrenic young adults.

The most challenging aspect of organization research is the study of organizational process. The study of processes in organizations requires longitudinal assessment of phenomena about which there is little understanding. The case study is the ideal design for these investigations. It provides the mechanism for following activities in an organization through time and for developing a detailed accounting of events. Two examples of studies that focus on the longitudinal assessment of organizational activities are the studies done of the management functions by Mintzberg[42] and the study of innovation by Milio.[43]

In Mintzberg's[42] comparative case study of five managers, there was sufficient consistency in the observational data to develop basic propositions characterizing managerial work activities and suggest a taxonomy. Milio's[43] four-year study illustrated the innovative process in which a neighborhood health-center project was successfully merged with a large community nursing agency in a metropolitan area. As the organization progressed through five stages, different strategies were employed by personnel for locating resources to support innovations.

DISPELLING THE MYTHS ABOUT CASE STUDY METHOD

In analyzing the criticism of case study methodology, one finds that the major disadvantage is the lack of rigor and control in the method and the consequent limited generalizability of findings. Critics have also raised questions about the time and money case studies require for the quality of information obtained. On the positive side, however, there are several myths about case study research that should be dispelled.

Myth 1: Case Study Method is Soft and Subject to Ambiguity and Bias

Using a case study to substantiate a preconceived position *will* result in a biased study. Lack of bias can be achieved if the investigator is open to contrary findings, which are then reflected in the study's conclusions. To further reduce bias, Yin advocates reporting preliminary findings during the data-collection phase, to two or three critics who are capable of offering alternative explanations and suggestions.[4]

There are specific steps in using the case study method that are somewhat different from the outline of a classical experimental-design.

1. Describe the objectives and purposes for conducting the study in behavioral terms.
2. Identify the unit of study as the individual, family, group, community, or organization.
3. List the characteristics, relationships, and processes that will be focused on in the investigation.
4. Review the literature.
5. Specify how the subject or unit of study will be selected.
6. Identify potential data sources.
7. Describe the data-collection plan and methods.
8. Outline a tentative scheme for organiz-ing the findings into a coherent, well-integrated description of the unit of study.
9. Project a plan for reporting results.
10. Suggest directions for future research based on findings.
11. Anticipate hypotheses for further study generated from the case study.

Examining these steps, one becomes aware of the approach employed in case studies. Hypotheses are generated from the findings, not formulated as part of the design.

Myth 2: A Case Study is Easy To Do

A case study is *not* an easy method. The demands of case study methodology on a person—intellectually, physically, and emotionally—may be far greater than that of any other research strategy.[4] For case studies, data-collection procedures are not routinized and data-collection activities are oftentimes more demanding than when one uses experimental and survey methods. Moreover, previous research experience is needed if the theoretical issues being studied and the data being collected are to be free from bias. It is not an undertaking for a novice.

To be successful in doing case study research, the investigator must be a good listener, able to answer questions, and capable of maintaining objectivity and flexibility throughout the study. Being a good listener involves two skills: observing and sensing any important covert messages, and assimilating large amounts of new information without bias. An investigator who is a good listener captures the mood and affective aspects of participants' reports of incidents, and is not blinded by his or her own ideologies and preconceptions.

Myth 3: The Case Study Method Can Be Mastered Without Difficulty

A prerequisite for undertaking case study research is to have an inquiring mind. When doing case studies the phases of data collection are not discrete. Posing questions for oneself, about why an event appears to have happened or is happening, is difficult but critical during all phases. There is a need too to balance adaptiveness with rigor, but to avoid rigidity. Few case studies end exactly as planned. If a major shift in direction is made, either because there is a need to pursue an unexpected lead, or because a new "case" emerges in the course of the study, a revised design needs to be formulated.[4]

Researchers who use case study methodology must have a clear understanding of the issues involved. Careful conceptualization enables the experienced investigator to focus on relevant events and structure information into manageable units of analysis. Data collection in a case study is not the mere recording of data. It involves interpreting the data as they are collected: ongoing interpretation is essential for making inferences about what actually is transpiring, particularly if sources of information contradict one another or if there is need to further validate interpretations.

Myth 4: The Case Method Has No Design or Protocol

The difficult part of case studies is developing the research design. Traditionally, case study research has been considered "soft," but paradoxically, the softer a research technique the harder it is to do.[4] Five components of a case study design, as with research using quantitative methods, are especially important: the study's question, its propositions, its unit of analysis, the logical linking of the data to propositions, and criteria for interpreting findings.

The heart of a protocol for a case study is a set of substantive questions reflecting the actual inquiry.[4] A case study protocol is a major technique for increasing the reliability of case study research. A carefully developed protocol reminds the investigator of what is being studied and provides guidelines for carrying out the case study. According to Yin,[4] the protocol should provide an overview of the case study including the study objectives, auspices, study issues, and relevant readings. Second, it should specify field procedures, the credentials of investigators, and the methods for gaining access to study sites. Third, the protocol should clearly state the specific questions the investigator will keep in mind when collecting data. Fourth, the protocol should provide a guide for the case study report.

The findings from case study research are limited in their generalizability. Is generalization a goal of all research? Clinical methodologists do not believe it is.[44–46] In survey research, a large sample may strengthen external validity, but it does not extend the range of generalizations beyond the parameters of the initial population. Since case study methodology oftentimes deals with an *N* of one, it differs from large-group surveys with respect to external validity—the inference of results to a larger population of subjects. Randomization of a selected sample of cases is difficult to achieve, but cross analysis of cases is possible.

ISSUES OF RELIABILITY AND VALIDITY

Case studies have unique problems with respect to reliability. It is often difficult to know whether the explanation derived from a study accounts for what is going on in the situation, and is in fact the correct explanation, or whether there are alternative explanations using other approaches.

Internal validity refers to the plausibility of a statement relating the variables of interest. In naturalistic settings, it refers to the believability of explanations about a phenomenon. No matter what type of research methodology is selected to answer an investigator's question, he or she must control or eliminate the effects of extraneous variables or provide alternative explanations.

Issue of Reliability

A major strategy employed to increase reliability of case study research is the protocol—a set of substantive questions reflecting the actual inquiry.[4] The questions are posed to the investigator and provide a structure for the investigation. Potential sources of information for answering each question are also identified. Miles and Huberman[47] describe how an investigator can develop an outline of specific sources of data that can be displayed in tabular form—a form they refer to as a "table shell."

Replication of single-subject research should also be attempted.[48] In replication studies, the setting should remain as constant as possible, and the protocol should be consistent across subjects.

Issue of Valid Inference

Even in well-controlled experimental research, threats to internal validity exist. The issue of valid inference is a critical one when using the case study method. Kazdin[10] addresses the varying dimensions that need to be considered when planning a case study, to strengthen interpretations of the data collected and to reduce threats to internal validity. The dimensions of a case study that need to be assessed include the design, type and collection of data, the number and type of subjects, and the study problem. Each of these dimensions are depicted in Table 28.2. The characteristics of each dimension for high and low levels of inference are discussed in the following section.

With respect to design, the first characteristic (if an organizational strategy or clinical intervention) is the independent variable, and if it is not directly manipulated the study design is known as ex post facto. Because the control over the independent variable is relatively low, the inferences one can draw are also low. In contrast, where the independent variable is controlled, the research is preplanned and the degree of inference is higher.[47–49]

Variation exists in the type of data that are collected for case studies, from self-reported or subjective impressions of events to formal objective data. For example, repeated time series interviews that are audiotaped and accompanied by objective rating scales or check lists, yield higher levels of inference than do subjective descriptions alone.

TABLE 28.2   Improving Internal Validity of Case Studies

Characteristics	Low Inference	High Inference
Design	Ex post facto	Planned
Type of data	Subjective	Objective
Data collection	Single measurement	Repeated measurement
Subjects		
Number	$N = 1$	$N > 1$
Type	Homogeneous	Heterogeneous
Problem	Acute	Chronic
Protocol	Nonstandardized	Standardized
Effect	No monitoring	Repeated monitoring
Integrity		
Impact	Single measure	Multiple measures
Follow-up	No formal measure	Formal measures assessment
Assessment		
Generalization		

Adapted from Kazdin AE. Drawing valid inferences from case studies. J Cons Clinic Psych 1981; 49:183–192.

Hersen and Barlow[8] note that in the conduct of a case study, continuous assessment measurement is desirable. These authors suggest that researchers choose measures that can provide repeated measurement throughout the study. Where a single measurement alone is used, inference is low.

Most case studies involve only one subject, but replicating a study using a number of subjects is desirable where the goal is to increase the validity of the study findings. A greater degree of inference can be drawn from data that show evidence of successful effects across several cases over time. The researcher can diminish threats to internal validity when a study addresses a problem occurring over time by using the case method repeatedly to assess subjects with diverse racial, social, or age characteristics.

Johnson and Pennypacker[49] advocate planning some type of monitoring to assess the accuracy and integrity of the independent variable throughout a study. This monitoring can be done by a periodic review of the standardized protocol or by engaging multiple observers to check adherence to the protocol.

Holm[50] describes how statistical procedures can be employed in an experimental case study of a single subject to increase validity. In Holm's study, the phases of base line, intervention, and reversal, for patients with hypertension, are analyzed in a single-subject experiment with diet as a treatment.

Credibility of the effect reported in case studies can be enhanced by using multiple measures to gather data on the variables of interest. A design for the development of cross-case analysis where data from several cases are collected and analyzed, is depicted in Figure 28.1.

WRITING THE FINAL REPORT OF A CASE STUDY

Grouping data, whether quantitative or qualitative, with respect to each of the questions in the protocol, facilitates the integration of evidence in the final report. Interview segments from different respondents, but on the same topic can also be clustered to enhance the analysis. One pitfall to avoid is spending too much time on note taking—on polishing subjects' narrative responses during data collection—instead of staying focused on the central questions in the protocol.

The problem of excessive field notes were surmounted in an organizational study entitled, *National Commission on Neighborhoods*,[51] which produced over 40 case studies of community organizations. The technique used in organizing data to write the final report involved formulating 60 open-ended questions, then responding to each question in short paragraphs using the evidence collected.

Case Study Research in Nursing Administration: State of the Art

One of the advantages of the case study is that it permits an investigator to understand the wholeness of complex phenomena by focusing, for example, on intergroup relationships and managerial processes. Moustafa[52] analyzed the contents of four leading nursing research journals over a five-year period between 1977 and 1981. The journals were *Nursing Research, Heart and Lung, Research in Nursing and Health,* and *Western Journal of Nursing Research.* Eighteen (or 4%) of the publications were classified as management studies. In examining the methodologies employed in these studies, not one of the management studies reported using case study methodology.

In a review I did recently of articles in the *Journal of Nursing Administration* (JONA) for 1975 to 1985, only one study was reported as a case study; it was entitled "Developing Criterion Measures of Nursing Care: Case Study of a Process" by Clinton, Renyes, and Goodwin.[53] Clinton and associates describe the process a team of nurse researchers ex-

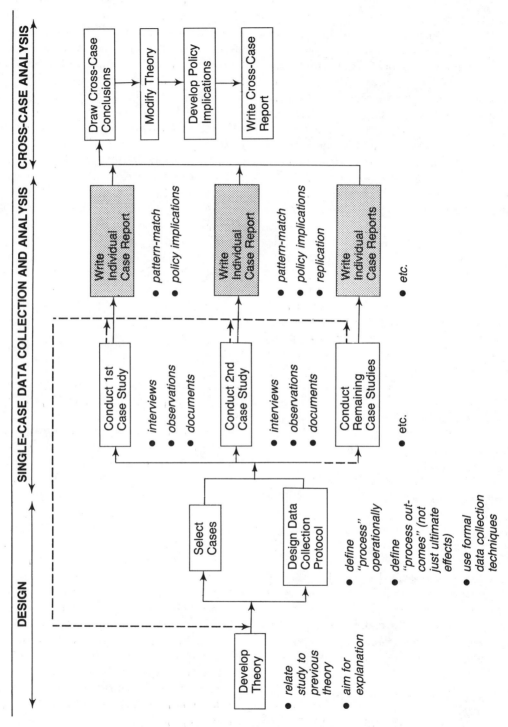

Figure 28.1 Design for Cross-Case Analysis. From Yin RK. Case study research: design and methods. Applied social research series, Vol 5. Beverly Hills: SAGE Publications, Inc., 1984, p. 51.

perienced in designing an instrument to measure nursing care. Although the unit of analysis and protocol questions are not described in the article, the study is a narrative of the events encountered by the team.

Using Kratochwill typology of case study methods, in JONA there are, however, a number of single-example cases that can be classified as descriptive case studies. The focus of these studies is often related to patient classification, cost containment measures, personnel development, and the function of nurse administrators.

Cross-Case Analyses: A Strategy for Theory Building

According to Lijphart,[54] case studies can be classified on the basis of purpose or function: in the history of science, theory testing and analyses of deviant cases have helped to explain, strengthen, or weaken existing theories. Cross-case analysis as a strategy to build theory is a worthy undertaking for future nurse researchers.

Nursing administration as a specialty of nursing is in need of theory. In examining existing studies, one finds few high-inference case studies. Can we consider undertaking multiple case studies, at various sites, and doing cross-case analysis?

An example of cross-case analysis in the care of children is Coty's study.[55] This investigator developed and tested a category system of coping behaviors that were manifested by hospitalized children. Using Lazarus's theoretical framework of coping, Coty analyzed 39 case studies of hospitalized children published in the *Maternal Child Nursing Journal* between 1972 and 1982. And Fry,[56] a nurse educator, undertook a cross-case analysis of recent court decisions in medical ethics cases, involving privacy related to contraception, procreation, abortion, and refusal of treatment. In analyzing the courts' decisions, Fry extrapolated themes from multiple cases.

When little is known about a phenomena, cross analysis of in-depth case studies can generate and test basic theory. Research that generates theory is desperately needed in nursing administration. Fawcett believes that research is neither more nor less than a vehicle for theory development.[57] Figure 28.1 graphically depicts how cross-case analysis contributes to the development of theory.

Linking Practice, Research, and Theory Building

Case study findings are an important source of hypotheses for future research. Moreover, case studies provide a way to keep research consistent with practice. By their reports, researchers assist practitioners to improve practice.

A major concern for researchers and practitioners is the generalizability of research findings to problems in the workplace. The researcher's concern for generalization and the practitioner's concern for applicability and effectiveness can be addressed through replication studies. Through replication, an intervention or innovation demonstrated to be internally valid in a particular study is given a further test of external validity in practice. Replication provides a feedback loop to researchers and practitioners showing how to improve on an intervention or innovation by adding necessary components or eliminating ineffective ones, "taking them back to the beginning point of research with a new research hypothesis."[58]

Just as conceptual models guide the construction and implementation of nursing education programs, conceptual systems of nursing administration can serve as guides in planning organizational structures in healthcare agencies. Conceptual models can provide criteria for standards of nursing practice, quality assurance, and nursing audit programs. For example, a case study of the process and outcomes of nursing practice and quality assurance measures, and the relationship of each to a department's philosophy could be linked together to form a conceptual framework of accountability.

Past to Future: Where Do We Go from Here?

Over a decade ago, Lindeman,[59] in a nationwide survey, identified 15 important areas for nursing research. Five of these are directly related to nursing administration: (1) determination of valid and reliable indicators of quality nursing care; (2) determination of valid and reliable methods for establishing nurse staffing; (3) assessment of the relationship between the quality of nursing leadership and the quality of nursing practice in institutions; (4) evaluation of the effectiveness of various approaches to peer review; and (5) determination of effective means of communicating, evaluating, and implementing changes in practice.

In a more recent survey, Henry and associates[60] reported on the judgments of experts in nursing administration as to research priorities. When asked to list and prioritize researchable questions for nursing administration, two themes were uppermost—cost and quality of care. In soliciting ideas about nursing administration research, the respondents stressed that investigations for the field be theory driven and theory generating.

The National Commission on Nursing formulated action plans in view of the forecasted rapid changes and developments in health care. One of the immediate goals highlighted by the Commission, for administrators and trustees is to examine organizational structures to ensure that nurse administrators are part of policy-making bodies in institutions. Case studies are needed that provide in-depth examinations of nurse executives' contributions to short- and long-term policy and operational changes in the workplace.

Stevens[7] believes that nursing practice is largely controlled by nurse administrators. Management, leadership, and nursing theories are commonly explored in educational programs for nursing administration. Case studies designed to focus on several nursing departments that are implementing a specific nursing theory could be undertaken to show how the outcome of nursing practice is changed.

Examining data from each single case and doing cross-case analyses will yield higher validity than where designs are limited to single subjects. In the 1980s, two overriding factors are affecting the delivery of health care, namely, administrative and clinical technology. Included in administrative technology are computerized staffing, productivity monitoring, and management systems. An in-depth analysis using case study methodology of how these technologies affect leaders, administrators, head nurses, and staff nurses would be useful. Investigation of ways to maximize the use of technological resources to transform nursing situations might be undertaken through a study of how head nurses relate computer technology to their patient populations. In an investigation, the researcher—through observation and interview—would analyze the relationship of changing technologies and patient populations.

Another area that could benefit from case study research is related to agencies supplying temporary nurses to hospitals. How has this arrangement, from the perspective of the nurse administrator, agency nurse, and staff nurse employee, affected the quality of care, cost of care, staff morale, and level of satisfaction?

External consultation services to nurse administrators are used to provide information on management techniques and offer guidelines for change. Case studies addressing how these services have changed management practices at the individual and departmental levels, in single and multiple institutions, are also worth undertaking.

Awareness of ethical decision making in management has been heightened in the 1980s. Nursing has been involved in meeting urgent demands for intensive care of clients. Staffing decisions have caused personal and professional conflicts about the equitable distribution of scarce resources. A planned case study of head nurses to examine the ethical and moral dimensions of their leadership role would delineate value priorities. A case study could document the scope of ethical conflicts. Issues of an interdisciplinary nature might emerge that would be hypothesis generating.

If single case studies were done in several hospitals on acuity levels, cross-case analysis could yield important findings with implications for planned changes in nursing services. Subsequent studies on strategies of change in nursing practice and acuity levels would provide direction for the development of a future theory of nursing administration, which in turn could be tested through intentionally replicated case studies in these same institutions.

Nurse Administrator's Commitment to the Advancement of Nursing Science

Parse and associates[62], in reflecting on the value of commitment to the advancement of nursing science wrote, "It is through the process of creative conceptualization, a tolerance for ambiguity, and watchful diligence that the growing edge of the field of nursing will be cultivated. The hope of the future of nursing rests with those who choose to cultivate the growing edge, which is the interface of what is and what is not yet." These statements have relevance for the research endeavors of nurse administrators.

Do nurse administrators believe case studies are appropriate for exploratory investigations? Do they view research methods in a hierarchic order? Do they think descriptive studies are the least valuable, and that experimental designs are the only answer for causal and exploratory questions?

The appropriateness of a hierarchic attitude is questionable when we examine the methodologies used by scientists in other disciplines. Historians, for example, undertake historiography for causal explanations of phenomenon. Yin[4] proposes a pluralistic view of research methodology as opposed to a hierarchic one. He advocates combining multiple methods in one design depending on the types of questions posed, the extent of control required, and the focus of an investigation.

In the 1930s, the case study was recognized as a worthwhile approach to systematic analysis of the problems of nursing. One hears relatively little about the value of case studies today., According to Hodgman,[63] the case study has been devalued over time in both research and education. Perhaps this occurred because of the deficits in analytical and documentation skills we observe today. Soundly conceived and well-developed case studies *are needed* for the future of nursing administration science.

REFERENCES

1. Donaldson S, Crowley D. The discipline of nursing. Nurs Outlook 1978;26:113–144.
2. Isaac S, Michael W. Handbook in research and evaluation. San Diego, CA: Edits, 1981.
3. Parse RS, Coyne B, Smith MJ. Nursing research qualitative methods, Bowie, MD: Brady Communication, 1985, pp. 95–104.
4. Yin RK. Case study research: design and methods, Beverly Hills, CA: Sage, 1984.
5. Glaser GB, Strauss AL. The discovery of grounded theory: strategies for qualitative research. 3rd ed. Chicago, IL: Aldine, 1970.
6. Glaser GB, Strauss AL. Anguish: a case history of a dying trajectory. Mill Valley, CA: Sociology Press, 1970.
7. Stevens B. Educating the nurse manager: case studies and group work, MD: Aspen Systems, 1982.
8. Hersen M, Barlow DH. Single-case experimental designs: strategies for studying behavior change. New York: Pergamon Press, 1976.

9. Kratochwill TR. Single subject research strategies for evaluating change. New York: Academic Press, 1978.
10. Kazdin AE. Drawing valid inferences from case studies. J Cons and Clinic Psych 1981;49:183–192.
11. Yin RK. The case study crisis: some answers. Adm Sc Quart 1981;26:58–65.
12. Runyan WM. In defense of the case study method. Am J Orthopsychiatry 1982;52:440–446.
13. Brewer MB, Collins BE. Perspectives on knowing: six themes from Donald T. Campbell. In: Brewer MB, Collins BE, eds. Scientific inquiry and the social sciences. San Francisco: Jossey-Bass, 1981, pp. 1–9.
14. Jick TD. Mixing qualitative and quantitative methods: trangulation in action. Adm Sc Quart 1979;24:602–611.
15. De Bakey L, De Bakey J. The case report: guidelines for preparation. International Journal of Cardiology 1982;4:357–364.
16. Shapiro MB. The single case in fundamental clinical psychological research. Br J Med Psych 1961;34:255–262.
17. Bolgar H. The case study method. In: Wolman, B, ed. Handbook of clinical psychology. New York: McGraw Hill, 1969, p. 28–39.
18. Barlow DH. Behavior therapy: the next decade. Behavior Therapy 1980;11:315–328.
19. Dukes W. N = 1. Psych Bull 1965;64:74–79.
20. Hayes SC. Single case experimental design and empirical clinical practice. J Consult Clin Psychol 1981;49:1932-211.
21. Kazdin A. Methodological and interpretive problems of single case experimental designs. J Consult and Clinic Psych 1978;49:183–192.
22. Levy RD, Olson DG. The single subject methodology in clinical practice: an overview. J Soc Serv Res 1979;3:25–49.
23. Thomas EJ. Research and service in single case experimentation: conflicts and choices. Soc Work Res and Abs 1978;14:20–31.
24. Shulman LS. Disciplines of inquiry in education: an overview. Ed Res 1981;10:5–12.
25. Smith LM. An evolving logic of participant observation, educational ethnography and other case studies. Rev of Res Ed 1979;6:316–377.
26. Stake RE. The case study method in social inquiry. Educ Res 1978;7:5–8.
27. Mintzberg H. An emerging strategy of "direct" research. Admin Sci Q 1979;24:582–589.
28. Yin RK. The case study crisis: some answers. Adm Sci Quart 1981;20:58–65.
29. Hersen, Barlow, 1976 (same as ref. 8).
30. Kratochwill TR. Time series research: contributions to empirical clinical practice. Behavior Assessment 1983;5:165–176.
31. Dougherty M. Becoming a woman in a rural black community. New York: Holt, Rinehart and Winston, 1978.
32. Blake F. Open heart surgery on children: a study innursing care. Washington, DC. Public Health Ser-

vice Publication No. 2075. U.S. Government Printing Office, 1964.
33. White M. Illness in an Appalachian family: a study of conflict management. In: Riffle, K, ed. Rehabilitative nursing case studies. New York: Medical Examination Co, pp. 96–100.
34. Baltes MM, Zerbe MB. Reestablishing self-feeding in a nursing home resident. Nurs Res 1976;25:24–26.
35. Martinson I. Home care for the dying child: professional and family perspectives. New York: Appleton-Century-Crofts, 1976.
36. Resio, Verhonick. Nursing research. Boston: Little, Brown, 1975.
37. Durand B. Failure to thrive in a child with Down's syndrome. Nurs Res 1975;24:272–286.
38. Leninger M. Barrers and facilitators to quality health care. Philadelphia: FA Davis, 1975.
39. Poulin MA. The nurse executive role. J of Nurs Adm 1984;2:9–14.
40. Kaluzny, Veney. Health service organizations. Berkeley, CA: McCutchan, 1980.
41. Wilson HS. Deinstitutionalized residential care for the mentally disordered: the Soteria House approach. New York, Grune & Stratton, 1982.
42. Mintzberg H. The nature of managerial work. New York: Harper & Row, 1973.
43. Milio N. Health care organizations. J Health & Soc Beh 1971;12,2:163–73.
44. Kennedy MM. Generalizing from single case studies. Eval Quar 1979;3:661–678.
45. Meir P, Pugh E. The case study: a viable approach to clinical research. Res Nurs Health 1986;9:195–202.
46. Starke RE. The case study method in social inquiry. Educ Res 1978;7:5–8.
47. Miles MB, Huberman AM. Analyzing qualitative data: a source book for new methods. Beverly Hills, CA: Sage, 1984.
48. Kratochwill TR. Time Series research: contributions to empirical clinical practice. Behavior Assessment 1983;5:165–176.
49. Johnson J, Pennypacker H. Strategies and tactics of human behavioral research. Hillsdale, NJ.: Eribaum, 1980.
50. Holm K. Single subject research. Nurs Res 1983;32:253–255.
51. National Commission on Neighborhoods. People building neighborhoods. Washington, DC. US Government Printing Office, 1979.
52. Moustafa N. Nursing research from 1977 to 1981. W J Nurs Res 1985;7(3):349–356.
53. Clinton J, Denyes M, Goodwin J. Developing criterion measures of nursing care: case study of a process. J of Nurs Adm 1977;7:41–45.
54. Lijphart A. The comparable cases strategy in comparative research. Comp Pol Stu 1975;8:158–177.
55. Coty S. Coping in hospitalized children: an analysis of published case studies, Nurs Res 1984;33(5):277–282.
56. Fry ST. Protecting privacy: judicial decision makingin search of a principle. Dissertation Abstracts International, 1986;46:10:3055A.

57. Fawcett J, Downs F. The relationship of theory and research. CN: Appleton-Century-Crofts, 1986.

58. Bellack A, Hersen M, (eds): Research methods in clinical psychology. New York: Pergamon Press, 1984 p. 74.

59. Lindeman CA. Delphi survey of priorities in clinical nursing research. Nurs Res 1975;24(6):434–441.

60. Henry B, Moody L, Pendergast J, O'Donnell J, Hutchinson S, Scully G. Delineating nursing administration research priorities. Nurs Res 1987, 309–314.

61. National Commission on Nursing. Summary report and recommendations. Chicago: The Hospital Research and Educational Trust, 1985.

62. Parse RR, Cayne AB, Smith MJ. The experience of aging: an ethnographic study. In: Parse RR, Cayne AB, Smith MJ, (eds) Nursing research: qualitative methods. Bowie, MD: Brady Communications Company, 1985.

63. Hodgman E. The Clinical nurse specialist as researcher. In: Hamric A, ed. The clinical nurse specialist in theory and practice. New York: Grune & Stratton, 1983, p. 76.

29

Some Approaches to the Analysis of Repeated Measurement Data

Jane Pendergast

THE INVESTIGATION of many research problems requires multiple measurements to be taken on each individual or animal—called an "experiment unit"—under investigation. These could be different measurements, such as various biological measurements, or responses to different questions on a questionnaire, or even the same measurement taken at different points in time or under various conditions. If different types of measurements have been collected and it is of interest to treat the set of responses as an outcome measurement (instead of analyzing each response separately), it is necessary to use a multivariate statistical technique—such as multivariate analysis of variance (MANOVA), factor analysis, cluster analysis, or canonical correlation analysis, to name a few. On the other hand, if multiple measurements have been made on the same variable, one might be able to use either a multivariate or univariate statistical technique, depending on the purpose of the analysis and on the assumptions that the researcher is willing to make regarding the underlying joint distribution of these measures.

The statistical procedures discussed in this chapter are limited to those applicable to "repeated measurement data," a term generally reserved for data measuring the same variable at several time points or under various conditions for each experimental unit. In these analyses, what is of interest is detecting or modeling changes over time or condition. It could also be applicable to determine if such patterns of change vary for different groups of subjects. For information on statistical techniques applicable to other types of multivariate data or for techniques intended to answer other types of questions, the interested reader is referred to texts such as those by Afifi and Clark[1], Harris[2], or for more mathematically oriented readers, Anderson[3] or Morrison.[4]

WHAT MAKES REPEATED MEASUREMENTS SPECIAL?

One might ask the question, "Why is it necessary to distinguish between repeated measurement data and data collected on different subjects at each time point?" The answer lies in the statistical concepts of independent and correlated data. If two variables are correlated, they tend to vary together. If the value of one is increased, the other will tend to increase (positive correlation) or decrease (negative correlation). On the other hand, if they are independent, a change in one of them implies nothing about a corresponding change in the other. In fact, by definition, independence implies no correlation.

At the heart of most statistical analyses and critical to the validity of resulting interpretations, is the assumption of a random sample, which implies independence of the sampled experimental units from some population of interest. In analyses of repeated measurement data, we assume the experimental units (e.g., patients in a medical study) are randomly sampled, and thus independent. However, the multiple (repeated) measurements taken on each experimental unit (e.g., measurements taken over time on a patient) will tend to be correlated, and thus cannot be assumed to be independent. For example, suppose a study was designed to examine the effect of one dose of a given drug on the blood pressure measurements of nonhypertensive patients over a fixed period of time. If an individual entered into the study with a base-line blood pressure on the high end of normal, we might expect that individual to have one of the higher blood pressures at the next time point as well, that is, we would expect a positive correlation between the blood pressures at the first two time points. Since the difference between two positively correlated random variables will have a smaller variance than that of two independent variables, it is important to acknowledge the correlation structure of the data when performing statistical analyses. Another way of stating this is that if we assume a positive correlation among the repeated measurement variables, we would expect the within-subject variability to be less than that between subjects.

CLASSIFYING VARIABLES USING STEVENS'S CLASSIFICATION SYSTEM

Before choosing a statistical technique to analyze repeated measurement data, it is important to identify the scale of measurement employed for each of the variables. One popular classification system is that proposed by Stevens,[5] in which variables are classified as "nominal," "ordinal," "interval," or "ratio."

Nominal variables have values that are not intrinsically ordered in any way, such as race.

Ordinal variables have levels that are intrinsically ordered, but the magnitude of the difference between one level and the next cannot be measured, and the difference is not necessarily considered to be uniform for each successive pair of levels. For example, a three-point scale of "mild," "moderate," and "severe" would be considered ordinal, without an assumption that the difference between "mild" and "moderate" is of the same magnitude as that between "moderate" and "severe." Sometimes nominal and ordinal variables are lumped together and called "categorical" or "discrete" variables.

An interval-valued variable also has a natural ordering, but the magnitude of the difference between any two successive values is a meaningful quantity, measuring the amount of change. An interval scale has the property that a given amount of change between any two values means the same at any point on the scale. For instance, temperature would be considered an interval scale, since the difference between 30° F and 40° F is the same amount of change as that between 40° F and 50° F.

A ratio-valued variable is an interval-valued variable with a natural zero point. A change of scale, such as from inches to centimeters, does not alter the zero point. For instance, temperature is not ratio-valued, since the zero point can be defined arbitrarily. However, time, length, or weight would be ratio-valued. Some interval or ratio variables may be described as "continuous" variables, which means that any value between the highest and lowest value on the scale is possible. Examples would include temperature, height, weight, distance, and time until a task is completed. Note that some variables may have an underlying continuous scale of measurement, but are recorded on an ordinal scale. For instance, weight might be recorded as "underweight," "normal," or "overweight."

DISTINCTION BETWEEN RESPONSE AND EXPLANATORY VARIABLES

The intent of repeated measurement analysis and how the data are collected may require a distinction between those variables considered to be explanatory in nature, and those considered to be responses. An explanatory variable, also called a "predictor" or "independent" variable, is used to model or explain variation in the response or outcome variable. Other names for a response variable include "predicted" or "dependent" variable. Note that the term "explanatory" connotes a causal model, which may not be applicable, depending on the design of the study.

Some statistical measures or procedures do not make a distinction between explanatory and response variables. Examples of these include correlation coefficients, or a chi-square test of association. Other procedures, such as analysis of variance or regression analysis, do make this distinction.

REPEATED MEASURES ANALYSIS OF VARIANCE

One of the more common analyses involving repeated measurement data is the repeated measures analysis of variance (repeated measures ANOVA). In this analysis, the response variable is a continuous repeated measurement variable. Its values are modeled as a linear function of at least two categorical predictor variables: an effect of the time point or condition under which it is measured, and an effect due to the subject. The simplest example would be the case where one group of subjects is measured at several time points and it is of interest to determine if the mean responses vary across time.

The One-Factor Repeated Measures ANOVA Model

Suppose an attribute Y was measured on each of n subjects at the same p time points. Let Y_{ij}

denote the measurement at time t_j on the ith subject, and let μ_{ij} be its corresponding mean (i.e., $E(Y_{ij}) = \mu_{ij}; i = 1, 2, \ldots, n; j = 1, 2, \ldots, p$ where E is the expectation operator and means "the expected value of" or "mean of"). We could write the model as

$$Y_{ij} = \mu_{ij} + \varepsilon_{ij}$$
$$i = 1, 2, \ldots, n; j = 1, 2, \ldots, p \qquad (29.1)$$

where ε_{ij} represents random error of measurement. One can think of μ_{ij} as the average response of subject i at time t_j if the study was replicated many times under the exact same conditions. However, the dependence of Y on time is not apparent in this formulation of the model, nor is the interdependence of measurements taken on the same individual. How Y changes across time and among subjects is modeled in the mean μ_{ij} from Equation 29.1 in a linear fashion:

$$\mu_{ij} = \mu + \pi_i + \tau_j + (\tau\pi)_{ij} \qquad (29.2)$$

where μ is the grand mean, π_i is an effect due to the subject, τ_j is an effect of the jth time point, and $(\tau\pi)_{ij}$ is the time by subject interaction effect.

Assumptions

The time factor is assumed to be a fixed factor, which means the resulting interpretations pertain only to the time points analyzed. These τ_j's measure the overall effect on the response variable attributable to the different time points, and are usually scaled so that they sum to zero.

The π_i's measure the contribution to the response attributable to the differences among subjects. If one subject tends to have consistently higher response values across time than another, his or her π_i value will be larger. Since each π_i is associated with a particular randomly selected subject, the π_i's are considered to be independent random effects. It is the assumed random nature of the subject effect that allows us to generalize to all subjects from which the sample was drawn, not just to the particular subjects in the study. The ANOVA model assumes these random subject effects are normally distributed with a common variance, scaled so that they have a population mean of zero.

The subject by time interaction term $(\tau\pi)_{ij}$ measures the deviation from the grand mean μ of the ith subject's response at time t_j beyond what can be explained by that subject's overall effect (π_i) and the effect of the time point (τ_j). Since these interaction effects are associated with randomly selected subjects just as the π_i's are, they too are considered to be random effects. The $(\tau\pi)_{ij}$'s associated with different subjects are assumed to be independent, but those associated with the same subject (at different time points) are assumed to be correlated. The model assumes they are normally distributed with a common variance, scaled so that their mean is zero across the population of all subjects, and independent of the subject effects.

The random error terms $(\varepsilon_{ij}$'s$)$ are also assumed to be normally distributed with mean zero and common variance, and independent of the subject and interaction effects.

Note that since μ_{ij} is modeled in Equation 29.2 as being partially comprised of random effects, it is a random variable itself. Let us now examine what these assumptions imply about the covariance structure of the p measurements taken on each subject.

The Variance-Covariance Matrix

First, consider two time points, t_j and $t_{j'}$, and the corresponding mean responses across the population of subjects, μ_j and $\mu_{j'}$. Since these means are comprised of observations on common subjects (that is, "within-subject" means), it is likely that they will be correlated. Denote that population correlation by $p_{jj'}$ and it follows that the covariance of these two means is

$$cov(\mu_j' \; \mu_{j'}) = p_{jj'} \; \sigma_j\sigma_{j'} \qquad (29.3)$$

where σ_j and $\sigma_{j'}$ represent the standard deviations of the true mean responses at times t_j and $t_{j'}$, respectively. That is,

$$\sigma_j^2 = E(\mu_{ij} - \mu_j)^2. \qquad (29.4)$$

We can depict the set of all variances and covariances at the p time points by constructing a pxp covariance matrix Σ where the ith row corresponds to t_i and the jth column corresponds to t_j.

Note that since $p_{ij} \; \sigma_i \; \sigma_j = p_{ji} \; \sigma_j \; \sigma_i$, the matrix is symmetric.

$$\Sigma = \begin{bmatrix} \sigma_1^2 & p_{12}\sigma_1\sigma_2 & \cdots & p_{1j}\sigma_1\sigma_j & \cdots & p_{1p}\sigma_1\sigma_p \\ p_{21}\sigma_2\sigma_1 & \sigma_2^2 & \cdots & p_{2j}\sigma_2\sigma_j & \cdots & p_{2p}\sigma_2\sigma_p \\ \cdot & \cdot & & \cdot & & \cdot \\ \cdot & \cdot & & \cdot & & \cdot \\ \cdot & \cdot & & \cdot & & \cdot \\ p_{i1}\sigma_i\sigma_1 & p_{i2}\sigma_i\sigma_2 & \cdots & p_{ij}\sigma_i\sigma_j & \cdots & p_{ip}\sigma_i\sigma_p \\ \cdot & \cdot & & \cdot & & \cdot \\ \cdot & \cdot & & \cdot & & \cdot \\ \cdot & \cdot & & \cdot & & \cdot \\ p_{p1}\sigma_p\sigma_1 & p_{p2}\sigma_p\sigma_2 & \cdots & p_{pj}\sigma_p\sigma_j & \cdots & \sigma_p^2 \end{bmatrix} \qquad (29.5)$$

Hypothesis Testing

Second, we wish to test the null hypothesis of no difference across time points,

$$H_0: \tau_1 = \tau_2 = \cdots = \tau_p = 0 \quad (29.6)$$

against the alternative H_a: at least one τ_j is not zero. To do this, we first need to estimate the various components of variability in the model, called "sums of squares." One such source of variability measures the differences among subjects averaged over time points (SS_{subj}), another measures differences among time points averaged over subjects (SS_{time}), and the third is a residual variability accounting for individual deviations from the overall pattern across time, that is, the time by subject interaction ($SS_{t\times s}$). With each source of variation is a measure of the accuracy of the estimate, called its degrees of freedom. Table 29.1 presents the computational formulas for this design. The last column of the table contains the mean squares of the three sources of variation, which are computed by dividing the sum of squares by its associated degrees of freedom.

The usual test of the hypothesis of the main effect of time given in Equation 29.6 is performed by forming the ratio of the mean square of time to that of the time x subject interaction

$$F = \frac{MS_{time}}{MS_{t\times s}} \quad (29.7)$$

and comparing the value obtained to that of an F distribution with $p - 1$ and $(p - 1)(n - 1)$ degrees of freedom. Whether this is an

exact or approximate test under the null hypothesis (Equation 29.6) depends on the assumptions made concerning the covariance matrix given in Equation 29.5. If for each subject, the variance of the difference between any two measurements is the same, regardless of which two time points are chosen, then the F test is exact. This is known as the "sphericity" assumption. Huynh and Feldt[6] have shown that this condition is equivalent to assuming that there is some constant λ such that

$$cov(\mu_{ij}, \mu_{ij'}) = 1/2\,(\sigma_j^2 + \sigma_{j'}^2) - \lambda \quad \text{if } j = j'$$
$$= 1/2(\sigma_j^2 + \sigma_{j'}^2) \quad \text{if } j \neq j' \quad (29.8)$$

where λ is the same for each subject (i) and each set of time points ($j \neq j'$). One special case in which Equation 29.8 holds is when the variances at each time point are equal and the correlation between any two time points is the same (i.e., $\sigma_j^2 = \sigma^2$ and $\rho_{ij} = \rho$ for all i and j). This structure on the covariance matrix is known as "compound symmetry." Terms such as sphericity and compound symmetry often show up on the output of statistical computing packages (e.g., *BMDP*[7], *SAS*[8], and *SPSS*[×9]), which provide the user with a test of this assumption. However, such a test tends not to be very sensitive with small sample sizes.

What if the condition in Equation 29.8 does not hold? Then the test will tend to be liberal, in that it will produce "significant" results too often (too many Type I errors). The work by Box[10] indicates that under the null hypothesis, $MS_{time}/MS_{t\times s}$ is distributed as an F with $(p - 1)\varepsilon$ and $(n - 1)(p - 1)\varepsilon$ degrees of free-

TABLE 29.1 One Group Repeated Measures ANOVA Table

Source of Variation	DF	Sum of Squares	Mean Square
Subjects	$n - 1$	$SS_{subj} = (2) - (1)$	$SS_{subj}/(n - 1)$
Time	$p - 1$	$SS_{time} = (3) - (1)$	$SS_{time}/(p - 1)$
Time × Subj	$(p - 1)(n - 1)$	$SS_{t\times s} = (4) - (2) - (3) + (1)$	$SS_{t\times s}/(p - 1)(n - 1)$
Total	$np - 1$	$SS_{total} = (4) - (1)$	

$(1) = (\Sigma_i\Sigma_j\,Y_{ij})^2/(np)$ $(2) = \Sigma_i(\Sigma_j\,Y_{ij})^2/p$ $(3) = \Sigma_j(\Sigma_i\,Y_{ij})^2/n$

$(4) = \Sigma_i\Sigma_j\,Y_{ij}^2$

dom. If the condition of Equation 29.8 holds then ε = 1. In the worst case, ε = 1/(p − 1). Therefore, a conservative adjustment to correct for this is to set ε to this lower bound and compare the *F* statistic in Equation 29.7 to an *F* distribution with 1 and *n* − 1 degrees of freedom. Another approach involves estimating the value of ε and adjusting the *df*'s accordingly. Two such estimates, one suggested by Greenhouse and Geisser[11] and another (less conservative) one by Huynh and Feldt,[6] are given in computing packages such as *BMPD*[7] and SAS.[8] For computational details, interested readers are referred to a textbook on experimental design, such as Winer[12] or Myers.[13]

Two-Factor Repeated Measures ANOVA, One Repeated Measurement

This design is very similar to the one-factor repeated measurement model, only now instead of modeling the responses of one group of subjects over time, we model the responses of two or more groups. Let the subject grouping factor (e.g., gender) be denoted as factor *A*, with levels $A_1, A_2, \ldots, A_a$ and groups sample sizes $n_1, n_2, \ldots, n_a$. As in the one group case, the two-factor model includes random effects due to subject, and the subject by time interaction. However, it is important that the model be written in such a way as to recognize that the kth subject in group A_1 is not the same person as the kth subject in group A_2. This structure is defined by saying that subjects are "nested" within groups. If the same subjects were in each group, we would say that subjects were "crossed" with groups.

A linear model for the response of subject *k* within group A_i at time point t_j can be written

$$Y_{ijkm} = \mu + \alpha_i + \pi_{k(i)} + \tau_j + \alpha\tau_{ij} + \tau\pi_{jk(i)}$$
$$+ \varepsilon_{m(ijk)}$$

$$i = 1, 2, \ldots, a; j = 1, 2, \ldots, p;$$
$$k = 1, 2, \ldots, n_i; m = 1; \quad\quad (29.9)$$

where μ is the overall mean, α_i is the effect due to group A_i, $\pi_{k(i)}$ is the effect of subject *k* nested within group A_i, τ_j is the effect of time t_j, $\alpha\tau_{ij}$ is the group by time interaction, $\tau\pi_{jk(i)}$ is the time by subject interaction (nested within group), and $\varepsilon_{m(ijk)}$ represents the experimental error, which is nested within an individual observation.

Assumptions

The assumptions of this design are an extension of those of the one-group case. Since *A* and the time factor are considered fixed effects, inferences can be drawn only to those particular groups and time points. These fixed effects are scaled so that $\Sigma_i\alpha_i$, $\Sigma_j\tau_j$, $\Sigma_i\alpha\tau_{ij}$ and $\Sigma_j\alpha\tau_{ij}$ all sum to zero. $\pi_{k(i)}$, $\tau\pi_{jk(i)}$, and $\varepsilon_{m(ijk)}$ are random effects, with the same distributional assumptions as in the one-factor model.

Variance-Covariance Matrix

Within each level of *A*, the variance-covariance matrix of the repeated measurements has the same structure as that listed in equation 29.5. Let $\Sigma_{A1}, \Sigma_{A2}, \ldots, \Sigma_{Aa}$ denote the group covariance matrices. In addition, this design assumes homogeneity of these group covariance matrices; that is, $\Sigma_{A1} = \Sigma_{A2} = \ldots = \Sigma_{Aa} = \Sigma$.

Hypothesis Testing

In the one-factor repeated measures ANOVA, we were interested in testing the null hypothesis of no time effect, that is, a flat response curve over time. In this two-factor extension of the one-factor design, there could be differences in the shape of the response curves among the groups that we would like to detect. The existence of these differences is investigated by testing for a group by time interaction

$$H_0: \alpha\tau_{ij} = 0 \quad i = 1, 2, \ldots, a; \\ j = 1, 2, \ldots, p. \quad (29.10)$$

The alternative hypothesis is that at least one $\alpha\tau_{ij}$ is not zero. If the data lack sufficient evidence to suggest such an interaction exists, we proceed as if the response curves are parallel across groups. The next question we might ask is "do these curves overlap?" This is known as the test of the main effect of group, which tests the null hypothesis

$$H_0: \alpha_1 = \alpha_2 = \ldots = \alpha_a = 0 \quad (29.11)$$

against the alternative that at least one α_i is not zero. This is tested by first computing an average across time for each subject and then comparing the means of these averages among groups. (Note that if two curves are parallel, the difference between the two is constant over all time points. Thus the difference between groups of the mean averages across time provides us with a measure of that constant difference.) Regardless of whether the main effect of group is significant or not, we might also be interested in determining whether the response curves are flat over time. This is the test of the main effect of time, with null hypothesis

$$H_0: \tau_1 = \tau_2 = \ldots = \tau_p = 0 \quad (29.12)$$

and alternative hypothesis that at least one τ_j is not zero.

The mean squares for the various sources of variability are computed in a manner similar to that in the one-factor design, and each test is performed by forming the appropriate F ratio. To test the group × time interaction (the hypothesis of Equation 29.10), the ratio of the A × time interaction mean square to that of the time × subjects within groups interaction is formed

$$F = \frac{MS_{A \times t}}{MS_{t \times subj(A)}} \quad (29.13)$$

and compared to an F distribution with $(a - 1)(p - 1)$ and $(p - 1)\Sigma_i(n_i - 1)$ degrees of freedom. If the Huynh-Feldt condition (see Equation 29.8) holds, this test is exact. If not, the Greenhouse-Geisser or Huynh-Feldt correction can be applied to adjust the degrees of freedom.

The test of the main effect of A (i.e., of Equation 29.11) is tested via the F ratio

$$F = \frac{MS_A}{MS_{subj(A)}} \quad (29.14)$$

and compared to an F with $(a - 1)$ and $\Sigma_i(n_i - 1)$ degrees of freedom.

The test of the main effect of time (i.e., as in Equation 29.2) is performed by comparing the ratio

$$F = \frac{MS_{time}}{MS_{t \times subj(A)}} \quad (29.15)$$

to an F distribution with $(p - 1)$ and $(p - 1)\Sigma_i(n_i - 1)$ *df*s. As with the test of the group by time interaction, this test is exact if the Huynh-Feldt condition holds. If not, the Greenhouse-Geisser or Huynh-Feldt correction to the degrees of freedom can be applied.

If the group by time interaction is significant, the main effect tests are not applicable because they average over dissimilar quantities. If the hypothesis of no time effect is of primary interest, it can be tested separately in each group. On the other hand, one might prefer to compare groups at each time point separately. Such main effect comparisons performed at each level of a factor are known as tests of simple main effects.

To test for a difference among time points in group A_i, the mean square for time is computed from the data in A_i only ($MS_{time\ at\ Ai}$) and an F ratio is formed by dividing it by $MS_{t \times subj(A)}$. The P value of the test is determined by comparing it to the same F distribution used for the main effect of time.

The test of a simple main effect of groups is an approximate test and requires more work. A ratio is formed by comparing the mean square for groups computed from the data at time t_j ($MS_{A\ at\ tj}$) to an approximate error MS. This denominator MS_{error} is a combination of both within- and between-subject variability:

$$MS_{error} = [SS_{subj(A)} + SS_{t \times subj(A)}]/$$
$$[p\Sigma_i(n_i - 1)]. \qquad (29.16)$$

The value of this ratio is compared to an F distribution with $(a - 1)$ and f degrees of freedom, where

$$f = \frac{(u + v)^2}{(u^2/f_1) + (v^2/f_2)} \qquad (29.17)$$

and $u = SS_{subj(A)} = df_{subj(A)} \cdot MS_{subj(A)}$
$v = SS_{t \times subj(A)} = df_{t \times subj(A)} \cdot MS_{t \times subj(A)}$
$f_1 = df_{subj(A)} = \Sigma_i (n_i - 1)$
$f_2 = df_{t \times subj(A)} = p\Sigma_i(n_i - 1).$

Other Multifactor Repeated Measures ANOVAs

Although the discussion thus far has been limited to two simple designs, the same concepts extend to multiple grouping factors and multiple repeated measurement factors. In general, these designs can be broken down into a mixture of within-subject and between-subject sources of variability. Care must be taken to construct the proper F ratios, since the denominator mean square will differ when testing different effects. The reader is cautioned that the default F ratios formed by many general ANOVA software programs may not be applicable to the repeated measures design. However, these programs should give the user sufficient information to compute the proper F statistic. For higher-order designs, the interested reader is referred to texts on statistical design of experiments, such as those by Winer[12] and Myers.[13]

MULTIVARIATE ANALYSIS OF VARIANCE (MANOVA)

The repeated measures ANOVA design is considered a "univariate" linear model analysis because *one* dependent variable is modeled as a linear function of various effects. The multiplicity of measurements over time on each subject, as I have described them, are handled by including a time factor in the model and acknowledging the correlation structure among the repeated measures. However, the Huynh-Feldt condition imposed a fairly strong assumption on the covariance matrix Σ in Equation 29.5 to get exact F tests of the factor effects.

In contrast, MANOVA models a "set" of *two or more* dependent variables as a linear function of the factor effects. In fact, these dependent variables need not even be measured in the same units. For instance, one could model heart rate, systolic blood pressure, and diastolic blood pressure, a set of three dependent measures, as a function of which drug a patient receives. For the purposes of this discussion, however, we will restrict ourselves to the situation where the set of dependent measures are the set of p repeated measures over time.

An arbitrary covariance structure among these dependent variables is allowed. However, we pay a price for such generality by needing larger sample sizes to obtain the same power to detect differences.

One Factor MANOVA

The simplest MANOVA model is comparable to the two-factor repeated measures ANOVA already discussed in that it has one grouping or treatment factor, factor A, with levels A_1, A_2, ..., A_a and sample sizes n_1, n_2, ..., n_a. It is of interest to determine if the mean responses over time differ among the a groups.

The model can be written in vector notation as follows:

$$
\begin{bmatrix} Y_{i1k} \\ Y_{i2k} \\ \cdot \\ \cdot \\ \cdot \\ Y_{ipk} \end{bmatrix} = \begin{bmatrix} \mu_1 \\ \mu_2 \\ \cdot \\ \cdot \\ \cdot \\ \mu_p \end{bmatrix} + \begin{bmatrix} \alpha_{i1} \\ \alpha_{i2} \\ \cdot \\ \cdot \\ \cdot \\ \alpha_{ip} \end{bmatrix} + \begin{bmatrix} \varepsilon_{i1k} \\ \varepsilon_{i2k} \\ \cdot \\ \cdot \\ \cdot \\ \varepsilon_{ipk} \end{bmatrix}
$$

or

$$
\underset{p \times 1}{\mathbf{Y}_{ik}} = \underset{p \times 1}{\boldsymbol{\mu}} + \underset{p \times 1}{\boldsymbol{\alpha}_i} + \underset{p \times 1}{\boldsymbol{\varepsilon}_{ik}} \qquad (29.18)
$$

where $\mathbf{Y}_{ik}$ = a column vector containing the p repeated measurements on subject k in group i,

$\boldsymbol{\mu}$ = a vector of overall means on the p measurements,

$\boldsymbol{\alpha}_i$ = a vector of the effects of the ith group, and

$\boldsymbol{\varepsilon}_{ik}$ = the vector of experimental random errors associated with the kth subject in group i.

Factor A is considered to be a fixed effect, with the α_i's scaled so that each component in the vector sums to zero. Note that we can denote the population vector of means in the ith group for the p time points as the sum $\boldsymbol{\mu}_i = \boldsymbol{\mu} + \boldsymbol{\alpha}_i$. Each row of the vector equation above is a univariate linear model (a one-factor, nonrepeated measures ANOVA), but if we analyzed each time point separately, we would lose the information provided by the correlation among the dependent variables and lose power to detect differences among groups.

Assumptions

As in the univariate ANOVA model, we assume the random errors are normally distributed, but this time with a multivariate normal distribution instead of a univariate one. This distribution is assumed to have a zero mean vector and covariance matrix Σ.

What does this Σ look like? Let σ_{ij}^2 denote the variance of the n_i measurements at time t_j in group i. That is,

$$
\sigma_{ij}^2 = E(Y_{ijk} - \mu_{ij})^2 = E(\varepsilon_{ijk}^2)
$$
$$
i = 1, 2, \ldots, a; j = 1, 2, \ldots, p. \qquad (29.19)
$$

The model assumes homogeneity of this variance for each of the i groups, that is, $\sigma_{1j}^2 = \sigma_{2j}^2 = \ldots = \sigma_{aj}^2 = \sigma_j^2$. Similarly, the correlation between measurements at times t_j and $t_{j'}$ is assumed the same in each of the a groups. If we denote this correlation by $\rho_{jj'}$, we see that the covariance structure in this model has the same form as Σ in (29.5). However, in this model, the Huynh-Feldt condition is not necessary.

Hypothesis Testing

To test the null hypothesis of no difference among groups, we need a test to determine if the $\boldsymbol{\alpha}_i$ are all equal. That is, we test $H_0 : \boldsymbol{\alpha}_1 = \boldsymbol{\alpha}_2 = \ldots = \boldsymbol{\alpha}_a = \mathbf{0}$ against the alternative hypothesis that at least two of them are different. This does not imply that the profiles over time are flat, only that they overlap.

In the univariate case, we formed an F ratio where the numerator was based upon the sum of squares measuring variability related to the hypothesis being tested and the denominator was based on the sum of squares of the appropriate error source of variability. The logical extension in the multivariate case is to form sum of squares matrices. The diagonal of these matrices corresponds to the univariate analyses for each component of the response vector of repeated measurements. The off-diagonals reflect the correlation among elements of the response vector. We cannot divide one matrix by another to form an F ratio, but we can multiply the numerator matrix (or hypothesis matrix, **H**) by the inverse of the denominator matrix (or error matrix, **E**). The more this resultant matrix ($\mathbf{HE}^{-1}$) differs from the identity matrix (i.e., a matrix with 1's on the diagonal and 0's elsewhere), the more evidence we have to reject the null hypothesis.

There are several different test statistics that are commonly used to test the above hypothesis of no difference among groups, known as Pillai's Trace, Hotelling-Lawley's Trace, Wilks's Criterion, and Roy's Maximum Root. They will not necessarily lead to the same conclusion, because each is based on a different way of measuring how different $\mathbf{HE}^{-1}$ is from the identity matrix. It is also not possible to give a general set of rules to specify which test would be best in any given situation. The distributions of these test statistics are complicated, so in most cases, the sampling distributions of the test statistics are approximated to get the P values.

It should be noted that in the special case when $p = 2$, Wilks's Criterion reduces to an exact test known as Hotelling's T^2. The resulting test statistic has an exact F distribution under the null hypothesis of no group effect.

Can we test the hypothesis that the shape of the response curves over time differ among groups? Are they flat? The answer to these questions is "yes," but in order to do so, we have to construct "contrasts" of the dependent variables. A contrast is a linear combination of variables such that the coefficients sum to zero. For instance, $c_1 Y_{i1k} + c_2 Y_{i2k} + \ldots + c_p Y_{ipk}$ where $\Sigma_j c_j = 0$ is a contrast of the dependent variables.

To test for differing response curves among groups (the group by time interaction), we would need $p - 1$ contrasts of the Y_{ijk}'s because the time effect has $p - 1$ degrees of freedom. Several different sets of contrasts might be used, but one set frequently chosen is the set that compares each time point to the first, possibly a base-line measure. For this set, we would create the vector $\mathbf{D}_{ik} = (D_{i1k},$

$D_{i2k}, \ldots, D_{i,p-1,k})'$ where $D_{ijk} = Y_{i,j,k} - Y_{i1k}, j = 2, 3, \ldots, p$. The test would then be performed exactly as described above for the main effect of groups, only this time the $\mathbf{D}_{ik}$ vector is used as the response vector instead of the $\mathbf{Y}_{ik}$ vector. Thus, we are looking to see if the pattern of change over the repeated measures differs among the groups.

The test of the main effect of time averages over groups, so it would only be of interest if we are willing to accept the hypothesis of no group by time interaction. It also uses the contrast vector $\mathbf{D}_{ik}$ instead of $\mathbf{Y}_{ik}$. Without a group effect the model becomes

$$\mathbf{D}_{ik} = \boldsymbol{\mu} + \boldsymbol{\varepsilon}_{ik}. \qquad (29.20)$$

If the null hypothesis of no time effect is true, then the response curve over time is flat, so the difference between any two time points will be zero (i.e., $D_{ijk} = 0$) within random error. Thus the test of the main effect of time is really a test of the hypothesis H_0: $\boldsymbol{\mu} = \mathbf{0}$ against the alternative that at least one component of $\boldsymbol{\mu}$ is not zero. This can be done in most standard computer software packages with a MANOVA routine by specifying a constant term on the right-hand side of the model and testing the magnitude of the effect associated with it as we did with the group effect. How this is accomplished varies among different packages, so care needs to be taken to specify it properly.

For further details on these tests and the MANOVA procedure in general, the interested reader is referred to a good introductory discussion by O'Brien and Kaiser[14] or multivariate textbooks such as that by Harris[2] or Morrison.[4]

NONPARAMETRIC METHODS

The techniques discussed so far have all been based on the assumption of underlying normal distributions. For some models, that assumption can be relaxed to allow other, possibly unspecified, distributions as well by applying a nonparametric test. At this time, we do not have general nonparametric analogues to all repeated measures ANOVA or MANOVA designs, but we do have a few procedures that can be used in special cases. The ones discussed here will be based upon a ranking of the data as opposed to the actual data.

The Friedman Test

The Friedman test is applicable to the one group case, where it is of interest to determine if the responses over time differ. The only assumptions of the test are that the subjects are randomly sampled from the population and that the response measures over time can be ranked from smallest to largest. The ranking is done as follows. For each subject, assign the value 1 to the smallest of the p response measures over time, the value 2 to the second smallest, and so on. Tied values are handled by assigning an average rank. For instance, if the second and third smallest values are the same, both would be assigned a value of 2.5. If the third, fourth, and fifth smallest were tied, each would be assigned a rank of 4. If the ranking was done properly, the sum of the p ranks for each individual should be $\frac{1}{2}p(p + 1)$.

The null hypothesis of the test is that each ranking is equally likely, which would be the case if there were no difference among time points. The alternative hypothesis is that at least one of the time points tends to have higher response values than at least one other.

The test is performed by forming a statistic that measures the difference among the average ranks at each time point to what would be expected if the null hypothesis is true. If all rank orderings are equally likely, the average rank across subjects at each time point should be close to the average rank of the first p integers, which is $\frac{1}{2}(p + 1)$. The further any of these average ranks gets from this value,

the larger this statistic becomes and the more evidence we have to reject the null hypothesis. For small sample sizes and numbers of time points, exact tables of critical values exist. (See, for example, Lehmann,[15] pages 262–265.) For larger samples, an approximate test can be performed by computing an asymptotically equivalent statistic and comparing it to an F distribution with $(p - 1)$ and $(p - 1)(n - 1)$ degrees of freedom. (See, for example, Conover,[16] pages 299–309.)

Aligned Ranks Test

The Friedman test suffers from a lack of sensitivity if the number of time points is small. We ranked within each subject separately because we expect a subject effect that results in some subjects' responses being consistently higher than others. The principle behind the use of aligned ranks is to subtract out a measure of the subject effect (and overall mean), leaving only an estimate of the time effects and making the resulting observations more comparable.

To perform this test, one first subtracts from each subject's measurements some estimate of the "middle," such as the subject's mean or median response over time. This will "align" the observations in such a way as to make the different subjects' values more comparable. The resulting deviations from this "middle" are then ranked across all subjects in the manner described above, using the ranks 1 through np. Under the null hypothesis of no treatment effect, one would expect the average of the aligned ranks at each time point to be about the same. Since the sum of the first np integers is $\frac{1}{2}np(np + 1)$, we would expect the sum at each time point to be about $\frac{1}{p}$ of that total, or $\frac{1}{2}n(np + 1)$ and the average over the n subjects at each time point to be about $\frac{1}{2}(np + 1)$.

As with the Friedman test, the test statistic is a measure of the squared deviations of the observed average ranks across subjects to what would be expected if there were no time differences. The form of the statistic as given in Lehmann,[15] pages 270–273, is compared to a chi-square distribution with $p - 1$ degrees of freedom.

CATEGORICAL DATA METHODS

In this section, methods that are applicable when the response variable is either nominal or ordinal are discussed. Some techniques take into consideration the ordinal nature of the data; others do not. Treating an ordinal variable as if it were nominal fails to acknowledge an important structure in the data, and the resulting tests can be less sensitive to "shifts" in responses over time. Models derived for ordinal data may require that fewer parameters be estimated than those designed for nominal data and then may be easier to interpret, which is also a benefit.

McNemar's Test

The first test is a very simple one applicable to a situation where the response variable is dichotomous, that is, where there are two possible outcomes, such as "success" and "failure" or "presence" and "absence" of a particular characteristic, and these outcomes are measured at two time points. If we assign the values 1 and 2 to the two responses, the data can be presented in a two-way contingency table as follows:

Time 2

		$Y = 1$	$Y = 2$	
	$Y = 1$	a	b	$a + b$
Time 1	$Y = 2$	c	d	$c + d$
		$a + c$	$b + d$	n

The test is looking for a change in the pattern of responses from time 1 to time 2. Note that the diagonal cells with a and d counts in them tell us nothing about a change, since those subjects responded the same at each time point. The null hypothesis being tested can be stated in terms of the off-diagonal cells. Let π_{ij} = the probability that a subject in the population of interest will fall into the ith row and j^{th} column of the above table. The null and alternative hypotheses can be written:

$$H_0: \pi_{12} = \pi_{21}$$
$$H_A: \pi_{12} \neq \pi_{21}. \tag{29.21}$$

The test statistic is usually written in the form

$$T = \frac{(b - c)^2}{b + c} \tag{29.22}$$

and for large values of the sum of the off-diagonal cell counts, $b + c$, is compared to a chi-square distribution with 1 degree of freedom. For small sample sizes, tables for an exact test are available. If $b + c \leq 20$, such tables can be found in Conover[16] using the statistic $T_1 = b$.

Another way of formulating the null hypothesis is in terms of marginal probabilities. Let $\pi_{i+} = \pi_{i1} + \pi_{i2}$ represent the population proportion of subjects in row i, and $\pi_{+j} = \pi_{1j} + \pi_{2j}$ represent the proportion of subjects in row j. By adding π_{11} to both sides of the equation in Equation 29.21 we can rewrite the hypotheses as:

$$H_0: \pi_{1+} = \pi_{+1}$$
$$H_A: \pi_{1+} \neq \pi_{+1}. \tag{29.23}$$

(Note that if $\pi_{1+} = \pi_{+1}$, then $\pi_{2+} = \pi_{+2}$.) Thus McNemar's test is a test of the equality of paired proportions. If we let n_{i+} denote a random variable representing the number of subjects with $Y = i$ at time 1, then n_{i+} has a binomial distribution with mean $\pi_{i+} n_{++}$ and variance $(\pi_{i+})(1 + \pi_{i+}) n_{++}$, where $n_{++} = n$ is the total number of subjects. Similarly, if n_{+j} is a random variable representing the number of subjects with $Y = j$ at time 2, then n_{+j}

has a binomial distribution with mean $\pi_{+j}n_{++}$ and variance $(\pi_{+j})(1 + \pi_{+j}) n_{++}$. Denote the sample estimates of the marginal probabilities by $p_{1+} = (a + b)/n$, $p_{2+} = (c + d)/n$, $p_{+1} = (a + c)/n$, and $p_{+2} = (b + d)/n$. The estimated variance of the difference $d_1 = p_{1+} - p_{+1}$ is:

$$s^2(d_1) = \frac{p_{1+}(1 - p_{1+})}{n} + \frac{p_{+1}(1 - p_{+1})}{n}$$

$$-\frac{2(ad - bc)}{n} \qquad (29.24)$$

which can be used to place an approximate confidence interval on the difference d_1.

Marginal Homogeneity

The concept of equal marginal probabilities can be extended to the case where the response measure is either ordinal or nominal, with $r \geq 2$ possible response categories. We again assume two time points. Using the notation introduced in the last section, let p_{ij} be the proportion of the n subjects in the ith row and j^{th} column; p_{1+} the marginal proportion in the ith row; and p_{+j} the marginal proportion in the jth column; $i = 1, 2, \ldots, r$; $j = 1, 2, \ldots, r$.

Time 2

	$Y = 1$	$Y = 2$		$Y = i$		$Y = r$	
$= 1$	p_{11}	p_{12}	.....	p_{1i}	...	p_{1r}	p_{1+}
$= 2$	p_{21}	p_{22}	.....	p_{2i}	...	p_{2r}	p_{2+}
$\vdots$	.	.	.....	.	...	.	$\vdots$
$= i$	p_{i1}	p_{i2}	.....	p_{ii}	...	p_{ir}	p_{i+}
$\vdots$	.	.	.....	.	...	.	$\vdots$
$= r$	p_{r1}	p_{r2}	.....	p_{ri}	...	p_{rr}	p_{r+}
	p_{+1}	p_{+2}	.....	p_{+i}	...	p_{+r}	

If we let π_{ij}, π_{i+}, and π_{+j} be the population analogues of p_{ij}, p_{i+}, and p_{+j}, respectively, then the condition of marginal homogeneity can be stated as $\pi_{i+} = \pi_{+i}$, for $i = 1, 2, \ldots, r$.

How can we test for marginal homogeneity? We need a statistic that measures the overall differences between the proportions of subjects with the same response at the two time points. Let us denote the difference in paired marginal proportions by $d_i = p_{i+} - p_{+i}$, $1 = 1, 2, \ldots, r$. Since the row and column marginal proportions must sum to 1, the sum of their differences must sum to zero, so we need only the first $r - 1$ of the d_i's to test for marginal homogeneity. Place these $r - 1$ d_i's in a column vector $\mathbf{d} = (d_1' \, d_2, \ldots, d_{r-1})'$ and let $\mathbf{V}$ be an estimate of the $(r - 1) \times (r - 1)$ covariance matrix associated with $\sqrt{n}\,\mathbf{d}$. The test statistic is essentially a measure of the squared distance of the vector $\mathbf{d}$ from the zero vector ($\mathbf{0} = (0, 0, \ldots, 0)'$) in $r - 1$ space (or $r - 1$ dimensions), where "distance" is measured in terms of standard deviations. Mathematically, the test statistic has the form

$$Q = n\,\mathbf{d}'\mathbf{V}^{-1}\mathbf{d} = n \sum_i \sum_j d_i d_j v^{ij} \qquad (29.25)$$

where v^{ij} is the element in the ith row and j^{th} column of the inverse of $\mathbf{V}$. (The inverse of the matrix $\mathbf{V}$ is a matrix $\mathbf{V}^{-1}$ such that $\mathbf{V}\mathbf{V}^{-1} = \mathbf{V}^{-1}\mathbf{V} = \mathbf{I}$, the identity matrix.) The elements of $\mathbf{V}$ are easy to compute, in that $v_{ij} = -(p_{ij} + p_{ji}) - (p_{i+} - p_{+i})(p_{j+} - p_{+j})$ if $i \neq j$, and $v_{ii} = p_{i+} + p_{+i} - 2p_{ii} - (p_{i+} - p_{+i})^2$. However, the elements of the inverse $\mathbf{V}^{-1}$ (the v^{ij}'s) require the use of a computer.

Under the null hypothesis of marginal homogeneity and for large samples, the Q statistic has a chi-square distribution with $r - 1$ degrees of freedom. This statistic was suggested by Bhapkar,[17] but others have been proposed as well. For further discussion of this test and other related tests, the more mathematically oriented reader is referred to Agresti.[18]

Multiple Response Categories and Time Points

If one has more than two response categories measured on an ordinal scale and two or more time points, the nonparametric rank tests described in the previous section can be used. However, because there is a limited number of categories, one would expect a considerable number of tied rankings. Because of this, an adjustment needs to be made to the test statistic to account for less variability in the rankings than would be expected if the response had been measured on a continuous scale. The references cited for those tests explain how to make the appropriate adjustments.

There are other procedures designed for nominal data that can be used, and computer software is available, but a discussion of such is beyond the scope of this chapter. The more mathematically oriented reader is referred to the papers by Grizzle, Starmer, and Koch,[19] and Koch, Landis, Freeman, Freeman, and Lehnen.[20]

In summary, when designing a study, it is important that the researcher be cognizant of the statistical methodology available to answer the study questions. How the data are to be analyzed can affect not only which questions can be answered, but also the way in which the data are collected and recorded. It would certainly be a pity to invest a considerable amount of time and money in a study, only to discover at the end that the statistical tools necessary to answer critical questions are not available. When possible, it is always a good idea to discuss the project with a statistician, to make sure that the proposed statistical methodology is both appropriate and powerful enough to meet the goals of the study, and to clarify the underlying assumptions of the methodology.

In nursing administration, research is often undertaken to assess the impact of a policy change. For example, has a new system for scheduling nurses increased their level of job satisfaction? Has the implementation of the Diagnoses Related Group (DRG) system reduced occupancy rate? Have changes in the Medicaid program improved the quality of care available to the elderly? Because it takes time to observe the full impact of a policy change, studies designed to assess the magnitude of such a change often collect repeated measurements over time. The statistical techniques presented in this chapter can be used to determine whether a policy change had an impact, and if so, to estimate the changes in the magnitude of that impact over time.

REFERENCES

1. Afifi AA, Clark V. Computer-aided multivariate analysis. Belmont, CA: Lifetime Learning Publications, 1984.
2. Harris RJ. A primer of multivariate statistics. New York: Academic Press, 1975.
3. Anderson TW. An introduction to multivariate statistical analysis. 2nd ed. New York: John Wiley and Sons, Inc, 1984.
4. Morrison DL. Multivariate statistical methods. New York: McGraw-Hill, 1976.
5. Stevens SS. Handbook of experimental psychology. New York: Wiley, 1951.
6. Huynh H, Feldt LS. Conditions under which mean square ratios in repeated measurement designs have exact F distributions. J Am Stat Assoc 1970; 65:1582–1589.
7. Dixon WJ, chief ed. BMDP statistical software manual. Berkeley: Univ of California Press, 1985.
8. SAS Institute, Inc. SAS user's guide: statistics, version 5 edition. Cary, NC: SAS Institute, Inc, 1985.
9. SPSS Inc. SPSS^x user's guide. New York: McGraw-Hill Book Co, 1983.
10. Box GEP. Some theories on quadratic forms applied in the study of analysis of variance problems. II. Effects of inequality of variance and covariance between errors in two-way classification. Ann of Mathematical Statistics 1954;25:484–498.
11. Greenhouse WS, Geisser S. On methods in the analysis of profile data. Psychometrika 1959;24:95–112.
12. Winer BJ. Statistical principles in experimental design. 2nd ed. New York: McGraw-Hill, 1971.
13. Myers JL. Fundamentals of experimental design. 3rd ed. Boston: Allyn and Bacon, 1979.
14. O'Brien RG, Kaiser MK. MANOVA method for analyzing repeated measures designs: an extensive primer. Psychol Bull 1985;97(2):316–333.
15. Lehmann EL. Nonparametrics: statistical methods based on ranks. Oakland, CA: Holden-Day, 1975.
16. Conover WJ. Practical nonparametric statistics. 2nd ed. New York: John Wiley & Sons, 1980.

17. Bhapkar VP. A note on the equivalence of two criteria for hypotheses in categorical data. J Am Stat Assoc 1966;61:228–235.

18. Agresti A. Analysis of ordinal categorical data. New York: John Wiley & Sons, 1984.

19. Grizzle JE, Starmer CF, Koch GG. Analysis of categorical data by linear models. Biometrics 1969;25:489–504.

20. Koch GG, Landis JR, Freeman JL, Freeman DH, Lehnen RG. A general methodology for the analysis of experiments with repeated measurements of categorical data. Biometrics 1977;33:133–158.

30

Quality Assurance

Katherine R. Jones

HOW TO assure health-care quality is one of the major issues in the health services industry. In nursing, the central goal is to make certain that care practices produce beneficial, acceptable patient outcomes. Positive outcomes do not happen by chance. They are the result of deliberate decision and action.[1]

What is quality health care? Quality health care consists of the appropriate application of medical science to patient care, with due regard to the risks versus the benefits associated with that care.[2] Quality assurance is the formal and systematic exercise of identifying problems in care delivery, designing activities to overcome the problems, and carrying out follow-up steps to ensure that no new problems have been introduced and that corrective actions have been effective. It is different than quality assessment, which is the act of detecting and measuring the difference between efficacy and effectiveness of health interventions that can be attributed to care providers, taking into account the environment in which the care is delivered.[3]

Quality assurance incorporates issues of accessibility to care, effectiveness of care, continuity of care, and cost containment. One of the major issues in health care today is how hospitals and other health-care agencies can change and adapt to increasing public demands and governmental regulations for both quality and cost containment. The emphasis on quality assurance that is now emerging is in part driven by opportunities that present themselves in the changing health care environment. Purchasers of care

are asking questions about quality as well as cost and access in their negotiations with providers.[4] Since health care practices are infringing upon other expenditure opportunities, major purchasers of health care services are seeking the best buy in terms of both cost and quality. Public policy should seek to achieve an acceptable balance between the collective expectations of the public as represented by the purchasers and providers of care, and the available resources.[5]

The call for greater accountability by providers mandates improvements in data collection, record keeping, and service provision.[6] Health care organizations that are national in scope and better capitalized (have more resources) should be developing computerized quality systems that are capable of providing clinicians with immediate feedback on management of their patients.[4]

Historically, quality assurance was linked to professional autonomy. Society expected health-care professionals to fulfill their obligation to the public for competent practice through self-regulation. Nurses traditionally have been granted less autonomy and have been accountable to physicians and to employing institutions. Some, however, claim that institutions have not been fully accountable; therefore, they are now expected to improve their accountability for quality control through standards mandated by voluntary agencies, most prominently the Joint Commission for Accreditation of Hospitals (*JCAH*, recently renamed the Joint Commission on Accreditation of Health Care Organizations JCAHCO), government entities

(Peer Review Organizations, for example), legal decisions, and consumer interest groups like the Silver-Haired Legislature and Business Coalitions. Pressures for improved accountability in many cases have put additional responsibility on hospital management and caused friction between the health professional and managerial groups.[7]

The principal mechanisms for ensuring quality of nursing care in the past were state licensing laws regulating qualifications for entry into practice; organizational policies and regulations, which controlled the selection, supervision, evaluation, and retention of nursing personnel; and legal and voluntary agencies such as the state department of health and JCAH, which regulated the physical facilities, equipment, and staffing of various health institutions.[2] The current demand for cost and quality control by legislative bodies, the public, and third-party payers have made additional nursing quality assurance programs a necessity.

Nurse administrators in health-care organizations are accountable for the coordination and conduct of quality-centered patient care activities.[8] A major challenge facing nurse administrators today is providing quality care in a cost-effective manner. Unfortunately, measuring quality is as difficult as measuring health-care costs. The integration of standards of practice in specific clinical services and national standards such as those emanating from the JCAH and the American Nurses' Association (ANA), with a well-defined quality assurance program, provide the opportunity for dynamic leadership in nursing.[9]

QUALITY ASSURANCE

According to Schmadle, quality assurance involves assuring the consumer of a specified degree of excellence through continuous measurement and evaluation of structural components, goal-directed nursing process,

and consumer outcomes; using pre-established criteria and standards and available norms; and following up with the appropriate alterations for the purpose of improvement.[10] Coyne and Killien[11] state that quality assurance is a process directed toward evaluating the quality of patient care provided in a particular setting, through standards for care, and implementing mechanisms for ensuring that the standards are met. Quality assurance activities provide evidence to a community that the health services its residents receive under the auspices of a health-care institution are of the highest quality and consistent with available resources.

The premise of the quality assurance model is that standards of care serve as the cornerstone for both care planning and care evaluation. Moreover, it is assumed that congruence between defined standards for giving care and criteria used for measuring care must exist, so that achievements and deficiencies of nursing practice can be clearly identified.[12]

Stevens[13] identified three essential components of a quality assurance system: standards, surveillance, and corrective action. Quality assurance in nursing requires successfully accomplishing the following: (1) identifying the characteristics that denote quality; (2) identifying the level of quality that can be produced at an acceptable cost for consumers; (3) translating the characteristics into measurable criteria; and (4) organizing the nursing division to ensure that the product of the organization (nursing care) meets the criteria.[14] The main thrusts of a quality assurance program should be to both measure and improve the quality of nursing care being delivered.[2]

An ideal quality assurance system provides usable information, guarantees cost effective care, and actively involves both nursing staff and administrators. Role responsibilities for nurses at all levels of the nursing organization must be specified, with identified reporting pathways and data-collection methods. Routine evaluation of the system, with appropriate modification to respond to changes in the practice of professional nursing and the delivery of patient care, is an important element of any quality assurance program.[14]

A quality assurance system provides continuous monitoring of nursing practice, and is an integral component of a comprehensive, hospitalwide, multidisciplinary quality assurance program. In many respects it is a self-evaluation system, in which results are fed back to nursing service to improve its effectiveness. A direct linkage between patient care evaluation activities and patient care planning is required, if the recommendations for change are to be implemented effectively.[12] The scope of a quality assurance program may range from a narrow focus on the technical correctness of direct patient care, to a broad focus on issues such as availability, acceptability, and appropriateness of the total patient care system.

The JCAH was a strong force in development of quality assurance programs. This agency developed and implemented a hospital quality assurance standard, effective January 1, 1981, which required a well-defined, organized quality assurance program with an ongoing objective assessment of important aspects of patient care and procedures for the correction of identified problems. Health agencies, consequently, need to implement a comprehensive and integrated quality program that demonstrates an ability to identify important or potential problems, determine the cause and the size of problems, implement a course of action to eliminate problems, monitor progress, and document the end result.[7]

The American Nurses' Association (ANA) likewise has developed a quality assurance model, based on beliefs about what constitutes good nursing care. These beliefs and values determine the standards and criteria used to judge quality, and identify acceptable levels of nursing care.[7] According to the ANA, quality review programs are intended to judge the quality of services provided by professional nurses and to contribute to the improvement of the delivery of nursing services by expeditious identification and correction of problems and deficiencies.[7]

Quality Assurance Program Components

A variety of methods should be incorporated into a quality assurance program, including concurrent and retrospective patient care audits, patient care profile analysis, and peer review. This array of methods enhances the likelihood of determining specifically which elements of nursing care produce optimal outcomes for each type of patient. With this determination, inefficiencies and ineffectual interventions can be replaced with more appropriate methods, through changes in the organization of services or through continuing education, for example.[2] The effectiveness or ineffectiveness of a particular nursing intervention refers to the extent to which certain pre-established outcomes can be attained through use of that intervention. The efficiency of a particular nursing intervention is its cost-benefit ratio, or the relationship between the monetary value of the resources expended and the monetary value of the results achieved.

A quality assurance system must take into account the structure in which care is given, the patient outcomes, and the process of care giving. The essential procedures are:

1. Establishing standards and criteria for structure, process, and outcome.
2. Auditing against standards and criteria, collecting data, and comparing standards to actual practice; evaluating results by analyzing and interpreting data.
3. Identifying strengths and weaknesses of nursing practice; evaluating staff performance.

4. Making recommendations for improvements of nursing process and patient outcomes; identifying courses of action; selecting and implementing actions to change practice.
5. Re-auditing for results; providing feedback about results of actions to personnel.

There are other major aspects of a quality assurance program.[1] One is to promote the ongoing or continuous monitoring of patient care. Another is to investigate the barriers to quality patient care that exist in an organization. A vitally important component is the improvement of patient care through nursing research and the implementation of research findings.

Quality nursing care is dependent on the accountability of individual nurses for the nursing process used in care delivery, and outcomes that result from care for individual patients. The individual nurse is answerable for the actions he or she takes based on predetermined standards of nursing practice. The nurse administrator is similarly accountable.[10] Health-care provider involvement in quality assurance activities stems from the responsibility of providers to society for self-regulation.

Quality assurance can actually be defined as an unwritten contract between the hospital or health-care agency, and society.[8] Since the single most important objective of a quality assurance program is to improve the quality of nursing care, the people who actually deliver the care must assist nurse administrators in determining what constitutes quality nursing care, how that care will be measured, how the care provided compares to standards, and what actions should be taken to correct deficiencies.[8] A professional nurse's philosophy is that quality assurance is the responsibility of every nurse and an integral part of each person's functioning. The nurse administrator can help the nursing staff assume more responsibility by using the following guidelines:[10]

1. Clarify responsibilities and standards of performance.
2. Make responsibilities realistic and progressive.
3. Evaluate progress on a frequent and continual basis.
4. Use the motivators of achievement, recognition, responsibility, advancement, and growth.
5. Help nurses meet their own needs in the process of achieving agency and department goals.
6. Be sure that nurses can handle their assigned level of responsibility and then hold nurses accountable.

Criteria and Standards

The values that exist in an institution determine how "quality patient care" is defined at any given point in time, and represent the agreed-upon level of excellence. These values are reflected in policies, procedures, statements of philosophy, and job descriptions. Values are also reflected, albeit more subtly, in organizational structures, services provided, special programs and projects, and budget allocations. Values are made explicit through the writing of standards of practice. Standards are professionally defined expressions of the range of acceptable variation for a criterion.

Standards express goals for nursing care, and vary in their specificity. Within an institution they form a consensus of professional thinking. Standards are based on research, expert opinion, and observation.[11] The setting of standards for a given patient group is the first step in structuring an evaluation system. There are two definitions of standard:

1. A criterion of excellence or attainment (optimal)

2. A base line against which to measure the event or behavior (minimal)

Standards should be realistic, appropriate for a given patient base, and reflect the level of nursing care for which resources are available. Standards should be written in simple language, be easy to apply, and easily interpretable.[13]

Evaluation instruments should be based on an institution's standards of nursing care and practice. Standards are found in many organizational mechanisms. For example, job descriptions outline the standards against which personnel performance will be measured. By standardizing the functions, responsibilities, and specific qualifications of a job, position descriptions also reflect that quality of care is being based on the standards set by an institution. Performance evaluations, thereby, are based on how well nurses achieve the organization's nursing care standards in actual everyday practice.

Standards are established and derived from a variety of sources—federal, state, and local units of government, licensing agencies, accrediting organizations (JCAH), professional organizations, trade associations, institutions (personnel policies), departments, patient care units, and individuals. Statements of standards must be readily available to personnel on patient care units. Standards are intended to provide a basis for measurement that is objective, achievable, practical, flexible, and acceptable. Realistic standards that are achievable lessen the likelihood of frustration, engender the motivation to perform well, and are more acceptable to practitioners.[6] Standards are not instruments of evaluation; they are too comprehensive and general in nature for such a use. Standards need to be broken down into elements of care called criteria; it is criteria that are used to measure performance and translate standards into actions. Each criterion is referenced by code to a specific standard.

Criteria are predetermined elements of health care against which the aspects of the quality of a medical service can be compared. They represent the intent of a related standard of care.[7] A criterion should be a reliable indicator of quality. It is a standard rule or test on which a judgment or decision can be based.[10]

The development of criteria is best accomplished by nursing management teams from each clinical service. Criteria should be written by nurses who are specialists in the particular area being addressed. A collaborative approach ensures that significant practice efforts and achievable outcomes are addressed.[2] A criterion should answer the question "What does a physician, nurse, or patient have to do or demonstrate in order to achieve satisfactory care or status?"

Sources of information for criteria development include nursing policies and procedures, patient satisfaction studies, and regulatory codes. Areas for criteria development include communication with the patient and family, environmental factors, response time or adaptive behavior on the part of patients, patient comfort and safety, patient physiologic status, self-care skills, and patient and family knowledge of health programs. Criteria should be specific rather than general; in order to obtain better information, allow only one interpretation, and clarify expectations of staff. Criteria must be clinically sound, and reflect current clinical practice and judgment: they represent the optimal nursing care for a patient with a specific condition under existing circumstances in a particular institution.[2] Criteria need to be concise, realistic, understandable, stated in behavioral terms, written in short, clear phrases, and achievable with a reasonable degree of effort.[2,15]

Two different kinds of criteria can be identified. Implicit criteria are the subjective opinions of the persons doing the evaluation. Professionals use internalized criteria of what they consider good practice. Implicit criteria are particularly helpful in complex cases where disease severity, comorbidity, genetics, or environmental factors complicate the management of care and make explicit review difficult. Explicit criteria are quantifiable, have greater reliability, and enable less well-trained individuals to conduct a review.[16]

Details of Quality Assurance Programs

Identifying a problem in the quality assurance context means discovering any deviation from expected occurrence. An appraisal system focusing on quality involves the collection of information about actual performance and the comparison of the fit between that performance and the standard that has been set. Each institution needs to decide specifically what is to be measured, how frequently, using what methods, and by which individuals.[11] Methods to compare actual versus desired performance include concurrent or retrospective audits, direct observations of nurse or patient performance, patient or nurse interviews, surveys or questionnaires, and knowledge testing. The selection of methods depends on the purpose of an evaluation and available resources.

Once a problem is identified, it is necessary to validate its existence and determine the extent of the problem: its nature, complexity, and characteristics. Accurately identifying a problem requires the use of many data sources: patient medical records, incident reports, infection control reports, committee reports, patient and staff surveys, audit results, and direct observations.

Once a problem's existence is verified and described in full, it is next necessary to determine the cause of the deficiency or the reason for noncompliance. Either could be related to a lack of knowledge (deficiency in theory or technical information); a gap in performance (deficiency in behavior or practice, in spite of appropriate knowledge); or a flaw in the

system (deficiency in organizational, administrative, or environmental factors that prevent appropriate practice).

Problem resolution is the next step, and requires determining the extent of a desired change given available resources, the practical limitations of any proposed change, and the impact of a proposed change on the practice of nursing. Target dates for resolving the problem need to be set, and responsible persons must be identified. Responding to what is found with respect to a problem is the means through which improvement in quality care takes place. Several types of responses to the identification of a problem can occur: at one end of the continuum there is recognition of progress if standards are being met or if improvement from the review has been made. In this case, positive feedback is important for maintaining quality performance. If standards are not being met, the response depends on the nature of the problem, the style of the organization and its management, and the resources available for further problem solving.[11]

There are three classical frameworks from which nursing care can be evaluated: structure, process, and outcome. The structural framework involves examining the physical setting in which care is delivered and the conditions in which care is administered. The relevant conditions include the philosophy of nursing service, organizational structure and objectives, financial resources, equipment, and institutional and professional licensure. Structural standards are directed toward assessing the protocols by which nursing care is organized and managed. Standards that pertain to structure are designed to identify the necessary environmental and organizational conditions for quality care. Structural standards describe the conditions under which it is likely that good nursing will take place; they do not, however, ensure that good care does in fact take place.[13]

The process framework involves the nursing process itself, including taking of a health history, performing a physical examination, making nursing diagnoses, determining nursing care goals, writing care plans, performing nursing tasks, measuring nursing care outcomes, and recording patient responses to treatment. Process standards relate to the activities of an individual nurse as well as to the interaction between a nurse and a patient. The process standard requires a professional judgment in determining whether a criterion has been met.[13]

The outcome framework involves measuring changes in patients' health status that result from nursing interventions. These changes include modification of patients' symptoms, signs, knowledge, attitudes, satisfaction, skill levels, and compliance.[2] Sanazaro[17] has identified four major categories of outcomes: (1) clinical outcomes measured as mortality, longevity, change in disease status and symptoms, and risk of adverse effects; (2) outcomes attributable to education, counseling, and caring, measurable as patients' knowledge and understanding of their condition and self-management; outlook and attitude toward their condition; satisfaction with their physician and with their medical care generally, and compliance with their treatment plan; (3) outcomes defining a patient's function as an individual, family member, or member of the community; and (4) the effects of incurring costs and undergoing hospitalization.

The JCAH has announced that it soon will begin using surgical mortality and complication rates as a central measure in the accreditation of agencies. The stated purpose of using morbidity and mortality rates is to judge whether each hospital provides care at least equal to local and national standards. The JCAH, while acknowledging the need to adjust for certain unique features of patients, is convening task forces to develop national norms for neonatal mortality, infection rates, and other measures for high-risk populations and procedures.

Successful outcomes are the ultimate achievement of nursing care. It is difficult, however, to identify all the factors that influence care, and to define outcome criteria that are attributable largely to nursing practice. Patient knowledge, behavior, and health state are influenced by many factors besides nursing care; the care given by other providers, particularly physicians, can be equally influential.[18] Many relationships are unclear, especially the linkage between specific processes and specific outcomes. Multiple variables exist in the patients' environment that are not controlled by nursing; human behavior is not consistent; all patients do not respond in the same ways, and desired results might be achieved without any nursing intervention at all.[8] Donabedian[16] states that serious questions can be raised about the traditional mortality and morbidity indices of quality hospital care because so many factors are involved. Consequently, measurement of outcome alone is not sufficient. All three perspectives—analysis of structure, process, and outcome—are necessary for valid problem-solving and as a basis for future planning.

In addition, interpersonal one-to-one relationships contribute to the quality of care in their own right, and are also the mechanisms through which technical care is planned and implemented. Attributes of interpersonal processes are important determinants of a patient's satisfaction with care—in one sense an outcome measure. Interpersonal elements are also a factor in care, a process to which both patient and practitioner contribute. Since patients are not expert in the technical aspects of care, they use evidence of personal attention, interest, and concern. Technical components of care include identifying a patient's problem, determining the objectives of care, and executing treatment. The purpose of a treatment strategy is to maximize the net expected benefit to be derived from care—in other words, to deliver the highest quality of technical care of which one is capable, given the state of medical science.[16]

Patient classification and quality assessment play an interactive role in the task of planning the delivery of nursing care. Patient classification systems are often used to determine nurse staffing requirements, while quality assessments provide feedback regarding the appropriateness and completeness of staffing patterns. A direct relationship between staffing and quality exists to the extent that resource allocation affects program performance. In the future, patient classification systems will also be useful in defining more specific process or outcome criteria, especially in the areas of cost and utilization.[19]

At the health delivery system level, quality assurance activities include measures of access to care, such as distance from organized services, available provider alternatives, transportation availability, hours of available care, and measures of patients' beliefs and attitudes about health care. Moreover, utilization review of admissions and lengths of stay is required by Medicare and Medicaid.[6] Feedback to nursing staff about the quality of system functioning is needed. Nurse administrators must decide how much information to provide, in what form, to which individuals, and with what frequency.

The most recent form of quality assurance program activity is monitoring. Monitors are required for different levels of organizational activities. Division-level monitors from which criteria can derive include discharge planning, care planning, and primary nursing. Unit-level monitors include such behaviors as patients' compliance with postmyocardial infarction exercise programs. Unit-level monitors could well be an effective means for bringing about long-term substantive improvements in patient care and could encourage professional behaviors because of greater staff nurse commitment, more acceptance of

accountability for practice, and a more professional environment. This in turn could lead to reduced staff turnover and better recruitment of new staff.[11]

There are four components to monitoring: (1) identification of an area of concern; (2) specification of standards related to the concern; (3) specification of criteria by which attainment of standards might be measured; and (4) development of methodologies specifying how data will be collected for each criterion. A statement of minimal level of acceptable performance for each criterion is expressed as a percentage or as a relative change in performance. It requires judgment based on knowledge of an institution, an institution's capacity for change, and the degree of quality expected in the community.[11] The JCAH requires ongoing review and monitoring of certain categories of patients and practices: antibiotic use, numbers of transfusions, infection control, patient safety, and medical records.

Management Aspects

"Quality control" is a management term. It involves activities that evaluate, monitor, or regulate the quality of services rendered to consumers and includes both managerial and clinical functions.

Nurse administrators are accountable—individually, professionally, and institutionally—for patient care. Managers of nursing care now operate in an environment of continuous and dynamic change. The most significant change could well be that the primary emphasis in health care is no longer characterized largely by professional altruism. Today's ethos is instead dominated by the economics of health services. Decisions by nurse administrators increasingly take place in competitive economic arenas. In this era of high demand for quality patient care and tightly controlled resources, assuring a comprehensive and effective quality assessment program is the nurse administrator's obligation to hospital administrators, to the boards of directors, and to the public.

Nurse administrators facilitate the integration of professional nursing practice in complex organizational structures. Organizations should be structured in such a way that staff nurses can give high-quality care to patients in environments that minimize conflicts related to the norms of professional freedom, the constraints of bureaucratic structures, and limited economic resources.

To accomplish these tasks, the nurse administrator begins by establishing a purpose for the department of nursing. The statement of purpose serves to define the unique contribution made by nursing to the organization's product—patient care. The guiding purpose of the nursing department should then be marketed by the nurse executive to internal groups, such as the medical staff, and to external groups, such as third-party payers and consumers. The identified purposes and goals of the nursing department also need to be clearly linked to the department's philosophy; this in turn serves as a key reference for the development of a comprehensive quality assurance program. With a firm foundation and commitment to quality assurance in the nursing department, integration of nursing with the total organizational quality assurance effort is greatly facilitated.[20]

A nursing quality assurance program should be flexible and broad based, yet focused to ensure that information from quality assurance activities can be used in daily decision making. The nurse administrator quantifies the resources available for quality assurance activities, sets priorities, recommends program design, and develops strategies for implementing quality assurance plans. Resources must be evaluated according to their accessibility, availability, appropriateness, and acceptability to nursing services. The quality assurance action plan is best determined after completion of a thorough assessment of resources.[20]

Professional nurses on each individual nursing unit have the obligation to monitor the quality assurance process on their respective units. The nurse executive coordinates these activities. When performance is identified as problematic, the professional group deals with the problem and reaches collective conclusions about the best mechanisms for corrective action. A peer evaluation system could be employed for identifying individual compromises in care. Thus, mechanisms for implementing new standards of practice or changes in practice behavior are monitored properly. Nursing management accepts the responsibility for implementation and monitoring. The responsibility for quality is shared by the institution and nurses. It is through shared responsibility and accountability that a higher level of participation and interaction in quality assurance is achieved. In addition, quality assurance becomes directed more specifically to care that can be measured, evaluated, and altered as necessary.[21]

A clearly delineated quality assurance program serves as the basis for short-, medium-, and long-range goals, which in turn determine the nursing budget.[22] Unit-level managers as well as executive-level nurses are responsible for promoting an investigational approach to patient care problems and demonstrating how patient care plans, orientation, and educational programs are all elements of the standards of care and of quality assurance programs. Quality assurance systems have enormous potential for hastening the building of a body of scientific knowledge for nursing, mandatory for elevating nursing to the level of a scientific discipline.[22]

Quality Assurance Tools

Patient care audits are perhaps the most common quality assurance tool, and are required by JCAH. Audits involve selecting an important element of performance and comparing the observed level of performance with predetermined criteria and standards.

There are several types of patient care audits: audits that focus on specific diagnostic categories, diagnostic tests and procedures, care problems, and certain care processes. An audit methodology can be employed either concurrently or retrospectively. A retrospective audit is an inspection of medical records to evaluate documentary reliability, completeness, and compliance with standards for nursing care as established by the nursing department and agency, and professional, governmental, and accrediting groups. A concurrent process audit is an inspection of the nursing process as carried out and documented by nursing staff to evaluate the extent of compliance in an agency with established standards of nursing practice. A currently popular method for assuring quality in hospital nursing departments is concurrent unit-based auditing. Results from these audits are reported upward but identification and resolution of problems are done on a unit basis.[1] Problems related to quality are identified in a variety of ways, including nursing rounds, incident reports, unit audit compliance assessments, patient satisfaction surveys, and personnel monitoring.[1] According to Fifer,[23] however, audits by themselves are not an effective mechanism for assuring quality, inasmuch as they could easily be complicated and compromised by observer bias.

An example of a retrospective process audit is the Phenauf Audit. The Phenauf approach uses a 50-item form framed to identify segments of the seven nursing functions contained in the statutes of licensure for nurses: application and execution of physician orders; observation of signs and symptoms; supervision of patients; supervision of others participating in care; reporting and recording; application and execution of nurs-

ing procedures and techniques; and promoting physical and emotional health.

The Slater Scale is an example of a concurrent audit. It rates nurse performance in the clinical setting by focusing on six general nurse-patient interactions: meeting the psychosocial needs of patients; meeting the psychosocial needs of patients as members of groups; meeting the physical needs of patients; meeting the combined physical and psychosocial needs of patients; communicating on behalf of patients; and fulfilling professional responsibilities.

The QualPac Scale developed by Wandelt and Agar was derived from the Slater Scale, and its 68 items measure the quality of care that patients receive either from direct nurse-patient interactions, or from interventions made on their behalf.[24] It is scored by nurse observers who rate items that describe observable nursing actions. The QualPac Scale concentrates on the process of care. The primary scientific bases that are reflected in the scale are related to the psychosocial, physical, communication, and professional implications of nursing care. QualPac can be applied in any setting where nurse-patient interactions occur. The standard for measurement is the care expected of a first-level nurse who is safe, adequate, and therapeutic.[25]

Utilization review, such as that mandated by Professional Standards Review Organizations (PSRO) legislation and JCAH, is a second quality assessment device. The purpose of utilization review is to assure that care given is necessary medically, conforms to acceptable professional standards, and is provided in the most efficient manner possible.[17] Utilization review involves concurrent review of the status of newly admitted and extended stay patients with the goal of minimizing unnecessary or inappropriate admissions, stays, tests, and procedures.

Risk management programs are another way of assuring that quality care is delivered.

Such programs include preventive measures as well as monitoring activities. Preventive strategies involve the selection, orientation, and training of personnel; documentation that clinical practice and administrative functions are carried out in accordance with established policies and procedures; and a centralized reporting system that identifies, evaluates, and resolves patient care problems in a timely fashion. Actual implementation of quality assurance measures involves thoroughly verifying current licensure, checking employment references and assessing skills. Certification to perform specialized procedures such as those involved with chemotherapy, intravenous medications, or advanced life support could be included.[26]

Professional credentialing is a formal method for controlling quality and involves statutory credentialing in the form of licensure, as well as professional credentialing in the form of certification and registration. Licensure is a process by which an agency of a state government grants permission to individuals accountable for the practice of a profession to engage in that profession, and prohibits all others from legally doing so. Certification is a process by which a nongovernmental agency or association certifies that an individual licensed to practice has met certain predetermined standards.[27] It is the states' attempt to certify competency; however, professional societies establish the standards and award the certificates.

Institutional credentialing involves statutory licensure and professional credentialing through accreditation. Accreditation is a process in which a voluntary, nongovernmental agency or organization approves and grants accredited status to institutions, programs, or services that meet predetermined structure, process, and outcome criteria.[27]

Credentialing alone is usually ineffective in assuring quality, since licensure standards are broad based, and licenses are infrequently revoked and often granted on a lifetime basis.

In addition, licensure lacks a performance evaluation data base. To function as an effective method for assuring quality, licensing systems will have to be supplemented with data systems that track professional competence throughout a practitioner's lifetime.

Mandatory continuing education has also been proposed in deliberations about quality assurance programs. However, there is little evidence of a direct relationship between continuing education and quality of care. Finally, peer review is yet another measurement approach. It involves selecting a random sample of patient medical records in order to make judgments as to the quality of care provided by colleagues.

Cost and Quality

One frequently overlooked aspect of assuring quality is its cost. Careful attention to cost is an integral and required component of all quality assurance studies. Brown[28] has identified cost effectiveness as a key link to quality assurance. She does not believe, however, that lower cost should necessarily be equated with lesser quality, nor that higher quality necessarily means higher cost.

Different programs and approaches to care can be compared by using cost-benefit or cost-effectiveness analysis. Which of these approaches is chosen depends on the purpose of the analysis—whether one wants to compare the cost-benefit ratio of several programs, or the relative costs of different alternatives to achieve the same goal. The outcome of such an analysis provides a measure of a program's comparative efficacy, effectiveness, and efficiency.

Efficacy is the ability of an intervention to produce an intended benefit to a defined population under ideal conditions. The benefit of a particular technology should be judged as comprehensively as possible, reflecting the positive and negative aspects for the consumer's physical and mental health. It is possible to weight probable outcomes and account for patient preferences for various states of ill or good health. Effectiveness is the extent of benefit achieved under usual conditions, and reflects performance under ordinary circumstances, by the average practitioner, for the typical patient. Efficiency is the extent to which a benefit is achieved with minimum expenditure of resources.[29]

There are two kinds of efficiency worthy of attention. Clinical efficiency refers to health care that avoids harm or redundancy; production efficiency refers to the system within which care is delivered. It is possible to improve the quality of care without increasing its cost by improving clinical efficiency, or to reduce the cost of care without reducing quality by improving production efficiency.[16]

Wennberg and his colleagues have developed a methodology known as small-area research that studies the appropriateness of medical practice as an outcome analysis. Specifically, Wennberg analyzes the differences in amounts of health-care resources consumed in specific, comparable geographic areas. Brook and Lohr[3] describe this approach as "variations in use," a term that refers to the different levels of per capita consumption of services—especially to hospital care, office visits, drugs, and specific procedures. Variations in consumption are of particular significance where all the usual explanations for usage—such as demographic, social, economic, and health status factors—have been controlled, leaving no obvious explanation for differences except those related to the practice styles of individual health-care providers.

Wennberg has studied many variables, including per capita usage of beds and personnel, and expenditures and reimbursements per capita. From such data he is able to construct an "index of discretion," the goal of which is to measure the efficacy and effectiveness of practice.

CONSIDERATIONS FOR THE FUTURE

Health assessment is both a conceptual and methodologic challenge. Constructing health measures is a complex task. The focus of health assessment needs to go beyond physiologic parameters, like extended lifespan, to the domains of physical, mental, and social functioning and well-being.[30]

We know next to nothing about the efficacy of "cognitive" practices, such as listening to, counseling, or reassuring patients. Yet these represent the art of nursing care. We need to know more about nurse-patient interaction and communication, and perhaps most importantly, how styles of interaction affect recovery.

Even less is known about effectiveness. We cannot be sure that what is learned in a best possible circumstance provides a reliable guide in ordinary every day practice. Basically, what is needed is an "epidemiology" of effectiveness: a routine collection of information that describes the outcomes of tests, drugs, procedures, and other services as used in everyday practice.[16]

It is also essential that appropriate outcomes be developed for both our aging population and the aging aged population in dealing with conditions such as senility, Alzheimer's disease, and depression. Other outcomes need to be defined to better assess new technologies like artificial organs and transplants.

Implementation of the diagnosis related group (DRG) based prospective reimbursement system also has implications for nursing and quality assurance. One of the challenges for nursing is the need to establish standards that promote cost-effective performance without sacrificing quality. We need studies that consider the relationship among nursing resources, nursing diagnosis, and DRG. In a society that holds health-care providers increasingly accountable for the cost of care, there is a need to develop valid, reliable tools that measure quality in relation to cost. Nurses must work together to develop classification schemes that identify homogeneous populations and develop evaluative criteria and related measurement tools for monitoring both quality and resource consumption.[9]

In the future, more attention needs to be paid to linking care processes with outcomes of care. We are unable to say with confidence that the services rendered to patients bear some plausible relationship to patients' subsequent health status. Establishing the clinical validity of process measures, that is, the degree to which process predicts outcome, is a significant area for future research.

The future of health services research, as it relates to quality of care assessment, will come from integrating the four areas of efficacy, effectiveness, variations in population-based rates of use, and quality of care, into an operational model for policy, planning, and evaluation. Such a model will better address the continuing problems in health care systems and organize a flow of information about all four concepts that is useful for evaluating and recommending future alternative strategies of health-care delivery.[3]

In conclusion, when thinking about quality, there are several perspectives as to what is most important. From a governmental viewpoint, efficiency and effectiveness are uppermost. For consumers, access and the acceptability of care are highly valued. From a professional perspective, the critical factors are competence and effectiveness.[6]

Professionals involved in the delivery of health care have a commitment to quality care. The challenge is to translate this commitment into programs that make the measuring of health-care quality a reality. Scientific knowledge, in combination with utilization guidelines, substantially supports and facilitates the operating of quality assurance programs. Research will help clarify the relationship between what is done in practice, and the outcomes of practice.[31]

Quality assurance needs to be an integral component of the role of each individual practitioner. The nursing profession has an obligation to assure that its practice is consistent with high standards, requirements of patients, and local needs. Nursing groups have the responsibility for defining levels of performance, setting standards of practice on which performance can be evaluated, and specifying the acceptable response to those standards. Nurse administrators have the responsibility to assure that professional staff members participate at all levels of a comprehensive quality assurance system.

REFERENCES

1. Sheridan DR, Bronstein JE, Walker DD. The new nurse manager: a guide to management development. Rockville, MD: Aspen Systems Corporation, 1984.
2. Gillies DA. Nursing management: a systems approach. Philadelphia: WB Saunders Company, 1982.
3. Brook RH, Lohr KN. Efficacy, effectiveness, variations, and quality: boundary—crossing research. Medical Care 1985;23(5):710–721.
4. Elwood PM, Paul BA. Commentary: But what about quality? Health Affairs 1986;5(1):135–140.
5. Smith CT. Commentary: high expectations versus limited resources. Health Affairs 1986;5(3):86–90.
6. Byers M, Phillips C. Nursing management for patient care. Boston: Little, Brown, 1979.
7. Sliefert MK. Quality control: professional or institutional responsibility. In: McClosky JC, Grace HK, eds. Current issues in nursing. Boston: Blackwell Scientific Publications, 1985.
8. Simms LM, Price SA, Ervin NE. The professional practice of nursing administration. New York: John Wiley & Sons, 1985.
9. Meisenheimer CG. Quality assurance: a complete guide to effective programs. Rockville, MD: Aspen Systems Corporation, 1985.
10. Ganong JM, Ganong WL. Nursing management. Rockville, MD: Aspen Systems Corporation, 1980.
11. Coyne C, Killien M. A system for unit-based monitors of quality of nursing care. J Nurs Adm 1987; 17(1):26–32.
12. Edmunds L. A computer-assisted quality assurance model. J Nurs Adm 1983;XIII(3):36–43.
13. Stevens BJ. First-line patient care management. Rockville, MD: Aspen Systems Corporation, 1983.
14. Ulrich B, Tredin N, Cavauras CA. Assuring quality through a professional practice approach. Nursing Economics 1986;4(5);272–287.

15. Althaus JN, Mardyck NM, Pierce PB, Rogers MS. Nursing decentralization: the El Camino experience. Wakefield, MA: Nursing Resources, 1981.

16. Donabedian A. Quality, cost, and clinical decisions. The Annals of The American Academy of Political and Social Science 1983;468:196–204.

17. Sanazaro PJ. Quality assessment and quality assurance in medical care. Annals Review Public Health 1980;1:37–68.

18. Bloch D. Evaluation of nursing care in terms of process and outcome: issues in research and quality assurance. Nursing Research 1975;24(4):256–263.

19. Giovannetti PBJ. Patient classification: implications for quality assessment. In: Luke RD, Kruger JC, Modrow RE, eds. Organization and change in health care quality assurance. Rockville, MD: Aspen Systems Corporation, 1983.

20. Lewis EM. Administrative support. In: Meisenheimer CG, ed. Quality assurance: a complete guide to effective programs. Rockville, MD: Aspen Systems Corporation, 1985.

21. Porter-O'Grady J. Creative nursing administration: participative management into the 21st century. Rockville, MD: Aspen System Corporation, 1986.

22. Kerfoot KM, Watson CA. Research-based quality assurance: the key to excellence in nursing. In: McClosky JC, Grace HK, eds. Current issues in nursing. Boston: Blackwell Scientific Publications Inc, 1985.

23. Fifer WR. Integrating quality assurance mecha-nisms. In: Luke RD, Krueger JC, Modrow RE, eds. Organization and change in health care quality assurance. Rockville, MD: Aspen Systems Corporation, 1983.

24. Froebe DJ, Bain RJ. Quality assurance programs and controls in nursing. St. Louis: The CV Mosby, 1976.

25. Fox RN, Ventura MR. Internal psychometric characteristics of the quality patient care scale. Nursing Research 1984;33(2):112–117.

26. Tehan J, Colegrove SL. Risk management and home health care: the time is now. Quality Review Bulletin 1986;179–186.

27. Hinsvark IG. Credentialing. In nursing: whatever happened to the credentialing center? In: McCloskey JC, Grace HK, eds. Current issues in nursing. Boston: Blackwell Scientific Publication Inc, 1985.

28. Brown B. Preface. In: Meisenheimer CG, ed. Quality assurance: a complete guide to effective programs. Rockville, MD: Aspen System Corporation, 1985.

29. Larson EL, Peters DA. Integrating cost analysis in quality assurance. Journal of Nursing Quality Assurance 1986;1(1):1–7.

30. Ware JE Jr. Commentary: monitoring and evaluating health services. Medical Care 1985;23(5):705–709.

31. Crane J, Horsley J. Research innovations in nursing: implications for quality assurance programs. In: Luke RD, Krueger, JD, Modrow RE, eds. Organization and change in health care quality assurance. Rockville, MD: Aspen System Corporation, 1983.

31

Outcome Indicators of Quality Care

Judy Luckenbill Brett

THE PURPOSE of this chapter is to present information about efforts to measure the most important aspect of nursing care, namely the results of practice. Patient outcomes, experienced as a result of nursing practice, reflect one key aspect of quality nursing care. This chapter begins with a discussion of the various attempts to define quality nursing care. A conceptual framework for measuring quality care is presented and the progress in attempts to measure quality are described. The importance of outcome indicators, as well as their limitations and relationships to other components of the quality nursing care model, are discussed in depth. The literature describing nursing-related outcomes is reviewed, and reported outcomes are classified and critiqued. Strategies for clarifying outcomes and their relationships to quality nursing care are provided, and a discussion of future implications of outcome indicators concludes the chapter.

QUALITY NURSING CARE

The concept of quality nursing care has been discussed and studied heavily, yet it remains poorly understood. Nursing care, even without reference to quality, is itself not well defined. The behavioral part of nursing care is observable, thus definable, and to some extent measurable. However, not all of nursing care is observable. A nurse sitting at a bedside, holding a patient's hand while explaining the patient's illness is an observable nursing action. But the sympathy, empathy, acceptance, and understanding transmitted in the nurse's action, or the message received and comfort experienced by the patient as a result, are not directly observable. Thus, part of the difficulty with identifying the quality in nursing is related to the difficulty of defining and measuring nursing itself. Despite this difficulty, much effort is currently being devoted to identifying precisely what quality is, when it exists, and what contributes to or results in quality. The marginal success of these efforts is due in part to the ambiguous nature of the term "quality".[1] Quality means various things to different people.[2]

Few authors provide formal definitions of the construct we call quality nursing care.[3] When definitions do exist, they are generally broad. For example, quality nursing care exists when the client has been assisted to attain and maintain an optimal state of functioning.[4] This and other definitions of "good health-care" are too general for practical application in the clinical setting.[5] Other authors' definitions are too narrow, those, for example, that are expressed in terms of measures or instruments used—a change in blood pressure[6] or a score range on a questionnaire.[7] Definitions as narrow as these are not transferrable to different patient groups. In addition, serious questions of validity are raised by the oversimplification of the obviously complex and multidimensional concept of quality care.

Lindeman, Hagen, and Kreuger's[8] defini-

353

tion of quality is more comprehensive. These authors define quality as the relative effectiveness of nursing care, conceptualized as a cluster of values and health status indicators, in maintaining or improving the health status of a homogeneous subset of recipients of care. This definition suggests that values and indicators are important to the measurement of quality, yet unique to specified subgroups of a population. The definition also reflects the three elements addressed in all discussions of quality: values, relativity, and standards or criteria.

Values

Values—societal, group, as well as personal—determine the definition of quality.[9,10] For example, if a society values preservation of life above all else with little regard for the quality of life, this value will be reflected in the definitions of quality nursing care in that society. However, if a subgroup in a society has values that conflict with the more general societal values, the definition of quality nursing care will be modified by that subgroup. Thus, no valid definition of quality nursing care can be developed without consideration of the values of the groups or subgroups involved as either recipients or providers of care.

Relativity

The second element in any discussion of quality nursing care is relativity, or the acknowledgment that an absolute definition of quality cannot exist. Since excellence reflects some specific point on a continuum, the point selected to represent excellence is merely a convenient operational definition[11] influenced by such factors as frame of reference, unit of analysis, expectations, and resources. Any definition of quality nursing care, therefor, varies depending on the client, agency, region, technology, and provider in-

volved.[12–13] In addition, definitions of quality nursing care are inherently dynamic since societal values change over time.[9] Given the variety of factors that need to be considered, and the infinite number of possibilities included for each of those factors, the formulation of a universal definition of quality, for even the simplest of situations, is virtually impossible.

Standards and Criteria

The third element of all discussions of quality is the need to identify standards or criteria for the measurement of quality nursing care.[6,14–17] Although Bloch[16] clearly differentiated between criterion (a value-free indicator) and standard (a value linked to an indicator), both the dictionary and common usage persist in interchanging the terms. Bloch ultimately incorporated the two terms into a "criterion referenced standard," which, as she explained, included an indicator and a level of the indicator that could be used to define the achievement of quality.[18] The attempt to separate the value from an indicator illustrates that although indicators (blood pressure, for example) may be the same for a variety of patients, the acceptable value of an indicator (120/80 for normal patients versus some other value for a hypertensive patient) may differ among patients. Most commonly today, criteria are treated as subdivisions of standards, or as discrete factors that are measurable and observable.[19] Regardless of the label (standard or criterion), or the distinction between the value and the indicator, some form of these parameters need to be decided on if discussions and definitions of quality are to be meaningful and utilitarian.

Where do standards and criteria originate? Donabedian suggested that standards are set by leaders in the field at any given time.[17] Diddie stated that the foundation for criteria is in sound principles of pathophysiology and clinical nursing as documented in medical literature that is less than six years old.[20] Observations of the norm—the most commonly occurring standard—or scientific testing of the validity of a specified standard can also be used to establish acceptable levels.[18] The most desirable origin of a standard is scientific testing, followed by systematic empirical observation, in combination with expert opinion. Regardless of their origins, standards enable us to quantify and measure the quality of nursing care. Unless quality nursing care can be measured, it cannot be tested.

In summary, authorities writing about quality nursing care consistently discuss these topics: values, criteria, or standards, and the lack of absoluteness of any definition. Differences in the authorities' discussions and definitions are due largely to their choice of terms rather than to disagreement about the essential components of quality care.

Defining quality nursing care continues to be a complex task. Although no absolute definition of quality nursing care can exist, and all definitions are value laden, a constitutive or theoretical definition can be formulated. Quality nursing care can be defined as the achievement of explicit standards or criteria that have been formulated by authorities, norms, or scientific testing, after consideration of the values and variables unique to a specific situation of nursing care. It is obvious that any operational definition of quality nursing care is of necessity relative to and dependent on the nature of the situation being evaluated. Consequently, each investigator must carefully and clearly define the desired quality for the situation being investigated.

Despite theoretical difficulties in defining quality, nurses obviously have opinions on when quality exists. In a study of reasons for working or not working, nurses had the perception that "high quality" existed when they were able to spend time with patients and provide "professional care."[21] These same nurses seldom used the term "low quality" when referring to "unsafe or inadequate care." They were also concerned about errors of omission or comission that could adversely affect the health of their patients.

A CONCEPTUAL FRAMEWORK FOR QUALITY

Any exploration of the dimensions of a concept like "quality care" should be grounded explicitly in theory, or, in the absence of theory, in a conceptual framework that has the potential for generating a theory.[22] Several conceptual frameworks of quality healthcare are potentially useful for guiding the study of nursing care quality.[23–25] However, Donabedian's systems perspective[26] has the widest application and is especially relevant for the study of nursing outcomes. Donabedian's framework also has the advantage of being simple yet comprehensive.

Donabedian first introduced his structure, process, and outcome framework in an attempt to organize the evaluation of quality medical care. Applied to nursing, the framework suggests that the varying dimensions of quality care be viewed as a structure, process, or outcome. All factors affecting, involved in, or resulting from quality nursing care can be classified using the three dimensions of this model. Propositions deriving from Donabedian's model assert that the process of care is related to the outcome of care, and that the structure in which the process of care occurs either enhances or hinders the effectiveness of care.

Structure

Many authors[5,11,26–31] have ennumerated the varying dimensions of structure. Included in these dimensions are: (a) the physical setting of an institution, its size, equipment, and facilities; (b) the philosophy and objectives of an institution; (c) personnel and their characteristics, such as attitudes, qualifications, and experience; (d) organizational arrangements, such as management structure, the organization of practice (primary, team, or functional nursing), and styles of supervision; (e) legal authority for the mission of the institution, licensure, and accreditation; (f) financing mechanisms; and even (g) the biopsychosocial condition of patients on entry into the system. Structure thus pertains to the setting in which care is given and encompasses a large variety of variables, some of which are controllable and some of which are not.

Structural variables have been the most commonly used to study quality nursing care. They are the easiest and least expensive to examine; information about structure can usually be gathered from observations, records or questionnaires.[28] The justification for using structural variables to study quality has been that adequate structures are a necessary condition of quality—without adequate buildings and policies, for example, the process of delivering care is impeded and outcomes are adversely affected.

Unfortunately, the relationship of structure to process and outcome is largely undetermined. It is not altogether clear which aspects of structure truly affect quality. Regulations are generally believed to enhance quality, but excessive regulations may inhibit innovation.[28] Similarly, personnel requirements that cannot be met by the available work force could prevent an institution from obtaining adequate numbers of qualified employees, thereby reducing quality. Quality of medical and nursing care may also be affected differently by certain aspects of structure.[32-33] Since the relationship of structure to quality nursing care remains speculative, structural variables isolated from process or outcome variables cannot be used as proxy assurances for quality nursing care.

Process

The process dimension of quality care measurement focuses on the activities, pursuits, and behaviors of nurses.[11] Behavior or lack of behavior—encompassing what is and what is not done, and what should or should not be done—is considered. Assessment, diagnosis, development of care plans, actual nursing interventions, and evaluation of their effectiveness constitute the process of quality nursing care. Patient behavior may also be included as a dimension of the process of care since the behaviors that patients display are a determinant of outcomes.[25] Some authorities[5,14,27,34] view compliance behavior not as a process, but as an outcome of patient education, for example. Part of the difficulty in measuring structure, process, and outcome is recognizing the level of analysis. Depending on whether the level of analysis is the patient, nurse, or organization, some elements of quality care can be measured as both process and outcome, or even as structure, process, and outcome. As with any morphogenic systems perspective, categorization of a variable as either structure, process, or outcome depends to some extent on one's measurement goals.

Process dimensions are generally readily available for study, via patient records or direct observation. Process is thus believed to be less expensive to measure than outcome, particularly when collecting outcome data involves following patients over a period of time.[28] Process indicators can also be measured concurrent with the care being provided, so that if problems become apparent, they can be immediately addressed.

Development of criteria to evaluate process is time consuming,[14] and often it is difficult to arrive at consensus about what the criteria should be. Peer judgments are thus frequently used in the evaluation procedure. One disadvantage of this practice is that unless explicit criteria are utilized, peer judgments of process are prone to wide intra- and interjudge variability.[28] Perhaps the most significant disadvantage of using process measures to evaluate quality nursing care is that the majority of nursing procedures lack objective proof of their value. A definite relationship between nursing process and change in health status has not been established.[27,35] Questions exist about the reliability of the most commonly used process instruments.[36–37] The problem of the reliability, however, is not unique to nursing.[38] Without scientific proof of which actions make a difference, standards or criteria must be based on norms or expert opinion; expert opinion may be inaccurate and norms may merely reinforce the status quo. Even the association of a process with an outcome may not describe causality.[30] Thus, measurement of process variables, in isolation from outcome variables, does not provide a valid assessment of quality care.

Outcome

Outcome variables are defined as the end result of care and have traditionally included mortality, morbidity, disability, social functioning, and satisfaction.[5] Outcomes have also been defined as a measured change in behavior, any alteration in health status, acquired knowledge or skill mastery, satisfaction, and compliance.[11] Outcomes are the combined result of several converging forces: the restorative process inherent in each individual; environmental and social factors; and the contributions of health professionals— nurses, physicians, and physical therapists, for example—and families.[34]

Outcome variables are the ultimate criteria by which structural and process measures are validated. Improved health status and consumer satisfaction are the stated goals of health-care providers.[4,25] Outcomes are the products of actions. Unless outcomes are measured, whether or not a goal has been

achieved remains unknown. Moreover, merely having the finest facilities and performing well does not necessarily mean that the facilities and services were necessary or appropriate in the first place.

Conversely, the sole use of outcomes to measure quality is also inadequate. Outcomes indicate good or bad care in the aggregate, but measurement of outcomes alone does not provide insight into the nature of assets and deficits to which outcomes might be attributed.[26] Outcomes are also difficult to measure due to the absence of end points or the sometimes long intervening time periods that must necessarily elapse before an outcome can be assessed.[5] Nursing outcomes are particularly difficult to measure. A female patient who survives a mastectomy provides evidence of a positive medical outcome. However, measurement of the outcomes of nursing interventions, which would be more related to the woman's adaptation to her mastectomy and to her continuation of a productive, well-adjusted life, are far more difficult to obtain—and they are most likely not the result of nursing interventions alone.[5]

Outcomes are also the most relative of the three components of quality nursing care since they vary widely for different patients. Due to the infinite number of factors that potentially affect outcomes, comparisons of outcomes cannot be done across a population unless the patients being assessed represent a fairly homogeneous subgroup.[28]

Outcome assessments are also generally more expensive to complete since the data must frequently be collected using an interview or repeat examination done after a patient has been discharged from the hospital.[28] Outcomes are also particularly sensitive to subjective value judgments. For example, whether mere prolongation of life is a positive outcome is highly questionable. Today, decisions about prolonging life are increasingly being made in light of people's expressed desire about the quality of life they

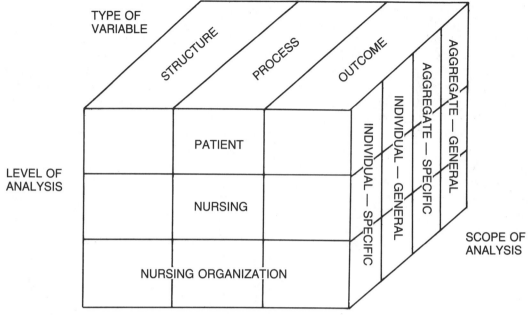

Figure 31.1.   Model of Quality Nursing Care.
Adapted from Donabedian A. Some basic issues
in evaluating the quality of health care. American Nurses Association Publication (G-124) 1976,
p. 4.

can experience.[28] It is difficult, therefore, to
arbitrarily decide exactly what is, or what is
not, a positive health outcome. Thus the
study of outcome dimensions, in isolation
from the study of process and structure dimensions, will not provide the answers
needed to completely describe quality nursing care.

Level and Scope of Analysis

In addition to the interrelationships of structure, process, and outcome, the level and
scope of analysis needs to be considered when
defining and measuring quality nursing
care.[12–13,19,25] A model of quality care is
depicted in Figure 31.1. Three levels of analysis are illustrated: patient, nursing, and
nursing organization. More analytic levels
may exist for nursing,[31] since they do exist
for other disciplines. Each of the three levels

is of interest to some nursing constituencies,
and more than one may be of interest to an
evaluator at any given point in time.[19,29,31]

Nursing organizations, for example, have
structure, nursing and managerial processes,
and outcomes.[39] The quality nursing care
model could be used to study organization
outcomes as an indication of effectiveness.
Hinshaw and Atwood's studies, evaluating
the cost and satisfaction outcomes of a structural staffing change, is an example of an
organization-level analysis.[7]

Nursing is the level of analysis whenever
specific aspects of nursing practice are tested
to measure their value. For example, changes
in the medical record form used to record a
nursing care plan represent a change in
structure. The process of doing a nursing
assessment and developing a nursing care
plan would remain unchanged, although the

Table 31.1 Standards for Patient, Nursing, and Organizational Levels of Analysis

	Structure	Process	Outcome
Patient	The amputee has the capacity, motivation, and opportunity to learn ambulation.	The diabetic patient accurately tests his or her urine for sugar and acetone.	Normal peristalsis returns by the second postoperation day.
Nursing care	The nursing process is applied in the derivation of patient care plans.	The nurse turns the unconscious patient every two hours.	A program for diabetic teaching is designed & implemented.
Organization	A fail-safe system for removing outdated supplies from nursing units exists.	The nursing division reassigns staff on each shift according to the classification-system data.	Absenteeism is reduced 50%.

Adapted from Stevens B. The nurse as executive. 3rd ed. Rockville, MD: Aspen Publishers, Inc, 1985.

form of documenting the plan would be different. The number of nursing care problems and diagnoses documented on the new form would be an outcome indicator using nursing as the level of analysis.

An assessment of patients engaging in self-care can also be done using the model, even in the absence of ongoing professional intervention. For example, the quality of self-care in a group of recovering myocardial infarction patients might be examined. The patients' health status, knowledge, experience, and past medical care would be considered aspects of structure. The patient's implementation of dietary changes, exercise protocols, and life-style changes to eliminate stress would be process variables. Measures of quality of life, adherence to changes, longevity, pain, and psychosocial well-being could be outcome measures.

Examples of different standards of structure, process, and outcome for patients, nursing, and the organization are illustrated in Table 31.1. Clear identification of the level of analysis also helps to eliminate the confusion over whether variables belong in the structure, process, or outcome category. Although often considered a process variable, patient compliance may be an outcome of a nurse's attempt to use information to change patient attitudes. Likewise, job satisfaction and employee turnover can be measured as out-

comes of an organizational change such as the implementation of primary nursing. Or they can be measured as aspects of structure in a study of the incidence of medication errors. Not only is quality relative, but structure, process, and outcome variables are also relative to the unit of analysis.

An additional consideration is the scope of analysis—the specificity and size of the target population. Examples of criteria reflecting attention to the scope of analysis are depicted in Table 31.2. An analysis may be specific or general, applying to single units or aggregates.

OUTCOME INDICATORS

The importance of outcomes for validating the process and structure of nursing care has already been highlighted.[5,29–30,40] In addition to validating nursing practice, defining and measuring outcomes is increasingly important as consumers and others involved in health care express their concern and interest in results. The Joint Commission on Accreditation of Hospitals (JCAH) has added outcome criteria to its accreditation survey. Mortality statistics of specific hospitals are being made public. The Health Care Financing Administration (HCFA) has announced that outcomes of nursing home care as opposed

Table 31.2   Criteria Reflecting the Scope of Analysis in the Measurement of Quality

	Individual	Aggregate
General	Patient understands discharge instructions.	Percent of patients understanding discharge instructions.
	Patient's blood pressure decreased.	Percent of patients experiencing a decrease in blood pressure.
Specific	Patient can state date and time of posthospital doctor's office visit.	Percent of patients stating date and time of posthospital doctor's office visit.
	Patient's blood pressure will be less than 160/100.	Patient's blood pressures will decrease by at least 5 points systolic and diastolic.

to structural arrangements will be emphasized.[41] Regulators are certainly focusing on outcomes as indicators of quality.

How will all of this emphasis on outcomes affect the nursing profession? Outcome indicators that are purely the end result of nursing care and not due in any part to some other aspect of the health-care delivery system are rare, or, at best, difficult to measure. For example, reasons for infections in central-line catheters include faulty insertion procedures on the part of the physician, faulty maintainence on the part of the nurse, or the supressed immune system of the patient. Similarly, it is difficult to assess how much of the recovery of a trauma victim is due to the surgeon who repaired the broken bones, to the nurse who assured skeletal alignment, or the patient's natural healing process.

The difficulty in identifying outcomes directly attributable to nursing lies not only in the interdisciplinary and complex nature of health care delivery, but also in the fact that the focus of nursing is holistic. Whole systems encompass far too many variables given our existing, primitive analytical methods. A nurse is not simply concerned with the patient's physical and physiological bone-mending processes or complications due to immobility. He or she is also concerned with the emotional, social, and cognitive sides of patients—their ability to cope with the life changes that trauma creates, to sleep at night, and to maintain their family support struc-

ture. The outcome of a physician's intervention is clear: the bone heals. But healing is not due to medical intervention alone.

Identifying and measuring all of the direct and indirect factors and their outcomes borders on the impossible. Nevertheless, direct and indirect measures do exist. Three forms of outcome measures are: goals and objectives, standards and criteria, and instruments.

Goals and objectives are an important measurement device in any organization.[39] Nursing organizations use goal and objective statements to provide direction and identify when success has been achieved.[42] Nursing care plans traditionally incorporate objectives of care, which are statements of the anticipated outcomes a nurse expects the patient will realize. A nursing diagnosis such as "alteration in nutrition; deficit related to loss of appetite," would most likely be accompanied by goals to improve the appetite, maintain current weight, or increase the patient's weight by a specified amount. If the statements of objectives are explicit and measurable, and if the objectives are achieved (the patient does in fact eat more, does not lose weight, or gains the specified amount of weight), then the assumption could be made that the identified interventions—for example, to provide small, frequent feedings; to arrange a dietary consult; to weigh the patient daily—were associated with the achievement of the objectives. It is important to understand, however, that in the absence of scientific proof of causality, which can only be

Table 31.3 Dimensions of an Outcome Instrument: Criterion Measures of Nursing Care Quality

Universal Dimensions	Health Deviation Dimensions
1. Air	9. IV & Wound Observation
2. Water	10. Health Deviation II
3. Food	11. Medications
4. Elimination	12. Therapeutic Diet
5. Rest/Activity/Sleep	13. Therapeutic Fluids
6. Solitude & Social Interaction	14. Exercises
7. Protection from Hazards	15. Physical Activity Restrictions
8. Normality	16. Recommended Rest
	17. Special Appliances
	18. Skin-Wound Care

Adapted from Horn B, Swain M. Criterion measures of nursing quality care. National Center for Health Services Research Summary Series. (DHEW Publication No. [PHS] 78-3187), U.S. Dept. of HEW. August, 1978.

obtained in a controlled experimental study, great "leaps of faith" must occur in linking the achievement of objectives and the interventions.[30]

Standards and criteria provide a second way in which outcomes can be measured. Nurses have a long history of involvement with standards and criteria, particularly process and structure standards.[43] Texts and articles explain how to write standards,[16,43–46] supply lists of ready-made standards and criteria,[47–51] and provide directions for the implementation of standards.[52–55] As with goals and objectives, to the extent that standards and criteria are explicit, measured, and achieved, intelligent assumptions can be made about the relationship of process and outcome.

Instruments that can be used to measure outcomes are fewer in number and newer than those for process and structure. Two instruments that offer particular promise for outcome measurement are the Patient Indicators of Nursing Care (PINC), developed by Majesky and associates, and the Criterion Measures of Nursing Care Quality.[15,34]

Data for the 24 items on the PINC are gathered using concurrent record reviews and patient observation. Three categories of indicators—infection, immobility, and fluid balance—were developed from literature reviews and empirical studies. Scoring is based on changes in the presence or absence of complications. The instrument was designed to provide a quick and easy global assessment, that could test outcomes across populations. Testing of the instrument has demonstrated inter-rater and split-half reliability, as well as content and construct validity.[15]

The Criterion Measures of Nursing Care Quality was developed by Horn and associates under a grant from the National Center for Health Services Research. Concurrent record review and patient observation are used to assess achievement of criteria derived from Orem's self-care conceptual framework. Nursing care is assessed using 8 universal and 10 health deviation dimensions (Table 31.3). Within these dimensions, a total of 539 criteria have been developed and can be selectively used to measure evidence that: (1) a requirement has been met, (2) the patient has knowledge to meet a requirement, (3) the patient possesses skills to meet a requirement, and (4) the patient has the motivation to meet a requirement. Extensive reliability testing of the instrument had been reported. All but 55 of the 539 items have demonstrated evidence of reliability. An intraclass coefficient of .99 for a small component of the instrument has also been reported.[35] Content validity for all instrument items has been established and data on construct validity is available. With the exception of the 55 untested criteria, this instrument represents the profession's most advanced effort in scientific measurement of outcome criteria.

Conditions that apply to the use of objectives and standards as indicators of outcomes also apply to the use of instruments. Instruments are more likely to have explicit and measurable criteria. Instruments should also be reliable and valid. One of the disappointing aspects of outcome instrument development has been the continued inability to demonstrate correlations of scores of outcome instruments with scores of process instruments.[35] Correlations between process instruments and outcome criteria have also been difficult to demonstrate.[32]

Nursing is not alone in its struggles to validate the outcomes of practice. Williamson claims that many medical practice outcomes are not truly validated.[38] As an example, he cites ligation of the internal mammary artery, a procedure that was widely used in the treatment of coronary artery disease during the 1950s. Outcomes attributed to the surgery included a dramatic increase in exercise tolerance and relief from angina, on the assumption that tying off the artery forced a greater blood flow through the coronary and nearby arteries. A randomized clinical trial, including a control group having surgery with exposure but no ligation of the artery, ultimately demonstrated the same outcomes for both the control and experimental groups. It is clear that all disciplines need to exercise caution in interpreting outcomes, particularly with respect to claims of causation.

Much effort has been directed toward finding associations between outcomes and nursing practice. The categories of outcomes that have been studied are listed in Table 31.4.

To demonstrate the contribution of nurse practitioners, outcomes of practice among this group of professionals have frequently been studied.[55] Comparisons of nurse practitioner outcomes to those of physicians pro-

Table 31.4 Categories of Measurable Outcomes

1. Patient satisfaction
2. Patient knowledge or understanding of disease or treatment
3. Functional health status
4. Clinical health status
5. Psychoemotional health status
6. Perceptions of patients, family, nurses, physicians
7. Disposition of patients
8. Negative results-complications
9. Discharge readiness of the patient
10. Patient compliance
11. Appearance of the patient

viding the same services,[56–57] and reports of before and after measurements following the addition of a nurse practitioner to a provider group[6,58–59] have been done. Outcomes that have been measured in regard to nurse practitioners include: patient satisfaction, compliance, and understanding; functional and clinical health status; patient perception of health status; and the cost of care. Although the study findings cannot actually prove that nurse practitioners make a difference, the studies have significant implications for all nurses. The increased consumer satisfaction and improved compliance that was typically associated with nurse practitioners in these studies may lead to long-term positive changes in health status, including less disability for diabetic children, reduced hearing loss from otitis media, and decreased rheumatic fever following tonsillitis. These examples of preventable problems are influenced by patient and family behaviors.[5] Although perhaps more finely tuned in nurse practitioners, skills that are believed to increase compliance and positively affect the behavior of patients are practiced by all nurses. Thus, the outcomes of the practice of nurse practitioners may well provide examples of outcomes that should be explored following the care provided by all nurses.

Perhaps the most frequently used outcome indicators of nursing care are measures of satisfaction and patient complaints. Satisfaction measurements of patients, families, physicians, and nurses have been widely undertaken.[60–64] Patient satisfaction is usually measured using a series of questions developed by an investigator in which the patient answers yes or no, or responds on a Likert-type scale. Evidence of reliability and validity for many of these measures is generally not provided. Two patient satisfaction with nursing care questionnaires do exist, however, that have been extensively tested and demonstrate evidence of validity and reliability. The La Monica Oberst Patient Satisfaction Scale (LOPSS) is a 41-item Likert-type scale developed for use with hospitalized patients.[62] Three subscales in the LOPSS have been identified using factor analysis: dissatisfaction, interpersonal support, and good impression. Hinshaw and colleagues[7,60] have frequently used an adapted version of the Risser Patient Satisfaction Scale.[65] This scale, too, uses a Likert-type format but has three different subscales measuring satisfaction: (a) technical-professional, (b) trusting relationship, and (c) education relationship.

It is important to note that patient satisfaction is frequently criticized as an indicator of quality nursing care.[66] The criticism is largely based on the assertions that patients cannot evaluate nurses or their care since they do not understand nursing practice and, as patients, they are hardly objective; thus their responses are automatically considered suspect. However, nurses generally believe that patient opinions are important, especially with regard to comfort and support.[67]

Patients' knowledge and understanding of their disease and treatment are frequently suggested as outcome measures.[68] Usually, questions are developed specific to the information given to a patient,[6,61,69] although one study[35] used the Horn and Swain[34] outcome criteria for patients' knowledge of medications. Typically, a pre- and post-test format with either paper and pencil tests, or a patient interview, are used. Prior to and following the implementation of a plan of care, patients are asked to identify the nature of their disease; normal values for blood pressure, blood glucose, or drug dosages; symptoms indicating complications; diet, or alterations in life style. Differences in scores before and after care are attributed to nurses' interventions.[69]

Measures of functional health status assess patients' physical and psychological capacity to perform activities of daily living.[68] Typically, an activity is measured at two points in time, and changes are noted. General scales such as the Katz Activities of Daily Living Scales have been widely used,[61] and a number of specific scales have been developed.[70] Consideration of a patient's age and social role has usually been included. Given and associates[6] measured functional status as changes in the performance of major everyday activities at work, school, or at home. Patients were initially classified as nonsymptomatic, symptomatic, reduced function but able to care for self, restricted from major activity, or bed disabled.

Clinical health status is generally measured in relation to some aspect of a patient's medical diagnosis. Physiological and physical signs and symptoms, can all be health status indicators. Measurements before and after interventions,[6] or comparisons of matched control and study groups are often done.[59,61,71] Health status variables may be easy to measure—changes in blood pressure, blood glucose values,[59] or weight loss,[72] for example. Or they may necessitate laboratory tests, such as those needed for the measurement of hypernatremic dehydration (serum sodium and blood urea nitrogen concentrations).[73] Instruments may be adapted for use: Kane adapted the California Pain Assessment Profile and the work of Melzak, which measures both the presence and intensity of pain.[61] Some researchers develop their own clinical measures. For example, Lewis developed a nausea and vomiting scale for chemotherapy patients[70]

Measurement of functional outcomes may also require sophisticated equipment for assessing changes in health status—inspirometers may be needed to measure respiratory function, a typical outcome of psychoeducational interventions with surgical patients,[63–64] or arthrographs may be necessary for measuring joint stiffness and mobility.[71]

Given and associates developed a weighted severity index of clinical outcomes[6] that included diastolic and systolic blood pressure, and end organ involvement in cardiac, optic, cerebrovascular, and renal systems. However, these investigators did not describe how the weights for the six indicators were determined.

Obviously a range of costs in terms of equipment and tests may be incurred in measurement of clinical outcomes. The results of measures of health status are generally reliable although validity is a separate issue, particularly if the outcome is being measured to validate a specific procedure. In the latter case a controlled, randomized experimental design is required.

Psychoemotional status is frequently used as an outcome indicator. Pre-existing scales that have been extensively tested for reliability and validity are available. Scales used in nursing studies include: State-Trait Anxiety Inventory, Multiple Affect Adjective List, S-R Inventory of Adjective List, Profile of Mood States,[63,64] CES-D Scale, and Rand Health Insurance Study General Well-Being Measure.[61] Observer ratings of cooperation, demanding behavior, well-being, psychological complications, apprehension and stress have also been reported.[64] Physiological indicators of psychoemotional status have been used on occasion. Palmar sweat tests, plasma fatty acids, eosinophils, vomiting, and pulse rates are examples of the indicators that are often measured.[63, 64] Lewis has developed a new

scale to measure how patients undergoing chemotherapy regard their bodies.[70]

Consumer and provider perceptions of quality of care can provide another measure of outcome. Patient opinion surveys typically are a mixture of items that call for a patient's judgment about the quality of care received and the resulting health status.[74–75] A careful examination of the items contained in survey questionnaires is necessary to discern whether the adequacy of a patient's knowledge or perceived satisfaction with care is being measured. Each of these phenomenon is quite different and calls for different questions.

Differences in perception exist among nurses, physicians, and patients about the characteristics of quality nursing care.[76] A patient may respond correctly to all questions testing the aquisition of information that a nurse believes is essential, yet not be satisfied that the knowledge gained was adequate or appropriate. Surveys designed to explore patients' perceptions of quality need to reflect the specific expectations of the developers. For example, after identifying nurses' perceptions of quality,[76] Hinshaw and colleagues used nurse perception of quality as an outcome indicator for a study of the effects of changes in staffing patterns.[7,60] Given and associates measured changes in patient perceptions of health status to explore the effectiveness of selected care processes.[6] Despite the difficulties inherent in developing and interpreting the results of opinion surveys, patient and nurse opinions and perceptions have been used as outcome indicators in a variety of situations.

Days at home versus days in hospital,[77,78] readmission or hospitalization rates,[59,79–80] length of stay,[61,63,64,79,81] days spent in intensive care units,[64] discharge to home or nursing home, and mortality rates[77,82,83] have been used as outcome indicators. Obviously, all of these indicators are influenced by multiple factors.

Negative results of care have also been investigated. Adverse drug reactions, infections, dehydration, falls, confusion, and decubitus ulcers have been measured or suggested as potential measures.[72–73,84] Majesky's PINC instrument is useful for concurrent measurement of preventable complications during hospitalization.[15] Another instrument still being developed by Vermeersch, will enable nurses to objectively identify confusion in hospitalized patients.[85] Identification of negative outcomes has led to development of risk-factor scales that assist the nurse to identify high-risk patients and begin early implementation of interventions specifically designed to prevent or minimize negative outcomes.[84]

Cost of care has also been used as an outcome indicator, particularly in studies where the organization is the level of analysis.[7,61,64,79,86] Cost is fairly easy to calculate when reductions in length of stay occur. Most hospital financial officers can provide a cost per hospital day, or use the DRG (diagnosis related group) payment rate divided by the average length of stay for the DRG. Once calculated, costs can be a powerful indicator of the value of a program or activity.

Discharge readiness has also been assessed,[78] as has patient compliance.[58] The appearance of the patient is a rather simple indicator, but one that is appropriate, particularly in long-term facilities. Appearance, for example, can be measured on a subjective cleanliness and neatness scale.[72]

It is evident that a wide range of outcome indicators exists. Although the nature, preciseness, ease, and cost of measurement of these indicators varies greatly, the sheer number of reports describing measurement of a wide range of variables indicates that nurses can and do measure outcomes. Reliability and validity for many of the outcomes reviewed have not been reported and may not exist. In some cases, evidence of reliability and validity may not be needed or warranted;

the accompanying cost may be prohibitive and greater than the benefit. Research is costly and research dollars are scarce. Resources must be invested wisely. Researchers and nonresearchers who talk about, explore, and investigate outcomes—systematically or otherwise—need to be cognizant of sound research principles and methods. They must be able to explain why certain research principles were not employed. Failure to do so will invalidate the meaning of the findings no matter how positive the outcomes.

Implications of Outcome Indicators

Defining quality is the first step in measuring its existence. Definitions of quality need to be carefully framed to reflect the values, standards, and criteria relative to each targeted situation and population.

Outcome indicators are necessary, but they are not sufficient in and of themselves. Unless aspects of the structure and process of nursing care are measured, and unless attempts are made to relate structural and process measurements to outcomes, the value of a system of care cannot be determined, fostered, or changed.

Regardless of how difficult it may be to validate the antecedents of outcomes, nurses are responsible for identifying what they expect and plan to achieve. Even in the absence of a universally accepted definition of quality nursing care, and where demonstrated relationships between varying aspects of structure, process, and outcome cannot yet be ascertained, attempts to identify and measure outcomes must nevertheless be made. Identification of outcomes using explicit goals, objectives, standards, and criteria, and continued efforts toward development of outcome instruments[92] are all highly useful and important activities. Assessing our standards and goals, as well as developing measurement instruments can demonstrate nursing's contribution to successful patient outcomes.

FUTURE DIRECTIONS FOR THE MEASUREMENT OF NURSING OUTCOMES

As the cost and quality consciousness of consumers increases, emphasis on outcomes as indicators of quality care will most likely also increase. It is evident that much work is needed to identify and define outcomes that are relevant, measurable, reliable, and valid, as well as affordable in terms of the time and resources consumed during measurement.

A starting place is to raise the consciousness of nurses about the vital nature of results— about the outcomes of care they provide. Without a doubt, nurses' actions make a significant difference. Our task is to measure and define that difference. This is not a task unique to nursing. Careful reviews of the outcomes and measurements in other disciplines, as well as in nursing, will stimulate thinking about how to apply existing measures in new ways, how to refine and adapt measures to changing circumstances, and how to create entirely new measures.

Some methods and areas of investigation worth considering include the following:

1. *Cross-sectional and longitudinal studies of the differences in individual and aggregated outcomes, within and between different groups.* Additional outcome measures need to be identified. Organizational studies focusing on the cost-benefit implications of specific outcomes should be a priority.
2. *Study of the relationship of patient outcomes and contiguous nursing processes, preferably in controlled, experimental designs.*[27,29,87] These studies will ultimately demonstrate that nursing interventions are valid and worthwhile.
3. *Study of the proximate and intermediate outcomes of care.*[88] Majesky has made a beginning by developing an instrument that can be used throughout the course

of hospitalization,[15] but more needs to be done.

4. *Studies of currently unidentified aspects of process that may better explain resulting patient outcomes.* Sullivan differentiates between "hard" and "soft" process variables.[89] Hard variables are the treatments, drug dosages, diet, and exercise regimens prescribed to "cure" an illness. Soft variables are the nonspecific aspects of patient needs, such as the need for continuity of care, affiliative bonding, communication, and participation in treatment. These variables may explain the increased effectiveness of nurse practitioners over physicians with respect to patient compliance, knowledge, and understanding. Other as of yet unidentified soft factors are, in all likelihood, more important to nurses than to physicians. Benner's explanation of how nurses acquire knowledge offers exciting promise for discovering what nurses do that changes results.[90]
5. *Documentation of outcomes, even those that can only be perceptions.* It is not enough to record what we do, but results of the doing also need to be recorded. The "impressions" of nurses need to be afforded respectability. Nurses treat human responses to actual and potential health problems.[91] If nurses "treat," then nurses, more than any others, should be the experts concerning the results of nursing practice. Patient's changed responses are our results. When a nurse writes "appears calmer," results have been observed. Nurses have not, however, been socialized to give these kinds of observations the respect they deserve, by writing, for example, "the patient *was* calmer," "was resting quietly," "had stopped pacing," "was sleeping," and so forth. All of these are indicators that the interventions to reduce anxiety—or something—worked.

Until it can be proven otherwise, that interventions have nothing to do with results, nurses can associate what they do—the nursing process—with outcomes of nursing care.

6. *Resolution of our search for pure nursing outcomes.* Physicians prescribe and pharmacists supply pain medications. Nurses hear the complaint of pain, assess the nature of pain, and choose and administer the pain-relieving intervention. It is the nurse's experience, knowledge, and observation that play a part in evaluating the timing and effectiveness of an intervention. Giving medication is supposedly a "dependent nursing function," one done under the authority of a physician. But what aspect of the process is actually dependent? How much of the medication giving above process is even interdependent? The outcome of this process—pain relief—its completeness, rapidity of onset, and duration result from the nurse's independent action.

Nurses play a key role in the delivery of health care. The nurse, therefore, as much as any other health team member should lead the way in monitoring outcomes, take appropriate professional credit when things go well, and implement corrections when they do not.

The concerns of nursing are clear: diagnosis and treatment of human responses to actual and potential health problems.[91] To achieve desired results, nurses frequently work through and with others—family support persons or other health care workers. It really should not matter who does whatever it is that produces the desired results. All that should matter is that the desired results—a fundamental concern of nursing—are identified, obtained, and replicated on demand.

Health care has entered a new era of cost and quality consciousness. Outcomes of care are a critical component of the cost-quality interface. The future of nursing in the total health-care delivery system may well depend on our sophistication—in our ability to define, measure, and influence the outcomes of care. Our skill and enthusiasm must not be found wanting.

REFERENCES

1. Curtin L. Quality, safety and the healthy hospital. Nursing Management 1987;18(2):7–8.
2. Strong V. Nursing products, primary components of health care. Nursing Economics 1985;3(1):60–61.
3. Chance K. The quest for quality. Image 1980;12(2):41–45.
4. Froebe D, Bain R. Quality assurance programs and controls in nursing. St. Louis: CV Mosby Co, 1976.
5. Bailit H, Lewis J, Hochheiser L, Bush N. Assessing the quality of care. Nurs Outlook 1975;23(3):153–159.
6. Given B, Given C, Simoni L. Relationships of processes of care to patient outcomes. Nursing Research 1979;28(2):85–93.
7. Hinshaw A, Scofield R, Atwood J. Staff, patient and cost outcomes of all-registered nurse staffing. J Nurs Adm 1981;11(11–12):30-36.
8. Lindeman C, Hagen D, Kreuger J. Targeted research: an empirical approach to defining quality of nursing care. In: ANA, ed. Issues in evaluation research. Kansas City: American Nurses Association, 1976, pp. 92–105.
9. Lang N. Issues in quality assurance in nursing. ANA Publication (G-124), 1976, pp. 45–76.
10. Nicholls M, Wessels V, eds: Nursing standards and nursing process. Wakefield, MA: Contemporary Publishing, 1977.
11. Schmadl J. QA: Examination of the concept. Nurs Outlook 1979;27:462–465.
12. Donabedian A. Some basic issues in evaluating quality nursing care. ANA Publication, (G-124), 1976, pp. 3–28.
13. Curtin L, Zurlagg C. Nursing productivity: from data to definition. Nursing Management 1986;17(6):32–41.
14. Zimmer M. Quality assurance for outcomes of patient care. Nursing Clinics of North America 1974;9(2):305–315.
15. Majesky S, Brester M, Nishio K. Development of a research tool: patient indicators of nursing care. Nursing Research 1978;27:365–371.
16. Bloch D. Criteria, standards, norms—crucial terms in quality assurance. J Nurs Adm 1977;7(7):20–30.
17. Donabedian A. Promoting quality through evaluating the process of patient care. Medical Care 1968;6:181–202.
18. Bloch D. Interrelated issues in evaluation and evaluation research. Nursing Research 1980;29:69–73.

19. Kitson A, Kendall H. Rest assured. Nursing Times 1986;82(35):28–31.
20. Diddie P. A general hospital meets the challenge. J Nurs Adm 1976;6:6–16.
21. Wandelt M, Hales G, Merwin C, Olsson N, Pierce P, Widdowson R. Conditions associated with registered nurse employment in Texas. Austin, Texas: Center For Research, School of Nursing, 1980.
22. Fawcett J. The relationship between theory and research: a double helix. Advances in Nursing Science 1978;1(1):49–62.
23. De Geyndt W. Five approaches for assessing the quality of care. Hospital Administration 1970;15(21):21–42.
24. Georgopoulos B. The hospital as an organization and problem-solving system. In: Georgopoulos B, ed. Organization research on health institutions. Ann Arbor: Institute for Social Research, 1972.
25. Starfield B. Health services research: a working model. N Engl J Med 1973;289(3):132–136.
26. Donabedian A. Evaluating the quality of medical care. Milbank Memorial Fund Quarterly 1966;44(3, Pt.2):166–202.
27. Bloch D. Evaluation of nursing care in terms of process and outcome: issues in research and quality assurance. Nursing Research 1975;24:256–263.
28. Palmer R. Quality assessment. In: Greene R, ed. Assuring quality in medical care. Cambridge: Ballinger, 1976.
29. Stevens B. The nurse as executive. 3rd ed. Rockville, MD.: Aspen Publishers, Inc, 1985.
30. Padilla G. Quality assurance programme for nursing. J Adv Nurs 1982;27(2):135–145.
31. Evans R, Brown B. A model for evaluating primary nursing. Nurs Adm Q 1981;5(4):93–100.
32. Hegyvary S, Haussman R. Correlates of the quality of nursing. J Nurs Adm 1976;6(9):22–27.
33. Neuhauser C, Andersen R. Structural comparative studies of hospitals. In: Georgopoulos B, ed. Organization research on health institutions. Ann Arbor: Institute for Social Research, 1972.
34. Horn B, Swain M. Criterion measures of nursing quality care. Washington, DC: U.S. Department of Health, Education and Welfare, 1978. DHEW Publication No. (PHS) 78-3187.
35. Ventura M, Hageman P, Slakter M, Fox R. Appraisal of quality of nursing care measures. In: Tilquin C, ed. Systems science in health care, Vol. 2, Proceedings of the International Conference on Systems Science in Health Care, Montreal, July 14–17, 1980. Toronto: Pergamon Press, 1981, pp. 1573–1578.
36. Smith R. Internal properties of the CASH nursing care evaluation instrument. Health Services Research 1975;10(2):135–145.
37. Ventura M, Hageman P, Slakter M, Fox R. Inter-rater reliabilities for two measures of nursing care quality. Research in Nursing and Health 1980;3:25–32.
38. Williamson J. Assessing and improving health care outcomes. Cambridge, MA: Ballinger Publishing Co, 1978.
39. Charns M, Schaeffer M. Health care organizations, a model for management. Englewood Cliffs, NJ: Prentice-Hall, 1983.
40. Openshaw S. Literature review: measurement of adequate care. International Journal of Nursing Studies 1984;21(4)295–304.
41. American Nurses' Association. Capital Update 1986;4(23):5+.
42. Kordick M. A quality assurance system based on management by objectives. Quality Review Bulletin 1983;9(3):83–85.
43. American Nurses' Association. A Plan for implementation of the standards of nursing practice. Kansas City: ANA, 1975.
44. Mason E. How to write meaningful nursing standards. New York: John Wiley & Sons, 1978.
45. Siegel M, Bullough B. Constructing and adapting protocols. American Journal of Nursing 1977; 77(10):1616–1618.
46. Hilger E. Developing nursing outcome criteria. Nursing Clinics of North America 1974;9(2):323–330.
47. Duke University Hospital Nursing Services. Guidelines for nursing care: process and outcome. Philadelphia, JB Lippincott Co, 1980.
48. American Nurses' Association. Standards of maternal and child health nursing practice. Kansas City: ANA, 1983b.
49. American Nurses' Association and American Association Neuroscience Nurses. Neuroscience nursing practice, process and outcome criteria for selected diagnoses. Kansas City: ANA, 1985.
50. Oncology Nursing Society and American Nurses Association. Outcome standards for cancer nursing practice. Kansas City: ANA, 1979.
51. Pigg J, Schroeder P. Frequently occurring problems of patients with rheumatic diseases. Nursing Clinics of North America 1984;19(4):697–
52. Nichols A, Wirginis M. Linking standards of care with nursing quality assurance—the SCORE method. Quality Review Bulletin, 1985;11(2):57–63.
53. Grant M. The implementation of cancer nursing standards. Quality Review Bulletin 1980;6(10):26–30.
54. Ng L, Warren J. A critical care approach to the implementation of the standards of cardiovascular nursing practice. Cardio-Vascular Nursing 1986; 22(3):13–18.
55. Fagin, C. Nursing as an alternative to high-cost care. American Journal of Nursing 1982;82(1):56–60.
56. Corbett M, Burst H. Nurse-midwives and adolescents, the South Carolina experience. Journal of Nurse Midwifery 1976;21(4):13–17.
57. Slome C, Wetherbee H, Daly M, et al. Effectiveness of certified nurse-midwives. A prospective evaluation study. American Journal of Obstetrics and Gynecology 1976;124(2):177–182.
58. Fink D, Greycloud M, Cohen M, Malloy M, Martin F.

Improving pediatric ambulatory care. American Journal of Nursing 1969;69(2):316–319.

59. Runyan J. The Memphis chronic disease program, comparisons in outcome and the nurse's extended role. Journal of the American Medical Society 1975;231(3):264–267.69.

60. Atwood J, Hinshaw A. Multiple indicators of nurse and patient outcomes as a method for evaluating a change in staffing patterns. In: Batey M, ed. Communicating nursing research, Vol. 10. Boulder, CO: Western Interstate Commission for Higher Education, 1977, pp. 235–255.

61. Kane R, Wales J. Bernstein L, Leibowitz A, Kaplan S. A randomised controlled trial of hospice care. Lancet 1984;April 21:890–894.

62. La Monica E, Oberst M, Madea A, Wolf R. Development of a patient satisfaction scale. Research in Nursing and Health 1986;9(1):43–50.

63. Hathaway D. Effect of preoperative instruction on postoperative outcomes: a meta-analysis. Nursing Research 1986;35(5):269–275.

64. Devine E, Cook T. Clinical and cost-saving effects of psychoeducational interventions with surgical patients: a meta-analysis. Research in Nursing and Health 1986;9:89–105.

65. Risser N. Development of an instrument to measure patient satisfaction with nurses and nursing care in primary care settings. Nursing Research 1975;24: 45–52.

66. Kitson A. The methods of measuring quality. Nursing Times 1986;82(35):32–34.

67. Marram G. Patients evaluations of nursing performance. Nursing Research 1973;22(2):153–157.

68. Wolff E. Systems management: evaluating nursing departments as a whole. Nursing Management 1986;17(2):40–43.30.

69. Johnson M, Mitch W, Sherwood J. Lopes L, Schmidt A, Hartley H. The impact of a drug information sheet on the understanding and attitude of patients about drugs. JAMA 1986;256(19):2722–2724.

70. Lewis F, Firsich S, Parsell S. The development of reliable measures of patient health outcomes related to quality nursing care for chemotherapy patients. In: Batey M, ed. Communicating Nursing Research, Vol. 11. Boulder, CO: Western Interstate Commission for Higher Education, 1978, pp. 52–53.

71. Beyers P. Effect of exercise on morning stiffness and mobility in patients with rheumatoid arthritis. Research in Nursing and Health 1985;8:275–281.

72. Institute of Medicine. Improving the quality of care in nursing homes. Washington, DC: National Academy Press, 1986.

73. Himmelstein D, Jones A, Woolhandler S. Hypernatremic dehydration in nursing home patients: an indicator of neglect. Journal of the American Geriatrics Society 1983;31(8):466–471.

74. Rosenman H, Jenkins M. A nursing staff designs its own system. Nursing Management 1986;17(2):32–34.

75. Simpson K. Opinion surveys reveal patients' perceptions of care. Dimensions in Health Service 1985;62(7):32–31.

76. Hinshaw A, Oakes D. Theoretical model-testing: Patients', nurses', and physicians' expectations for quality nursing care. In: Batey M, ed. Communicating Nursing Research, Vol. 10. Boulder, CO: Western Interstate Commission for Higher Education. 1977, pp. 163–187.

77. Master R, Feltin M, Jainchill J, et al. A continuum of care for the inner city. N Engl J Med 1980;302: 1434–1440.

78. Parkes C. Terminal care: evaluation of an advisory domiciliary service at St. Christopher's Hospice. Postgraduate Medical Journal 1980;56(660):685–689.

79. Jones K. Study documents effect of primary nursing on renal transplant patients. Hospitals 1975;49(24): 85–89.

80. Mortensen M, McMullin C. Discharge score for surgical outpatients. American Journal of Nursing 1986;86(12):1347–1349.

81. Bursten B. Posthospital mandatory outpatient treatment. American Journal of Psychiatry 1986;143(10): 1255–1258.

82. Saunders R, Hickler R, Hall S, Hitzhusen J, Ingraham M, Li L. A geriatric special-care unit: experience in a university hospital. Journal of the American Geriatrics Society 1983;31(11):685–693.

83. Stark A, Gutman G. Client transfers in long-term care: five years' experience. American Journal of Public Health 1986;76(11):1312–1316.

84. Janken J, Reynolds B, Swiech K. Patient falls in the acute care setting: identifying risk factors. Nursing Research 1986;36(4):215–219.

85. Vermeersch P. Development of a scale to measure confusion in hospitalized adults. Doctoral Dissertation. Case Western Reserve University, Cleveland: 1986. UMI Publication No: 87-01011.

86. Ancona-Berk V, Chalmers T. An analysis of the costs of ambulatory and inpatient care. American Journal of Public Health 1986;76(9):1102–1104.

87. Donabedian A. Needed research in the assessment and monitoring of the quality of medical care. Washington, DC: U.S. Dept. of Health, Education and Welfare, 1978, DHEW Publ. no. (PHS) 78-3219.

88. Brook E, Davies-Avery A, Greenfield S, et al. Assessing the quality of medical care using outcome measures: an overview of the method. Medical Care 1977; Supplement to 15(9):1–165.

89. Sullivan J. Guest editorial. American Journal of Public Health 1982;72(1):8–9.

90. Benner P, Tanner C. How expert nurses display their intuition. AJN 1987;87(1):23–34.

91. American Nurses' Association. Nursing: a social policy statement. Kansas City: ANA, 1980.

92. Lang N, Clinton J. Assessment of quality nursing care. In: Werley H, Fitzpatrick J, eds. Annual review of nursing research, Vol. 2. 1984.

32

Productivity Measurement

Sandra R. Edwardson

Everybody knows what productivity signifies generally. When productivity is reported to be higher here than there, or now than before, those here or now are pleased.[1] (p. 12)

MOST health-care managers would agree that improving productivity is central to the success and survival of health-care facilities. Nurses contemplating the future of their profession express a closely related concern: the urgent need to demonstrate the real contribution of nursing services to the health and well-being of citizens. Yet the term productivity is so closely associated with programs to reduce costs and eliminate waste that there is a widespread fear that productivity is the enemy of quality.

The measurement of productivity serves several purposes. It can measure progress in the production of a good or service, answering questions about whether or not an organization is improving its efficiency and the nature or quantity of its output. Productivity measurement can also provide explanations for progress in production—whether improvements in efficiency or output are due to better selection and use of inputs or to changes in the production process. Finally, productivity measurement can provide a criterion for the distribution of resources among organizations or organizational units.[1]

In their pioneering review of the literature on nursing productivity, Jelinek and Dennis identified several reasons for being concerned about productivity measurement. First, nursing services account for a large proportion of the budget of most health-care facilities. As a result, even small efficiencies can have a major impact on the cost of care. Second, the chronic shortage of qualified nursing personnel makes it important that available personnel are used wisely. Finally, difficulties encountered in measuring nursing output make it tempting to use simplistic standards such as nurses per bed and hours per patient day.[2] Inappropriate standards can result in inappropriate allocation of resources and, ultimately, in diminished quality of care.

A WORKABLE DEFINITION OF PRODUCTIVITY

Among the most difficult problems encountered in productivity measurement is finding a workable definition of the concept. The basic economic definition of productivity as the ratio of output per input is really a family of concepts that includes almost any comparison of output with input. All organizations use multiple inputs in doing their work but may produce one or many outputs. Productivity may refer to the relation between one or more outputs and all inputs, between output and one input holding all others constant, or between output and all other inputs holding one constant.

The clarity of the concept of productivity seems to vary according to the sector of the economy under consideration. In the industrial sector, and especially in firms manufacturing only a few discrete products, such as automobiles or computers, the quality and quantity of inputs can usually be measured in physical units such as number and properties of raw materials and personnel. Output can also be measured in physical terms using quantity, directly observable quality, and market-clearing prices.

Health-Care Productivity

The service sector of the economy, and health care in particular, present major problems in productivity measurement. Chief among these is the fact that health-care organizations produce services rather than physical products. Moreover, production and consumption of a service are usually simultaneous events, creating major management and analytic problems.

From the management point of view, services, unlike physical products, cannot be produced during periods of slack demand to be stored for use or sale in periods of peak demand. Nor can the provision of services be postponed due to excessive demand for service or a shortfall of inputs. Characteristics such as these mean that high productivity depends on complex systems for expanding and contracting productive capacity. In acute care settings, productivity (as conventionally measured) may be attenuated unavoidably by a need for standby capacity to meet an unexpected demand for services such as maternity and emergency care.

Measuring the productivity of service organizations also presents analytic problems. Manufacturing firms frequently produce a variety of products, varying in quality, materials, and purpose. But few firms produce the range and complexity of outputs generated by hospitals and other health-care facilities. Berry observed: "Hospitals are in fact an extreme case of multiproduct firms and, unfortunately, a classic example of firms for which it is virtually impossible to differentiate completely among the several services produced."[3]

The output of hospital services has most frequently been measured in terms of patient days. Other outputs that have been considered are specific hospital services, episodes of illness, end results, health levels, and intermediate inputs.[4] Of these, end results and health levels have the greatest intuitive appeal since they capture the ultimate purpose for providing health-care services. Chen and Bush, for example, define output as the difference between the stock of health (or value of input) before treatment and the stock of health (or value of output) after treatment.[5]

Yet using outcomes and health levels as the output presents problems. First, there are no widely accepted measures of health status.[6] Second, health-care services are but one of several possible factors contributing to the status of people's health. In addition to the quality and quantity of health care, outcome and health status can be affected by the patient's basic biologic capacity and willingness to comply with prescriptions, by the level of economic development and public health measures in the community, and by events that intervene between the provision of the service and the patient's ultimate outcome. As a result, hospital services can be viewed as an intermediate input into the production of the highest attainable level of health; these services make a marginal or "value-added" contribution to health status.[4]

Lacking an available and meaningful indicator of health status or outcome for use as a measure of output of hospital services, analysts have chosen instead to use intermediate outputs such as hospital days and number of procedures performed. Recently, two important modifications of these outputs have been introduced. First, outputs are increasingly conceived of as incorporating consideration of the quality, as well as quantity of services produced.[7] Productivity evaluation, therefore, requires measures of inputs, outputs, and quality.

The second change in output evaluation is the trend toward using the concept of case mix. "Case mix" is the term used to describe the combination of inpatient care treatments produced by hospitals.[8] Interest in case mix derives from the well-known fact that patient days are not homogeneous units but vary in nature and in the numbers and types of resources required to produce them.

Berki observed that patient stays are associated with three types of services: (1) admission-specific services that are independent of the diagnosis on admission or discharge and of the length of stay, (2) stay-specific services, such as routine nursing care and hotel-type services, determined by length of stay and largely independent of the diagnosis, and (3) diagnosis-specific services determined by suspected or defined diagnosis, modified by case severity. Berki asserted that cost variations for the first two services can be adequately captured by unweighted patient days, but that diagnosis-specific services require the use of case-mix weighted patient days.[4]

Current conceptualizations of case mix rely on a definition of hospital output as treated cases where treatment is the combination of services expected to result in a positive outcome, given patient illness characteristics and the current state of knowledge. "Instead of measuring the actual change in health status, we assess the degree to which the hospital provides the inputs that can be expected to lead to the desired change in health" in each case mix category.[9]

Case-mix measurement methods have become an important public policy issue since Medicare's shift to prospective payment based on one case-mix measure, Diagnosis Related Groups (DRGs). Prospective payment reflects the change in the goal of health-care policy in the seventies "from getting the most health benefit for each health-care dollar to limiting the total number of dollars spent."[6] During the sixties and early seventies, policy makers were preoccupied with constraining health-care cost inflation by defining hospitals' output and explicating cost

functions. Since then, the goal has changed from controlling costs per unit of output, to controlling total expenditures.

Because the results of these strategies focusing on per unit cost control were considered inadequate, the focus subsequently changed to refining output by applying case-mix methods to create more homogeneous output units. Although the DRG method is currently in use by the Medicare program, there is a common expectation that it will be modified or supplanted by other case-mix measurement strategies. Leading contenders include the patient severity index,[10] disease staging,[11] and patient management categories.[12]

To summarize at this point, productivity assessment in health-care organizations is complicated by the fact that services are produced and consumed at the same time and that it is difficult to identify a useful and acceptable definition of output. Because many factors in addition to health-care services contribute to health status and a patient outcome from an episode of care, outputs of any particular health-care service can be viewed as an intermediate output and as an input into the production of health. Various case-mix measures are currently under investigation to identify more adequately the output of hospitals.

Nursing Productivity

Most investigations of nursing productivity have concentrated on nursing services delivered in hospitals. My discussion will continue in that vein.

Jelinek and Dennis were among the first to attempt a comprehensive review of the existing knowledge regarding nursing productivity.[2] Although they found a multitude of published papers and studies related to one or more of the elements possibly related to productivity, they found no organizing conceptual framework for understanding all the related elements. Consequently, these investigators proposed a systems model of nursing productivity in which the inputs for nursing services are transformed by technology (processes) into outputs. Consistent with system theory, they also included important contributing environmental factors.

Jelinek and Dennis chose a systems rather than the more traditional economic model for productivity evaluation because of their belief that the structure and operation of nursing-care delivery is not appreciably explained by marketplace perspectives.

I have selected an economic frame of reference, which concentrates on the input-output ratio, for this discussion, however, because of the clear and growing need for nurses to justify the expenditure of resources in quantitative terms.

Using economic terms, productivity is viewed as a relative concept meaning that it is "good" or "bad" only in relation to past performance or the performance of comparable producers. High productivity is preferred to low productivity, assuming that the outputs are of the desired quality and the level of productivity can be sustained over a period of time.

To focus on inputs and outputs is not to denigrate the importance and usefulness of a systems model. In an economic model, the process and environment components are simply thought of somewhat differently—as variables that permit or hinder improvements in productivity. Process, therefore, will be discussed with respect to how it can affect the level of output obtained from a given level of input.

The environment of an organized nursing service can be as near as the other hospital departments or as remote as the federal government. While nurses can and should seek to alter environmental factors to enhance the delivery of nursing care services, they can frequently do so only in the long run. For that reason, this presentation restricts productivity evaluation to those inputs and outputs under the more-or-less direct and short-term control of nurse practitioners and managers.

Inputs

The concept of inputs into nursing service production is conceptually simple but analytically problematic. Inputs include the raw materials, personnel, supplies, and equipment used to provide care. The contribution of supplies and equipment to the production of nursing services has received considerable attention by investigators in the service setting. Supplies and equipment have also been included as an integral element of nursing actions in a number of research studies.

The concept of raw materials is more difficult to incorporate, however. For human service organizations, patients and clients are the principal raw material. Unfortunately, patients and clients do not come in homogeneous units, and, as some of the case-mix research suggests, they may not even come in homogeneous groupings. Hence, a major measurement problem in doing productivity evaluation is how to account for variations in patient characteristics so that productivity ratios can be adjusted for differences in inputs when comparisons are made.

The hospital case mix measures I described earlier are designed to use information available only at the time of discharge. While conceptually consistent with efforts to classify patients into homogeneous groups at the start of service, these measures need to be modified to standardize the measurement of inputs, especially when they are used to analyze specific patient groups or patient care units. Disease staging methods, for example, applied at the time of admission, might well provide useful information for standardizing patient types on medical diagnosis.

Patient classification systems developed for personnel staffing purposes are the principal tools used to differentiate patient types with respect to nursing care. Based on direct measurements of the time required to provide care to patients, patient classification can provide valid and reliable estimates of the total time (and expense) required to give nursing care in a given setting. These systems were developed out of a recognition that two patients with the same medical diagnosis or of the same age may have significantly different care requirements due to differences in severity of illness, coexisting and complicating conditions, motivation, and other factors.

Patient classification systems are usually developed to be institution specific. As Levine and Phillip noted, the optimum number and mix of nursing personnel will vary with the range of services provided, the physical layout of the facility, the degree of automation, institutional routines, prevailing wage rates, turnover levels, and the amplitude of fluctuations in patient arrivals.[13] Because classification systems are customized for each setting, and because most systems predict time, but not personnel skill requirements, any two organizations' systems are unlikely to provide comparable data.

The use of patient classification data to standardize the patient-characteristic portion of inputs into nursing care need to be carefully considered for another reason as well. One of the chief purposes of classification systems is to predict shift-to-shift variations in personnel work load: a patient's requirement for nursing care at the time of admission is not necessarily predictive of total care requirements for the hospitalization because of the increase or decrease in level of function that may result from hospital treatments. Patient classification data, therefore, may be valuable if collected retrospectively for the total length of stay. Such modifications of an input measure would mean that the input is not entirely independent of the process of care, in that nursing interventions, or the lack thereof, may have influenced the amount of nursing care required during the hospitalization.

Outputs

Although there are issues related to the measurement of nursing inputs, the study of nursing productivity has suffered more from two other constraints: lack of an adequate output measure and lack of an adequate model of the production of nursing services.[14–15] Because of difficulties in measuring health status outcomes, Jelinek and Dennis concluded that output in the nursing productivity framework should be the nursing process, operationally defined as the nursing service rendered, including personnel outcomes, such as absenteeism, and patient outcomes.[2] Implicit in their conclusion, Jelinek and Dennis adopted the intermediate output approach used by analysts of overall hospital productivity.

In her critique of the Jelinek and Dennis model, Aydelotte questioned their choice of output variables. She spoke specifically of the inclusion of variables such as employee satisfaction and turnover in the definition of output, asserting that nursing output should be related to institutional purposes of care, teaching, and research. "The output of a subsystem should be related to the overall purposes of the institution and the mandate it has been given from society."[16] Aydelotte also maintained that components of productivity should be described operationally as processes or outcomes in terms that are understandable by persons other than nurses.

If nursing adopts the intermediate output approach to evaluating nursing output, then output is probably best defined operationally as the nursing services rendered. Nursing services rendered could include patient days, hours of care, procedures, visits, and other activity measures. As in the measure of overall hospital productivity, however, these output indicators are not necessarily homogeneous. Case-mix measures, therefore, are also important for creating more homogeneous nursing care outputs.

Ever since the introduction of DRGs, nurses around the country have questioned whether DRGs are an adequate measure of the variability of nursing resource consumption. A large number of papers have been published in the past four years demonstrating that some DRG-created groupings may adequately estimate nursing care requirements. But these same studies have also found that the resources required by patients in other DRGs vary wildly and that the DRG system fails to capture this variability.[17–20] Having demonstrated this shortcoming, it is important that nurses continue to search and lobby for case-mix measures that more adequately represent the resources required to provide acceptable care.

Improved case-mix measurement will help in investigating the efficiency of nursing services but it does not address the effectiveness issue. The effectiveness of the output can be understood as the safety, appropriateness, and excellence of care, and as encompassing changes in health status, patient outcome, and patient satisfaction.[7] Although efficiency has always been an ingredient in productivity analysis, incorporating the concept of quality of the output is more recent and presents greater problems. Part of the difficulty has already been addressed—namely, the problem of identifying acceptable health status and outcome measures.

But a closely related problem is the presumption among many health-care providers that efficiency is the enemy of quality. Reilly and Legge conjectured that, because of the high degree of uncertainty present in the health-care process, providers may be unable to consider technological trade-offs that are common in other sectors of the economy. "Because medical certainty is frustrated by the idiosyncratic nature of the individual patient, refinements in the technology became

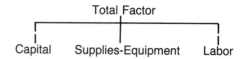

Figure 32.1 Types of Productivity Evaluation.

necessary to account for these variables."[21] It is probably correct to say that both physicians and nurses have adopted the notion that more care is better care in an attempt to deal with the complexity of the problems and the uncertainty a caseload of patients presents.

Jelinek and Dennis dealt with the effectiveness issue by defining productivity as "the relationship between the amount of acceptable output produced and the input required to achieve that output."[2] Accepting this definition implies that the goal of nursing services is not necessarily to achieve the best possible outcome or maximal health status, but an acceptable level of outcome or health status. The analytic task for productivity evaluation, therefore, is to identify and develop operational definitions of acceptable output. It is beyond the scope of this paper to describe what this definition might be. But it is likely to be different from the idealistic standards set by professional associations, and more likely to correspond to the modest operational standards and guidelines used in many service settings.

LABOR PRODUCTIVITY IN NURSING

The study of productivity is generally of two types: total factor and labor productivity. As shown in Figure 32.1, total factor productivity evaluates the contributions of all types of inputs to the output of a firm. Labor productivity analysis is more commonly used, and, in a service occupation such as nursing, this form of analysis is also more important.

Figure 32.2 proposes that labor productivity in nursing is a function of the characteristics of personnel, the technology employed, and management practices. In the discussion

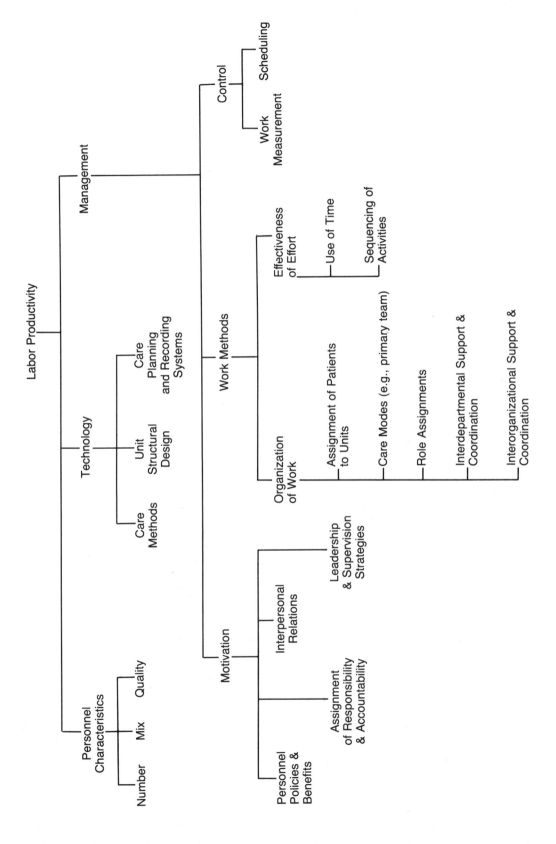

Figure 32.2 Factors Affecting Labor Productivity.

that follows, each of the variables identified in the figure is defined, and a brief synopsis of some of the relevant theoretical and empirical findings is presented. The literature discussed is not intended to be an exhaustive review; moreover it relies heavily on the excellent 1981 review of nurse staffing by Young, Giovannetti, Lewison, and Thoms.[22]

Personnel Characteristics

Personnel variables correspond to the factors that are traditionally included as the inputs of productivity models. Personnel inputs are best measured in terms of the number of physical units such as full-time equivalents (FTEs) or number of hours worked. These units may not be homogeneous, however, due to individual differences in educational preparation and skill level. Therefore, personnel units have been defined to include the number, skill mix, and quality of personnel.

Number of Personnel

Research into the effects of the number of nursing staff employed has produced mixed results. Although the size of nursing staff is assumed to affect the process of care, Di-Marco and associates found that the quality of nursing care plans and a total quality score, composed of measures of the care plan, patient record, and nursing care, were negatively correlated with the number of full-time and part-time registered nurses (R.N.s) employed in the medical-surgical units of one hospital.[23]

Skill Mix

Research and evaluation into the skill mix of the nursing staff have also produced contradictory results. A high proportion of professional nurses has been found to be related to better coordination;[24] lower omission rates of required nursing tasks;[25] performance of a greater number of tasks, and a larger proportion of professional tasks;[26] and an increased number of patient problems identified and documented.[27] New and associates, on the other hand, found that professional nurses did not increase the time they spent with patients when the ratio of registered nurses was increased.[28]

Others have questioned whether the substitution of nonprofessional for professional nursing personnel—a commonly used cost cutting strategy in nursing—can produce gains in efficiency. Cost savings are believed to be attenuated because less-skilled workers are less flexible, require more supervision, and have more nonproductive time than professional nurses.[29–31]

Most empirical studies of all R.N.s, or predominantly R.N. staffs, have suffered from methodological problems. Some have been uncontrolled case studies.[27,32–33] Other investigators have evaluated the simultaneous introduction of an enriched staff mix and primary nursing, making it impossible to differentiate the changes attributable to skill mix from those due to the mode of organizing care.[34–37] In addition, few of these studies have established the equivalence of units being compared in terms of the nature of clients served, salary rates, occupancy rates, quality of leadership, and the nature of patient outcomes.[22]

Methodological problems like these suggest the need to conduct studies that are either input- or output-oriented. Input-oriented studies have as their goal minimizing inputs rather than maximizing outputs; they manipulate inputs rather than process or output. Output-oriented studies, on the other hand, seek to maximize the quantity or quality of output by altering the way given resources are used. Confusion arises when both inputs and processes are manipulated in the same study.

Quality of Personnel

The quality of nursing personnel has been studied most frequently in relation to the educational preparation of nurses.[38–42] Young and associates conclude that studies of the educational preparation of nursing personnel suffer from such methodologic problems as the lack of attention to sample size, sample selection, and response rate. Although the studies reviewed by Young, Giovannetti, Lewison, and Thoms demonstrated observable differences among educational levels on selected performance characteristics, none explicitly addressed the relevance of education to staffing, organizational mode, and other staffing issues.[22]

Harbison used the concept of human capital formation in discussing the productivity of modern industrial societies. Human capital formation is the process of acquiring and increasing the numbers of people with skill, education, and experience that are strategic for the development of the country. This human capital can be imported into the country, developed in employment, or developed through training and educating a new generation of workers. In his research conducted in the decade after World War II, Harbison found that the increase in high-level workers in the 50 companies studied was related to innovation, especially among companies that developed new products, or designed new systems of administration. He also found that a greater use of professional and managerial employees resulted in an increase in fixed and overhead costs but that the greater use of high-level employees was primarily associated with dynamism and progress, rather than the expansion of bureaucracy.[43]

Technological Factors

Technology is understood to be equivalent to Perrow's concept of techniques as the activities used to transform raw materials into products. In nursing, technology refers to the nursing care practices intended to comfort and improve patients' health status. Three indicators of technology are care methods, unit structural design, and care planning and recording systems.

Care Methods

Care methods include the numerous interventions employed by nurses to carry out a patient's plan of care. Piper divided these interventions into three categories: (1) daily essential activities that are common services nurses provide to all patients, (2) physician-dependent interventions, those that are ordered by doctors as part of the medical plan of care, and (3) independent functions, those activities identified on the basis of nursing assessment and diagnosis.[44]

Productivity is likely to be affected by each of these types of interventions. Citing the general disregard for independent nursing interventions, Snyder recently compiled a description of these independent functions.[45] Much of the existing clinical nursing research can be used in future studies of productivity. Research examining the clinical efficacy of interventions would be even more useful if investigators measured cost and other resource-use data along with the variables of primary interest.

Unit Structural Design

Another variable included in the technology category is the structural design of units. Design refers to the physical layout of inpatient units and includes such physical structures as linear, circular, spoke, and Friesen arrangements, as well as total work area, area per bed, number of beds, and availability of equipment. The literature review by Young and associates found travel time to be generally lower in circular and radial units. No attention, however, had been given to other factors that affect productivity, such as the organizational mode of nursing and the characteristics of patients.[22] Other factors likely to be affected by unit design are the availability of supplies, communication devices, and assistance from other personnel—all factors that can be expected to affect the efficiency and effectiveness of work.

Care Planning and Recording Systems

A final technology variable is care planning and recording systems. Nurses have shown a good deal of interest in both planning and recording systems. In addition to the numerous care planning and charting guides that have been published, development of computerized information systems that incorporate care planning and documentation suggest that nurses hope to improve both the quality and efficiency of care.[46–48]

Management Factors

Management includes the planning, organizing, directing, and controlling activities used to accomplish organization objectives. Operationally, the variables that are hypothesized to affect labor productivity most directly are motivation, work methods, and control.

Motivation

Motivation in management is concerned with what mobilizes human behavior, what directs behavior toward a goal, and how such behavior is sustained over time.[49] Although nursing has been found to be an occupation with high motivating potential,[50] most studies of motivation have attempted to understand factors believed to be associated with decreased motivation or with management practices that enhance or interfere with motivation.

Levels of motivation are hypothesized to be influenced by personnel policies and benefits, assignment of responsibility and accountability, interpersonal relations, leadership, and supervision strategies. One or more of these motivation factors has been investigated in each of the numerous studies of job satisfaction and turnover among nurses.[51–54] Although the results of these studies are mixed, the preponderance of evidence seems to suggest that nurses are more likely to be satisfied by achievement, responsibility, greater job scope, and recognition than by work conditions, salary, and status. Much research remains to be done to determine which if any of these factors have differential effects on the quality or efficiency of nursing services.

There is good reason to think that recognition, responsibility, and the like make a difference in productivity. Describing the United States economy as a whole, Moore and Moore observed that quantum leaps in productivity have been made through technical invention, development, and improvement, and that gains in productivity are possible only where there is recognition of opportunity, the freedom to experiment, and the right to fail.[55]

Katzell, reporting the experience of several companies in which productivity improved, concluded that productivity is associated with one or more of the following conditions:

1. Mechanisms exist by which employees participate in decisions that affect their work,
2. The scope of duties of rank-and-file workers has been enlarged,
3. Managers and supervisors participate in decisions that affect both their own and related operations,
4. Channels of communication and of authority have been reduced in number and in length,
5. Pay increases are related to increases in performance and responsibility, and
6. Improved supervision, work methods, and technology have reduced worker

frustration and increased overall effectiveness.[56]

Work Methods

Work methods include two broad categories of variables: organization of work and effectiveness of effort. Organization of work has received a great deal of attention. Beginning with the first attempts to organize patients according to primary diagnosis or type of service required, assignment of patients to units best suited to meet their special needs has become a major method for assuring the efficiency and effectiveness of hospital services. In recent years, the most rapid growth has been in intensive care units (ICUs). Evolving from postoperative recovery rooms in the 1940s, ICUs were increasing at the rate of 5 to 6% by the early 1980s.[57,58] Questions have been raised about whether these units have improved survival rates and quality of life, and whether or not they are worth the associated high cost.[59, 61] Since nursing services are a major component of the cost of these units, the use of ICUs is an example of an organizational issue that could have a significant impact on nursing productivity.

The organizational mode of nursing care delivery is another widely studied subject. The four dominant modes that have evolved are, in historical order, the case method, the functional mode, team nursing and primary nursing. Variations have included total patient care and modular nursing.

The Young and associates literature review found that primary nursing is superior to team nursing in virtually all comparisons. But as noted earlier, studies evaluating the costs and benefits of primary nursing often have been done in conjunction with interventions altering the ratio of professional to nonprofessional staff as well. Because of the problems of sorting out the independent contribution of organization mode and staff mix, the findings of these studies are questionable.[22]

Another way to study work methods is to consider the effectiveness of effort, an approach that has received relatively little attention. Data about the use of time and sequencing of activities are frequently a byproduct of work measurement studies used to develop patient classification systems. Christman and Clark compared the degree to which registered nurses and nursing assistants stayed occupied. They found that nursing assistants were busy only 65 to 73% of the time, while registered nurses were occupied 92 to 100% of the time.[30–31]

Role Assignments

Roles are behavioral patterns that have established norms,[62] include a set of prescribed behaviors, and provide an area of choice with respect to activities, methods, and styles. Role expectations are of two types: self-expectations and others' expectations, each of which may vary in importance as motivators. Organizational role expectations are defined by the systematic properties of an organization as a whole, the subsystem in which a person is located, and the particular position occupied by both a focal person and role set.[63] Studies of role perception and stress among hospital employees, including nurses, have revealed that there is an association between role perception and stress.[64–66] Educational strategies have been used successfully with nurses to produce positive effects on role perception and role assumption.[67–68]

Interdepartmental and interorganizational support refers to the amount of instrumental assistance provided by personnel and organizational units other than a focal work-group. Coordination among departments and organizations means the extent to which these units work or act together harmoniously. While the potential influence of both support and coordination on productivity seems obvious, these variables have been subjected to little systematic investigation. An exception is the work of Munson and associates. The investigators hypothesized that coordination is likely to be especially important in situations that are complex and where the patient population is variable and subject to unpredictable changes in condition. Munson and associates also suggested that the need for nursing personnel will vary with the availability of support services.[69]

Control

The final management variable is control, defined here to include such activities as work measurement and scheduling. Work measurement is a set of methods for determining the characteristics of work activities under stable conditions through a time device and performance rating adjustments. Examples include time study, motion study, micromotion work sampling, and predetermined motion-time study.[70] Since the first patient classification systems for predicting nurse staffing requirements were introduced in the 1950s, patient classification has grown to be a common feature in virtually all hospitals. In addition to assisting with staffing and scheduling decisions, the data generated by classification have been useful in identifying nursing costs for individual patients, for planning nursing assignments, and for assigning patients to units.[71] But the patient classification systems are only as good as the methods used to develop and maintain them. The challenge ahead for managers is to continually monitor the classification systems for validity and reliability to assure that their accuracy and credibility is maintained.

FUTURE DIRECTIONS

The problem of productivity measurement is complex because (1) measuring the outcome of nursing care is difficult and often controversial, (2) the relationships between care processes and nursing outcomes are not al-

ways well understood, and (3) the most efficient combination of resources for performing many care processes is not known. Finding solutions to these problems suggests a large number of topics for future research. Solutions also require creative coordination of efforts by researchers and practitioners.

What should productivity evaluation be designed to do? To paraphrase Lipscomb's specification of health program evaluation, productivity evaluation should: (1) allocate resources so as to maximize the health status to clients, (2) simultaneously link information about the process of care with information about the structure and outcome of care, and (3) classify a target population into relatively homogeneous groups with respect to the variables associated with their needs for nursing care, such as severity of illness and degree of functional impairment. These mandates imply a need for information about the following:

1. types of resources potentially able to meet health-care needs of a target population,
2. the effective availability of each resource,
3. alternative intervention strategies at each clinically defined stage of each disease at which programs might be directed,
4. the amount of each resource required to undertake each alternative intervention strategy, and
5. the expected impact of each strategy on the health status of each subpopulation in a target population.[72]

To accomplish these tasks, nurses are needed who are able to overcome their suspicion of productivity management. Since management engineering was first applied to hospitals in the early 1900s, nurses have sometimes feared that careful analysis of work threatened the quality of care. In part, nurses' apprehension may stem from a tendency to confuse increased service intensity with improved quality.

Fear that increased productivity automatically signals decreased quality can be removed only by ensuring that output indicators are adjusted for quality, or that outputs are explicit measures of quality. While increasing productivity, by definition, will lower cost, the use of quality-adjusted output measures assures that the quality of nursing care will not be compromised.

Jelinek and Dennis proposed a definition of nursing productivity over 10 years ago. It continues to summarize our collective thinking today.

The concept of productivity encompasses both the effectiveness of nursing care, which relates to its quality and appropriateness, and the efficiency of care, which is production of nursing output with minimal resource waste.[2]

REFERENCES

1. Fabricant S. Meaning and measurement of productivity. In: Dunlop JT, Diatchenko VP, eds. Labor productivity. New York: McGraw-Hill, 1964, pp. 12–26.
2. Jelinek RC, Dennis LC. A review and evaluation of nursing productivity. Washington, DC: U.S. Department of Health, Education and Welfare, 1976, DHEW publication no. (HRA) 77-15.
3. Berry RE. Cost and efficiency in the production of hospital services. Milbank Memorial Fund Quarterly 1974;52:291–313.
4. Berki SE. Hospital economics. Lexington, MA: DC Heath, 1972.
5. Chen MW, Bush JW. Maximizing health systems output with political and administrative constraints using mathematical programming. Inquiry 1976;13:215–227.
6. Marmor TR, White WD. Increasing the productivity of health personnel: labor market issues. In: National Council on Health Planning and Development. Productivity and Health—Papers on Incentives for Improving Health Productivity. Washington, DC: U.S. Department of Health and Human Services, 1980, DHHS publication no. (HRA) 80-14025. p. 32.
7. Applied Management Sciences, Inc. Productivity and health: hospital productivity—a synopsis of the literature. Washington, DC: U.S. Department of Health and Human Services, 1980, DHHS publication no. (HRA) 80-14028.
8. Klastorin TD, Watts CA. On the measurement of hospital case mix. Medical Care 1980;18:675–85.
9. Hornbrook MC. Hospital case mix: its definition, measurement and use: Part I. The conceptual framework. Medical Care Review 1982;1:1–43.
10. Horn SD, Chan C, Chachich B, Clopton C. Measuring severity of illness: homogeneous case mix groups. Medical Care 1983;21:14–30.
11. Gonnella JS, Goran MJ. Quality of patient care—a measurement of change: the staging concept. Medical Care 1975;13:467–73.
12. Young WW, Swinkola RB, Zorn DM. The measurement of hospital case mix. Medical Care 1982;20:501–12.
13. Levine JD, Phillip PJ. Factors affecting staffing levels and patterns of nursing personnel. Bethesda, MD: U.S. Department of Health, Education and Welfare, 1975, DHEW Publication no. (HRA) 75–6.
14. Aydelotte MK. Nurse staffing methodology: A review and critique of selected literature. Washington, DC: U.S. Department of Health, Education and Welfare, 1973, DHEW publication no. (NIH) 73-433.
15. Griffith JR. Measuring hospital performance. Chicago: An Inquiry Book, 1978.
16. Aydelotte MK. The model and description of variables. In: Jelinek RC, Dennis LC, eds. A review and evaluation of nursing productivity. Washington DC: U.S. Department of Health, Education and Welfare, 1976, DHEW publication no. (HRA) 77-15. p. 342.
17. Riley W, Schaefers, V. Costing nursing services. Nurs Manag 1985;4:40–43.
18. Mitchell M, Miller J, Welches L, Walker DD. Determining cost of direct nursing care by DRGs. Nurs Manag 1984;15:29–32.
19. McKibbin RC, Brimmer PF, Clinton JF, Galliher JM, Hartley SS. DRGs and nursing care. Kansas City: American Nurses' Association, 1985.
20. Sovie MD, Tarcinale MA, Vanputee AW, Stunden AE. Amalgam of nursing acuity, DRGs and costs. Nurs Manag 1985;16(3):22–42.
21. Reilly BJ, Legge JS. The embattled hospital: cost control measures versus imperatives for expansion. Journal of Health Politics, Policy and Law 1982;7:254–70.
22. Young JP, Giovannetti P, Lewison D, Thoms ML. Factors affecting nurse staffing in acute care hospitals: a review and critique of the literature. Hyattsville, MD: Department of Health Education and Welfare, 1981, publication no. (HRA) 81-10.
23. DiMarco N, Castels MR, Carter JH, Corrigan MK. Nursing resources on the nursing unit and quality patient care. International Journal of Nursing Studies 1976;13:139–52.
24. Georgopoulous BS, Mann FC. The Community Hospital. New York: Macmillan, 1962.
25. Miller SJ, Bryant WD. A division of nursing labor: experiment in staffing a municipal hospital. Kansas City: Community Studies Inc, 1965.
26. Marram G, Flynn K. Abaravich W, Carey S. Cost-effectiveness of primary and team nursing. Wakefield, MA: Contemporary Publishing, 1976.

27. Hinshaw AS, Scolfield R, Atwood JR. Staff, patient, and cost outcomes of all-registered nurse staffing. J Nurs Admin 1981;11(11):30–6.
28. New PK, Nite G, Callahan J. Too many nurses may be worse than too few. Mod Hosp 1959;93(4):104–9.
29. Fettler MD. Manpower substitution in the hospital industry: some causes and implications. Hosp Admin 1972;17:26–42.
30. Christman L. A micro-analysis of the nursing division of one medical center. Nurs Digest 1978;6(2):83–7.
31. Clark EL. A model of nursing staffing for effective patient care. J Nurs Admin 1977;7(2):22–7.
32. Burt ML. The cost of all-RN staffing. In: Alfano G, ed. All-RN nursing staff. Wakefield, MA: Nursing Resources, 1980, pp. 87–90.
33. Miller PW. Staffing with RNs. In: Alfano G, ed. All-RN nursing staff. Wakefield, MA: Nursing Resources, 1980, pp. 91–5.
34. Dahlen A. With primary nursing, we have it all together. Am J Nurs 1978;78:426–8.
35. Marram G, Barret MW, Bevis EM. Primary nursing: a model for individualized care. St. Louis: CV Mosby, 1974.
36. Osinski EG, Powals JG. The cost of all RN staffed primary nursing. Supervisor Nurs 1980;11:16–21.
37. Nenner VC, Curtis EM, Eckhoff CM. Primary nursing. Supervisor Nurs 1977;8(5):14–6.
38. Reichow RW, Scott RE. Study compares graduates of two-, three-, and four-year programs. Hospitals 1976;50(14):95–100.
39. Davis BG. Clinical expertise as a function of educational preparation, Nurs Res 1972;21:530–4.
40. Davis BG. Effects of levels of nursing education on patient care. Nurs Res 1972;23:150–5.
41. Nelson LF. Competence of nursing graduates in technical, communicative, and administrative skills. Nurs Res 1978;27:121–5.
42. Hogstel MO. Associate degree and baccalaureate graduates: do they function differently? Am J Nurs 1977;77:1598–1600.
43. Harbison F. High-level manpower, productivity, and economic progress. In: Dunlop JT, Diatchenko VP, eds, Labor Productivity. New York: McGraw-Hill, 1964, p. 332–335.
44. Piper LR. Accounting for nursing functions in DRGs. Nurs Manag 1983;14(11):46–8.
45. Snyder M. Independent nursing interventions. New York: John Wiley & Sons, 1985.
46. Saba VK, McCormick KA. Essentials of computers for nurses. Philadelphia: JB Lippincott, 1986.
47. Study Group on Nursing Information Systems. Computerized nursing information systems: an urgent need. Res Nurs Health 1983;6:101–5.
48. Werley HH, Grier MR, ed: Nursing information systems. New York: Springer, 1981.
49. Dossett DL. Motivating staff. In: Sullivan EJ, Decker PJ, eds, Effective Management in Nursing. Menlo-Park, CA: Addison-Wesley, 1985, p. 99–129.
50. Joiner C, Johnson V, Chapman JB, Corkrean M. The motivating potential in nursing specialties. J Nurs Admin 1982;12:26–30.
51. Duxbury ML, Armstrong GD, Drew DJ, Henly SJ. Head nurse leadership style with staff nurse burnout and job satisfaction in neonatal intensive care units. Nurs Res 1984;33:97–101.
52. Everly GS, Falcione RL. Perceived dimensions of job satisfaction for staff registered nurses. Nurs Res 1976;25:346–8.
53. Slavitt DB, Stamps PL, Piedmont EB, Hasse AMB. Nurses' satisfaction with their work situation. Nurs Res 1978;27:114–20.
54. Slocum JW, Susman GI, Sheridan JE. An analysis of need satisfaction and job performance among professional and paraprofessional hospital personnel. Nurs Res 1972;21:338–42.
55. Moore LB, Moore CB. Productivity and organization management In: Dogramaci A, ed. Productivity analysis—a range of perspectives. Boston: Martinus Nijhoff, 1981.
56. Katzell ME. Productivity: the measure and the myth. New York: AMACOM, 1975.
57. Draper EA. Benefits and costs of intensive care. Image 1983;15:90–4.
58. Hook EW, Horton CA, Schaberg DR. Failure of intensive care unit support to influence mortality from pneumonococcal bacteremia. JAMA 1983;249:1055–57.
59. Knaus WA, Draper EA, Wagner DP. The use of intensive care: new research initiatives and their implications for national health policy. Milbank Memorial Fund Quarterly 1983;61:561–83.
60. Thibault G, Mully AG, Barnett HE, et al. Medical intensive care: indications, interventions, and outcomes. NEJM 1980;302:938–42.
61. Wagner DP, Knaus WA, Draper EA, Zimmerman JE. Identification of low risk-monitor patients within a medical-surgical intensive care unit. Med Care 1983;21:425–34.
62. Kelley JA. The role of top level nurse administrators. In: University of Minnesota proceedings—nursing administration: issues for the '80's—solutions for the 70's. Minneapolis: University of Minnesota, 1977.
63. Katz D, Kahn RL. The social psychology of organizations. New York: John Wiley & Sons, 1966.
64. Oaklander H, Gleishman EA. Patterns of leadership related to organizational stress in hospital settings. Admin Sci Quarterly 1964;8:520–32.
65. Rickson RE. Insulation from role-induced strain in three hospital organizations. Dissertation. Seattle: University of Washington, 1967.
66. Corwin R. The professional employee: a study of conflict in nursing roles. Am J Sociology 1966;66:604–15.
67. Kramer M. Reality shock—why nurses leave nursing. St. Louis: CV Mosby, 1974.
68. Weiss SJ. The effect of transition modules on new graduate adaptation. Res. Nurs. Health 1984;17:51–9.

69. Munson FC, Beckman JS, Clinton J, Kever C, Simms LM. Nursing assignment patterns user's manual. Ann Arbor, Michigan: AUPHA Press, 1980.

70. Johannides DF. Cost containment through systems engineering. Germantown, MD: Aspen, 1979.

71. Giovannetti P. Patient classification systems in nursing: a description and analysis. Hyattsville, MD: U.S. Department of Health, Education and Welfare, 1978, DHEW publication no. (HRA) 78-22.

72. Lipscomb J. Health resource allocation and quality of care measurement in a social policy framework. Policy Sci 1978;9:19–43.

33

Survey Methodology

Diane R. LaRochelle

EACH time we gather information to assess or "size up" a situation we are conducting an informal survey. Despite the limitations of these quick and nonsystematic assessments, they often provide sufficient data on which to base subsequent decisions, if those decisions are of a small magnitude with limited impact. For example, a vice-president for nursing might informally question head nurses at a management council meeting to obtain their opinions about a proposed procedural change. This is a somewhat limited survey procedure but one, nonetheless, that is likely to result in a positive outcome.

Major decisions, which affect either policies or programs, however, warrant the systematic collection of data that meet the scientific standards of reliability and validity and are acceptable to all parties concerned. When administrative decisions are made in the absence of data that have been systematically collected, it is common to rely on rules of thumb, intuition, and past experience, or to replicate decisions that seem to have worked for others in similar situations. For example, I asked a group of nursing administration students how they thought the adoption of a strict no-smoking policy in a hospital would affect patients' attitudes. The students reasoned that patients who smoked would probably choose to go to another hospital if the no-smoking policy were instituted.

The issue of whether to implement a no-smoking policy actually did form the basis for a survey that was conducted at the University of Minnesota Hospitals, where researchers attempted to identify the attitudes of patients and employees about eliminating all smoking.[1] The study sample consisted of 100 randomly selected individuals from a pool of discharged patients, 100 employees randomly selected using hospital payroll records, and 100 faculty members randomly selected from a list of the medical school faculty. The method chosen for data collection was a telephone interview conducted by trained interviewers.

It is interesting to note that the responses from hospital employees and faculty who participated in the survey were identical to those of my nursing administration students. The responses from patients, however, were strikingly different: only 10% of the patients surveyed had negative views about a smoke-free hospital. In fact, 88% of the patients believed a smoke-free hospital was a good way to eliminate the health hazards of smoking, and 83% believed it would be an important improvement in patient care.[1]

This example points out why intuitive approaches and similar unsubstantiated approaches are often insufficient for decision making. Health-care organizations are too sophisticated and complex for managers to rely solely on data gathered informally and nonsystematically. Our competitive and complex health-care system demands that credible data sources be identified and used appropriately to improve the effectiveness of administrative judgments. Survey research, as well as the judicious use of existing survey data, offer administrators valuable mechanisms for enhancing the effectiveness of decisions.

In this chapter I will first provide a brief historical overview of survey research. Next, I will describe survey research methodology, including its strengths, weaknesses, and significance. To provide the reader with an insider's perspective on the various elements of survey research, several published surveys have been selected to illustrate major points. My aim is to enhance the ability of nurse administrators to critically evaluate survey data and to design surveys for use in the management of nursing services.

OVERVIEW OF SURVEY RESEARCH

Surveys are a specialized form of empirical social research designed to elicit information about people, including their attitudes, perceptions, opinions, plans, and ideas.[2] Babbie[3] points out that there are many different types of surveys such as public opinion polls, market research studies of consumer preferences, and academic studies.

The best way of collecting survey data is to go directly to a selected group of individuals whose attitudes or ideas regarding the specific issues being studied are needed for decision making. These individuals are contacted directly through telephone or personal interviews, or mailed questionnaires. Obtaining data directly from persons through interviews and questionnaires is the first major distinguishing feature of survey research. The second is the use of large samples and specialized sampling methodologies to ensure that subjects possess those characteristics representative of the population of interest. The third distinguishing feature of surveys relates to the type of research design that is used, which is typically cross-sectional or longitudinal.

The value of conducting survey research lies in the rich descriptive and statistical data that surveys provide. Because survey data are

generated by the subjects themselves, the information obtained by this method often has more validity than information obtained by other research methods, such as observation or review of existing documents. For example, if we wanted to determine nurse administrators' opinions about leadership, one might have more confidence in a study that used a survey design with a large sample of head nurses, supervisors, and directors in hospitals of various size[4] than in another study that merely surveyed the attitudes of students in a nursing administration program and did not account for the level of management and size of institution that students represented. The same principle holds true for research involving patients. For instance, Jonas[5] described the discrepancies in data about patients' complaints that became evident only when the information obtained directly from patients was compared to the data reported by physicians.

Surveys are conducted to obtain a better understanding of people and their behavior. The major objectives of survey research are to provide descriptions and explanations, and to explore assertions about selected populations. In relation to health care, surveys are typically conducted using patients and their families to determine their attitudes, preferences, and opinions about various aspects of health care delivery.[6-9] Another common type of survey is aimed at identifying and describing factors associated with health and illness behaviors, including compliance.[10-15] Additionally, surveys are conducted to assess patients' satisfaction with their care;[16,17] to identify factors associated with illness and coping,[18,19] and to elicit responses of patients related to health-care needs.[20-22]

Survey instruments developed for patient studies are sometimes adapted for simultaneously polling nurses and other health-care providers so that the responses of the various groups can be compared.[1,23] Finally, institutional surveys may be conducted to obtain data associated with an organization, and the distribution and allocation of patient services.[24–26]

Fink and Kosecoff point out that surveys have become a major means of collecting data to answer questions about our "health, social, economic, and political life."[2] Surveys tend, therefore, to be instituted for very specific reasons. Babbie notes that "there are as many different reasons for conducting surveys as there are surveys."[3] Patient surveys are usually undertaken because there is a lack of information from the patient's perspective relative to a decision of consequence that needs to be made. From an administrative perspective, surveys provide data useful for policy and program decisions related to planning and establishing an environment conducive to the delivery of quality patient services.

Because survey research can be both costly and time consuming, some investigators[27,28] suggest that the potential use of other data sources be thoroughly explored before deciding to conduct a survey. In addition, it is recommended that the following four questions be answered prior to embarking on a survey. First, is it desirable to obtain data from a large probability sample to reduce selection bias? Second, is there a need to use standardized measurements to ensure comparability of information? Third, is there a need to obtain information directly from informants? Finally, are the analysis requirements such that a special data set needs to be obtained to test hypotheses or to satisfy statistical assumptions?[28] If the data required for an administrative decision do not correspond positively with any of the four conditions described in the questions, then the time and effort of conducting a survey cannot be easily justified.

A final introductory note about survey research is that a survey refers to both the method of data collection—the administration of questionnaires and the conduct of interviews to elicit data directly from subjects—as well as to the research design, that is, to the overall plan, structure, and strategy for data collection. In survey research, the research plan—a written blueprint that directs the study; the structure—the conceptual framework used for selecting and defining variables; and the strategy—the methods used to gather and analyze data, are somewhat different than in other types of investigations. But surveys must be conducted with the same amount of rigor as other types of research to assure the validity, reliability, and generalizability of the data, as well as to convince decision makers of the credibility and usefulness of the findings.

METHODOLOGY OF SURVEY RESEARCH

Historical Background

Survey research is a method that is aimed at "collecting original data for describing a population too large to observe directly."[29] Babbie noted that the value of survey research was recognized as early as 1880 when Karl Marx mailed questionnaires to 25,000 French workers to elicit their opinions about the extent to which they were being exploited by their employers.[3] However, survey research, in the social scientific sense, is a twentieth-century development.[30] In the United States, the Bureau of Census is the major initiator of survey research, conducting the decennial census and sample surveys that provide demographic and economic data.[3]

A census is the collection of data on every individual in a population. The collection of census data, therefore, is expensive and complicated, and is usually limited to obtaining data of a general nature that can be placed into broad categories, such as level of income. Surveys, on the other hand, use a representative sample of the population of interest. They are designed to elicit specific information that focuses on a narrow topic of concern. The principle advantage of sample sur-

Table 33.1 Design Components of Survey Research

Purpose	Research Design	Population
Describe	Cross sectional	Census
Compare	Longitudinal	Sample survey
Explain	Cohort	
Relate	Panel	
Predict	Comparison group	
Explore	Experimental	
Evaluate	Quasi-experimental	

Data Collection	Variables of Interest
Telephone survey	Social characteistics
Mail questionnaire	Demoraphic characteristics
Face-to-face interview	Attributes
	Attitudes
	Perceptions
	Opinions
	Perceived needs
	Beliefs
	Values
	Ideas
	Feelings
	Plans
	Motivations
	Behaviors (past & present)
	Intentions
	Aspirations

veys lies in the large amount of standardized data that can be collected. Also, because a survey is usually designed to address a specific problem or issue, the results can be particularly useful to decision makers involved in the everyday operation of organizations.

Over the past several decades, methodological developments, and the refinement and application of rigorous research procedures have enhanced the quality, reliability, and validity of survey research. The Census Bureau is credited with developing and field testing standardized definitions of sampling. Stouffer and Lazarsfield are recognized for their rigorous application of empirical research methods. And the Gallup, Roper, and Harris polling firms are acknowledged for their contributions in the areas of probability sampling and questionnaire development. Additionally, institutions such as the Institute for Social Research at the University of Mich-

igan are recognized for their experiments with survey research methods, their apprenticeship training for social researchers, and collaboration with government and industry in the conduct of surveys aimed at collecting data on special problems.[3]

Types of Surveys

Surveys can be classified according to their purpose, design, population, data collection procedures, and variables of interest. Each of the components of survey research are depicted in Table 33.1.

Surveys are generally undertaken to generate statistical descriptions about a sample of subjects that can be generalized to a specific population. They are also used to explore and explain the relationships among variables and to compare selected populations. Thus, surveys can provide decision makers with relevant data such as whether or not differences discovered between groups are in fact statistically significant.

I have selected two studies from the literature to illustrate descriptive and relational surveys. When reading about them, note the purpose of the surveys, their design, population, method of sample selection, data collection procedures, variables of interest, and results.

A descriptive survey by Ailinger[31] entitled, *"Hypertension Knowledge in a Hispanic Community,"* is an excellent example of a study that generated descriptive data generalizable to the population of interest. Ailinger assessed the knowledge of hypertension for 330 people in a 6000-member Hispanic community. Ten census tracks were selected using 1970 census data, from which 330 households were identified. One person from each household was included in the study. Bilingual interviewers were trained by the investigator to collect data pertaining to participants' perceptions of the definition, etiology, diagnosis, associated risk factors, treatment, prognosis, and sequelae of hypertension.

Results highlighted the cultural similarities and differences of perceptions about hypertension between Hispanics and others. Of all the subjects, 36% had inadequate knowledge of hypertension, a figure consistent with surveys of the general public. Hispanics, however, were much better informed than the general public with regard to medication treatment and the relationship of hypertension to strokes. Major knowledge deficits were a lack of understanding of hypertension and associated risk factors. Ailinger pointed out that her survey findings supported the importance of conducting assessments of each person's knowledge of a disease prior to the development and implementation of a plan of care to avoid basing care on faulty assumptions.

By contrast, Burckhardt's correlational study,[32] "The Impact of Arthritis on Quality of Life," explored the impact of physical, psychological, and social factors on the perceptions of quality of life for individuals with arthritis. Ninety-four subjects, 74 women and 20 men who were 27 to 98 years of age, were selected from the rosters of a private clinic and a senior citizen organization. Potential subjects were first approached by telephone to determine if they met the criteria for participation. Those who did were scheduled for an interview and were asked to respond to the items on a set of survey instruments.

Using a complex method for data analysis, Burckhardt first hypothesized a causal model, selecting those variables that had the greatest potential for explanation relative to quality of life. Specific hypotheses were then developed and tested using path analysis to define and explain the complex relationships depicted in her model. The results of this survey were important because they corroborated the findings of earlier surveys that showed self-esteem, a sense of personal control, and supportive relationships to be critical factors affecting perceptions of the quality of life for persons with arthritis. Burckhardt's survey lent support to the use of cognitive frameworks for explaining the effect of chronic illness, and suggested potentially fruitful avenues for experimental studies aimed at testing nursing strategies that decrease functional impairment and pain, thereby improving the quality of life.

Steps in Survey Research

The design of survey research involves the same general considerations as other types of research: problem identification, sample selection, choice of instrumentation, data-collection procedures, techniques for data analysis, and the format for reporting results. Beyond these, survey research is unique and requires specific decisions and judgments. Some of the major design considerations that need to be addressed in survey research are summarized in Table 33.2. A review of the

Table 33.2   Design Considerations in Survey Research

1. Problem Identification
   a. Describe the purpose of the survey
   b. Identify major objectives
   c. Isolate variables of interest
2. Sample Selection
   a. Decide on the sample frame and unit of analysis
   b. Determine if a probability sample is required
   c. Determine time frame for the study
   d. Choose sampling procedures
   e. Decide on sample size and acceptable response rate
3. Instrumentation
   a. Choose existing questionnaires or select content for new questionnaires or interveiw schedules
   b. Test and refine content
   c. Determine acceptable levels of reliability and validity
4. Data Collection Procedures
   a. Explore advantages and disadvantages of mailed questionnaires, telephone interviews and face-to-face interviews
   b. Choose procedures for distribution and collection of questionnaires
   c. Develop protocols and training sessions for data collectors
   d. Follow human subjects guidelines outlined in the Federal Code of Regulations
5. Data Analysis
   a. Choose appropriate descriptive statistics and other statistical techniques to reflect design decisions
   b. Format the data and inspect for accuracy and consistency
   c. Consider all sources of error in relation to the total research design
6. Reporting Results
   a. Decide on a format for reporting results
   b. Choose methods for presentation of data including charts and graphs.
   c. Report all relevant judgments pertaining to the type of survey, instrumentation, sample selection, data-collection, and analysis procedures that affect the quality of data and errors in the data

items in this table highlights the need for technical knowledge and survey research expertise. Inexperienced researchers may unknowingly make methodological errors that erode the quality of data and decrease its value for decision making.

Planning Survey Research

When information is needed about an identified group of people, conducting a survey to obtain the desired information is usually the first solution that comes to mind. In fact, surveys have become so commonplace in our society, that we tend to forget that this kind of research must be executed with the same rigor as other types if it is to hold up to scientific scrutiny. Contrary to popular opinion, survey research when done properly is neither "quick" nor "easy."

The quality of survey research is highly dependent on the quality of the sampling technique, the reliability and validity of instruments, and the preciseness of data-collection procedures. As with all research, there is a wide variation in the quality of reported surveys. Fowler[28] emphasizes the importance of quality in sampling, validating, and developing a credible data set. He notes that if there is a major compromise or weakness in any step, it is not sensible to make major investments in other steps of the research. For example, if the instruments selected for the survey do not have acceptable validity and reliability, it makes no sense to mail them to a large number of subjects with the aim of decreasing sampling error.

Fowler introduced the notion of "custom design" for survey research, meaning that "a researcher should go down the list of design options carefully, assess the alternatives, assess the cost of potential for error, and make decisions about which compromises make sense and which do not."[28] One design consideration, which is of particular importance in survey research, is the training of interviewers. If one takes the time, for example, to develop a credible interview schedule to elicit the opinions of a special group on an issue, then it is prudent to train all interviewers about how to probe subjects for incomplete answers in a neutral way. Without such training, there is no assurance that the personal interpretations and explanations provided by interviewers are unbiased. A decision not to train interviewers may be too costly in terms of the numerous sources of bias that can affect the credibility of the study.

The remainder of this section on planning survey research focuses on cross-sectional and longitudinal research designs and how they are used. Also, major components of the research plan are discussed from the standpoint of researcher decisions. Finally, selected methodological issues are identified and addressed. As previously stated, the quality of the research and credibility of the data are directly related to the number and type of methodological errors incurred.

Design Considerations

One should not undertake a survey if there is another way to obtain the data that are needed. However, once it is determined that a survey should be conducted, the researcher should clarify the purpose of the undertaking and the intended use of the data set. He or she should also identify the variables of interest and the target population that must be reached, then carefully select the instruments, and work out the sampling and data-collection procedures.

Surveys may use any one of several designs. The two most frequently used are cross-sectional and longitudinal. In a cross-sectional survey, "data are collected at one point in time from a sample selected to describe some larger population at that time."[3] The research by Klegan, Kingstrom, and Gregory[33] entitled, "Ambulatory Health Care Centers: Image and Preference Among Consumers," is an example of a cross-sectional survey. Klegan and associates mailed a self-administered questionnnaire to 291 individuals who lived near a newly constructed health-care center. The purpose of the survey was to determine consumer perceptions of health centers. Subjects were asked to rate selected characteristics of health centers in relation to physicians' offices. One-hundred and thirty-seven people (47%) responded. Respondents rated health centers higher than physicians' offices with respect to the availability of care during off hours and the cost of care. The centers were rated lower than physicians' offices in terms of personal atmosphere, seeing a physician of choice, and physicians' attitudes. Those individuals who indicated a preference for receiving care at a center had a positive image of health centers in relation to patient-physician relationships, office atmosphere, and quality of care. The survey showed that mere awareness and availability of a health-care center is not a sufficient inducement. The data provided by the survey are representative of the information needed by professionals involved in planning, organizing, and marketing of health-care services.

Longitudinal surveys "permit the analysis of data over time: either descriptive or explanatory."[3] Longitudinal studies, however, are often not done because of the length of time needed to attain results, the expense involved, and the numerous problems that can arise when data are collected over an extended period of time. One example of a longitudinal study is a client-satisfaction survey conducted by Dankot, Pandiam, and Gordon.[16] This survey consisted of a questionnaire that was mailed to a sample of clients receiving therapy on a monthly basis in a community mental health center. Forty-five questionnaires were mailed each month until a sample of 279 clients was obtained. The purpose of the survey was "to obtain information from current and past clients, input a computerized data base, and generate reports for therapists, program managers, center directors, and state agency directors."[16] To accomplish this objective, the investigators maximized the utility of clients' perceptions over time by merging clients' responses with selected case-management information, as well as with diagnostic, demographic, and programmatic data.

This study demonstrated the value of collecting patient-survey data on a regular basis for self-evaluation, program planning, and development. In addition, an important unexpected outcome of the study was the observation that clients would provide reliable data and respond to queries about their care in sufficient numbers to assure an acceptable response rate.

There are two variations of the longitudinal survey—cohort and panel studies. A cohort study "focuses on the same specific population each time data are collected, although the samples studied may be different."[3] An example of a cohort study is the work by Wolinsky, Moseley, and Coe entitled, "A Cohort Analysis of the Use of Health Services by Elderly Americans."[24] Panel studies, on the other hand, "involve the collection of data over time from the same sample of respondents."[3] Panel surveys are typically used to monitor changes in a select group of individuals over a period of months and years. Typically used to identify trends, an example of a panel study is the survey by Coulton and Frost entitled, "Use of Social and Health Services by the Elderly."[35]

Instrumentation

Survey research usually involves the development of one or more questionnaires to elicit accurate and uniform data from respondents that are also relevant to the problem being studied. Data collected with one particular instrument may provide information on patients' satisfaction with care provided by nurse practitioners. But the same instrument will not necessarily explain under what circumstances a patient will decide to use a nurse practitioner rather than a physician. Special questions need to be developed to obtain each unique piece of information. It is beyond the scope of this chapter to discuss the specifics of instrument development. One of the standard research texts detailing the steps in questionnaire development, including the selection of content, choice of scales, testing and refining of questions, and establishing psychometric properties, should be used.

It is a challenge to the researcher to develop survey questions that are interpreted in the same way by all subjects and that consistently provide adequate, credible, and usable data for decision making. Three documents that should be used in the development of a questionnaire are the statement of purpose for the survey, the list of variables to be measured, and the plan for data analysis.[28] The statement of purpose and list of variables provide a reference point for the inclusion or exclusion of specific questions. The analysis plan identifies the subgroups targeted for special estimates.

The researcher uses all three of these documents to refine his or her ideas in relation to the variables that must be measured. According to Fowler the researcher should clarify the following:[28] (1) which variables are dependent and which measures of central tendency are to be estimated; (2) which variables are independent; and (3) which variables may be needed as control or intervening factors to explain the patterns that are observed and to check out competing hypotheses.

Sampling Procedures

When conducting a survey, there is a choice of using either probability or nonprobability sampling. Probability sampling should be used for large-scale general surveys where a representative sample of the target population is needed to obtain a credible data set. Fowler[28] stresses that samples should be evaluated by examining the process by which participants were selected, as opposed to merely assessing the characteristics of the individuals studied. The techniques most commonly used to obtain samples are simple random sampling, stratified random sampling, and random cluster sampling.

Nonprobability sampling techniques include systematic sampling, purposive sampling, and accidental or convenience sampling. One of the special texts on survey research should be consulted when decisions pertaining to sampling are made during the design phase of a project. This is especially necessary to avoid the omission of a subgroup of interest.

Another consideration is the size of a sample. It is imperative that the researcher not guess what sample size is adequate but rather make this determination based on the estimated minimal sample sizes needed for the smallest sampled subgroups.[28] In addition, sampling error should be estimated to assure that the sample is representative of the population from which it is chosen. The smaller the sampling error, the more representative the sample will be. Fowler[28] points out that one of the major strengths of survey research is the possibility afforded by the method to calculate sampling error.

Data-Collection Procedures

The data-collection procedures used most often in the conduct of survey research are telephone interviews, mail questionnaires, and face-to-face interviews. Researchers may also choose to use a combination of methods, such as the administration of a questionnaire followed by a face-to-face interview.

If people are employed to collect study data, protocols should be developed for the data collectors to follow. Interviewers should be trained in interviewing techniques, such as how to initiate and terminate an interview. They should also be instructed to handle the various problems that may occur. The quality of study data is dependent on the systematic implementation of data-collection procedures and handling the problems that arise in a consistent manner. Fowler[28] warns us that "many of the shortcomings of data collection stem from faulty execution of details rather than a lack of understanding" by those involved. Considerations like these are especially important for patient surveys.

There is little guidance in the literature pertaining to when or how to best survey patients' opinions. In general, investigators have obtained substantially higher response rates with interviews than with self-completion questionnaires.[35] It is also interesting to note that there is no strong basis for the assertion that the response rate is higher for hospital rather than for home-based surveys. Despite the fact that the mean response rate for hospitalized patients is slightly greater than the mean response rates of patients' surveyed in their homes, the differences are not as great as one might expect. Moreover, the gap has been shown to narrow when participant suitability, eligibility, and availability are taken into account.[35]

The assumption that home-based studies are preferred because they assure greater privacy and diminish patients' fear of repercussions from hospital employees, is unfounded.[36] In fact, it has been shown that patients are more willing to voice criticism while in the hospital than they are after they return to their home.[36] In relation to timing, the available evidence strongly suggests that the survey be instituted as close to the relevant events about which information is sought as possible.

PATIENT RELATED SURVEYS: EXISTING DATA SETS

In the area of patient surveys, the federal government has taken the lead, providing a vast source of easily retrievable data for decision makers. These surveys fall into two major categories: vital statistics and utilization of health services.

Vital Statistics

Vital statistics are collected by a variety of agencies at various government levels, from local and state public health departments to the National Center for Health Statistics (NCHS). In 1979, the NCHS established a National Death Index (NDI) for the purpose of facilitating prospective studies "to determine the relationship between chronic degenerative diseases such as cancer and environmental, occupational, medical, and life-style factors."[5] The NDI classifies mortality data according to the Ninth Revision International Classification of Diseases Adapted for use in the United States (ICDA-9). The ICDA-9 Clinical Modification (ICDA-9-CM) is an extension of the ICDA-9 all hospitals receiving federal funds are required to use. Differential death rates by age, color, and gender are reported in the following U.S. government publications: *Monthly Vital Statistics Report, Vital Statistics of the United States, The Statistical Abstract, and special studies published in Vital and Health Statistics, Series 20.*[5]

In addition to data on deaths, morbidity data are available from several different federal reports. For example, the Center for Disease Control publishes reportable communicable disease data in the *Morbidity and Mortality Weekly Report.*[5] Additionally, the NCHS periodically publishes the Health and Nutri-

tion Examination Survey (HANES), which is published in Vital and Health Statistics, a survey that includes persons selected via household interviews who then participate in a detailed medical and nutritional history and clinical exam. Data provided by this survey include dietary intake, physical measurements, biochemical characteristics, and demographic and socioeconomic characteristics.[5] The Health Records Survey is also published in Vital and Health Statistics. This survey consisted of three reviews of nursing home patients and personnel conducted in 1963, 1964, and 1969.[5]

Other studies are published in both *Vital Statistics* and the *Monthly Vital Statistics Report.* The Hospital Discharge Survey (HDS), reports morbidity and mortality rates in hospitals, thus providing an illness profile of the nation's hospitals.[5] The Health Interview Survey provides data on "personal and demographic characteristics, illness, injuries, impairments, chronic conditions, and other health topics" based on questionnaires sent to selected households.[5] Also, the National Ambulatory Medical Care Survey reports data obtained from a questionnaire distributed to a stratified random sample of allopathic and osteopathic physicians in private practice. These data include patient demographics, morbidity, utilization, and selected practice characteristics.[5]

Utilization of Health Services

Patterns of health-care utilization is another area of importance to health-care planners and decision makers. An excellent source for these data is the National Medical Care Utilization and Expenditure Survey (NMCUES), cosponsored by the National Center for Health Statistics (NCHS) and the Health Care Financing Administration (HCFA). This is a comprehensive four-part survey of a national probability sample of 8000 households, a sample of 4000 medicaid households from four states, a medical provider survey, and an administrative records survey. These surveys were designed to:[5] (1) provide a statistical base for the federal health-care cost-containment effort; (2) provide updated comparable measures of utilization and expenditures for monitoring national health insurance programs; and (3) provide data on trends and costs over time of health-care services for different population subgroups—the poor, the elderly, and the uninsured, most notably.

The Health Interview Survey, previously mentioned, provides data on the utilization of ambulatory services from the patient's perspective. The major sources of data on utilization of ambulatory services from the provider's perspective are the National Ambulatory Medical Care Survey (NAMCS) and *Hospital Statistics*, an annual publication of the American Hospital Association (AHA).[5]

Pertaining to the utilization of hospital services, major resources are *Hospital Statistics* (mentioned above) and "Hospital Indicators," which appears monthly in *Hospitals, the Journal of the American Hospital Association*. Additional data on utilization appear in the government publications, *Health Resources Statistics*, and *Health: U.S.*, which appears annually.[5]

In conclusion, a common criticism leveled at nurse managers is that too often their decisions are made in the absence of valid and reliable data. The use of survey data overcomes this problem because research provides a credible data set for certain types of management decisions, particularly those related to patients. In this chapter I have shown why data derived from patient surveys is a particularly valuable resource for nurse managers involved in the planning, organizing, marketing, and monitoring of patient care. In addition, I have presented the major design components of survey research and the essential steps to consider in both the evaluation of existing data and in the conduct of patient surveys. Nurse managers should

consider the use of surveys as a basis for product-line development, selection of health-care delivery sites, determination of staffing patterns, health teaching, and evaluating client outcomes.

The challenge to nurse administrators is to know when and how to use survey data. The quality and effectiveness of management decisions will be directly tied to the comprehensiveness, accuracy, and credibility of data elicited from patients, prospective patients, and their families.

REFERENCES

1. Kottke E, Hill C, Heitzig C, Brekke M, Blake S, Ameson S, Caspers C. Smoke-free hospitals. Minnesota Medicine 1985; 68 (1):53–55.
2. Fink A, and Kosecoff J. How to conduct surveys. Beverly Hills: Sage Publications, 1985.
3. Babbie EK. Survey research methods. Belmont, CA: Wadsworth Publishing Co, Inc, 1973.
4. LaRochelle DR. An analysis of the effects of education on the leadership perceptions of nurse managers. Unpublished Doctoral Dissertation, 1978, University of Connecticut.
5. Jonas S. Health care delivery in the United States. 2nd ed. New York: Springer Publishing Co., 1981.
6. Craft M. Preferences of hospitalized adolescents for information providers. Nursing Research 1981; 30(4):205–211.
7. Kaemmerer CJ. Twin cities consumers' attitudes on health care. Minnesota Medicine 1985;68(1):57–60.
8. Knauer VH. Health care delivery in the 1980s: the consumer's perspective. Hospital Progress 1980; 61(3):56–59, 72.
9. Wolinsky FD, Kurz RS. How the public chooses and views hospitals. Hospital and Health Services Administration. 1984;29(6):58–67.
10. Chang BL, Uman GC, Linn LC, Ware JE, Kane RL. Adherence to health care regimens among elderly women. Nursing Research 1985;34(1):27–31.
11. Hallal JC. The relationship of health beliefs, health locus of control, and self concept to the practice of breast self-examination in adult women. Nursing Research 1982;31(3):137–142.
12. Laffrey SC. Normal and overweight adults: perceived weight and health behavior characteristics. Nursing Research 1986;35(3):173–177.
13. Lauck BW, Bigelow DA. Why patients follow through on referrals from the emergency room and why they don't. Nursing Research 1983;32(3):186–187.
14. Muhlenkamp AF, Sayles JA. Self-esteem, social support, and positive health practices. Nursing Research 1986;35(6):334–338.

15. Muhlenkamp AF, Waller MM, Bourne AE. Attitudes toward women in menopause: a vignette approach. Nursing Research 1983;321:20–23.
16. Damkot DK, Pandiani JA, Gordon LR. Development, implementation, and findings of a continuing client satisfaction survey. Community Mental Health Journal 1983;19(4):265–278.
17. Ventura MR, Fox RN, Corley MC, Mercurio SM. A patient satisfaction measure as a criterion to evaluate primary nursing. Nursing Research 1982;31(4): 226–230.
18. Derdiarian AK. Informational needs of recently diagnosed cancer patients. Nursing Research 1986; 35(5):276–281.
19. O'Rourke MW. Subjective appraisal of psychological well-being and self-reports of menstrual and non-menstrual symptomatology in employed women. Nursing Research 1983;32(5):288–292.
20. Cranley MS, Hedahl KJ, Pegg SH. Women's perceptions of vaginal and cesarean deliveries. Nursing Research 1983;32(1):10–15.
21. Schlueter LA: Knowledge and beliefs about breast cancer and breast self-examination among athletic and nonathletic women. Nursing Research 1982; 31(6):348–353.
22. Walsh VR. Health beliefs and practices of runners versus nonrunners. Nursing Research 1985;34(6): 353–356.
23. Lauer P, Murphy SP, Powers MJ. Learning needs of cancer patients: a comparison of nurse and patient perceptions. Nursing Research 1982;311:11–16.
24. Kirchhoff KT. A diffusion survey of coronary precautions. Nursing Research 1982;31(4):196–201.
25. Lorenz CJ, Jr. Three hospitals join forces for survey. Hospitals 1980;54(16):129–131.
26. Sund K, Ostwald SK. Dual-earner families' stress levels and personal and life-style-related variables. Nursing Research 1985;34(6):357–361.
27. Burns JA. Knowledge is power: how to develop effective market surveys. Health Care Marketing 1985/1986;3(2/3):99–112.
28. Fowler FJ Jr. Survey research methods. Beverly Hills: Sage Publications, 1984.
29. Babbie EK. The practice of social research. Belmont, CA: Wadsworth Publishing Co, Inc, 1983, Survey research, p. 208–242.
30. Kerlinger FN. Foundations of behavioral research. (2nd ed). New York: Holt Rinehart & Winston, 1973.
31. Ailinger RL. Hypertension knowledge in a Hispanic community. Nursing Research 1982;31(4):207–210.
32. Burckhardt CS. The impact of arthritis on quality of life. Nursing Research 1985;34(1):11–16.
33. Klegan DA, Kingstrom PO, Gregory DD. Ambulatory health care centers: image and preference among consumers. Journal of Ambulatory Care Management 1982;5(4).
34. Wolinsky FD, Moseley R II, Coe M. A cohort analysis of the use of health services by elderly americans. Journal of Health and Social Behavior 1986;(27): 209–219.
35. Coulton C, Frost AK. Use of social and health services by the elderly. Journal of Health and Social Behavior; 1982;(23):330–339.
36. French KBA. Methodological considerations in hospital patient opinion surveys. Int. J. Nurs. Stud 1981;(18):7–32.

34

Evaluation of In-Service Effectiveness

Elizabeth A. Hefferin

TODAY'S nurse administrators are expected to promote and support the functioning and stability of organizations. They also bear the complex responsibility of assuring that their own discipline, nursing, is represented optimally to top management and to clients, and that nursing services are provided by competent practitioners.

This latter responsibility requires a continuing awareness that the quality of services provided depends not only on the knowledge and skill of practicing nurses, but also on the decision-making, communicating, and other management abilities of nurse managers—including in-service education directors. Nurse administrators are empowered to select in-service educators and invest them with the task of providing educational opportunities needed by nursing personnel to perform reliably.

As managers of in-service, nurses are expected to oversee the development and provision of staff education programs—classes, courses, and workshops, for example—a process that involves planning, organizing, directing, and evaluating.[1] An important part of the in-service director's evaluation responsibility is to gather and interpret pertinent information, and analyze critical instruction-related efforts; make decisions about an existing program or any of its components;[2] and make reasoned judgments about the need for a new program and that program's relative worth.[3] Exercise of this evaluation function enables in-service educators to respond appropriately when problems related to nursing practice surface and in-service is asked to provide remedial instruction.

To illustrate the relationship of program evaluation and decisions about whether remedial instruction is necessary, take the case of a staff-development department asked to provide a pharmacology course to reduce the incidence of nurses' medication-related errors.[4] An investigation reveals that the problem is due not to the need for remediation, but primarily to nurses' unfamiliarity with patients' problems and to the unstandardized methods used to verify orders and administer medications. Following the introduction of a program of primary care, the incidence of medication errors drops significantly, and a costly remedial programming activity is averted.

Perhaps heard even more often than the demand for remedial programs are complaints that what nursing personnel have learned is not put into practice.[5] In this era of cost containment, educators must somehow determine whether these situations reflect a need for retraining, more in-depth education, or an intervention that is *not* within the purview of in-service.

How can educators identify the conditions that give rise to the expectation that more in-service education will "cure" the problem? If the following circumstances exist, then in-service education is needed: (1) there is documentable evidence of deficits in staff knowledge; (2) other departments are performing up to established standards; (3) institutional policies and procedures are written clearly and adequately; and (4) problems disappear when policies or procedures are changed, or when a task is carried out appropriately by a staff member.[4]

When these circumstances do *not* exist, however, it is more likely that an administrative intervention is needed. Consequently, collaborative efforts on the part of management and education are essential for the effective resolution of problems.

Once it has been determined that there is, in fact, a training problem, formulating an in-service offering as an educational solution requires that (1) specific, written performance standards be established; (2) methods for assessing individual learning needs be developed; and (3) determinations be made as to whether performance deficiencies are related to actual learning needs, lack of practice opportunities, or the disregard of already established standards.[6] The last requirement is especially important; separating training from nontraining problems can help to control in-service costs by reducing the number of unnecessary training hours. In attempting to account for instructor time and other program costs, staff educators must also document the efficacy of in-service offerings in terms of whether attendees achieve the expected levels of knowledge and performance competence in line with the parameters that reflect course objectives.

Based on their belief in the importance of staff education, nurse administrators have traditionally allocated a significant portion of their available resources—money, space, and personnel—to in-service departments. Because of this long-standing support, many have come to assume that there is a large and continuing need for training activities. Certainly, as an integral component of the nursing department, in-service educators often participate in the activities of the service,

explore problems, and delineate the probable costs and benefits of strategies for resolving problems.

However, merely enhancing the image of in-service productivity does not automatically guarantee improvement either in personnel performance or in client outcomes. To the contrary, increases in the amounts of time that staff spend away from nursing units engaged in educational activities may actually increase costs and decrease productivity because of the overuse of nonproductive time.[7] Too little emphasis has been placed on validating the worth of educational activities to nurses, clients, and organizations.

Hospital management has a vested interest in promoting the cost-efficiency of in-service education. Executives are concerned as well with whether the in-service program operates effectively in support of the hospital's mission to provide quality care. Consequently, educating nurses to provide safe therapeutic care, in line with current knowledge and in cost-effective ways, is a vital function of in-service educators.

Obviously, determinations of the effects of educational strategies depend on how accurately personnel learning needs are assessed and how well learners incorporate into their practice what they are taught. However, because the assessment of staff performance is usually the prerogative of nurse managers, educators are generally unable to directly appraise the degree to which training contributes to the desired changes in personnel behaviors. Nevertheless, it is the responsibility of nurse educators to obtain subjective and objective information about learning problems. In-service staff can then make use of this information to sharpen the focus of in-service programs by developing explicit program objectives and outcome criteria.

As part of their management control responsibility, nurse educators also can go beyond assessing the relative worth of individual programs to evaluating the overall effectiveness of their total in-service effort. The entire in-service program can be evaluated in terms of its objectives, resources, services, and results as well as in terms of the relationships between each of these elements.[8] For example, together with an analysis of the costs and benefits of the program operation, program criteria can be applied to staff learning needs and organizational expectations to define the purposes, objectives, and structure of the in-service program.

Program monitoring criteria can be used to evaluate the scope of the program, the population served, and the relevance of the program. Program impact criteria can be used to evaluate individuals or groups and a variety of intended and unintended outcomes. Economic criteria can be developed to examine the costs and benefits of using certain resources compared with the cost and benefit of other mechanisms using different resources.[9] Relationships between the program components can be explored in terms of whether the objectives adequately address problems and whether the resources used are adequate for providing the training experiences that are needed.[8]

Because managers need information with which to make decisions, program evaluation may be undertaken for a number of reasons. For administrative purposes, evaluation may be used to assess the appropriateness of a program's operation, to identify ways of broadening the functions of the program staff, or to meet the requirements of a regulatory agency. Managers of education programs use evaluation for planning and policy making and to decide whether to expand, modify, or delete selected program activities. Evaluations are also undertaken to assess the epidemiology of problems, the comparative worth of similar products and techniques, and the outcomes of new services. Whether an evaluative component is built into a program initially or just tacked on as an after-

thought, accountability for assuring that programs are evaluated lies with the in-service program manager.

Viewed narrowly, it might appear that whether or not an in-service program is termed successful may well be conditioned by the director's personal perspectives on what is important, what is measured, and what needs to be reported.[10] For example, an educator may use only select evaluative information to improve, modify, or even justify the continued provision of a particular in-service course. This might be done despite available countervailing information about a lack of interest among personnel, or despite the existence of a similar program. However, when the program purposes, objectives, services, and anticipated effects have been clearly delineated, the inclusion of a properly constructed evaluation component permits the educator to obtain some definitive answers about whether or not a program "works." A well-done system of evaluation reduces the likelihood of inappropriately perpetuating programs that do not "work;" it also identifies the important factors that contribute to or inhibit effectiveness.[11]

PERSPECTIVES FOR EVALUATING IN-SERVICE

There are perhaps as many definitions of the term "program evaluation" as there are evaluators. Because program evaluation is a multifaceted process, the interpretations, scope, and impact of program evaluation vary as widely as the disciplinary perspectives of the persons involved. Given that the goal of in-service is to promote the quality of patient services by providing personnel with training appropriate to their responsibilities, the variance in application of program evaluation is no less widespread among in-service managers. Variation exists because educators must appraise unique information, make value judgments and cognitive decisions about program activities aligned with the special needs in each organization, and use a range of evaluative measures which reflect not only their understanding of organizational objectives but also their beliefs about nursing practice.[12]

To reiterate, program evaluation is complex. It involves using a number of approaches to obtain valid, reliable, and useful information about programs and their outcomes. Careful efforts, however, enable in-service managers to account for the utility of their program operations, to make decisions about the significance of outcomes, to understand the factors contributing to or hindering those outcomes, and to plan improvements.[13]

Theoretically, the application of evaluation techniques should improve the design of in-service programs by focusing advanced attention on selected learner outcomes. However, the demand for clear-cut evidence of positive program outcomes may force in-service educators to rely almost exclusively on summative evaluative practices, some of which are neither rational nor cost effective. Prescribing the desired benefits of in-service education, then monitoring outcomes for prespecified benefits, can easily result in measuring only a limited number of outcomes produced by narrowly construed teaching programs.[14]

The complexity of evaluating in-service education can perhaps be seen most clearly by examining the relationships among four basic problems described by intervention theory: (1) identifying and classifying individuals and their learning needs in order to plan, implement, and evaluate an educational intervention; (2) defining the rationale underlying the purposes or outcomes of interventions and the possible means for accomplishing them; (3) selecting the optimal means for planning and implementing an intervention; and (4) determining how to evaluate the various aspects of an intervention.[9, 15]

Identifying and Classifying Individuals and Their Learning Needs

The intervention model suggests that when staff learning needs are not clearly differentiated by learner level, decisions about learning processes and outcomes are not likely to be appropriate. Similarly, if the process and outcome of a program are not identified before a program is implemented, program-planning activities also have no relevance. Consequently, the use of otherwise valid and feasible measures to evaluate learner outcomes becomes illogical, and summative evaluations of program effectiveness are meaningless.[14]

In contrast, when evaluative techniques are used appropriately to examine the various aspects of planning and implementing in-service interventions, many of the factors that influence a program's effectiveness can be identified. Program modifications can then be introduced early to assure that the planned in-service activities will clearly contribute to improved patient care. A few examples are offered to illustrate the types of in-service–related information usually associated with the intervention model, the interrelationships among the elements in the model, and some of the implications for evaluating in-service interventions.

In dealing with the problem of identifying and classifying the learning needs of nursing staff, in-service educators can develop and use a number of needs assessment approaches. These include questionnaires—to elicit staff interest, self-perceived knowledge, and skill inadequacies; reviews of quality assurance audits of patients' charts and other patient-care records—to identify documentation problems; analysis of incident reports—to identify safety problems; and discussions with staff at various levels—to explore the need for training reviews.[12,16–17] Information related to nursing practice problems may also be obtained from reports of special studies or investigations, surveys of patients' opinions and observations, individual staff and unit-based performance appraisals, and periodic administrative reviews. Where in-service is expected to provide programs aimed at resolving specific problems, surveys of staff knowledge and first-hand observation are often useful.

Hence, at the first hint of a need for an in-service program, in-service educators should use various investigative techniques to explore the nature of a reported deficiency and determine the appropriate outcomes and possible means for resolving the problem. Examples of deficiencies include medication-related errors by staff nurses, or a lack of correlation between patient teaching activities noted in care plans and the documentation found in patients' medical records. Examples of mechanisms for resolving problems include working with nurse administrators to develop a standardized patient teaching checklist or medication procedure, or providing educational interventions to different staff groups to increase their level of knowledge relative to their patient teaching and documentation.

Obviously, input from both staff and administration is essential not only to clarify the possible differences between "reported" and "real" problems, but also to determine which staff levels or groups are involved and which administrative or educational interventions are most likely to result in practical yet acceptable resolutions.[4] The efficacy of an in-service offering thus depends on the degree to which the expected program outcomes and the strategies used to plan, implement, and evaluate a selected educational intervention appropriately reflect the unique learning needs of a specified group.

Defining the Rationale for Interventions

A second major focus in the intervention model is on the quality of the rationale underlying selection of a particular strategy or intervention. The rationale should identify and operationally define the three elements contained in the intervention model—the problem, the intervention, and the expected outcome. The rationale should explain the assumed causal, intervention, and action relationships among these elements, so that the problem, or need for the intervention, can be related to an intended outcome.[9]

By way of illustration, the intervention model assumes that a causal relationship exists between an identified problem and an observed undesirable condition or behavior—that supervisor inattention to staff needs is directly related to or causes staff dissatisfaction, for example; or that a lack of staff knowledge or skill causes performance inadequacies. The intervention model next assumes that a selected intervention strategy will reduce or eliminate the causal problem—that a leadership program will increase supervisor awareness of staff needs, for example, or that an in-service training program will enhance staff knowledge and skill. Finally, in the action relationship, the intervention model assumes that a desirable outcome can be linked directly to implementing an intervention—that teaching leadership skills to supervisors produces increased staff satisfaction, or that a staff in-service program decreases performance inadequacies.

Underlying each intervention are a number of principles that address the causes of problems, the processes of intervention, and the probable outcome. Although often not described in detail, these principles outline the nature, scope, and activity of an intervention.[14]

A consistent and practical rationale incorporates ideas from a number of theoretical and empirical sources, presents these ideas in an organized format, and suggests a spectrum of relationships that can exist among each of the elements. The careful spelling-out of the elements in a conceptual framework improves understanding of theory and practice, encourages focusing systematically on essential factors, and serves as a map for visualizing an entire set of intervention principles.[18] A conceptual framework also expedites the interpretation of factors contributing to a problem and the processes integral to the intervention. It helps assure that certain considerations are not under- or overemphasized, and it answers evaluative questions concerning the what and how of relating knowledge to practice.[19] Initiating this evaluative activity before implementing an intervention also helps to clarify the nature of possible conflicting interests—agency and client expectations, educator and staff concerns, for example—that may compromise an intervention.

It should be noted, however, that because of the abstract nature of a conceptual framework, transforming an intervention rationale into a tangible, workable series of steps for the planning and implementation of an educational intervention tends to be time-consuming. The time, however, is well spent, and, guided by a theoretical model, progress is orderly.

Planning and Implementing an Intervention

Many of the measures currently in use for assessing the various aspects of in-service–related problems have only limited validity and reliability. Additionally, there are usually a number of forces that impose practical limitations on in-service interventions—for example, societal mandates for agency support and resources, policies and unwritten precedents, competency standards, resistance to change, and staff motivation and availability.

Such practical and methodological issues appear and reappear throughout the intervention, planning and implementation phases of in-service programs. By way of illustration, when it becomes apparent that a nursing practice deficiency might be resolved through in-service education, the educator first assesses and classifies the problem and then determines which remedial activities and new behaviors will most likely resolve the problem.

The educator must then ascertain that performance standards have been established against which the proposed behaviors can be measured and used as evidence that the educational objectives have been attained. In securing administrative support for a program, the educator must consider agency policies, justify the need for resources, plan program sessions to accommodate the hours that staff work, and arrange for staff attendance. Problem-solving techniques are used throughout the planning and implementing stage to deal with various types of difficulties. During the program implementation period, the educator appraises the staff's learning, identifies successes and difficulties, varies teaching methods, and modifies the program to promote understanding and appropriate behaviors.

Not reflected in this overview of the planning and implementing process is the large number of expectations that influence an intervention. Managers' and educators' expectations may tend to limit the teaching content to the learners' current developmental levels, or expand the teaching design so that learners achieve beyond a basic level.[14]

Also not reflected is the fact that, although administration expects in-service to produce a positive return on its investment in terms of sustained changes in nursing practice, only rarely are educators able to engineer the systematic application of learning that is needed, either through direct monitoring or through line manager reinforcement. While immediate post-test feedback can be obtained from attendees on the perceived value of an educational offering and on the attendees' accomplishment of a program's stated learning objectives, feedback from line managers on the efficacy of the instruction is usually verbal and nonsystematic.

It seems axiomatic that, if all of the various administrative and educational expectations, resources, and other antecedent factors essential for the success of educational interventions are not identified and operationalized throughout the planning and implementing phases, then the relationships between antecedent conditions, interventions, and outcomes may, at best, be only partially determinable. Moreover, where information concerning the factors that influence planning and implementing programs is disregarded or is inaccessible, summative evaluations of interventions may be based primarily on limited outcome assessments or on other types of narrowly circumscribed data.

Evaluating Interventions

Although there continues to be a strong emphasis on evaluating the outcomes of interventions because of the increasing demand for accountability, other aspects of interventions clearly need to be evaluated. For example, determinations must be made concerning the extent to which the need for an educational intervention was objectively assessed, and to justify how it was proposed that instructional activities would account for individual and group differences in achieving a program's stated outcome. These determinations are essential not only for assessing the validity of impact evaluations, but also for a priori judgments about whether the anticipated benefits of a proposed intervention have the potential for outweighing the costs of developing a program and analyzing vast amounts of data to verify an intervention's efficacy.[20]

Qualitative determinations need to be made about whether the rationale for the intervention is logical, whether the underlying principles have been tested empirically, and whether the projected outcomes and available measures provide appropriate indicators of intervention efficacy. Other factors that need to be investigated are whether the intended steps of the program actually took place and whether unintended external or internal events occurred that could have interfered with the program and influenced program outcomes.

When evaluation is seen as an activity that begins at the first hint of an educational need, continues through the planning and implementing phases, and extends beyond the completion of the program back into the practice arena, evaluation serves its purpose—to validate program effectiveness and improve future programs.[21] An important consideration must be to assure that the database that supports the need for a program and serves as the basis for planning the program content and learning experiences also guides the evaluation procedures. It should be self-evident that the only way to determine whether staff have changed their behavior as the result of an educational intervention is to observe this behavior both before and after an intervention. Premeasures and postmeasures should be selected that (1) can be interpreted without educator bias (objectivity); (2) can adequately sample the behaviors being measured (reliability); and (3) provide factual evidence of the desired behaviors (validity).[22]

The recommendation that a variety of strategies be used for program evaluation has been made frequently in the literature.[9,12,22–27] By way of example, after the need for an intervention has been verified, a range of yardsticks has been recommended that can be applied throughout the planning and implementing of a program to answer questions about aspects of the program that need to be modified (formative evaluation);[28] about learner accomplishment of specified objectives (summative evaluation);[29] about learner perceptions of program value (participant satisfaction);[30–32] and about changes in learner performance following program completion (impact evaluation).[33–35] Types of program data useful for cost-benefit analysis have also been suggested.[36–38] Because evaluative questions specify the kind of information that needs to be collected, in-service managers can use program evaluation to justify the benefits of training programs.

When the in-service department is viewed as a system with its own objectives, the totality of the program's structure and function can be evaluated.[39–43] It should be remembered, however, that from a practical point of view, evaluation of the total in-service program is an extremely complex endeavor. The systematic scrutiny of all activities and factors associated with the department's total operation is involved, including as well, the full range of interrelated factors that influence the department's effectiveness.

Although the need for total program evaluation has been addressed in the literature, many discussions have emphasized only summative descriptions.[44–45] More recently, there is interest in using conceptual models for the evaluation of total programs. One such model, which posits a logical consistency between program antecedents, processes, and outcomes, has been described that appears to have considerable potential for use in the evaluation of university-based programs.[46–48] Another conceptual model for evaluating a total in-service program has focused on the decision-making process used in staff education programs.[49] Although these models offer a holistic approach to evaluating complex in-service programs and permit evaluation to take place at any stage of a program, all evaluators are encouraged to develop their own methodologies for obtaining information, using their own standards and judgments.[50]

TRENDS IN IN-SERVICE EVALUATION

The origins of nursing in the United States, and of in-service education, can be traced to the late 1800s. At the turn of the century, an increasing number of hospitals had to be opened to house the flood of sick victims among the immigrants who poured into urban areas. Many hospitals opened nursing schools, more to provide care than to educate nurses. The rapid expansion of nursing schools between 1890 and 1930 was directly associated with the increasing numbers and types of hospitals. Except where trained nurses were needed to manage wards and supervise nursing schools, in-service activities were not emphasized because most of the direct nursing care was provided by students.[51–52]

Nevertheless, because of complaints about the poor instruction in many nursing schools, and because of nurses' desire to keep up with changes, nurses' associations began holding meetings and providing seminars as early as the 1890s. Postgraduate courses also were offered by some teaching hospitals.[53] Nurses who seriously accepted the dual responsibility of caring for the sick and teaching students were just as intent on finding ways to expand their knowledge. Many quietly sought further training in their schools, or initiated new programs.[54]

By the 1930s, although many staff education programs operated unobtrusively, only a few were described in the literature.[55–56] In-service program descriptions, even through the 1940s, tended to be reported broadly and nonanalytically. In a 1946 description of in-service instruction in a university-based hospital, for example, new staff reportedly received an extensive 10-day orientation, followed by in-service training designed to meet their instructional and experiential needs.[57] There are few, if any, descriptions in the literature that discuss the relative effectiveness of program efforts, or the ways in which evaluative measures were developed.

Although it is quite probable that general assessments were made of at least some aspects of in-service effectiveness, and perhaps even of certain program operations, no formal reports of such evaluations were reported in the literature until the late 1940s. Possibly the first broad-scope study of nursing service and nursing education that included in-service activities was published in 1948 by Brown. The findings of this seminal study indicated that there was a critical need to improve the performance of all nursing personnel.[58] Reflecting their awareness of problems, nurse leaders in the 1950s and 1960s worked diligently constructing valid and reliable criteria for appraising the quality of nursing. Methods for designing criterion measures applicable to nursing practice were proposed, and guides were developed to identify the major components of care.[59-61] Another activity undertaken during this time was the first attempt to assess the effect on patient welfare of an in-service intervention designed to increase the quality of care provided by nurses.[62] Although the findings of these and other studies contributed much in the way of suggested approaches for evaluating in-service, objective tests were meager.

Because of the many changes that have taken place in national and state economies during the 1970s and 1980s, considerations related to cost containment have become pivotal for all educational decisions. Ever-spiraling operating costs have forced hospitals to reallocate their resources to accommodate new technologies and specialized services. Budgetary constraints have increasingly compelled nurse executives to do more with less, and to simultaneously improve quality and productivity.[63] Educators have come to rely on in-service as a means for informing nurses at work about prevailing ideas and for stimulating them to accept responsibility for their own competency. In-service educators have also developed conceptual frameworks and rational guidelines for the design, implementation, and evaluation of in-service programs. Consequently, a more structured approach to in-service has redirected educators' attention away from trying to meet all of the staff's "wants," and toward more cost-effective efforts to meet specific learning "needs"—carefully determined deficiencies in knowledge and skill.[17,26,64,65] The long-recommended use of behavioral objectives and performance criteria also has been given increasingly serious consideration.[7,27,36,66]

To determine whether definable trends could be observed in the methods used to evaluate in-service education programs, I reviewed the various in-service studies and reports published since 1950. The review is less complete than I intended because of the increasing number of such reports in recent years. Using manual and computer searches, reports in prominent nursing journals with titles using terms such as "continuing education" and "staff development" were included, when it could be ascertained that the programs being described were provided by health service agencies specifically for their employed personnel. Continuing education programs provided by universities or governmental agencies for broad distribution were excluded, as were general orientation and learn-on-the-job, in-service training programs.

Of the 213 program reports found, 69 met the above criteria for inclusion. Seven were published in the 1950s, 18 in the 1960s, 22 in the 1970s, and 22 between 1980 and 1986. Information obtained from these reports and abstracted in Table 34.1 was categorized as follows: (1) determination of need for the program; (2) focus and program structure; (3) evaluative measures used; and (4) outcomes of the educational intervention.

With respect to identifying the need for

Table 34.1 Selected Nursing In-Service Education Programs and Evaluative Measures Used

Study	Determination of Need	Focus and Structure of Program	Evaluative Measures Used	Reported Outcomes
Delabarre (1951)	Educator-perceived need for program	Neurologic Nursing: 2 phases, 64 hrs. initial orientation, + 20 2-hr. multidisciplinary ward conferences on problems	Postprogram evaluation on participant-perceived value of program	Most nurses rated program as valuable; suggested program be lengthened
Burnett and Greenhill (1954)	Educator decision to provide program; state funded	Mental Health Training: hospital RNs & CHNs of local-state health departments; 8–10 day programs in local settings in 2 states	Various evaluation formats: pre-post test on terms or interpret action in film; follow-up questionnaire in 1 state; pre-post supervisor-observations; post-self-evaluations	Objectives for evaluation formulated after data collected; positive changes noted in nurse behaviors with patients; uncontrolled variables & data inconsistencies
Rutan (1956)	Hospital need to prepare head nurses for role in new building	Head Nurse Training Course; 3 1-hr. sessions/wk. for 6 wks. + 40 hrs. with nurse-aide instructor + 8 hrs. in central service	Postprogram evaluation of perceived content value	Nurses learned policies, role practices & group-activity functioning
Bowe (1957)	Agency-perceived need for staff training	Tuberculosis Nursing: nonstructured weekly conferences, all topics	Staff group discussions & determination of new learning needs	Improved relationships among staff & between patients & staff; multidisciplinary involvement
Blumberg and Busche (1957)	Agency decision on staff need	Human Relations Training: 2 hrs./wk. for 10 wks.; supervisory nursing personnel	Postcourse evaluation; follow-up questionnaires at 4½ mos., followed by group interviews	Increased nurse participation in staff conferences; increased use of role play, counseling & communication skills
Hiner (1957)	Agency decision to aid RN professional development RN survey to determine topics	Selected topical meetings (e.g., pharmacy, diabetes, coronary disease, etc.): 1-hr. sessions monthly; 9 mo. program, all RN staff	Postprogram questionnaire for opinions on learning needs met, new topics, preferred meeting times	Nurses profited through knowledge gained or refreshed, expanded understandings of some topics
Poole (1958)	Agency decision to provide program	Disaster & First Aid: films & instruction; team & individual practice; all staff levels	Individual & group assessment of own learning during & after practice drills	Continuous program; promoted effective multirole functioning of all staff levels
Aydelotte and Tener (1960)	Educator-perceived need to help nurses improve patient care quality	Principles & Techniques of Patient Care: Examined effect of increasing staff without increasing patient care workload	Systematic work activity studies pre-post staff increases & pre-post in-service program	No improvement in patient welfare postprogram & none resulted from combined staff increases and in-service program

Source	Reason for Program	Program Description	Evaluation Measures	Outcomes
Hays (1960)	Agency need to prepare psychiatric nurse leaders	Staff Development in Psychiatric Nursing: 8-wk. course; focus on psychiatric principles, individual & group therapeutic interaction, patient & staff teaching; head nurses & potential head nurses	Precourse EPPS & psychiatric situations test; self- & program evaluations weekly; Post-self-met objectives, NLN achievement test, psychiatric situations; 6-mo. self- & supervisor evaluations	Improved RN ability to assume therapeutic role, patient & staff relations, conduct in-service sessions. Program-selected patients "seem to have benefited"
Rosenberg and Drew (1961)	Agency decision to provide program PHN list of questions related to topic	Dental Anatomy, Pathology & Hygiene: series of lectures for PHN staff of local health department	Post-program checklist; number of requests by PHNs to hear tapes of missed lectures	Increased PHN abilities to teach preventive dental care to patients & family & on fears & attitudes
Fine and Vavra (1962)	Agency-perceived need to develop an in-service program (also, opened a new hospital building)	Centralized & area programs & sessions on equipment & procedures, team nursing, patient teaching; staff & administrative sessions on all shifts	No measures described	Staff nurses & head nurses taught other personnel; group planning helped to improve morale and teamwork
Corona and Black (1963)	Agency-perceived need to reinforce team nursing concept. Staff survey showed limited knowledge of team nursing roles	Team Nursing Principles & Practice; series of 5 1-hr. weekly sessions; expanded to 6, and held on all shifts to accommodate all nurses	Postprogram evaluation of objectives met; follow-up opinions from supervisors on pre-post staff team behaviors; administrative observations of staff	Better communications among staff, more detail in care assignments, improved care plans and team conferences
Ritvo (1963)	Educator-perceived need for hospital supervisory staff to improve interpersonal & leadership skills	Human Relations Training: 2 hr. meetings weekly for 15 wks.	Anonymous postsession evaluations; formal interviews at 6-mos. postcourse; informal discussions	Although difficult to assess, insights were gained; observations showed "new" relationships between participants
Marshall (1964)	Educator decision to provide nursing process program & to explore follow-up methods	Nursing Care Plan Workshops: series of 4 1-day sessions on care plans, discharge planning, counseling & interviewing, ward teaching	Postprogram follow-up by supervisor & instructor; informal ward rounds, care plan & chart checks, discussions with head nurse & staff	Supervisory expectations and encouragement of staff RN implementation of workshop content
Frye (1965)	Agency-perceived need for closer ward supervision of nursing aides	On-the-job review of nursing procedures for night duty aides by charge nurses during a 3-mo. period	Subjective nurse evaluation of aide performance; head nurse subjective evaluations of patients' conditions in a.m., and review of patient comments	Increased awareness of night nurses concerning aide functioning and care practices

Table 34.1 (cont.)

Study	Determination of Need	Focus and Structure of Program	Evaluative Measures Used	Reported Outcomes
Loder (1965)	Supervisor decision to provide "in-service" to evening shift staff	Group meetings on evening shift on psychiatric patient care: 3 meetings/wk. to cover all staff on same topics	Record of topics presented	Improved intergroup relationships, interaction with patients, expression of staff feelings & opinions
Mercadante (1965)	Educator decision to develop program	Team Nursing Seminars, varying topics: 2 meetings/wk. off-duty time, RN team leaders	No measures described	Increased sharing of staff knowledge & problem-solving skills
Holliday (1967)	Educator decision to explore staff reactions to research-related in-service	Goals & Techniques of Data Collection (participant observation) on SCI Bowel-Training Project	Subjective evaluations by staff about participating in study-related activities	RNs felt had learned new facts about patients; aides felt increased self-worth
Baziak (1968)	Agency change in philosophy & management of psychiatric patients	Patient-centered, Colleague & Therapeutic Community Concepts: weekly meetings for 3 mos. with nursing director	Pre-post series of rating scales, observations, interviews, & transcriptions of group meetings	RNs less rigid, more expressively active due to instruction & support of nursing director
Goldman and Freund (1968)	Agency-perceived need to orient staff to new service department	Procedures related to Inhalation Therapy Department: 6 nursing divisions randomly assigned to 3 teaching approaches	Pre-post tests on knowledge; observations of errors in requests for inhalation therapy over 2-mo. period	No difference in knowledge gain per teaching method; programmed learning group made fewest errors
Hall and Mueller (1968)	Educator decision to explore training-related mental health attitude changes in NAs	Advanced Training in Psychiatric Nursing: 10-wk. course for 2 groups experienced NAs; new NA group received 12-wk. introductory training program	Pre-post test on mental illness ideology for new + 1 experienced group; 2nd group tested twice, 10-wks. apart, then given training	New NAs less custodially oriented after course; no postcourse attitude changes in experienced NA groups
McKinley (1968)	Agency-perceived need for staff leadership program	Management Principles & Nursing Service: 30 hrs. in weekly 2-hr. sessions, repeated for p.m. nurses; mixed teaching methods	Written case-method problem solving near course end; individual projects; postcourse interviews with selected nurses	Increased appreciation of good communications & personnel relationships; "thus effecting better nursing care"
Naber (1968)	Agency-perceived need by head nurses for role preparation program	Head Nurse Leadership Development: seminar series, range of topics, optional preceptored practice; selected head nurse candidates only	Postprogram anonymous, subjective feelings on program aspects & applicability of content	Program "yielded improved managerial skills, communication, and patient care"

Puleo (1968)	Educator decision to test teaching methods	Ward Management for Quality Patient Care: 1-hr. lecture vs. programmed module (2 wks. to complete) on-duty & at-home; 3 randomly selected RN groups	Pre-post tests on knowledge; records of time needed to complete module by on-duty & at-home groups	Use of programmed module involved less time & resulted in higher scores than lecture method
Diers and Johnson (1969)	Agency change from custodial to therapeutic environment; Staff-expressed role inadequacies & ambivalence	Psychiatric Nursing Workshop: 2 wks. on therapeutic nursing; individual + small & large group meetings; nurse-patient clinical practice sessions; workshop repeated at 1 yr.	Ongoing in-group evaluation of effectiveness; postworkshop subjective evaluations of learning	Staff learned to express their feelings & to elicit and understand patients' feelings; increased staff feelings of self-confidence
Nusinoff (1970)	Agency survey of staff problem situations and frustrations pre- & post (10 mos.) new change-of-shift in-service program	Interpersonal Relations in Nursing (+ charting, care plans, shift reports, talking with patients, leadership): 1-day institute/mo. for 10 mos.; some repeated to permit staff attendance at all 3 institute series	Informal observations; postsession evaluation of content & presentations	Progression from mixed menu to organized inservice plan decreased staff dissatisfactions & increased continuity of patient care
LaFontan (1971)	Educator decision to train all staff rotating through CCU	Coronary Care Course: 40 hrs. of formal classes + 1 wk. supervised practice; variable format to accommodate RNs on all shifts	Survey of coronary care attitudes and self-perceived skills at 2 yrs. pre- & 2 yrs. postprogram	In-house progam judged more successful than regional or other programs for meeting particular needs of own RN staff
LeCompte, Butts, and Busch (1972)	Eductor decision to test reliability of RN recordings of observed patient behavior-activity	Documentation of Observed Patient Behavior: 1-wk. workshop, videotaped patient situations observed by 3 randomly selected RN groups	Analysis of dictated observations of patient behaviors-activities & time-length of activity	Generally high agreement in all groups of behaviors observed; less agreement on timing of activities
McMahon and Neuman (1972)	Agency change in patient care procedure	Nursing Process Related to Postural Drainage: content + practice sessions (no other structure information given)	Postcourse procedure demonstration; self-evaluation of further learning needs	New evaluation tool designed to obtain staff and supervisor assessment of content application; no results presented
Neuman (1973)	Educator-perceived need of RNs for help in developing managerial abilities	Management Development Program: 2-2½ hrs. weekly (to 40 hrs.) presented yearly for first-line administrative RNs; structure modified in response to evaluations	Self-evaluations of progress & needs; supervisor evaluations of staff progress; chart audits, analysis of nursing & patient care incidents	Primary focus on program problems and subsequent program changes; no results presented

Table 34.1 *(cont.)*

Study	Determination of Need	Focus and Structure of Program	Evaluative Measures Used	Reported Outcomes
Sanborn, Sanborn, Seibert, Welsh, and Pyke (1973)	Educator-perceived opportunity to provide program	Doctor-Nurse Lecture Series: weekly for 9 wks.; lectures at 1 hospital were transmitted via interactive TV to a 2nd hospital	Postseries opinions of program & preferences for teaching methods; evaluation of TV medium by staff at 2nd hospital	No difference in opinions about program content; both groups ranked formal courses as most-preferred teaching method
Bunning (1975)	Small hospital & nursing home–perceived problems in providing adequate range of in-service programs to their staff	Multitopic periodic in-service programs provided by community college to 14 health-care facilities (rural) on contract basis: 2 sessions/day on monthly basis to each of 10 towns in 9-mo. school yr; same content in each town	Record of content & attendance at each session	Although generalized content did not meet institutional needs, was felt to be valuable addition to each institution's own in-service program
Distefano and Pryer (1975)	Agency-perceived need for staff understanding of mental health problems	Psychiatric Nursing Knowledge: 6-wk. program for RNs, LVNs, NAs; NA-matched control group	Pre-post tests on psychiatric nursing knowledge & opinions about mental illness	Psychiatric knowledge increased in all nursing groups; experimental NA group less restrictive than NA control group
Parker, Pierce, and Sturm (1975)	Agency decision to implement POR; staff-expressed need for more detailed information than had received previously	Problem-Oriented Record: series of 1-day workshops for nurses	Pre-post knowledge test; postworkshop attitude survey to compare pre-post feelings about POR (anonymous responses)	Significant gain in knowledge from workshop; nurse attitudes more favorable toward POR
Eckvahl (1976)	Agency-perceived need for management training program for selected nursing personnel	Management Training On-The-Job: 8-mo. series of lectures, clinical assignments, & seminars (2/3 time in clinical assignments)	Administrative evaluations (subjective) of the trainees' progress on a "periodic" basis	Large, cooperative nursing management team found to be needed to ensure program success
Linton and Marshall (1976)	Agency-perceived need to foster continuing RN learning. Survey of RN interest in specialty topics	Pulmonary Problems & Nursing Care: 2 hrs./wk. for 8 wks. (3/wk. to cover all shifts); interdisciplinary inputs into content (for RNs and LPNs)	Postcourse opinions about program (subjective); post-test on knowledge	Course felt to be of value to practice; post-test on knowledge felt to be threatening, anxiety-provoking
Monaco (1976)	Educator-perceived lack of programs for outpatient staff. Interviews with RNs to determine desired topics	Multitopic program: 30–45 min. sessions 2/mo.; repeated sessions to permit greater attendance; focus change to nurse presentations on own clinics & related topics	Program-evaluation tool developed at end of 1st year (to obtain separate RN & NA subjective evaluations of programs-presentations)	Nurses did not want more interviews to determine own learning needs; felt ongoing program adequate; NAs wanted to attend but not participate in programs

del Bueno (1977a)	Educator decision to provide program & study effects	Pharmacology Review & Nursing Applications: 10-hr. 4–6 wk. course in 10 hospitals (50 experimental & 50 control RNs)	Pre-post assessment of RN ability (knowledge) to question MD medication orders; pre-post observations of RN provision of medication-related information to patients	Improved RN ability to question medication orders, but no increase in RN provision of medication-related information to patients
Huckabay, Cooper, and Neal (1977)	Educator decision to explore effects of different teaching methods	Principles of Grief & Loss in Patient Care: 1-hr. class in each of 15 hospitals; 4 groups using lecture or filmstrip & discussion	Pre-post tests on knowledge transfer; post-test on feelings about program	Knowledge increase all groups; highest with filmstrip + discussion & lecture + discussion groups; these methods also most preferred by all groups
Jensen (1977)	Educator-perceived need for NAs to recognize-report patients' symptoms	Care of the Stroke Patient: 1-day workshops given by 1 hospital for NAs & for NAs at 17 local nursing homes	Postworkshop opinions of NAs about program; postprogram evaluation of NA performance improvement at 6 mo. by supervisors	NAs enjoyed workshop; supervisors felt that NA care-related performance had improved
Bille (1978)	Staff requests for information on alcoholism; 10% RN sample surveyed to determine topics	Care of the Alcoholic Patient: all-day workshop	No measures described	Use of staff interests & concerns led to high voluntary attendance
Boyer (1978)	Agency decision to provide program to change staff's rudeness/attitudes	Transactional Analysis in Customer Treatment: slide-tape program shown to all nursing personnel	Post-test on knowledge & opinions on program format	Staff enjoyed the program & learned the concepts, but did not change rudeness behaviors; no administrative reinforcement
Hennessy and Reavis (1978)	Educator-identified need for program based on nursing audit results & discussions with RNs & MDs	Acute Care of the Medical-Surgical Patient: 2-day sessions/wk. for 5½ wks. for RNs	Pre-post test on knowledge; course opinion form; follow-up individual interviews at 3 mos. on application of skills in practice	Increased RN use of assessment skills & patient-education activities
Adams (1979)	Agency-perceived staff need for instruction on emotional problems; chart audit showed "sporadic" reference to patients' mental status	Care of the Depressed Client: self-instructional module to be completed in 2 wks.	Pre-post chart audits (5 each RN); pre-post test of knowledge; case study	Improved nurse sensitivity to and charting of depression in clients

Table 34.1 *(cont.)*

Study	Determination of Need	Focus and Structure of Program	Evaluative Measures Used	Reported Outcomes
Bille (1979)	Educator decision to involve staff RNs in in-service planning; RNs explored learning needs of coworkers	Patient Teaching: 1-day workshop; 3 1-hr. preplanning sessions by representative staff RNs	Workshop opinion form; self-evaluation of skills use at 1 mo. postworkshop	Felt that learner motivation to use skills was increased due to participation in program development
McGugin, Merkel, and Hofing (1979)	Agency decision to implement POR	Problem-Oriented Record: 5 self-instructional modules + 1 hr. group session/wk. for 5 wks. for practice & discussion	Pre-post test on knowledge, skills & attitudes on POR; opinions about program; chart audit in ICU during 6 mo. period postprogram	Significant increase in knowledge, skills & positive attitudes on POR in groups with & without prior POR experience
Vendura (1979)	Staff-expressed dissatisfaction with 36-hr. LPN Pharmacology course + 2 mo. head nurse observation period; high number drug errors by RNs & LPNs	3-Phase Pharmacology Course (theory, math, roleplay & clinical assignments): a competency-based, variable-length program for all new RN & LPN employees	Pre-test on theoretical & math knowledge; post-tests at end of each phase-step of program; course opinion form	Medication error decrease among LPNs and new RNs during 1st yr.; no decrease in errors among RNs who did not take the course
Evenson (1980)	Educator-perceived need for staff nurse increase in quality assurance skills	Quality Assurance Teaching Program: 5 1-hr. sessions in one hospital; 4 1-hr. sessions in 2nd hospital	Pre-post test on knowledge; course value opinions; informal follow-up assessments of knowledge use	Staff knowledge increased in both hospitals; one hospital very active in evaluating patient care program; other hospital focused on evaluating selected patient-care practices
Hansell & Foster (1980)	Educator-perceived need to facilitate ongoing critical care in-service program at reduced cost	Critical Care Inservice Program; 3-wk. structured format vs. 3-wk. self-instructional modules; randomly selected RN experimental & control groups	Pre-post tests on knowledge, anxiety, professional values; comparison of costs per method	Self-instructional modules proved less costly & more satisfying to staff
O'Leary and Holzemer (1980)	RNs self-perceived need & request for course; policy developed to require venipuncture certification every 2 yrs.	Venipuncture Certification: 2-hr. workshops, repeated to permit attendance by all RNs over 6-mo. period	Post-test at 2–8 mo. to assess skill retention by randomly selected RNs: 6 on patient arm, 8 on simulated arm & 10 control RNs (untrained) on simulated arm	No difference in trained RNs on patient or simulated arm; control RNs scored poorly on simulated arm; validated use of simulated arm for venipuncture training

Source	Need/Rationale	Program	Evaluation	Findings
Puntillo and Duncan (1980)	Educator decision to provide program for ICU nurses & to test teaching approach	Assessment of Cardiopulmonary Interventions: 5 weekly 2-hr. seminars + 6 hrs. independent study on self-selected subtopics; ICU nurses	Pretest on knowledge; posttest option: on knowledge or use of nursing process forms; subjective feelings about program	Seminar format promoted discussion of self-learning; course content judged too extensive
Stetler, Garrity, Macdonald, and Smith (1980)	Agency-perceived need for management training for nurse middle managers; learning needs assessed through interviews, skills inventory, & study of critical incidents	Management Orientation Program: 3-day session on concepts; series of 10 instructor-guided modules; 12-mo. program with top nursing management involvement	Evaluation of 3-day program not described; modules involved pretests and in-class debriefings to present-discuss results of assignments	Nurses perceived content & method to be applicable in the clinical units; positive response to formal program & module sessions
Turkeltaub (1980)	Investigator-selected topic	Patient Teaching & Documentation in Diabetes Mellitus: 2-day course for experimental RN group; 1-hr. general diabetes documentation information for control RN group; double-blind study	Pretest chart audits & pretests on knowledge; post-test chart audits at 8 weeks	Increased chart-audit scores were accepted as evidence of improved care quality; no correlations between knowledge increases & chart-audit scores
Cox and Baker (1981)	Agency-perceived need for PHNs to meet newly developed behaviorally written practice standards	Role Expansion Program: 3-wk. university course for PHNs of local county health dept.; nonrandom experimental & control (untrained) groups	Pre-post tests on knowledge for both groups; 7 reinforcement-evaluation sessions for experimental group; chart audits before + 6 mos. after for experimental group only	Knowledge & chart score gains for experimental group; 86% judged competent in new skills; educational preparation affected knowledge gain
Heick (1981)	Agency-perceived need for CHN staff to be prepared for maternal child health role	Community Health Nursing Care of the Childbearing Family: university-provided 1-day sessions for 12 wks. at 4 community sites for state-employed CHNs; 1-day follow-up workshop at 4 mos. for CHNs & their supervisors	Follow-up survey at 2 mo. of CHNs & supervisors to assess MCH practice changes; resurvey at 8 mos. of CHNs & supervisors to reassess MCH practices & needs	Improvements in CHNs' MCH practices noted to varying degrees in respective agencies; further problem situations and other CHN learning needs identified
Kasprisin, Kasprisin, Marks, Yogore, and Williams (1981)	RNs' expressed need for more information about transfusion therapy	Blood Component Therapy Course: 6 1-hr. sessions	Pretest on various areas of transfusion therapy information; data used to develop course content	Course effect not described; precourse RN knowledge base described to document need for course

Table 34.1 *(cont.)*

Study	Determination of Need	Focus and Structure of Program	Evaluative Measures Used	Reported Outcomes
Buechler (1982)	Agency & staff concern about abilities to handle "CODE" situations effectively	Inservice sessions to show videotapes of mock and real CODE expectations: 10 sessions in 24-hr. period; mock CODE tape reviewed on each unit immediately after practice sessions-drills	Post-testing by 39 mock CODEs (13 units, 3 shifts) using established criteria & written & oral critiques postdrills; mock CODEs repeated at 12 mos. & re-evaluated on criteria	Improvement in staff abilities to handle mock CODEs; annual CPR reviews & semiannual mock drills improved staff response to real CODE situations
Holloran (1982)	Agency change of policy due to attrition from male NA catheterization team	Teaching Male Catheterizations: 3-mo. program for all RNs; 30 "trainers" given course on human sexuality & catheterization procedures. Mass program: 15 1½-hrs. sessions to reach all RN staff; film, lecture, simulation catheterizations (20 mins.), & other GU care approaches	Initial needs assessment on GU patient care program; feedback during "trainer" training; formative feedback on added approaches; post-training feedback on staff anxieties, MD reactions; pre-post tally of catheterizations by RNs	Involvement of RN staff group in planning facilitated development & implementation of program; anxieties overcome; reduction in nosocomial UTIs
Fogelsong (1983)	Educator decision to present course; audit of random charts to determine RN postsurgical patient care practices	Use of Medications for Effective Relief of Postoperative Pain: no information provided on course structure	Reaudit of postoperative charts 3 to 4 wks. after class	RNs gave more pain medicines after class, especially in 8–16 hrs. period postoperatively; pain relief documentation also increased
Lesher and Bomberger (1983)	Audit after prior 22-hr. class showed low care-plan completion; no feasible time period for holding repeat classes	Roving In-service Approach: weekly bulletin board placement of hypothetical patient situation for care plan development; instructor feedback on care plans for each nursing unit	Program evaluation form (subjective reactions)	No data presented; staff were "unanimous in favor of the roving in-service"
Parker, Alkhateeb, and Rosen (1983)	Educator decision to provide program; survey of all levels of nursing staff on 3 medical-surgical floors to assess attitudes & felt competencies	Patient Education Techniques-Methods for Nurses: no information provided on program structure	No measures described	Nurse attitudes toward patient education more positive; used greater variety of teaching aids; found no single answer to patient teaching problems

Author	Need/Rationale	Program Description	Evaluation	Results
Ellson (1984)	Agency-perceived minimal effect of prior 30-min. class on charting of care goals & patient teaching; base-line chart & kardex audit	Goal Writing/Patient Teaching Workshop: 5 1-hr. sessions at each of 5 VNA agency offices; 30-min. review at 6 wks; 45-min. review at 6 mos.	Subjective evaluations of each sesison; postaudit of 10 charts & kardexes at 6 mos. in each VNA office	Improved documentation on setting & updating of care goals; less improvement in documentation of patient teaching
Lang and Slayton (1984)	Agency-perceived need for role-context training for newly created charge nurse positions	Management Approaches (role & duties, priority-setting, decision making, communication, etc.): program structure not described	Evaluative questions listed; information on tools and obtained results not provided	Narrative focuses on inputs considered; effects of program not described
Oliver (1984)	Educator decision to provide CHN course on physical assessment skills	Adult Health Screening Workshops: 5-day courses on physical assessment skills (general + cardiopulmonary) held in 26 rural & urban state health dept. agencies; attendee & nonattendee groups	Pre-post records analysis (during 1 year before & after); postworkshop client home visits to observe CHN use of assessment skills (during 1-year postworkshop)	Slight improvement in record keeping among attendees; need for reinforcement of assessment skills by CHN supervisors
Shamian and Lemieux (1984)	Agency-perceived public concern about use of restraints; explored current criteria for & prevalence in use of restraints	Assessment & Interventions with Confused Patients, & Policies & Procedures in Use of Restraints: 2 sessions, 2 teaching methods (2 classes vs. preceptor + 1 formal class); random assignment of 14 nursing units	Post-test on knowledge at end of 2nd session; questionnaire at 3 mos. to RNS with preceptor, RNS who had 1 or 2 classes & RNs who did not attend program	Preceptor group retained more knowledge at 3 mos. than formal class group; control group results not reported
Dickinson, Holzemer, and Nichols (1985)	Agency (VNA)-perceived lack of arthritis knowledge in basic preparation of PHNs	Arthritis-Related Problems & Nursing Interventions: 2 2-hr. sessions 1 wk. apart for 2 randomly selected PHN groups	Post-test on arthritis experience & knowledge; chart audit at 4 wks. postprogram for 1st group & immediately preprogram for 2nd group	Program led to increased charting of arthritis-related nursing interventions
Sullivan and Decker (1985)	Agency-perceived need for program to train new nursing manager staff	Behavior Modeling Workshops on Different Topics (performance appraisals, counseling, employee complaints, etc.): 6–8 hrs. of lecture-discussion + role play with video feedback reinforcement	No measures described or inferred (recommended self-reinforcement or reinforcement by external source, e.g., supervisors)	Nursing management practice reportedly improved; head nurses felt more confidence in roles

Table 34.1 *(cont.)*

Study	Determination of Need	Focus and Structure of Program	Evaluative Measures Used	Reported Outcomes
Lifson and Cantlon (1986)	Agency-perceived need for trianing of charge nurses; development of charge nurse learning-needs assessment tool	Charge Nurse Leadership Program: 2-day seminar + ½-day follow-up session at 4 wks. to review individual progress in implementing leadership-oriented "projects"	Postcourse self-evaluation of objectives met and content areas, plans for knowledge use; post-program surveys among participants and supervisors at 1 yr.	Increased knowledge, self-confidence, & collegial relationships among participants; long-term effects perceived: higher-level functioning, greater job satisfaction, positive changes in performance ratings
Vogelberger (1986)	Agency-perceived need for program to alleviate care plan deficits	Nursing Care Plan Program: 1-hr. formal session on nursing diagnosis & goal setting, followed by unstated number of small group practice sessions on all shifts for all nurses; 2nd 1-hr. formal session at 8 wks, + more practice sessions; 3rd formal session at unstated period focusing on planning, implementing, & evaluating aspects of nursing process; another review session after approval of new chart-care plan form	1st session post-test on ability to make nursing diagnoses; individual & small-group feedback from practice sessions; quality assurance chart & care plan reviews for nursing diagnoses & goals; "random" chart reviews by education department	Staff response "positive" at end of 1st session; nurse difficulty in identifying goals at 2nd and subsequent sessions; head nurses developed own approaches to reduce care plan problem in own areas; efforts to improve care plans "are continuing"

PHN = public health nurse; EPPS = Edwards Personal Preference Scale; NLN = National League for Nursing; SCI = spinal cord injury; NA = nursing aides/assistants; CODE = call for emergency; UTI = urinary tract infection; GU = genito-urinary.

in-service programs, four programs were described that evolved because staff asked for new knowledge; 38 reflected an agency-perceived need for an in-service program; and 28 reflected a decision by academicians or in-service educators to provide a program.

As anticipated, the focus of programs varied widely, and the evaluative measures used varied with respect to how the need had been determined and the program was structured. A "happiness index" to obtain participants' perceptions of a program's value was described in 30 of the reports; 20 programs assessed knowledge on a pretest and post-test basis, three on a pretest basis only, and 9 on a post-test basis only. Participant self-assessments of knowledge or skills were noted in 12 reports; nine reports included formal or informal supervisor observations; and educator observations were reported in six publications. Pre-audits and post-audits of various records were reported for six programs; one described only a preprogram audit. The sole documentation described for two programs consisted of a list of the topics presented together with the number of people who attended.

Evaluation instruments were not identified in eight reports. Outcomes reported for 44 of the educational interventions indicated that program objectives were given appropriate consideration when the evaluative measures were selected.

There was a scattering of experimental studies; 14 reports included sufficient detail to support replication studies. In 10 of the publications, however, the reported outcomes reflected the program intent but the evaluative measures seemed to assess something other than the stated objectives and projected outcomes of the programs. Because this reporting deficit occurred more often in publications prior to the 1970s, one suspects that the omission of such important detail may have been related to an editorial preference for "briefed" reports and for informa-

tion primarily about the focus and structure of programs rather than for measurement— a preference that prevails even today.

Missing in many reports were descriptions of pilot testing and attempts to resolve problems in estimating the validity, reliability, and sensitivity of the data collection instruments. For example, the effects of some programs were measured through the use of subjective participant self-report questionnaires instead of through systematic observations of desired behaviors. While the latter type of measurement may not have been feasible, the validity of self-reports of one's own practice is always subject to question.

On the other hand, although systematic observations of practice are strongly recommended today by many experts, observational studies require observer training, which is time-consuming and costly, and therefore often impractical. Nursing audits have been found useful for highlighting educational needs and are often effective as follow-up measures of performance against established standards. However, because audits do not measure the nursing care actually being given, skill-utilization checklists could test such practices if applied objectively and at randomly selected time periods.

Efforts to determine the value of programs, in terms of knowledge gained and retained, may be thwarted because of high staff-attrition and nonresponse rates, and any measurement of knowledge that is used is usually conditioned by many factors. Problems arise, too, in attempts to address program costs. Estimates of the direct costs of personnel and supplies often can be determined more accurately than can indirect costs. Information related to administrative and other indirect costs, both fixed and variable, is difficult to obtain in most institutional settings.

Although it is generally accepted that the impact of an educational program may not be immediately determinable, a major shortcoming in many of the reports was the seeming unconcern for measuring the long-term or even the intermediate-term effects. A modification in attitudes or practices may take place in three to six or more months following an educational intervention. Moreover, in the evaluation of educational outcomes, it is usually essential to account for the effects of extraneous factors, including variations in management approaches and work climates. For example, one study demonstrated that community health nurses who received postprogram support and reinforcement from their immediate supervisors continued to incorporate their newly learned practice skills in their clinical setting. Community health nurses who did not receive support from supervisors tended to practice their new skills less consistently.[16]

Despite the broad mix of measures used for evaluating in-service education programs over the years, some clear trends can be identified. In the earliest reports, the success of an educational endeavor often tended to be judged in terms of the numbers of nurse staff who attended the training sessions provided. While attendance data continue to be a significant factor in justifying many in-service efforts, the reasons for attendance as a justification are different. In today's in-service offerings, staff interest and the relevance of content to practice are important considerations. In earlier times, nurses had limited opportunities to attend even the few educational programs that were available.

In the ensuing years, as nurses have been able to choose from an array of in-service programs, nurse educators have begun using a "happiness index" to assess nurses' satisfaction with content and methods of presentation. The end-program measurement of satisfaction continues to be used in many contemporary in-service offerings, and sometimes still serves as the only form of program evaluation.

Because satisfaction with in-service pro-gramming, in isolation from other factors, has not been directly associated with readily discernable improvements in nursing practice, nurse educators have initiated more frequent use of post-, pre-post, and follow-up testing of personnel knowledge and competency. Social and economic pressures for accountability have contributed to the emergence of such quality assurance measures as procedure reviews and records audits, and have furthered the development of realistic, achievable nursing standards of practice. Although there is evidence of increasing use of one or more of these more sophisticated approaches to evaluating contemporary in-service, reports in the current literature indicate that multidimensional measures are still not being used to assess the facets of in-service education. To generate results that are meaningful and useful for in-service efforts, evaluative methods need to be consistent with program and teaching strategies, and related to program objectives.

DEVELOPING AN EVALUATION PLAN

To demonstrate accountability, the manager of an in-service department must be able to do more than just document that a program provides orientation and on-the-job training for new employees and that various other educational endeavors enhance the end-program knowledge and skill repertoires of already-employed nurses. Nurse administrators who believe that their in-service departments should function in support of overall organizational goals are responsible for ensuring that practical yet systematic evaluation strategies are developed and operationalized, so that the effectiveness of in-service can be studied and the tangible benefits can be identified.[7]

Unfortunately, there is little evidence in the literature that broad-based analyses of in-service functioning have been attempted. Moreover, guidelines for conducting such total program evaluations are conspicuously absent. In the still widely used traditional model for evaluating educational courses,[22] emphasis is on the development and use of valid and reliable outcome assessments to determine whether the stated behavioral objectives of a single, specific educational offering have been met.

Using this model, the educator defines what knowledge and skill outcomes are expected and applies the selected outcome measures at the end of a program to assure that learning effects can be attributed in large measure to in-service training. This evaluative approach is direct and clear and lends itself well to quantification, but it does not take into account the range of antecedent personal characteristics of learners—their previous patient care and decision-making experience, motivation, and willingness to change—and work environment factors, such as peer pressure, supervisor expectations, available facilities, and the mix of patients— all of which can influence not only the application of new knowledge but the total learning process.

More important, the traditional evaluation model is simply not designed to permit appraisal of the various ways the overall in-service activity contributes materially to such qualitative goals as the enhancement of employee productivity and morale. Nor can inferences be made as to how the in-service department contributes to quality care.

In considering the many activities associated with the effective functioning of an active in-service education department, it is obvious that no single evaluation strategy can adequately address this complex entity. In-service programs are essentially qualitative in nature—the cognitive changes they bring about in people are usually changes manifest in behavior or performance occurring at some future point in time. Because efforts to evaluate the efficacy of qualitative programs are usually addressed with quantitative methods, in-service managers increasingly are attempting to quantify their various short- and long-term goals and to identify those aspects of in-service education that defy quantification.

To facilitate new ways of thinking about program evaluation, it is perhaps best to begin by constructing a conceptual model that outlines the overall purpose, process, structure, and outcomes of an in-service program. In short, a model needs to be constructed that provides a parsimonious picture of the program which can facilitate evaluation by specifying the factors to be studied. Using such a model, evaluation plans can be developed that define, in advance of program implementation, those goals, outcomes, and effects against which the progress of each major aspect can be systematically measured; and sampling, data collection, and analysis procedures can be undertaken that are appropriate for each aspect of the program.

Two theoretical perspectives that are particularly useful for evaluating in-service programs are the goal attainment and systems approaches. Goal attainment focuses on the intended consequences of a selected program and considers the processes for achieving specified goals and outcomes. The systems approach takes into account the total environment of a program and the many extraneous activities related to the attainment of goals. In the open-system approach, factors that are external to the program but that influence the program processes and outcomes are considered.

Due to the heterogeneous character of in-service, the questions needing answers are complex. Consequently, an evaluation plan most appropriate for determining in-service effectiveness may well combine the systems and goal approaches.

Nurse administrators who promote forward-thinking and on-the-job education expect in-service programs to encompass far more than training. Documentation of in-service accountability requires the development of a measurement system that taps as many aspects of in-service effectiveness as possible, with an evaluative process that is a part of an organization's overall operation. For in-service to be viewed as a continuing worthwhile investment, information derived from the in-service evaluation should be up-to-date, reflect involvement in the total organization, and serve as a vital aspect of quality patient care.

REFERENCES

1. Longest BB. Management practices for the health professional. 2nd ed. Reston, VA: Reston Publishing Inc, 1980, pp. 39–49.
2. Shortell SM, Richardson WC. Health program evaluation. St. Louis: CV Mosby, 1978, p. 8.
3. Suchman EA. Evaluative research. New York: Russell Sage Foundation, 1967, p. 31.
4. Sovie MD. Investigate before you educate. J Nurs Adm 1981;11(4):15–21.
5. Copp LA. Inservice education copes with resistance to change. J Cont Educ Nurs 1975;6(2):19–27.
6. del Bueno DJ. Accountability in staff education. AORN J 1975;22(4):538–541.
7. del Bueno DJ. Nursing staff development: critical times, critical issues. J Nurs Staff Develop 1986; 2(3):94–97.
8. Clemenhagen C, Champagne F. Quality assurance as part of program evaluation: guidelines for managers and clinical department heads. Qual Rev Bull 1986;12(11):383–387.
9. Rossi PH, Freeman HE, Wright SR. Evaluation: a systematic approach. Beverly Hills, CA: Sage Publications Inc, 1979.
10. Faulk LG. Continuing education program evaluation for course improvement, participant effect and utilization in clinical practice. J Nurs Educ 1984; 23(4):139–146.
11. Arney WR. Evaluation of a continuing nursing education program and its implications. J Cont Educ Nurs 1978;9(1):45–51.
12. Betz CL. Needs assessment and evaluation: methods used in nursing continuing education programs. J Cont Educ Nurs 1984;15(2):39–44.
13. Franklin JL, Thrasher JH. An introduction to program evaluation. New York: John Wiley & Sons, 1976.
14. Adelman HS. Intervention theory and evaluating efficacy. Eval Rev 1986;10(1):65–83.
15. Chen HT, Rossi PH. Evaluating with sense: the theory driven approach. Eval Rev 1983;7(3):293–302.
16. Cox CL, Baker MG. Evaluation: the key to accountability in continuing education. J Cont Educ Nurs 1981;12(1):11–19.
17. Koonz FP. Identification of learning needs. J Cont Educ Nurs 1978;9(3):6–11.
18. Yura H, Torres G. Educational trends which influenced the development of the conceptual framework within the curriculum. In: Faculty-curriculum development, Part III: conceptual framework—its meaning and function. New York: National League for Nursing, Department of Baccalaureate and Higher Degree Programs, 1975, p. 9–16, NLN publication no. 15-1558.
19. McKay RP. The conceptual framework as a component of curriculum development. In: Faculty-curriculum development, Part III: conceptual framework—its meaning and function. New York: National League for Nursing, Department of Baccalaureate and Higher Degree Programs, 1975, p. 31–40, NLN publication no. 15-1558.
20. Thompson MS. Benefit-cost analysis for program evaluation. Beverly Hills, CA: Sage Publications Inc, 1980.
21. Kibbee P. Developing a model for implementation of an evaluation component in an orientation program. J Cont Educ Nurs 1980;11(5):25–29.
22. Tyler RW. Basic principles of curriculum and instruction. Chicago: University of Chicago Press, 1950, pp. 68–81.
23. Dixon J. Evaluation criteria in studies of continuing education in the health professions: a critical review and suggested strategy. Evaluation and the Health Professions 1978;1(2):39–56.
24. Donovan HM. Inservice programs and their evaluation. Nurs Outlook 1956;4(11):633–635.
25. Epstein I, Tripodi T. Research techniques for program planning, monitoring, and evaluation. New York: Columbia University Press, 1977.
26. Mitsunaga B, Shores L. Evaluation in continuing education: is it practical? J Cont Educ Nurs 1977; 8(6):7–14.
27. Reilly DE. Behavioral objectives in nursing: evaluation of learner attainment. New York: Appleton-Century-Crofts, 1975.
28. Bille DA. An experience with formative evaluation. J Cont Educ Nurs 1976;7(4):25–30.
29. Alexander M. Evaluating the behavioral objectives. J Cont Educ Nurs 1985;16(2):63–64.
30. Chatham MA. A continuing education program for nursing aides: communication skills, self concept, and problem solving. J Cont Educ Nurs 1978;9(5): 26–29.
31. Goodykoonz L. Evaluating a continuing education program. J Cont Educ Nurs 1980;11(4):25–28.
32. Mezoff B. How to get accurate self-reports of training courses. Training and Develop J 1981; 35(9):56–61.
33. Corbett TC. Evaluation of post-implementation strategies and systems. In: Murphy KAJ, ed. The evaluation of continuing education for professionals: a systems view. Seattle: University of Washington Press, 1979:345–349.

34. Derby VL. Learners and course goal congruence: impact on learning outcomes. J Cont Educ Nurs 1982;13(4):16–25.
35. Marshall MH. Inservice programs require effective follow-up. Nurs Outlook 1964;12(8):42–44.
36. Boyer CM. Performance-based staff development: the cost-effective alternative. Nurse Educator 1981; 6(6):12–15.
37. Prescott PA, Sorensen JE. Cost-effectiveness analysis: an approach to evaluating nursing programs. Nurs Adm Quart 1978;3(1):17–40.
38. Shipp T. Cost-benefit/effectiveness analysis for continuing education. J Cont Educ Nurs 1981;12(4):6–14.
39. American Nurses Association. Guidelines for staff development. Kansas City: American Nurses Association, 1976.
40. Calkin JD. Let's rethink staff development programs. J Nurs Adm 1979;9(6):16–19.
41. Rufo KL. Guidelines for inservice education for registered nurses. J Cont Educ Nurs 1981;12(1): 26–33.
42. Stevens BJ. The nurse as executive. 2nd ed. Wakefield, MA: Nursing Resources Inc, 1980, pp. 327–351.
43. Stopera V, Scully D. A workable organizational model for staff development departments. J Cont Educ Nurs 1972;3(6):14–19.
44. Arndt C, Huckabay LMD. Nursing administration. St. Louis: CV Mosby, 1975, pp. 136–151.
45. Tobin H, Yoder-Wise PS, Hull P. The process of staff development: components for change. 2nd ed. St. Louis: CV Mosby, 1979.
46. Stake RE. The countenance of educational evaluation. In: Worthen BR, Sanders JR, eds. Educational evaluation: theory and practice. Belmont, CA: Wadsworth Publishing Co, 1973, pp. 106–128.
47. Yoder-Wise PS, Cox H. Evaluating a continuing nursing education program. J Cont Educ Nurs 1984;15(4):117–121.
48. Fojtasek G. A model for evaluating a staff development program. J Cont Educ Nurs 1985;16(2):58–62.
49. Puetz BE. Evaluation in nursing staff development. Rockville, MD: Aspen Systems Corporation, 1985.
50. Worthen BR, Sanders JR, eds. Educational evaluation: theory and practice. Belmont, CA: Wadsworth Publishing Co, 1973.
51. Matheny RV. Historical perspectives. In: Abdellah FA, Beland IL, Martin A, Matheny AV, eds. New directions in patient-centered nursing. New York: Macmillan, 1973, pp. 151–159.
52. Roberts MM. American nursing. A history and interpretation. New York: Macmillan, 1954.
53. Cooper SS, Hornback MS. Continuing nursing education. New York: McGraw-Hill, 1973.
54. Pfefferkorn B. Improvement of the nurse in service: an historical review. Am J Nurs 1928;28(7):700–710.
55. Beck MB. Staff education programs. Am J Nurs 1934;34:(9):901–907.
56. Densford K. An "in-service" program of staff education. Proceedings of the National League of Nursing Education, 35th annual report. New York: National League of Nursing Education, 1929, pp. 115–124.
57. Holtzhausen EA. Nursing service in a teaching hospital. Am J Nurs 1946;46(8):1–5.
58. Brown EL. Nursing for the future. New York: Russell Sage Foundation, 1948.
59. Abdellah FG. Criterion measures in nursing. Nurs Res 1961;10(4):21–26.
60. Abdellah FG. Methods of identifying covert aspects of nursing problems. Nurs Res 1957;6(2):4–23.
61. Nite G, Willis F. Nursing care of the hospitalized cardiac patient. New York: Macmillan, 1964.
62. Aydelotte MK. The use of patient welfare as a criterion measure. Nurs Res 1962;11(1):10–14.
63. Spitzer R. Catch the wave of nursing in the '90s. Nursing 87 Career Directory, 1987:8–10.
64. McMahon J, Neumann MM. Tool for evaluating the impact of an inservice program for nursing care. J Cont Educ Nurs 1972;3(2):5–7.
65. Thomas L. Prescriptive education. Nurs Outlook 1973;21(7):450–452.
66. Mundinger M. CE: Current contradictions in inservice. Nurs Adm Quart 1978;2(2):65–71.
67. Delabarre HC. An in-service program in neurologic nursing. Am J Nurs 1951;51(8):498–500.
68. Burnett FM, Greenhill MH. Some problems in the evaluation of an inservice training program in mental health. Am J Public Health 1954;44(12):1546–1556.
69. Rutan EL. A cooperative program of inservice education. Nurs Outlook 1956;4(9):522–524.
70. Bowe AB. Inservice education in tuberculosis nursing. Nurs Outlook 1957;5(8):472–475.
71. Blumberg A, Busche MJ. An inservice program in human relations. Nurs Outlook 1957;5(12):703–705.
72. Hiner B. Inservice education for good service. Nurs Outlook 1957;5(8):218–219.
73. Poole D. Preparing hospital nursing staffs for disaster service. Nurs Outlook 1958;6(10):586–589.
74. Aydelotte MK, Tener ME. An investigation of the relation between nursing activity and patient welfare. Iowa City: Nurse Utilization Project Staff, State University of Iowa, 1960.
75. Hays JES. A staff development program in psychiatric nursing. Nurs Outlook 1960;8(4):210–211.
76. Rosenburg A, Drew DM. An inservice program on dental health. Nurs Outlook 1961;9(2):85–87.
77. Fine RB, Vavra C. Content and consequences of an inservice education program. Am J Nurs 1962; 62(1):54–56.
78. Corona DF, Black EA. One hospital's approach to team nursing. Nurs Outlook 1963;11(7):506–507.
79. Ritvo MM. Human relations training for supervisory personnel in hospitals. Nurs Forum 1963;2(3):98–112.
80. Frye LB. An on-duty inservice experiment for aides. Nurs Outlook 1965;13(8):60–61.

81. Loder EE. "Group" inservice with the evening shift. Nurs Outlook 1965;13(7):31–33.

82. Mercadante LT. Leadership development seminars. Nurs Outlook 1965;13(9):59–61.

83. Holliday J. Clinical research training and subjective reactions of nursing service staff to the study process. Nurs Res 1967;16(3):219–227.

84. Baziak AT. Influencing nursing practice in changing hospital settings. Nurs Res 1968;17(2):146–154.

85. Goldman J, Freund LE. Implementation of a change. Nurs Res 1968;17(3):268–269.

86. Hall EL, Mueller BS. Effect of training on the mental illness ideologies of nursing assistants. Nurs Res 1968;17(2):172–174.

87. McKinley JE. Inservice education for leadership. Nurs Outlook 1968;16(9):47–49.

88. Naber M. A development program for head nurses. Nurs Outlook 1968;16(6):48–49.

89. Puleo MP. Comparison of on-the-job and at-home use of programmed instruction and the lecture method in an inservice education program. Nurs Res 1968;17(4):356–360.

90. Diers D, Johnson JE. How workshops prepare nurses for the therapeutic role. Nurs Outlook 1969;17(6):30–34.

91. Nusinoff JR. A structural approach to inservice education. J Cont Educ Nurs 1970;1(4):21–27.

92. LaFontan L. An approach to ICU nurse education in a small, rural, community hospital. J Cont Educ Nurs 1971;2(5):32–37.

93. LeCompte WF, Butts SV, Busch DE. Effects of training on behavioral observations by nurses. Nurs Res 1972;21(5):448–452.

94. Neuman MM Developing nurses' ability to manage . . . A program design. J Cont Educ Nurs 1973; 4(6):28–33.

95. Sanborn DE, Sanborn CJ, Seibert DJ, Welsh GW, Pyke HF. Continuing education for nurses via interactive closed-circuit television: a pilot study. Nurs Res 1973;22(5):448–451.

96. Bunning RI. Nursing inservice education in rural America: one proposal for meeting the need. J Cont Educ Nurs 1975;6(2):28–30.

97. Distefano MK, Pryer MW. Effect of brief training on mental health knowledge and attitudes of nurses and nurses' aides in a general hospital. Nurs Res 1975;24(1):40–42.

98. Parker B, Pierce M, Sturm I. Evaluating a workshop method for teaching the problem-oriented record to nurses. J Cont Educ Nurs 1975;6(3):34–39.

99. Eckvahl VR. On-the-job training. J Nurs Adm 1976;6(3):38–40.

100. Linton CB, Marshall FM. A hospital-based graduate nurses specialty institute: a continuing education program. J Cont Educ Nurs 1976;7(1):5–9.

101. Monaco RJ. Out-patient nurse involvement—An answer to success. J Cont Educ Nurs 1976;7(1):10–17.

102. del Bueno DJ. Continuing education. Spinach and other good things. J Nurs Adm 1977;7(4):32–34.

103. Huckabay LM, Cooper PG, Neal MC. Effect of specific teaching techniques on cognitive learning, transfer of learning, and affective behavior of nurses in an inservice education setting. Nurs Res 1977;26(5):380–385.

104. Jensen DL. A continuing education opportunity for nursing assistants. J Cont Educ Nurs 1977;8(5): 12–14.

105. Bille DA. Planning staff development: Theory X, or theory Y? J Cont Educ Nurs 1978;9(6):10–15.

106. Boyer CM. The answer doesn't always come prepackaged. Nurse Educator 1978;3(2):17–18.

107. Hennessy EC, Reavis R. Acute care of the medical-surgical patient: a program for non-critical care nurses. J Cont Educ Nurs 1978;9(4):29–32.

108. Adams R. A study of changes in client care activities of registered professional nurses following planned continuing education instruction. Dissertation. Tallahassee, FL: College of Education, Florida State University, 1979.

109. Bille DA. Successful educational programming: increased learner motivation through involvement. J Nurs Adm 1979;9(5):36–42.

110. McGugin M, Merkel S, Hofing A. An andragogical approach to teaching the problem-oriented method of recording. J Cont Educ Nurs 1979; 10(1):7–11.

111. Vendura N. Pharmacology program produces results. J Nurs Adm 1979;9(9):34–39.

112. Evenson BO. Teaching quality assurance. Nurse Educator 1980;5(2):8–12.

113. Hansell HN, Foster SB. Critical care nursing orientation: a comparison of teaching methods. Heart and Lung 1980;9(6):1066–1072.

114. O'Leary M, Holzemer WL. Evaluation of an inservice program. J Nurs Adm 1980;10(3):21–23.

115. Puntillo K, Duncan J. An alternative learning experience for intensive care unit nurses. J Cont Educ Nurs 1980;11(3):44–50.

116. Stetler CB, Garrity J, Macdonald ME, Smith S. A modular approach to management development. J Nurs Adm 1980;10(12):19–24.

117. Turkeltaub MRK. A study to determine the impact of a continuing education course for registered nurses on knowledge and skills utilized in providing patient care. Dissertation. Baltimore: School of Nursing, University of Maryland, 1980.

118. Heick MA. Continuing education impact evaluation. J Cont Educ Nurs 1981;12(4):15–23.

119. Kasprisin CA, Kasprisin DO, Marks D, Yogore MG, Williams HL. Quality assurance beyond the blood-bank. Supervisor Nurse 1981;12(5):45–48.

120. Buechler D. Code blue evaluation. Nurs Management 1982;13(5):25–28.

121. Holloran SD. Teaching male catheterization: an application of change theory for an entire nursing staff. Nurse Educator 1982;7(1):11–14.

122. Fogelsong DH. The impact of a staff development offering on nursing practice. J Cont Educ Nurs 1983;14(6):12–15.

123. Lesher DC, Bomberger AS. The roving inservice— An innovative approach to learning. J Cont Educ Nurs 1983;14(3):19–22.

124. Parker MC, Alkhateeb WA, Farkash Rosen DL. A nursing inservice curriculum for patient education. Nurs and Health Care 1983;4(3):142–146.

125. Ellson SK. Inservice education: it can improve your patient records! J Cont Educ Nurs 1984;15(3):78–81.

126. Lang MJ, Slayton LA. Inservice education: a way to manage job stress using a decision-making model. J Cont Educ Nurs 1984;15(3):82–84.

127. Oliver SK. The effects of continuing education on the clinical behavior of nurses. J Cont Educ Nurs 1984;15(4):130–134.

128. Shamian J, Lemieux S. Inservice education. An evaluation of the preceptor model versus the formal teaching model. J Cont Educ Nurs 1984;15(3):86–89.

129. Dickinson GR, Holzemer WL, Nichols E. Evaluation of an arthritis continuing education program. J Cont Educ Nurs 1985;16(4):127–131.

130. Sullivan EJ, Decker PJ. Using behavior modeling to teach management skills. Nurs and Health Care 1985;6(1):41–45.

131. Lifson LT, Cantlon C. Developing a leadership program for charge nurses. J Nurs Staff Develop 1986;2(4):138–143.

132. Vogelberger ML. A new approach to the care-plan problem. J Nurs Staff Develop 1986;1(3):120–125.

35

Assessing Decision-Making Style with Type Theory

Cynthia Freund

MANAGERS and executives spend a great deal of time and energy making decisions. No matter what the activities are called—budgeting, staffing, planning, evaluating, and so forth—all involve making decisions.[1-3] There are many different types of decisions made by managers and executives (nurse administrators) and many different ways in which those decisions are made. Some decisions are made by one person. Other decisions are made by a group; some groups are led to their decision by the nurse administrator, while other groups come to a decision on their own. Some decisions are made by administrators after having received input or opinions from others. Some decisions are final at the level at which they are made; others are subject to review at different levels in an organization.

There are many decision-making models available to help managers make better decisions. Linear programming and simulation models are quantitative models in which extensive computer programs are used to account for multiple variables involved in a decision. Normative and descriptive decision models, such as decision-tree models, help identify the variables or factors involved in a decision situation, estimate the probability of outcomes associated with alternative choices, and forecast the positive and negative consequences of alternative decisions.[4-6] Since many of these models involve extensive and time-consuming analyses, simplified models have been proposed for use on a daily basis

for those situations in which time does not permit comprehensive analysis.[7]

Reduced to its barest fundamentals, decision making involves two essential cognitive processes: taking in information, and acting on or drawing conclusions about that information. From early childhood on, individuals develop certain styles, predilections, or preferences regarding these two cognitive processes, and quite naturally, all styles and preferences have their strengths and limitations.[8] Since cognitive style and predilection are firmly rooted in early childhood development—and since cognitive processes are fundamental to decision making—decision models, tools, and techniques are only useful to the extent that they enhance one's cognitive style.

In helping managers improve their decision making, an important question, therefore, is, how do we help individuals identify their cognitive preferences and styles so that they can capitalize on their strengths and minimize their limitations? Further, how do we help new managers identify the cognitive styles of others so that they can put together effective decision-making groups? Jung's theory of psychological type, and the interpretation of his theory by Myers and Briggs, provide a basis for helping nurse administrators identify cognitive styles in decision making.

This chapter reviews Jung's theory, and Myers and Briggs's type theory; it describes the Myers-Briggs Type Indicator (MBTI), a tool to measure cognitive style as well as various uses of the MBTI; and, it describes how type theory and the MBTI can be useful in teaching decision making to nurse managers.

TYPE THEORY

Type theory refers to Jung's theory of psychological type as interpreted by Myers and Briggs, and operationalized through the Myers-Briggs Type Indicator. It is important to note, however, that type theory does not encompass all of Jung's theory of personality; it does not, for example, include such aspects of the theory as the animus, anima, and archetypes. Although many authors have described type theory, only three authors, who are the original, primary sources on type theory and the MBTI, will be cited in this section.[8–10] The reader is referred to the bibliography for additional references.

Jung observed patterns in the way people prefer to perceive and make judgments, and these patterns he called "psychological types." According to Jung, all conscious mental activity involves four cognitive processes: two perception functions—sensing and intuition, and two judgment functions—thinking and feeling. Everyone uses all four processes, but individuals differ in their preference for and skill in each process. Since many of the words used in type theory have meanings that differ slightly from the common understanding of these words, it is important to define the terms as used in type theory.

FOUR COGNITIVE PROCESSES

Perception

Perception is the process of becoming aware of something—of people, things, events, or ideas. It involves finding out what a problem or situation is and what the various things are that might be done. It includes gathering information and selecting the information to which one will attend. Thus, perception is the process of taking information into consciousness, either by sensing or by intuition.

"Sensing" is perception of the observable by use of the "senses"—sight, sound, touch, and so forth. Sensing attends to experiences available to the senses and to the facts of a situation, bringing to awareness that which is occurring in the present. Those who use sensing as their predominant perception process (sensing types) have an acute power of observation, a memory for details, an awareness of present experiences, and a sense of realism. Soundness, common sense, and accuracy are valued by people who are sensing types.

"Intuition" is perception of meanings, possibilities, and relationships by way of "insight." Intuition attends to what might be done about a situation, bringing to consciousness future possibilities rather than attending to the present. Intuitive types, who use intuition as their predominant perception process, have a capacity to deal with complexity, an ability to see abstract and theoretical relationships, a future-oriented perspective, and a sense of creativity. Imagination and a grasp of complexity are valued by intuitive types.

Judgment

Judgment is the process of making a decision about what has been perceived. It is the process of coming to conclusions and involves analysis, evaluation, choice, and selection of an action. Judgment is the process of conscious decision making by way of thinking or feeling.

"Thinking" involves coming to conclusions on the basis of "logic." It involves making decisions by ordering choices in terms of cause and effect, logical connections, and impersonal analysis. Thinking types, who prefer thinking to feeling as a primary judgment process, are objective, analytical, and critical, and they focus on relationships be-

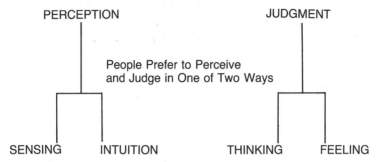

Figure 35.1 Perception and Judgment Preferences

tween the past, present, and future. Thinking types value fairness and justice.

"Feeling" involves coming to conclusions on the basis of "relative values." It involves making decisions by ordering choices in terms of personal values and the effect of decisions on others. Feeling types are subjective, warm, and compassionate and attend to what matters to others. Feeling types value harmony and affiliation. (See Figure 35.1.)

TYPE DEVELOPMENT

As noted above, all conscious mental activity involves perception and judgment, and all persons use both sensing and intuition for their perception functions and both thinking and feeling for their judgment functions— but not at the same time, and not with equal preference and skill. Individuals differ in their preference for and skill in using the four processes. Type theory assumes that children are born with a predisposition toward one of the four processes and that during childhood the preferred process is used most often. Consequently, highly differentiated skill is developed in the use of the preferred process; continued use of this process then leads to increasing competence with it. And constant reinforcement leads to the development of a dominant process.

During early childhood, while the preferred cognitive process is being developed

and refined, there is relative neglect of the opposite process. For example, if sensing is preferred, the opposite perception function—intuition—is neglected; if intuition is preferred, sensing is neglected. The same is true if the preferred process is one of the judgment functions. If thinking is preferred, feeling is neglected; if feeling is preferred, thinking is neglected. The neglected process, which is the opposite of the dominant process—sensing if intuition is dominant, intuition if sensing is dominant, thinking if feeling is dominant, and feeling if thinking is dominant—is called the inferior process; it is the one that is not fully developed until midlife or later, if at all.

In order to avoid developing a one-dimensional personality or cognitive style, an auxiliary process is also developed during childhood. Dominance occurs in one function—either perception or judgment, but since all mental activity involves both functions, the auxiliary process is in the other nondominant function. For example, if sensing or intuition is dominant (a perception function), the auxiliary process will be either thinking or feeling (a judgment function); if thinking or feeling is dominant (a judgment function), the auxiliary process will be either sensing or intuition (a perception function). The auxiliary process is always formed in the function where the dominant process is not. (See Table 35.1).

Table 35.1   Dominant and Auxiliary Processes

Dominant		Auxiliary
Sensing	*with*	Thinking
Sensing	*with*	Feeling
Feeling	*with*	Sensing
Feeling	*with*	Intuition
Intuition	*with*	Thinking
Intuition	*with*	Feeling
Thinking	*with*	Sensing
Thinking	*with*	Intuition

During youth, then, the primary objective is to develop command over the perception and judgment functions by developing mastery of one's dominant and auxiliary processes. While individuals are striving for excellence in their dominant and auxiliary cognitive processes during early life, they should also be developing at least passable skill in the other, less-preferred third and fourth processes. Greater command over the less-preferred approaches is a developmental objective of midlife. However, even though greater skill with the less preferred approaches can be developed, the dominant process remains so, continues to be preferred, and is the most highly developed. Likewise, the auxiliary process continues to be an individual's second best and second preferred. And individuals use their dominant and auxiliary processes most often. Only a very few exceptional people achieve a stage of individuation where they can use all four processes with equal ease and skill as the situation requires.

Not all people like the notion of a dominant cognitive process, preferring to think of themselves as equally skillful with all four. Jung noted, however, that lack of preference for one or two processes results in minimal development. Optimal use of the four processes "is not to be obtained through a strict level of equality, but through selective development of each [process] in proportion both to its relative importance to the individual and to its useful relationship to the other

processes."[8] (p. 15). Therefore, adequate development of conscious mental functioning requires the development of excellence in a favorite dominant process and adequate, though not equal, skill in an auxiliary process. Further, recognition of the least-developed processes is necessary so that these processes can be minimally developed and called to use, even if sparingly, when needed. Finally, adequate development requires the ability to use each of the four processes for that which it is best suited, even when the four are not equally mastered.

ROLE OF THE FOUR PROCESSES

The four mental activities serve different purposes in the many ways one becomes aware of people, things, events, and ideas— perception, and in the ways one comes to conclusions about what has been perceived— judgment. With sensing, the goal is the fullest experience of what is immediate and real; with intuition, the broadest view of what is possible and insightful. Thinking involves rational order by impersonal logic; feeling involves rational order through harmony among personal values.

When the different dominant processes are combined with the various auxiliary processes, eight different patterns of how individuals look at the world and live in the world result, as seen in Table 35.1. These combinations are referred to as types. When sensing is dominant and thinking is auxiliary, a person is considered a sensing, thinking type. Such people focus on the practical facts that are readily subject to logical analysis. Sensing, feeling types focus on the practical aspects of human needs. Intuitive, thinking types look for ingenious inspirations and subject these ideas to logical analysis; while intuitive, feeling types look for insight and explanations for understanding people and values. Thinking, sensing types apply their system of logic to the practical matters of the world; while thinking, intuitive types apply their logic and analysis to the theoretical matters of the world. Feeling, sensing types focus on harmonious relationships with practical helpfulness. Feeling, intuitive types focus on understanding people and their possibilities.

The differences between these types, described in very general terms here, are subtle but meaningful. All sensing types tend to focus on facts as opposed to possibilities, and all intuitive types tend to focus on possibilities rather than facts; but the way they use the facts or possibilities they perceive depends on which of their judgment functions is auxiliary, that is, whether they evaluate and make conclusions about the facts or possibilities they perceive on the basis of logical analysis or concern for personal values.

The same is true for those types whose dominant process is a judgment function—thinking or feeling. All thinking types use impersonal logic, and all feeling types use logic based on harmony and personal values. However, the impersonal or personal logic is applied only to that information that has been taken in—either facts or possibilities, depending on which perception function is auxiliary. Further, if the dominant process is a perception function, perception will be more attended to than judgment, and if the dominant process is a judgment function, judgment will be more attended to than perception.

These two dimensions of cognitive structure, perception and judgment, with the various combinations of the four mental processes according to their dominant and auxiliary role, form the basis for identifying eight different patterns or types of conscious mental activity. In addition to these two cognitive dimensions, however, Jung described a third dimension of personality structure, extraversion and introversion, or attitude toward life; and a fourth dimension, orientation to the outer world. These third and fourth dimensions expand the eight sets to

16, which are referred to by Jung as preference types, and by Myers and Briggs as psychological types, and—in the context of decision making—patterns of cognitive style.

ATTITUDE TOWARD LIFE

Jung gave the terms "extraversion" and "introversion" quite specific meanings, which have been somewhat distorted in common usuage. In common parlance, extravert means sociable and introvert means shy. Jung's and Myers and Briggs's concepts are much broader. Specifically, extraversion means outward-turning and introversion means inward-turning.

Like sensing-intuition and thinking-feeling, extraversion and introversion are opposite poles or attitudes. And like the perception and judgment processes, individuals demonstrate both attitudes, extraversion and introversion, but not simultaneously and not with equal preference or skill.

Extraversion

In the extraverted attitude, attention and energy flows out to the objects and people of the environment. There is a desire to act on and in the world. People who prefer the extraverted attitude are action oriented, get their stimulation and energy from events and people in the environment, and tend to be social.

Introversion

In the introverted attitude, attention and energy is focused on the inner world of ideas and concepts. There is a desire to turn into oneself and reflect. People who prefer the introverted attitude are contemplative, get their energy from their own inner world of thoughts and ideas, and enjoy privacy and solitude. (See Figure 35.2.)

People Direct Their Favorite Process

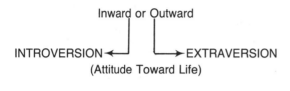

People Have a Favorite Function

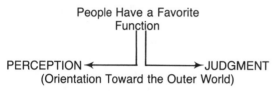

Figure 35.2 Extraversion-Introversion and Judgment-Perception Preferences

The Extraversion-Introversion Preference

People who use their dominant mental process primarily in the outer world are extraverts; those who use their dominant mental process primarily in their own personal world of inner thoughts are introverts. For example, extraverted individuals who use thinking as their dominant process and intuition as their auxiliary process, use their logical analysis and objectivity to organize and manage people, events, and the world around them. In contrast, introverted thinkers whose auxiliary process is intuition want to use their dominant process (thinking) in their inner world, striving for logical and orderly minds and ideas. Thinking, intuitive introverts use their auxiliary process (intuition) in the outer world, giving others the "impression" that intuition is their dominant process.

In other words, extraverts use their dominant process in the outer world, and consequently, show their best to the world. Introverts, on the other hand, show their second best, their auxiliary process, to the world, reserving their best for their most preferred place—their own inner world. Thus, intro-

verts are less well known and are often underestimated because they show their second-best, not their best function.

It is important not to assume that extraverts never like to be alone and introverts never like to be with others, or that extraverts are all action without reflection and introverts are all reflection with no action. Everyone must live as both extraverts and introverts. Many individuals achieve competence as both, but every individual prefers one attitude. Extraverts are most interested in and satisfied with the external world of action, but can, when necessary, deal with ideas and reflection. Likewise, introverts are most satisfied with their inner world, but can deal with the outer world when necessary.

By developing both dominant and auxiliary cognitive abilities, individuals are able to function in both their outer and inner worlds. By using their best and most highly developed skill (dominant process) in their favorite attitude (extraversion or introversion), individuals develop one area of significant strength and competence. By using their second-best skill (auxiliary process) in the opposite attitude, individuals achieve balance—the ability to function as both extraverts and introverts using both perception and judgment.

ORIENTATION TOWARD THE OUTER WORLD

Just as individuals have a preference for either sensing or intuition, thinking or feeling, and for extraversion or introversion, they also have a preference for either a perceptive or judging attitude. This latter preference, the fourth dimension of personality or type structure, reflects a preferred way of dealing with the outer world. Individuals live in the outer world with either a perceptive or a judging orientation. (See Figure 35.2.)

Perceptive Orientation

When a perceptive orientation is used to run one's outer life, one strives to keep things open, to receive new and additional information. Sensing types with a perceptive orientation are attuned to immediate realities, while intuitive types with a perceptive orientation are attuned to new possibilities. Regardless of the favored perception process (sensing or intuition), those who live in the outer world with a perceptive orientation are characteristically spontaneous, flexible, and curious and they strive to keep plans to a minimum; they want to understand and adapt to life.

Judging Orientation

When a judging orientation is used to run one's outer life, one seeks closure, organization, and decisions. Thinking types with a judging orientation base decisions and plans on logical analysis; feeling types with the same orientation base decisions and plans on human factors. All persons who live in the outer world with a judging orientation, whether they are thinking or feeling types, desire plans, organization, order, purposefulness, and decisiveness; they want to regulate and control their lives.

Use of the Orientations

In any new endeavor, the first step is to use a perception function—either sensing or intuition—to take in information about or to observe a situation. The second step is to use a judgment function—either thinking or feeling—to decide on the appropriate action or to arrive at a conclusion. Those whose orientation is a perceptive one usually remain longer in the perception process, always open and ready for new input, while those whose orientation is a judging one tend to move quickly through perception and jump to the judgment process, eager to bring closure.

It is important to note that a judging orientation does not imply that an individual is judgmental. A judging orientation means that individuals live in the outer world in a planned, orderly, and organized fashion with a desire for closure and conclusions.

The perceptive-judging orientation works differently with extraverts and introverts. Extraverts' preferred or dominant process is directed toward their favorite place—the outer world. Thus, an extravert's favorite process governs his or her orientation toward the outer world. If an extravert's favorite process is perception, he or she uses a perceptive orientation, characterized by openness and adaptability. If an extravert's favorite process is judgment, he or she uses a judging orientation, characterized by orderliness and a desire for closure.

Introverts' favorite process is also directed toward their favorite place—in their case, the inner world. Thus, their outer-world orientation is governed by their auxiliary or second-favorite process. If the introverts' favorite process is a perception process, they use a judgment orientation. Outwardly, they live in an orderly and planned fashion, reserving their flexibility and openness for their inner world. Likewise, if the introverts' favorite process is a judgment process, they live in a spontaneous and open fashion, using a perceptive orientation. (See Figure 35.3.)

To summarize at this point, Jung described four dimensions of psychological type based on his observations of individual differences. His work was subsequently expanded on by Myers and Briggs in their theory of psychological type. According to Myers and Briggs, all mental activity involves two functions: perception (taking in information) and judgment (coming to conclusions). There are two ways of perceiving—sensing and intuition, and two ways of judging—thinking and feeling. The perception and judgment functions are the first and second dimensions of psychological type.

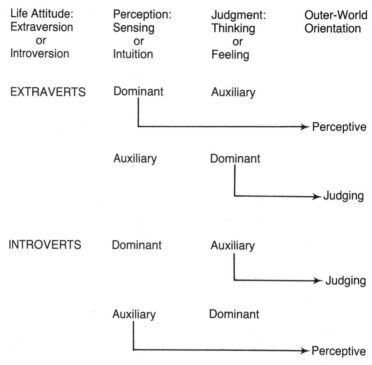

Life Attitude: Extraversion or Introversion	Perception: Sensing or Intuition	Judgment: Thinking or Feeling	Outer-World Orientation

Figure 35.3   Perceptive-Judging Orientation
Toward the Outer World

At some time or another, all individuals use all four processes, but not simultaneously, or with equal skill. In other words, when perceiving, individuals are not using a judgment process, and when judging, individuals are not using a perception process. Further, when using a sensing process, individuals do not use an intuition process at the same time; likewise, when using a thinking process, individuals do not use a feeling process at the same time. Thus, in consciousness, only one cognitive process is used at a time, although different ones can be used at various times.

Because of an inherent preference for one of the four processes, individuals use the preferred most often and develop greatest skill with this favored process. The favored process becomes dominant. To achieve balance in cognitive processes, individuals develop a second-best and second-favored proc-

ess, which is auxiliary. If the favored and dominant process is one of the perception processes, the auxiliary process is one of the judgment processes; if the favored and dominant process is one of the judgment processes, the auxiliary process is one of the perception processes.

All individuals also develop a preferred attitude, extraversion or introversion. Extraverts use their preferred process in the outer world, while introverts use their favorite process in the inner world.

All individuals also develop an orientation toward the outer world that describes the characteristic way in which they live in the world—either with a perceptive or judging orientation. For extraverts, their outer-world orientation is based on their dominant process. The outer-world orientation of introverts is based on their auxiliary process.

The four dimensions of psychological types are based on concepts of polarity and balance. All four dimensions have polar opposites: there are two opposite basic mental functions, perception and judgment; two opposite perception processes, sensing and intuition; two opposite judgment processes, thinking and feeling; two opposite attitudes toward life, extraversion and introversion; and two opposite orientations toward the outer world, perception and judging. Along each dimension, strength and competence are developed in one of the polar opposites, while the other is less well developed. The four dimensions put together in 16 combinations represent a complex set of dynamic relationships between the four mental processes, attitude toward life, and orientation toward the outer world. These 16 combinations are known as psychological types, which describe cognitive structure; the way people prefer to use their minds to take in information and draw conclusions; and the way people prefer to live in the world.

THE MYERS-BRIGGS TYPE INDICATOR

The Myers-Briggs Type Indicator, known as the MBTI, is an instrument designed to test Jung's theory of psychological type and put it to practical use[8] (p. 11). The four dimensions of type (introversion-extraversion, sensing-intuition, thinking-feeling, judgment-perception), and the description of the 16 types, which are derived from various combinations of the four dimensions, are the result of the lifelong work of Myers. With Briggs, Myers developed the MBTI over a 20-year period.[11]

Although the instrument was originally used as a research instrument, Myers and Briggs noted that its ultimate purpose was to make the theory of psychological type understandable and useful in practical applications. The MBTI is not like other personality instruments. It is based on a specific theory and consequently, the theory must be understood to understand the instrument and its results. Most important, it is not a diagnostic or evaluative tool. The results do not indicate that respondents are more or less normal, based on some standard of normalcy.

The objective of the MBTI is to identify basic preferences for one of the poles of the four type dimensions. The MBTI does not measure traits or behaviors. As noted in the MBTI manual,

The intent is to reflect a habitual choice between rival alternatives, analogous to right-handedness or left-handedness. One expects to use both the right and left hands, even though one reaches first with the hand one prefers. Similarly, every person is assumed to use both poles of each of the four preferences, but to respond first or most often with the preferred functions or attitudes.[8] (p. 3)

Thus, the MBTI is not a test with right or wrong answers or with good or bad, sick or well profiles. It is an indicator that shows important patterns and preferences in the way people take in information and make decisions.

RELIABILITY AND VALIDITY OF THE MBTI

Myers and Briggs began developing the Indicator in 1942, and the final version was completed in 1977. Over that time, extensive work was done on construction of the items and scales and on the reliability and validity of the instrument. Similar work continues. Consequently, there is an impressive amount of evidence on the MBTI's reliability and validity. The MBTI manual[8] (p. 140–223) and the scientific literature on the theory of psychological type, contain large amounts of data and reports of reliability and validity. The reader is referred to these sources for a detailed discussion, which will be briefly summarized here.

Throughout the process of developing the MBTI, extensive item analyses were conducted "to ensure that items (a) discriminated between the poles of a preference and (b) made a useful contribution to only one of the four indices"[8] (p. 146).

Both split-half and test-retest estimates of reliability have been obtained from many different samples, including high-school and college students, medical students, and teachers. From the samples of college-age and older subjects, internal-consistency reliability estimates range from .80 to .87 on split-half procedures and from .64 to .83 on test-retest procedures[8] (p. 164–174).

Extensive work has also been done on the validity of the MBTI, most of it directed at establishing construct validity. Two studies will be summarized. The MBTI is derived from Jungian theory of type development related to preferences for perception and judgment. Another instrument, the Gray-Wheelwright Psychological Type Questionnaire, developed by two Jungian analysts, is also designed to identify Jungian types. The two instruments, the MBTI and the Gray-Wheelwright, were administered to a sample of college students; correlations between the two, for three of the scales (the Gray-Wheelwright only measures three dimensions) were .79, .60, and .58. The investigators concluded that both instruments measured the same thing—the Jungian types they were designed to identify.[12] In the second study, investigators hypothesized that the constructs or preferences reflected in the MBTI should be recognizable by mates, persons psychologically close to one another. When subjects' types, as determined by MBTI responses, were compared to their mates' ratings, a significant agreement between subject responses and mate ratings was found.[13]

A considerable number of other studies have been conducted to assess both construct and predictive or criterion-related validity, and many of these are reported in the MBTI manual. In most of the studies, MBTI scores were compared to scores from other tests measuring similar or related traits to determine whether the match between comparison test scores were in the direction predicted by MBTI type. The comparison tests used included the Strong-Campbell Interest Inventory, California Psychological Inventory, Edwards Personality Preference Survey, Minnesota Multiphasic Personality Inventory, Sixteen Personality Factor Questionnaire, Allport-Vernon-Lindsey Study of Values, and Rotter's Internal-External Locus of Control. There has been considerable consistency in findings from the studies of validity: subjects' scores on comparison tests and other nontest variables fell within the range predicted by Jungian theory and MBTI results. McCaulley concluded that a sizeable body of evidence exists supporting the validity of the MBTI.[14]

THE TYPE FORMULA

Results from the MBTI are always reported in a standardized format—the type formula, which shows preferences in a fixed order. In addition, each preference has a standard abbreviation. Types are reported as follows: ENTJ, ISTP, or ESFP. In other words, in the type formula:

- the first letter indicates a preference for *E* or *I* (*E*xtraversion or *I*ntroversion, attitude toward life);
- the second letter indicates a preference for *S* or *N* (*S*ensing or i*N*tuition, the perception function);
- the third letter indicates a preference for *T* or *F* (*T*hinking or *F*eeling, the judgment function); and
- the fourth letter indicates a preference for *J* or *P* (*J*udgment or *P*erception, orientation toward the outer world).

The type formula identifies an individual's preference in each of the four-type dimensions: attitude toward life, perception and judgment functions, and orientation toward the outer world.

The type formula also identifies the dominant and auxiliary processes. The first step is to look at the fourth letter of the formula—this indicates which function is used in and shown to the outer world. If the fourth letter is *J*, the preferred judgment function (thinking or feeling) is extraverted, or shown to the outer world. If the fourth letter is *P*, the preferred perception function (sensing or intuition) is extraverted. For extraverted "types" (the first letter *E*) the extraverted "function" is the dominant process. For introverted types (the first letter *I*) the extraverted function is the auxiliary process.

Just as the fourth letter of the formula identifies the function that will be extraverted or shown to the outer world, the other preferred function will be typically introverted. For example, if the fourth letter is *J*, thinking or feeling is extraverted and either sensing or intuition will be introverted; if the fourth letter is *P*, sensing or intuition is extraverted and thinking or feeling will be introverted. For extraverted types the introverted function is the auxiliary process. For introverted types the introverted function is the dominant process.

In looking at a type formula, the *JP* preference (the fourth letter of the formula indicating orientation to the outer world), points to the dominant process for extraverts and the auxiliary process for introverts. Because extraverts prefer the outer world, they use their most preferred process, their dominant process, in the outer world, reserving their auxiliary process for the inner world. In contrast, introverts prefer the inner world and use their most preferred process—their dominant process, in their most preferred place—the inner world. Thus, introverts show their second-favorite process, the auxiliary process, to the outer world. Figure 35.4 illustrates the type formula.

Combining one of two preferences for each of the four dimensions of type theory results in sixteen different MBTI types. Descriptions

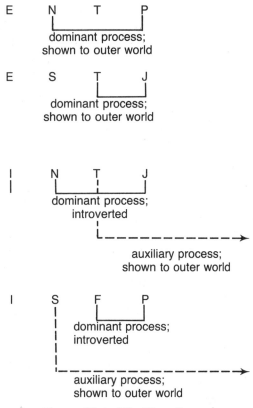

Figure 35.4   The Type Formula

for the extraverted and introverted version of each function can be found in the *Introduction to Type*.[15] The descriptions begin with the characteristics of the dominant process in either the extraversion or introversion preference, followed by the characteristics of the auxiliary process as related to the dominant process and the introversion-extraversion preference. It is important to realize that the 16-type descriptions are not merely the result of adding together the *EI*, *SN*, *TF*, and *JP* preferences. Rather, the descriptions are a reflection of the dynamic nature of type theory and of the interaction between preferences, dominant and auxiliary processes, attitude toward life, and orientation toward the outer world.

APPLICATIONS OF THE MBTI

Although the MBTI was originally seen as a research instrument, in recent years it has been used in a variety of ways. Since almost any human activity involves either perception or judgment in action or ideas, the potential applications of the MBTI cover a broad range of human experiences and situations. The MBTI and type theory have been used for individual, family, and group counseling; career guidance; education; and work situations involving cooperation and teamwork, to name but a few.

In all instances, the objectives are to help individuals understand and accept their own type preferences, learn how to use their type preferences appropriately, and appreciate and understand the "valuable" similarities and differences between themselves and others. In family situations, couples can learn to value each other's differences and to communicate more effectively and satisfactorily with each other, particularly if they are of different types; parents can learn how to foster and enhance type development in their children. In career guidance, various careers or professions can be examined to determine the skills most used in a given field and decide whether the demands of that field relate to one's most preferred and most developed or least preferred and least developed modes of perception and judgment.

In teaching situations, the MBTI can be used to assess student learning styles and to help teachers design teaching methods for different types of students. Some general tendencies of students can be predicted by their type. For example, extraverts will be more stimulated by group work and interaction with others, while introverts will prefer to work by themselves. Judging types will value the structure of the classroom and defined assignments that they can follow and complete, whereas perceptive types will find structure confining and will value the freedom to define the specifics and parameters of assignments and projects. At the same time, teachers have their own preferences and tend to teach and run their classrooms on the basis of their preferences. Sensing-type teachers will emphasize facts and practical applications; intuitive-type teachers will emphasize concepts and relationships; thinking-type teachers will focus on objective performance; whereas feeling types will focus on praise, support, and student feelings and reactions. Thus, teachers need to be particularly aware of their own type, its effect on their teaching style, and, most important, its effect on students, particularly those of the opposite type.[11]

Type theory and the MBTI have also been used in a variety of work situations to help people learn how to "talk the language" and work with different types, to create a climate where differences are seen as valuable rather than as problematic, and to construct working groups with sufficient diversity to solve problems and learn from each other. Ultimately, type theory and the MBTI can be used in almost any situation.

... to help those who work or live together to understand how previously irritating and obstructive differences can become a source of amusement, interest, and strength.[8] (p. 4)

APPROPRIATE USE OF THE MBTI

Unfortunately since the MBTI has become popular, it has been misused or used inappropriately. Because of this, the Association of Psychological Type, a professional association of persons interested in psychological-type theory, developed a Code of Ethics for the administration and interpretation of the MBTI.[16]

Two issues are worth emphasizing. First, the MBTI should be administered only by those qualified to administer it. One becomes qualified to administer the MBTI either through formal training or by taking a series of qualifying workshops, such as those offered by the Center of Applied Psychological Type (Gainesville, Florida). Second, the results of the MBTI should be provided in a face-to-face situation where the interpreter and respondent can interact.

The beauty of type theory is that its general principles can be summarized in such a way that most people who do not have extensive or formal training in psychological theory can understand it. However, type theory is not simple; it is complex and dynamic. MBTI results are meaningless to a respondent unless an explanation of the theory is provided. Anyone interpreting the MBTI needs to understand the theory in all its complexity so that the explanation can be both accurate and tailored to an individual's or group's needs, questions, and problems.

In addition, the MBTI is a psychometric tool. As such, accurate interpretation of results is dependent on an understanding of psychometric instruments in general and of the psychometric properties of the MBTI in particular. Interpretation of quantitative scores (as opposed to the type formula) is not recommended although they do provide information for an interpreter about the accuracy and importance of a respondent's preference[8] (p. 58). The quantitative scores, though, may be misinterpreted if an interpreter does not understand how the scores were derived; that is, if he or she does not understand the psychometric properties of the MBTI.

Verification of MBTI results ultimately rests with the respondent. In other words, an individual's type, as determined by the MBTI, should be confirmed by an individual's own sense of him- or herself. This verification, however, does not come about automatically. For some people, there is instant recognition of the accurateness of the MBTI results. For others, there may be doubts—doubts caused by confusion or a lack of appreciation for the preferences. Negative

connotations associated with some terms—for example, assuming that introversion implies neurotic, judgment implies judgmental, or feeling implies overemotional—may cause some people to reject those preferences. A current life crisis or confusion between the demands of work and one's preferences may affect an individual's responses to the MBTI. Thus, a valid interpretation of the MBTI and an understanding of type theory cannot be provided by merely giving someone his or her type results, or by providing written material. Interpretation and verification, to be meaningful and useful, are dependent on a thorough understanding of type theory, knowledge of the psychometric properties of the MBTI, and interpreter-respondent interaction.

ASSESSING MANAGERIAL DECISION-MAKING STYLE

Decision making is frequently included as a topic of study in educational programs for managers and executives, and most often the emphasis is on quantitative decision tools and normative and descriptive decision models. Examination of individual decision-making style and preference is rarely included. Although an understanding of various tools and models is important, so too is an understanding of one's own cognitive style. Type theory and the MBTI provide a useful framework for the study of individual decision-making and for examining problems that are important to nurse administrators. For example, they are useful for examining how an individual works with subordinates, peers, and superiors; how one delegates; and how one assembles effective working groups.

In using type theory and the MBTI, the first step is to administer the MBTI, give respondents their results, and explain type theory. An understanding of type theory is a prerequisite to any discussion of its applications. It is important to recognize, however, that practice in applying the theory in a variety of ways enhances understanding of the theory. An understanding of the theory is necessary before the theory can be used in a meaningful way, and application of the theory is necessary before the theory can be fully understood and used. Therefore, both theoretical explanations and exercises in application are important in teaching type theory.

ASSESSING DECISION-MAKING STYLE

Once an individual identifies and confirms his or her own type, it is useful to look at the strengths and weaknesses associated with each type. Although it is quite human to recognize the strengths associated with one's type, it is also natural to be reluctant to admit and accept the weaknesses. However, in decision situations it is important for managers to realize that given their type preferences they will have a tendency to process only certain kinds of information, to attend to certain kinds of data, and to draw conclusions based on certain kinds of criteria. Alert to these tendencies, they can either draw upon others of opposite type to supplement their thinking, or they can make a conscious effort to attend to the kind of information they would not naturally attend to and consider additional criteria in drawing their conclusions.

The mutual usefulness of opposite types is an important concept for decision makers. A sensing type focuses on the present, pertinent facts, essential details, and realism; an intuitive type focuses on the future, signs of change, the big picture, and possibilities. Each does what he or she does well, but seldom sees what another sees. They need each other to see what the other does not. The same is true for thinking and feeling types. Feeling types need thinkers to help them analyze, organize, weigh the facts and evidence, hold consistently to a policy, and fire people if necessary. Thinkers need feeling types to persuade others, conciliate, and assess how others will feel and react.

Opposite types can complement each other. However, too much oppositeness makes it difficult for people to work together. They see the world too differently and cannot understand each other. If they have two or three preferences in common, they have a basis for understanding and communicating with each other, while at the same time respecting their differences and learning from each other.

In assessing decision-making style, the most important consideration is to examine the strengths and weaknesses associated with one's type and preferences. Based on this, decision makers can assess which kind of decisions they can make well and with confidence, which kind of decisions they should "think twice" about, and when they should seek the input of others, preferably those who are different from themselves.

WORK RELATIONSHIPS WITH OTHERS

Type theory can be useful in helping managers work with others—subordinates, peers, and superiors. People of the same type, or those with three preferences in common, quite naturally understand each other. However, frequently there is friction between people of opposite types—they do not naturally understand each other, they talk a different language and see the world differently. Understanding another's type can lessen the friction. Knowing that someone thinks differently, not because he or she is being willfully contrary or obstinate, but because he or she is of a different type, can lessen irritation and friction.

Identifying the type preferences of others is not easy and needs to be done with caution. Even though the MBTI is a reliable and valid measure of type, each individual is the ultimate verifier of his or her own type. Likewise, even though with practice individuals may develop skill in identifying the type of others by observation, observation is a less reliable and valid measure.

The key to accurate interpretation is deliberate effort. It cannot be done spontaneously, sporadically, randomly, or in a cursory fashion. It needs to be done in a systematic manner. The observer must keep in mind the characteristics of all of the preferences, ruling in and ruling out preferences based on observation of "consistent" patterns and tendencies. The observer must also keep in mind the dynamic nature of type theory, remembering that for introverts, the auxiliary process is the most observable and that their orientation toward the outer world points to their second-favorite function. In work settings, a further caution must be considered: observable patterns and tendencies may be more a reflection of the demands of the work situation than of true preferences.

Even though identifying the type of others is not easy, requires time and effort, and is not firm, knowledge of the type of others can be very useful. As noted, it can reduce interpersonal friction and irritation. It can also help managers delegate more appropriately. For example, extraverts can be given jobs that involve variety and many people, but not long, slow jobs; introverts can be given jobs that require concentration, working alone, and considerable time to complete. Judging types do better when they can plan their work and follow the plan; perceptive types do better in situations that require flexibility and adaptability and prefer not to be bound to a plan. At the same time, judging types will follow a plan through to completion, but tend to ignore interruptions, even urgent ones. On the other hand, perceptive types may take on too many things at once and have difficulty completing any of them, tending to all interruptions, even insignificant ones. Thus, knowledge of subordinates' type preferences and the characteristics associated with various

types helps managers match the requirements of a job with the strengths of individuals.

Knowledge of type can also help in dealing with one's superior(s). The success of a proposal for a new program or project or a budget request can be enhanced by presenting the proposal or request in terms that appeal to a superior's preferences. If, for example, the person acting on the proposal is a feeling type, emphasis can be placed on the program's effect on the people served by the organization. Of course, any proposal should be complete in its analysis and justification.

WORKING GROUPS

Critically important to executives and managers is an effective managerial and working team. "Good teamwork calls for recognition and use of certain *valuable differences* between members of the team"[17] (p. 72). The value of the differences between team members is that they each bring something different to a problem, situation, or project, and what they bring in sum is more than the same number of people of the same type would bring. They will see quite varied aspects of a situation and direct action toward different ends. What would be boring and dull to some types (and thus not done well) will be interesting and rewarding to other types, and thus handled well. A variety of types on any team will contribute to greater effectiveness, more informed decisions, and greater satisfaction.

Teams of opposite types can run into difficulties, however. Opposite types often disagree on what, if anything, should be done and how it should be done. Forceful members, particularly judging types, are likely to maintain that they are right, while less forceful members resent being overpowered. Communication may suffer because what seems a perfectly reasonable and clear statement to one type may seem meaningless and preposterous to another type. Morale and effectiveness may be at stake in teams composed of opposite types.

Morale and effectiveness will survive, however, if team members recognize that both kinds of perception and judgment are necessary for sound problem-solving, if they respect and value each other's differences and learn to tailor their communication to others of opposite type. There are no "golden rules" about the proportion of team members that should be of the same or similar type (three or four preferences in common), near-similar type (two preferences in common), and opposite or near-opposite type (one or no preferences in common). It is probably important that the "head" of the team have at least one preference in common with all team members and that he or she have three preferences in common with several members. It is also important that members of the exact same type not be a majority.

The goal is to achieve a balance between introverts and extraverts, sensing and intuitive types, thinking and feeling types, and judging and perceptive types. However, the balance for some of the preferences may be tipped depending on the nature and purpose of the team. For example, an executive team might have more thinking than feeling types or more judging than perceptive types. On the other hand, a team concerned with patient care would probably need more feeling types. In any case, there are no formulas. The objective is to have all type preferences represented in relative proportion to the nature and purpose of the team.

In summary, type theory can be useful to managers and executives. Type theory describes how people use their minds—how they perceive or take in information and how they use information or draw conclusions. Type theory can enhance a nurse administrator's decision-making, which represents a large part of what a manager does. Knowledge of one's own type can help an individual capitalize on strengths and minimize weak-

nesses. And knowledge of the type of others, in combination with an understanding of type theory, can help increase effectiveness in working with people throughout an organization. With so much emphasis today on productivity, cost, and quantitative measurement—all of which are important—type theory and its application provides a relatively inexpensive way of maximizing human resources and increasing effectiveness.

APPENDIX A: DESCRIPTION OF TYPES

Extraverted Thinking Types: ESTJ and ENTJ

Extraverted thinkers use their thinking to run as much of the world as may be theirs to run. They organize their facts and operations well in advance, define their objectives and make a systematic drive to reach these objectives on schedule. Through reliance on thinking, they become logical, analytical, often critical, impersonal and unlikely to be convinced by anything but reasoning.

They enjoy being executives, deciding what ought to be done, and giving the necessary orders. They have little patience with confusion, inefficiency, halfway measures, or anything aimless and ineffective, and they know how to be tough when the situation calls for toughness.

They think conduct should be governed by logic, and govern their own that way as much as they can. They live according to a definite formula that embodies their basic judgments about the world. Any change in their ways requires a deliberate change in the formula.

Like other judging types, they run some risk of neglecting perception. They need to stop and listen to the other person's side of the matter, especially with people who are not in a position to talk back. They seldom find

From Myers I. Introduction to type. 3rd ed. Palo Alto, CA: Consulting Psychologists Press, Inc., 1980. Reprinted by permission of the publisher.

this easy, but if (repeat, *if*) they do not manage to do it, they may judge too hastily, without enough facts or enough regard for what other people think or feel.

Feeling is their least developed process. If they suppress or neglect it too long, it can explode in damaging ways. They need to make some conscious use of feeling, preferably in appreciation of other people's merits,—an art that comes less naturally to thinkers than to feeling types. Thinkers can, if they will, "make it a rule" in their formula to mention what is well done, not merely what needs correcting. The results will be worthwhile, both in their work and in their private lives.

ESTJ: With Sensing as Auxiliary

Look at things with their sensing rather than their intuition. Hence are most interested in realities perceived by their five senses, which makes them matter-of-fact, practical, realistic, factually-minded, concerned with here and now. More curious about new things than new ideas. Want ideas, plans and decisions to be based on solid fact.

Solve problems by expertly applying and adapting past experience.

Like work where they can achieve immediate, visible and tangible results. Have a natural bent for business and industry, production and construction. Enjoy administration and getting things organized and done. Do not listen to their own intuition very much, so tend to need an intuitive around to sell them on the value of new ideas.

ENTJ: With Intuition as Auxiliary

Look at things with their intuition rather than their sensing, hence are mainly interested in seeing the possibilities beyond what is present or obvious or known. Intuition heightens their intellectual interest, curiosity for new ideas, tolerance for theory, taste for complex problems, insight, vision and concern for long range consequences.

Are seldom content in jobs that make no demand on intuition. Need problems to solve and are expert at finding new solutions. Interest is in the broad picture, not in detailed procedures or facts. Tend to choose like-minded intuitives as associates. Also tend to need someone with sensing around to keep them from overlooking relevant facts and important details.

Introverted Thinking Types: ISTP and INTP

Introverted thinkers use their thinking to analyze the world, not to run it. They organize ideas and facts, not situations or people unless they must. Relying on thinking makes them logical, impersonal, objectively critical, not likely to be convinced by anything but reasoning. Being introverts, they focus their thinking on the principles underlying things rather than on the things themselves. Since it is hard to switch their thinking from ideas to details of daily living, they lead their outer lives mainly with their preferred perceptive process, S or N. They are quiet, reserved, detachedly curious and quite adaptable—till one of their ruling principles is violated, at which point they stop adapting.

If (repeat, *if*) they do not develop their perception, they will have too little knowledge or experience of the world. Their thinking will have no real relationship to the problems of their time, and not very much will come of it.

In the field of ideas they are decisive, though socially they may be rather shy except with their best friends. Their special problem is to make their ideas understood. Wanting to state exact truth, they tend to state it in a way too complicated for most people to follow. If they will use simple statements, even if they think the point is too obvious to be worth making, their ideas will be much more widely understood and accepted.

Feeling is their least developed process. They are not apt to know, unless told, what matters emotionally to another person. They should recognize that most people do care about having their merits appreciated and their point of view respectfully considered. And they should act accordingly. Both their working life and personal life will go better if they take the trouble to do two simple things—say an appreciative word when praise is honestly due, and mention the points where they agree with another person *before* they bring up the points where they disagree.

ISTP: With Sensing as Auxiliary

See the realities. Great capacity for facts and details. Good at applied science and at mechanics and the properties of materials and things. With nontechnical interests, can use general principles to bring order out of masses of confused data and meaning out of unorganized facts. May be analysts of markets, sales, securities or statistics of any kind.

Likely to be patient, accurate, good with their hands, fond of sports and outdoors, and have a gift of fun.

Great believers in economy of effort, which is an asset if they judge accurately how much effort is needed, and do efficiently what the situation demands. If not, economy of effort can become mere laziness and little will get done.

INTP: With Intuition as Auxiliary

See the possibilities. Value facts mainly in relation to theory. Good at pure science, research, math, and the more complicated engineering problems. With nontechnical interests, make scholars, teachers, abstract thinkers in economics, philosophy, psychology, etc.

Apt to have insight, ingenuity, quick understanding, intellectual curiosity, fertility of ideas about problems. More interested in reaching solutions than in putting them into practice, which others can do as well.

Need to check out even their most attractive intuitive projects against the facts and the limitations these impose. Otherwise may squander their energies in pursuing impossibilities.

Extraverted Feeling Types: ESFJ and ENFJ

Extraverted feeling types radiate warmth and fellowship. Reliance on feeling gives them a very personal approach to life, since feeling judges everything by a set of personal values. Being extraverts, they focus their feeling on the people around them, placing a very high value on harmonious human contacts. They are friendly, tactful, sympathetic, and can almost always express the right feeling.

They are particularly warmed by approval and sensitive to indifference. Much of their pleasure and satisfaction comes not only from others' warmth of feeling but from their own; they enjoy admiring people and so tend to concentrate on a person's most admirable qualities. They try to live up to their ideals and are loyal to respected persons, institutions and causes.

They are unusually able to see value in other people's opinions. And even when the opinions are conflicting, they have faith that harmony can somehow be achieved and often manage to bring it about. Their intense concentration on other people's viewpoints sometimes makes them lose sight of the value of their own. They are best at jobs that deal with people and any situation where the needed cooperation can be won by good will. They think best when talking with people and enjoy talk. It takes special effort for them to be brief and businesslike.

Being judging types, they like to have matters settled and decided, but they do not need or want to make all the decisions themselves.

They have many "shoulds" and "should nots" and may express these freely. They are conscientious, persevering, orderly even in small matters, and inclined to expect others to be the same.

If (repeat *if*) they do not develop their perception, they will, with the best of intentions, act on assumptions that turn out to be wrong. They are especially likely to be blind to the facts when there is a situation that is disagreeable or a criticism that hurts. It is harder for them than for other types to see things they wish were not true. If they fail to face disagreeable facts, they will sweep their problems under the rug instead of finding good solutions.

ESFJ: With Sensing as Auxiliary

Look at things with their sensing, which makes them practical, realistic, matter-of-fact, concerned with here and now. Appreciate and enjoy their material possessions and details of direct experience. Like to base plans and decisions upon known facts.

Enjoy variety, but usually adapt excellently to routine.

Compassion and awareness of physical conditions often attract them to nursing (where they provide warmth and comfort as well as devoted care) and to health professions in general.

ENFJ: With Intuition as Auxiliary

Look at things with their intuition rather than their sensing, hence are mainly interested in seeing the possibilities beyond what is present or obvious or known. Intuition heightens their understanding, long-range vision, insight, curiosity about new ideas, love of books and tolerance for theory.

Likely to have a gift of expression, but may use it in speaking to audiences rather than in writing. Interest in possibilities for people attracts them often to counseling in the fields of career choice or personal development.

Introverted Feeling Types: ISFP and INFP

Introverted feeling types have a wealth of warmth and enthusiasm, but may not show it till they know you well. Reliance on feeling leads them to judge everything by personal values; being introverts, they choose these values without reference to the judgment of others. They know what is important to them and protect it at all costs. Loyalties and ideals govern their lives. Their deepest feelings are seldom expressed, since their tenderness and passionate conviction are masked by their quiet reserve.

Their feeling being introverted, they conduct their outer lives mainly with their preferred perceptive process, either sensing or intuition. This makes them open-minded, flexible and adaptable—until one of the things they value most deeply seems in danger—at which point they stop adapting. Except for the sake of their work they have little wish to impress or dominate. The friends who mean most to them are the people who understand their values and the goals they are working toward.

They are twice as good when working at a job they believe in; their feeling puts added energy behind their efforts. They want their work to contribute to something that matters to them—human understanding or happiness or health, or perhaps to the perfecting of some project or undertaking. They want to have a purpose beyond their paycheck, no matter how big the check. They are perfectionists wherever their feeling is engaged and are usually happiest at some individual work involving their personal values.

Being idealists, they measure their accomplishments against an inner standard of perfection, instead of what is actually possible. They may suffer from too great self-demand, feeling that the contrast between their inner ideal and outer reality is somehow their fault. They need to find something they really care about, and then work to achieve it. With an ideal to work for, and good development of perception to help them recognize realistic difficulties and possible solutions, they can achieve a high degree of self-confident drive.

If (repeat *if*) they do not find a way to use their energies in the service of an ideal, they tend to become oversensitive and vulnerable, losing confidence in life and in themselves. If their perception is undeveloped, they may have so little realism that they aspire to the impossible and achieve frustratingly little.

ISFP: With Sensing as Auxiliary

See the realities. Mildly resemble ESFP, especially in seeing and meeting the need of the moment. Can pay close, unbroken attention for long periods, when work requires monitoring or close observation.

Show their warmth more by deeds than words. Compassionate toward all helpless creatures. Work well at jobs requiring devotion. Gentle, considerate, retiring. Consistently underestimate and understate themselves. May find satisfactory outlets in fields where taste, discrimination and a sense of beauty are of value.

INFP: With Intuition as Auxiliary

See the possibilities. Mildly resemble ENFP, especially in liking to concentrate on projects and disliking details not related to a deep interest. Understanding, tend to have insight and long-range vision. Curious about new ideas, fond of books and language. Apt to have skill in expressing themselves.

Ingenious and persuasive on the subject of their enthusiasms. Especially interested in possibilities for people. Enjoy counseling and teaching. With high ability, may excel in literature, art, science or psychology.

Extraverted Sensing Types: ESTP and ESFP

Extraverted sensing makes the adaptable realists, who good-naturedly accept and use the facts around them, whatever these are. They know what the facts are, since they notice and remember more than any other type. They know what goes on, who wants what and who doesn't. And they do not fight those facts. There is a sort of effortless economy in the way they deal with a situation, never taking the hard way when an easier one will work.

Often they can get other people to adapt, too. Being perceptive types, they look for the satisfying solution, instead of trying to impose any "should" or "must" of their own, and people generally like them well enough to consider any compromise that they suggest "might work". They are unprejudiced, open-minded, and usually patient, easygoing and tolerant of everyone—including themselves. They enjoy life. They don't get wrought up. Thus they may be very good at easing tense situations and pulling conflicting factions together.

Their expert sensing may show itself: (a) in a gift for machinery and the handling of tools and materials for craft or artistic purposes, or in ability to recognize quality, line, color, texture or detail; (b) in a capacity for exact facts, even when separate and unrelated, and the ability to absorb, remember and apply them; (c) in a continuous awareness, an ability to see the need of the moment and turn easily to meet it.

They are strong in the art of living, appreciate and enjoy their material possessions, and take the time to acquire and care for these. They value enjoyment, from good food and good clothes to music, art and all the products of the amusement industry. Even without these helps, they get fun out of life, which makes them fun to be with.

Being realists, they get more from first-hand experience than from study, are more effective on the job on written tests, and doubly effective when on familiar ground. Seeing the value of new ideas, theories and possibilities may well come a bit hard, because intuition is their least developed process.

Their net effectiveness depends on whether they develop their judgment to the point where it can balance their easygoing sensing and give some direction to their lives. If (repeat, *if*) their judgment is not good enough to give them any character or stick-to-it-iveness, they may adapt mainly to their own love of a good time, and become lazy, unstable and generally shallow.

ESTP: With Thinking as Auxiliary

Like to make decisions with their thinking rather than their feeling. Hence are more aware of the logical consequences of an act or decision.

Thinking gives them more grasp of underlying principles, helps with math and theory and makes it easier for them to get tough when the situation calls for toughness.

ESFP: With Feeling as Auxiliary

Like to make decisions with their feeling rather than their thinking. Feeling gives them tact, sympathy, interest in people, ease in handling human contacts, and may make them too easy as disciplinarians.

Feeling also makes for artistic taste and judgment, but is no help with analysis.

Introverted Sensing Types: ISTJ and ISFJ

Introverted sensing types are made particularly dependable by their combination of preferences. They use their favorite process, sensing, in their inner life, and base their ideas on a deep, solid accumulation of stored impressions, which gives them some pretty unshakable ideas. Then they use their preferred kind of judgment, thinking or feeling, to run their outer life. Thus they have a complete, realistic, practical respect both for the facts and for whatever responsibilities these facts create. Sensing provides the facts. And after the introvert's characteristic pause

for reflection, their judgment accepts the responsibilities.

They can remember and use any number of facts, but want them all accurate. They like everything kept factual, clearly stated, not too complex. Not till you know them very well do you discover that behind their outer calm they are seeing the facts from an intensely individual, often delightfully humorous angle. Their private reaction, the way a thing will strike them, is quite unpredictable.

But what they actually do about it will be sound and sensible because what they do is part of their outer life and so is governed by their best judgment. No type is more thorough, painstaking, systematic, hard-working, or patient with detail and routine. Their perseverance tends to stabilize everything with which they are connected. They do not enter into things impulsively, but once in, they are very hard to distract, discourage or stop. They do not quit unless experience convinces them they are wrong.

As administrators, their practical judgment and memory for detail make them conservative, consistent, able to cite cases to support their evaluations of people and methods. They will go to any amount of trouble if they "can see the need of it," but hate to be required to do anything that "doesn't make sense." Usually it is hard for them to see any sense in needs that differ widely from their own. But once they are convinced that a given thing does matter a lot to a given person, the need becomes a fact to be respected and they may go to generous lengths to help satisfy it, while still holding that it doesn't make sense.

Their effectiveness depends on their developing adequate judgment for dealing with the world. If (repeat, *if*) judgment remains childish, the world is not dealt with, the person retreats into silent preoccupation with inner reactions to sense-impressions, and not much of value is likely to result.

ISTJ: With Thinking as Auxiliary

Mildly resemble the extraverted thinking types.

Thinking stresses analysis, logic and decisiveness.

In their personal relationships, they may need to take extra pains to understand and appreciate. They will then be in no danger of overriding people less forceful than they are, and will find themselves richly repaid both in their work and in their private lives.

ISFJ: With Feeling as Auxiliary

Mildly resemble the extraverted feeling types.

Feeling stresses loyalty, consideration and the common welfare.

They are sympathetic, tactful, kind and genuinely concerned, traits which make them very supportive to persons in need of support. They are often attracted to fields where systematic attention to detail is combined with a care for people, as in the health professions.

Extraverted Intuitive Types: ENTP and ENFP

The extraverted intuitives are the enthusiastic innovators. They are always seeing new possibilities—new ways of doing things, or quite new and fascinating things that might be done—and they go all out in pursuit of these. They have a lot of imagination and initiative for originating projects, and a lot of impulsive energy for carrying them out. They are wholly confident of the worth of their inspirations, tireless with the problems involved, and ingenious with the difficulties. They get so interested in the current project that they think of little else.

They get other people interested too. Being perceptive types, they try to understand people rather than to judge them; often, by putting their minds to it, they achieve an uncanny knowledge of what makes a given person tick, and use this to win support for their project. They adapt to other people in the way they present their objective, but never to the point of giving it up. Their faith in their intuition makes them too independent and individualistic to be conformists, but they keep a lively circle of contacts as a consequence of their versatility and their easy interest in almost everything.

In their quieter moments, their auxiliary gives them some balancing introversion and adds depth to the insights supplied by their intuition. At its best, their insight, tempered by judgment, may amount to wisdom.

Their trouble is that they hate uninspired routine and find it remarkably hard to apply themselves to humdrum detail unconnected with any major interest. Worse yet, even their projects begin to seem routine and lose attraction as soon as the main problems are solved and the rest seems clear sailing. They may discipline themselves to carry through, but they are happiest and most effective in jobs that permit of one project after another, with someone else taking over as soon as the situation is well in hand.

If their judgment and self-discipline are *not* developed, they will throw themselves into ill-chosen projects, leave them unfinished, and squander their inspirations, abilities and energies on unimportant, half-done jobs. At their worst, they will be unstable, undependable, fickle and easily discouraged.

ENTP: With Thinking as Auxiliary

More independent, analytical and critical of their inspirations, more impersonal in their relations with people, more apt to consider only how others may affect their projects and not how the projects may affect others.

May be inventors, scientists, trouble-shooters, promoters, or almost anything that it interests them to be.

ENFP: With Feeling as Auxiliary

More enthusiastic, more concerned with people and skillful in handling them. Much drawn to counseling, where each new person presents a fresh problem to be solved and fresh possibilities to be communicated.

May be inspired and inspiring teachers, scientists, artists, advertising or sales people, or almost anything that it interests them to be.

Introverted Intuitive Types: INTJ and INFJ

The introverted intuitives are the great innovators in the field of ideas. They trust their intuitive insights as to the relationships and meanings of things, regardless of established authority or popular beliefs. They trust their vision of the possibilities, regardless of universal skepticism. And they want to see their ideas worked out in practice, accepted and applied.

Consequently, they have to deal firmly with the outer world, which they do by means of their preferred kind of judgment, either T or F. Thus they back up their original insight with the determination, perseverance and enduring purpose of the judging types. When they are driving to turn an inspiration into a reality, problems stimulate rather than discourage them. The impossible takes a little longer—but not much.

Certain dangers arise from their single-minded concentration. They see their goal so clearly that they may not even look for the other things they need to see—the things that conflict with their goal. They may not take the trouble to learn the details of the situation they propose to change. Since sensing is their least developed process, they can easily overlook relevant facts and the limitations these facts impose.

They may not consider the opposition they will meet, its strength or source or probable grounds. They may not consider the possibility that something is wrong with their idea. In scientific research or engineering design, a trial of their boldly ingenious ideas will visibly succeed—or fail and show where the idea *has* to be revised. They need to be particularly alert for flaws in their ideas in those fields where their insights cannot be tested so clearly.

Their auxiliary process, if adequately developed, can supply needed criticism of their ideas. Judgment can be used to foresee difficulties and decide what needs to be done about them. Most original inspirations need to be modified in the light of facts. Ideas need to be worked out and perfected to lessen objections. The best ideas still need to be presented to the world in terms understandable to other types.

If (repeat, *if*) their judgment is *not* developed, they cannot criticize their own inner vision, and they tend to reject all judgments from outside. As a result, they cannot shape their inspirations into effective action. Their ideas will go to waste, and they may be regarded only as visionaries or cranks.

INTJ: With Thinking as Auxiliary

Most individualistic and most independent of all the types.

Resemble extraverted thinkers in organizing ability and a tendency to ignore the views and feelings of those who don't agree with them.

Logical, critical, decisive, determined, often stubborn.

Tend to drive others almost as hard as they drive themselves.

Apt to be effective, relentless reorganizers. Can be efficient executives, rich in ideas.

INFJ: With Feeling as Auxiliary

Less obviously individualistic, more apt to win cooperation than to demand it.

Resemble extraverted feeling types in their

sympathetic handling of people and in a tendency to ignore harsh and uncongenial facts.

May apply their ingenuity to problems of human welfare on their own and in their own way.

Can be successful executives, especially where affairs can be conducted on a personal basis.

APPENDIX B: CODE OF ETHICS

Association for Psychological Type Code of Ethics

Preamble

APT members are dedicated to the use of psychological type theory to honor and enhance the dignity and individuality of people. They are committed to increasing their own and others' knowledge of psychological type theory and to use this knowledge to promote individual and social welfare. As practitioners of the theory of psychological type, APT members therefore conduct themselves according to the following principles:

Principle I.   Administration and dissemination of results
Principle II. Guidelines for interpretation of results
Principle III. Practitioner competence
Principle IV. Legal and professional responsibilities

Principle I.
Administration and Dissemination of Results
Information about a person's type should be acquired and used so as to be of maximum benefit to the individual.

1. The respondent to a type indicator should in all instances be informed of the purpose and intended use of results prior to

From Bulletin of the Association of Psychological Type. Association of Psychological Type, 1987. Reprinted by permission of the publisher.

taking the instrument. Taking the instrument should be voluntary.

2. Identified type results (as distinguished from grouped data) may not be given to a person other than the individual taking the instrument, without that individual's prior permission.

2a. In an organizational context, type information should be used to enhance individual and group satisfaction, rather than to restrict or limit individual or group functioning.

3. In providing type results to respondents, adequate information about psychological type theory and the individual's own indicated type, should be provided in a face-to-face setting. Results should not be given in impersonal ways, such as through the mail.

3a. Information regarding psychological type theory and type results may be given individually or in a group setting. However, individuals should be given an opportunity to clarify their indicated type with the practitioner. Practitioners are encouraged to provide, at a minimum, a full written description of the indicated type, such as is contained in *Introduction to Type.*

3b. In situations where type data are being used for research purposes only, individual results to respondents is not required. However, researchers are encouraged to provide the option for feedback based on individual request.

Principle II.
Guidelines for Interpretation of Results
Both the letter and spirit of psychological type theory as oriented toward the appreciation and positive utilization of individual differences, should characterize the interpretation of type results to individuals and groups.

1. Type attributes should be described in nonjudgmental or positive terms, and as tendencies rather than imperatives. Words like "preference," "tendency," "strength," "inclination," are consistent with psychological

type theory. Explicit reference should be made to the inherent value of all types.

2. Respondents should be informed that psychological type theory reflects an individual's preferences, and not abilities, intelligence, or likelihood of success. Consequently, the practitioner should not counsel a person toward or away from a particular career, activity or personal relationship, based solely upon type information.

3. The individual receiving type results is considered the judge of whether the type description "fits" or not. Where the individual disagrees with the description associated with reported scores, the practitioner should help the person identify the most suitable type description.

4. In providing information about psychological type theory to individuals and groups, care should be taken not to state or imply that type explains everything, but rather that it is one important component of very complex human personalities.

5. Interpreters of psychological type should be sensitive to their own biases. They should exert every effort not to communicate type biases to respondents.

6. Practitioners should interpret type information within the limits of currently available knowledge. They should be careful not to make inferences regarding type or the scores on any type indicator which go beyond the data.

7. Practitioners should not use psychological type indicators whose reliability and validity have not been demonstrated, or use parts of demonstrably reliable and valid type indicators unless the parts themselves have been demonstrated to be reliable and valid.

8. Data collection for the purpose of demonstrating the reliability or validity of a psychological type indicator or part of a psychological type indicator is acceptable provided that the experimental nature of the use is clearly communicated to the respondents, and in all reporting of the results.

Principle III.
Practitioner Competence
Practitioners of psychological type theory do so within the confines of their own knowledge, competence and roles.

1. In using psychological type theory, practitioners should accurately represent their competence and experience to clients.

2. Due to continuing advances in the understanding and application of psychological type theory, practitioners are strongly urged to update their knowledge and experience through reading, conference and workshop attendance, or other available means.

Principle IV.
Legal and Professional Responsibilities
Practitioners of psychological type theory assume specific professional and legal obligations and responsibilities.

1. APT members do not violate copyright laws by reproducing, in whole or in part, published instruments and materials related to psychological type theory.

2. APT members as practitioners of psychological type theory abide by federal and state laws relating to the conduct of professionals using psychological instruments.

3. Membership in the Association for Psychological Type may not be used to imply professional competence or qualifications.

4. The use of the APT Membership Directory is not permitted for advertising or sales purposes without obtaining prior written permission from the APT administrative assistant, according to board policy.

5. APT members as practitioners of psychological type theory accept the obligation to educate others who misrepresent or otherwise misuse the concepts of psychological type theory to the detriment of others.

6. APT members welcome and encourage theoretical diversity in their continuing exploration of psychological type theory, and avoid stating or implying that any particular theoretical preference is "correct."

Code Enforcement

A major function of APT is to encourage the ethical and appropriate use of psychological type theory by providing education, training and research results to members. Where an apparent violation of the present code of ethics occurs, one may initially assume inadequate knowledge as a possible factor. Therefore, as stated in Principle IV, Number 5, members should attempt to educate the individual involved by providing information relevant to the alleged inappropriate activity or use.

Where such personal effort fails to resolve the issue, a member should bring the matter to the attention of the Ethics Committee.

The Ethics Committee will provide a standard form for recording the alleged violation. Should the committee determine that the matter requires its attention, the member alleged to be in violation of the Code of Ethics will be contacted so that clarification of the issue and ultimate satisfactory resolution may occur.

Should no resolution occur after all avenues have been explored, and the member involved indicates that he/she will persist in the violation, the Ethics Committee, by a 2/3 vote of committee members, will request that the member resign from the Association for Psychological Type.

REFERENCES

1. Hall RH. Organizations: structure and process. Englewood Cliffs, NJ: Prentice-Hall, Inc, 1982, pp. 176–183.
2. Katz D, Kahn RL. The social psychology of organizations. New York: John Wiley & Sons, Inc, 1978, pp. 487–522.
3. Hage J. Theories of organizations. New York: John Wiley & Sons, Inc, 1980, pp. 92–121.
4. Vroom VH, Yetton PW. Leadership and decision-making. Pittsburgh: University of Pittsburgh, 1973.
5. Cyert RM, March JG. A behavioral theory of the firm. Englewood Cliffs, NJ: Prentice-Hall, Inc, 1963.
6. Vroom VH, Jago A. Decision-making as a social process: normative and descriptive models of leader behavior. Decision Sciences 1974;5(4):743–769.
7. Sullivan EJ, Decker PJ. Effective management in nursing. Menlo Park, CA: Addison-Wesley Publishing Company, 1985, pp. 145–147.
8. Myers IB, McCaulley MH. A Guide to the Development and use of the Myers-Briggs type indicator. Palo Alto, CA: Consulting Psychologists Press, 1985.
9. Myers IB, with Myers PB. Gifts differing. Palo Alto, CA: Consulting Psychologists Press, 1980.
10. Myers IB. Manual: the Myers-Briggs type indicator. Princeton, NJ: Educational Testing Service, 1962.
11. Lawrence G. People types and tiger stripes. Gainesville, FL: Center for the Application of Psychological Type, Inc, 1982, p. 5.
12. Stricker LJ, Ross J. A description and evaluation of the Myers-Briggs type indicator. Research Bulletin 62-6. Princeton, NJ: Educational Testing Service, 1962.
13. Cohen D, Cohen M, Cross H. A construct validity study of the Myers-Briggs type indicator. Educational and psychological measurement 1981;41(3):883–891.
14. McCaulley MH. Introduction to the MBTI for researchers. Gainesville, FL: Center for Application of Psychological Type, Inc, 1980.
15. Myers IB. Introduction to type. 3rd ed. Palo Alto, CA: Consulting Psychologists Press, 1980.
16. Association of Psychological Type. Code of ethics. Bulletin of the Association of Psychological Type 1987;7–8.
17. Myers IB. Type and teamwork. Gainesville, FL: Center for Applications of Psychological Type, Inc, 1974.

BIBLIOGRAPHY

Carlyn M. An assessment of the Myers-Briggs type indicator. Journal of Personality Assessment 1977;41(5):461–473.
Center for Applications of Psychological Type, Inc. Bibliography: the Myers-Briggs type indicator. Gainesville, FL: Center for Applications of Psychological Type, Inc, 1985.
Comrey AL. An evaluation of the Myers-Briggs Type indicator. Academic Psychology Bulletin 1983;5:115–129.
Haber RA. Different strokes for different folks: Jung's typology and structured experiences. Group and Organizational Studies 1980;5:113–119.
Hirsh SK. Using the Myers-Briggs type indicator in organizations: a Resource book. Palo Alto, CA: Consulting Psychologists Press, 1985.
Hoffman JL, Betkowski M. A summary of Myers-Briggs type indicator research applications in education. Research in Psychological Type 1981;3:3–41.
Kirton MJ. Adaptors and innovators: a description and measure. Journal and Applied Psychology 1976;62:622–629.
Lawrence GD. A synthesis of learning style research involving the MBTI. Journal of Psychological Type 1984;8:2–15.

McCaulley MH. The Myers longitudinal medical study (Monograph II). Gainesville, FL: Center for Applications of Psychological Type, Inc, 1977.

McCaulley MH. Application of the Myers-Briggs type indicator to medicine and other health professions (Monograph I). Gainesville, FL: Center for Applications of Psychological Type, Inc, 1978.

Mitroff II, Kilman RH. Stories managers tell: a new tool for organizational problem solving. Management Review 1975;64(7):18–28.

Yeakley FR. Communication stype preferences and adjustments as an approach to studying effects of similarity in psychological type. Research in Psychological Type 1982;5:30–48.

IV

Introduction: Nursing Administration Education

Ann Marriner-Tomey

THE PURPOSE of the Nursing Administration Education Section is to explore the evolution of education for nursing administration across levels—baccalaureate, master's, and doctorate; to identify issues facing the field of administration of nursing services and academic administration that must be considered when designing educational programs; to explore emerging paradigms; and to apply the use of a model in a practicum experience.

In Chapter 36, Simms presents the evolution of education for nursing administration from an apprentice model to scientific nursing, noting that the education of early nurse executives, Nightingale and Wald, combined a liberal education with nursing. Administration is presented as an essential component of professional nursing, as are research, education, and clinical practice. All professional nurses need nursing, research, and leadership knowledge. According to Simms, master's-prepared nurses should work from a strong science base to provide responsible leadership as clinical managers in a variety of settings. Doctorally prepared nurses are the emerging nurse executives, who can conduct independent research and assume leadership in education, health service systems, professional organizations, and other health-related enterprises. These executives are the nucleus of a new well-prepared leadership in nursing, successfully integrating clinical knowledge, research, teaching, and administrative practice.

Norton continues the historical theme in Chapter 37 by focusing on curriculum development. She parallels baccalaureate nursing education curriculum development with the five main approaches to curriculum development used in general education. Herbart, a late nineteenth-century German philosopher, advocated activity analysis technique to systematically select and organize subject matter. Dewey, the father of progressive education, recommended selecting learning activities that are sequenced to build on existing skills. He stressed integrating interaction and continuity with lateral and longitudinal aspects of experiences. His humanistic and experiential philosophy valued reflective thinking. Charters and Bobbitt stressed efficient and effective curriculum and a scientific approach. Charters introduced Taylor's job analysis as a means for developing and implementing the curricular objectives. Bobbitt used analysis technique to determine the most desirable activities and behaviors for educational experiences. In the late 1940s, Tyler developed a rational model for curriculum and instructional development that incorporated progressive education, a scientific approach, and behavioral psychology.

More specifically, Norton traces the historical curriculum development of nursing education, leadership, and management and addresses current and future curricular issues. Among other points, she stresses the increasing importance of critical thinking, leadership, management, and use of models and theories from nursing and relevant disciplines.

Moving to master's programs in nursing, in Chapter 38 Carroll outlines the roles and functions of nurse executives and middle- and first-line level nurse administrators as identified by the American Organization of Nurse Executives and the American Nurses' Association (ANA). She addresses curriculum content as identified by the ANA certification examination for nursing administration and nursing administration-advanced, and by the Council on Graduate Education for Administration in Nursing. Attention is given to both theory and experiential elements. Carroll traces the history of the pendulum-swing from a focus on functional preparation to advanced clinical practice and now back to an increasing awareness of the need for well-prepared nurse administrators. She emphasizes the importance of the faculty philosophy about the placement of nursing administration in graduate nurses programs. At one extreme, faculty may focus solely on clinical specialization. A major focus in clinical nursing with a minor in the functional area of nursing administration may be an option when faculty recognize the importance of role development. A nursing administration major may be possible where faculty believe nursing administration is a nursing specialty.

Progressing to doctoral programs in nursing, Singleton, in Chapter 39, continues the theme of synthesizing theoretical knowledge from the nursing and management in nursing service administration programs. She stresses the importance of looking at the environment in which the role will be enacted before designing educational programs. She notes there is currently an increase in competition among health-care agencies, in number of interdisciplinary relationships, in outside influences such as government and insurers, and in research emphasis. Singleton identifies types of doctoral programs and presents a review of selected aspects of existing doctoral programs as gleaned from bulletins obtained from programs identified in a 1983–84 listing of doctoral programs. Policies reviewed include admission requirements, licensure, prerequisite courses, experience, other requirements, length of program of study, committees and examinations, program objectives, and course work. Other curriculum research findings are also reported. Singleton concludes by discussing future needs.

Huckabay more specifically addresses the issues facing the field of administration of nursing services that must be considered when designing educational programs in Chapter 40. She gives an overview of the megatrends in health care affecting nursing and discusses nurse practice, cost containment, nursing education, colleagiality, and ethical-moral issues in nursing. Huckabay identifies technology, oversupply of physicians, shift from institutional help to self-help, increasing medical costs, and increasing older population as megatrends that must be addressed. She describes nursing practice issues identified from a review of the literature and discusses their implications on the role of the nurse executive.

Nursing practice issues identified include control over practice, entry into practice, changing demographics of the patient population, emphases on self-care and promotion of health, and forces related to collective bargaining. Huckabay stresses the importance of cost containment in health care and costing out nursing services. She identifies the development of a consistent core curriculum, adding to the scientific knowledge base, and the problem of declining student enrollment as major nursing education issues. The importance of doctor-nurse and service-education colleagiality is discussed. Six ethical-moral issues are identified and discussed: (1) standard of care, (2) terminal illness, (3) relationships issues, (4) patient rights, (5) congenital anomalies, and (6) setting priorities.

Froebe focuses in Chapter 41 on issues of academic administration and the way nursing's unique disciplinary problems combine with the general problems in higher education. She identifies declining enrollments, shortfalls in funding, increasing external controls, and aging faculties as common problems. Froebe identifies administrative concepts that are common to both nursing service and nursing academic administration and discusses governance, structure, communication technology, coordination, personnel, enrollment, fiscal impact, and external forces.

In Chapter 42, Reinhart addresses emerging paradigms of nursing administration education. She related paradigms, traditions, norms, myths, and theories. She uses a jigsaw puzzle analogy to describe paradigms and their component theories. Organizational paradigms direct policies, set standards, and establish shared meaning. Consequently, it is important for the administrator to be able to articulate the organizational paradigm. Paradigms tend to shift when fundamental assumptions are challenged or component theories are corrected. Reinhart traces paradigm shifts through the orthodox and neo-orthodox to the emerging nonorthodox organizational paradigms.

Lowenstein uses the Charns and Schaefer model in Chapter 43 for managerial assessment of a nursing unit for a practicum experience. It is geared toward a microanalysis of health-care organizations but can be adapted for microanalysis of units or departments. The eight major elements identified for assessment include external environment; mission, purpose, and goals; work-direct, management, and indirect support work; structure; coordination; people—individuals and groups; management technologies; and managerial processes. The model elements are placed into three decision-making categories: (1) interface of the organization with its external environment, which contains two elements—external environment and mission, and purpose and goals; (2) organizational design, which includes four elements—work, structure, coordination, and people; and (3) managerial strategies, which covers management technologies and managerial process. These are examined over two time frames—operational decision making and strategic decision making. The model is based on contingency theory. Therefore, prescriptions cannot be universally appropriate. Applications of the model are described.

36

The Evolution of Education for Nursing Administration

Lillian M. Simms

EDUCATION for nursing administration has never been under complete ownership by nursing. Early physicians saw the advantage of nurturing the development of trained nurses, identifying key individuals who could become matrons or superintendents capable of keeping the "reins well in hand." Nurses in the late 1800s and for much of the early 1900s were taught by physicians. The success of any hospital was dependent on nursing administration and still is in the late twentieth century. In new health-care environments, numerous care modalities are not necessarily housed in the same facility but may be guided by the same nursing administrative structure.

As society is jet propelled toward the twenty-first century with all of its promise of new space stations and other worlds, nursing administration is coming into its own, still sturdily linked with medicine, but with a clearly identifiable component of knowledge. The purpose of this chapter is to present an evolutionary perspective on the transformation of education for nursing administration from an apprentice model to a fully recognized component of scientific nursing.

CRITICAL ISSUES IN THE EDUCATION OF ADMINISTRATORS

Times have changed since the early days of Wald and Nightingale. Then it was possible for expert nurses to know all of the knowledge in a particular area of their field and it was possible for key people to be trained to practice nursing with on-site experiential learning. Education could be safely left in the hands of the expert practitioner.

Today, however, nursing as a profession has achieved scientific status. The rise of scientific nursing is comparable to the rise of scientific medicine, and the search for societal approval and recognition is over. The mandate for integration of the professional role is now obvious to many, but not yet widely acclaimed in all schools of nursing. Administration is no more of a specialty in nursing than is research. The discipline is *nursing* and the components of professional nursing include administration, research, education, and clinical practice.

The visiting nurse movement in this country began during the late-nineteenth century—a time dominated by immigration, industralization, urbanization, and infectious disease. History will say that the scientific nurse movement began during the late-twentieth century—a time dominated by the elder boom; advances in enabling technology and information systems; decline of formal organizations; overwhelming emphasis on participative management; arrival of the knowledge worker; and new definitions of wellness on this planet and in space.[1–2]

A Role in Transition

The nurse administrator today is a business professional practicing as a top-level administrator in a rapidly changing technological environment. There is demand for a staggering amount of nursing knowledge blended with financial and business knowledge. Much time is spent in long-range planning and developing productive relationships with physicians and the community.[3] The administrator is confronted with complex ethical issues and questions in patient care and policy making in addition to difficult budget and personnel decisions. Institutional ethics committees are a relatively new phenomenon in health-care institutions, and nurse administrators are in a crucial position to advocate for development and evaluation of these committees as an institutional response to complex ethical issues and questions in patient care and policy setting.[4]

Rapidly changing technology, consumer interest in self-care, government regulations, and economic decline have all had an impact on professional nursing as well as on other components of the health-care delivery system.[5] Nursing has come closer to a professional definition of practice and now reflects the influence of nursing theory and research. The American Nurses' Association (ANA)[6] defines nursing as the diagnosis and treatment of human responses to actual or potential health problems. This definition implies phenomena of concern to nurses, independent nursing action, theoretical bases for action, and evaluation of the effects of nursing actions. Nursing has matured and become recognized as part of the health-care system.

With clarification of the professional nursing role, expectations for nursing education have undergone continuing redefinition. Inadequacies in schools of nursing have been identified in terms of qualified faculty. Faculty participation in nursing services in any clinical setting is both sporadic and informal and nursing service administrators have little influence on nursing curricula. Solutions proposed by the American Academy of Nursing[7] include not just faculty practice but bringing together the collective expertise of the profession in shared practice, education, and research models, as well as administrative models.

A Crisis in Leadership

The Institute of Medicine report[8] describes a leadership crisis in nursing with a critical shortage of nurse administrators at all levels with the political, psychological, and social management skills needed to cope with today's changing world. Nurses are unprepared or unwilling to assume leadership roles. Women are not socialized to assume leadership roles, nor do existing nursing programs address the need to prepare nursing leaders who are effective administrators. Chaska[9] speaks of the nursing profession as being in a state of "mist," with conflicting understanding about professionalism or professional practice. Clifford in Aiken[10] describes leadership as the essential ingredient in professional practice in which professional nurses control both the performance of professional tasks and the environment in which tasks are performed. This view is supported by Stevens.[11]

As a clinical practice discipline, nursing needs to accept responsibility for and have authority over its education and practice.[12] In supporting this thesis, the National Commission Report gives high priority to the development of leadership roles. Advanced degrees are especially emphasized as preparation for clinical specialization, administration, and research. The American Academy of Nursing report on magnet hospitals[7] also supports advanced preparation for nurse executives. This report describes able nurse administrators as master's, if not doctorally prepared, with high-quality leadership skills.

Nurse administrators in service and education play a unique role in creating the environment in which professional practice can occur and endure. Yet for many years preparation for a clinical nursing specialty has been a major goal of graduate education, and graduate students have had few opportunities to specialize in administration. These years of decreased emphasis in administrative education are now evident in the paucity of nursing administrators with the broad knowledge base and sophisticated skills that are necessary to influence the scope and direction of health-care delivery systems.[13]

A similar situation exists in educational settings where deans and department directors come to the position with inadequate or no preparation for administering a school or department. Partridge[14] describes the decanal role as a dilemma of academic leadership. Finneran[15] cited the results of investigations that describe trends in evaluation of the performance of deans. Deans are expected to be knowledgeable in their area of expertise, have a strong research background, and be able to manage a business enterprise. Their performance as business managers receives the greatest emphasis in their performance.

Nurses who have sought advanced degrees in business administration have found themselves shortchanged and deficient in their major field. Business schools across the nation are under sharp criticism[16] for preparing M.B.A. graduates with limited ability to function in real-world institutions. Too much emphasis is placed on quantitative analysis and not enough on qualitative factors, thus producing individuals who lack creativity or entrepreneurial attitudes. The crisis in leadership in nursing suggests the need for nurses prepared at the master's and doctoral level who are well grounded in clinical and administration knowledge.

There is widespread belief among hospital administrators and long-term care administrators that nurse administrative colleagues could make the delivery of care more cost effective if they had better education in financial management and in human resource management.[8] Nurse executives should be able to contribute to executive management decisions beyond nursing services; they are in a unique position to influence cost containment, while maintaining good standards of care. Special courses and short-term workshops are insufficient to prepare individuals for the responsibilities of high-level administrative positions. Nurse executives need the same fundamental knowledge of management practice as their colleagues in other departments. The complexity of today's health-care settings requires nurse managers who are skilled in nursing as well as managing personnel and budgets.

HISTORICAL PERSPECTIVES

Early Executives in Hospitals and Settlements

By all accounts Nightingale was a remarkable woman. She is best remembered as a pioneer of nursing and a reformer of hospitals. In reality, Nightingale was the first nurse executive.[17] In addition to advancing the cause of medical reform, she helped to pioneer the revolutionary notion that phenomena could be objectively measured and subjected to mathematical analysis. She knew nothing about modern research methodology, but fully understood the importance of collecting and analyzing data. According to Cohen,[17] Nightingale not only instituted sanitary reforms in the hospitals at Scutari, she recognized the importance of medical statistics as a tool for improving medical care in military and civilian hospitals. She systematized the chaotic record-keeping practices and developed several graphical representations of statistics. She invented polar-area charts, in which the statistic being represented is proportional to the area of a wedge in a circular diagram. These charts, which she called "coxcombs," were used to dramatize the number of preventable deaths in the Crimea campaign.[17]

Although Nightingale was far ahead of her time regarding accurate record keeping, she was less able to appreciate clinical advances of her day. She showed no interest in the new germ theory of disease and its implications for the treatment of contagious diseases. Her clinical efforts were confined to improvements in ventilation, heating, sewage disposal, water supply, and kitchens. Her statistical charts and diagrams, however, were an important part of the Royal Commission Report, which was widely distributed in Parliament, the government, and the army. This document had an important effect on the improvement of environmental conditions in hospitals.

Nightingale's education was a combination of a liberal education and a training program for nurses in a hospital and orphanage near Düsseldorf, Germany, run by a Protestant order of "deaconesses." She served an apprenticeship at another hospital operated by the Sisters of Mercy in St. Germain in Paris. Her liberal education prior to nurses training was very unusual. Her father believed women should be educated, an unusual idea in the nineteenth century. He personally taught her Italian, Latin, Greek, philosophy, history, writing, and mathematics. In those days women in the highest circles of English society did not attend universities and certainly did not pursue professional careers.[17]

Nightingale's first "situation" was an unpaid appointment as superintendent of a London "establishment for gentlewomen during illness." Her responsibilities were to supervise the nurses and functioning of the physical plant as well as guarantee the purity of the medicines. She did not stay long in this post; her most famous work took place in the British military hospital at Scutari. Her efforts as a skilled administrator are recorded in nursing and world history as she effectively circumvented military authorities who re-

sisted any suggested changes that might point to their incompetence.[17]

Not always recognized as a nurse administrator, Wald, a public health nurse graduated from New York Hospital School of Nursing in 1891. Unhappy with her scant nursing knowledge, she enrolled in Medical School at Woman's Medical College in New York.[18] Using her nursing and entrepreneurial skills, Wald, along with Brewster, established a nurses' settlement house in one of the slum sections of the Lower East Side. As is true of today's nurse executives, they wore modest suits with black ties. By 1909, the East Side Settlement moved to Henry Street and became known as the Henry Street Settlement. The settlement numbered 37 nurses, 5 of whom held administrative posts with all others giving direct nursing care. The supervisors and 10 staff nurses lived in the Henry Street headquarters. Nurses kept two records, a bedside chart with notes for the physician and a work record for the superintendent of nurses. The Henry Street business included first-aid homes in densely populated sections of the city, small surgical offices for dressings, and a small obstetrical service. The Henry Street Settlement had grown from two nurses living on the top floor of a tenement house to a highly organized social enterprise with many departments. These innovative efforts are the hallmark of excellent administration and leadership.

These early superintendents of nurses had to be able nurses who knew training methods. They were responsible for the work of nurses and students and had authority to select and discharge them. In both hospitals and visiting nurse agencies, they purchased supplies and established rules and procedures for conducting the work of the organization. They not only supervised nursing care, they often gave it. Richards, "America's first trained nurse," describes working night duty with especially serious cases while doing regular work during the day.[19] Robb made daily rounds and taught students at the bedside.

The teaching responsibilities were deemed as important as the clinical and administrative responsibilities. In those days, research and the scientific base for practice were unknown. Most of the early administrators lived in the hospital or settlements they directed and knew the nursing and medical staff extremely well.

The evolution of nursing homes did not match the evolution of hospitals as sites for expert care. Early on, nursing homes and long-term care facilities became segregated from enlightened health care. Care was predominately custodial and inexpensive. The Social Security Act and other federally funded programs encouraged a sharp rise in long-term care beds in private for-profit nursing homes, and consequently the need for able administrators arose.

Early directors of nursing were retired and widowed nurses who took elders into their own homes to supplement their income. With the sharp increase in private for-profit institutions during the years 1945–1965, nursing had an unprecedented opportunity to develop nursing practice in a setting almost entirely controlled by nurses. Lodge[20] notes that early history does not reveal any nurse leaders in long-term care.

Changes in thinking about care in nursing homes did not occur in nursing until the recognition of geriatric nursing. The early leaders in gerontological nursing began their work in the 1960s. With the mushrooming number of older people, it seems logical that gerontology needs to be a curriculum component in all administration programs. Clinical care, knowledge, and personal leadership development over the life span require a gerontological orientation.

Nursing Administration Education Over Time

Erickson[21] described the historical evolution of nursing administration education in a paper presented at the Council for Graduate Education for Administrators in Nursing, Philadelphia, 1983. The following chronology is summarized from that work and Kalisch and Kalisch.[18]

Before 1873   No formal academic preparation for nursing administration; only the school of "hard knocks."

1873   First three Nightingale schools established bringing about the need for superintendents of nurses. Superintendent education meant observing administrative practice in another hospital; no academic preparation.

1899   First educational program for nursing administration and collegiate graduate education for nurses at Teachers College, Columbia University. Supported by the American Society of Superintendents of Training Schools for Nursing who were concerned about lack of uniformity in the systems of instruction in the rapidly multiplying schools of nursing. A two-semester program in administration in the Department of Domestic Science was established including:

- Physiology and hygiene
- Ethics
- Psychology in teaching
- Psychology
- Bacteriology
- Household chemistry
- Hospital and training school management
- Home sanitation and management
- Social reform management

This program was designed to prepare capable nurses for advanced responsible positions in hospital work and "thoroughly trained" superintendents who were capable of taking charge of small hospitals and training schools. In 1905, the course of study was extended to two years and included courses in:

- Training school administration
- Hospital administration
- Hospital construction
- Hospital laundries
- Hospital planning
- Food production and chemistry
- Hospital economics.

1920	Master's degrees in nursing initiated.
1935	Areas of graduate study for nursing included: • Supervision of schools of nursing • Administration in hospitals • Administration in public health nursing.
1934	The first educational program for hospital administration initiated at the University of Chicago.
1943	The second program in Hospital Administration at Northwestern University School of Commerce.
1950s	The W. K. Kellogg Foundation allocated 5 million dollars to 13 universities to assist development of graduate programs preparing administrators for hospital nursing services.
1956	Only 2 of the 13 participating universities still allowed specialization in administration at the baccalaureate level.
1960–70	ANA statement supported the need for clinical orientation in master's programs. Leadership became separated from administration.
1970s	Recognition of nursing administration as a practice area established through the certification program. Sharp decline in the number of people enrolled in administration; increase in clinical specialization.
1974	64 universities with master's programs in nursing; 58 with clinical majors and 24 with majors in administrations; extremely strong emphasis on clinical nurse specialists in contrast to former times when role models were head nurses and supervisors.
Late 70s	Disenchantment with nursing administration and general blame on nurse administrators for problems in nursing departments' low status. Kellogg support for development of joint programs in schools of business and public health.[22]
1980s	Turnaround again; tremendous interest in nursing administration. Most schools attempting to include administration in curriculum. Considerable variation in the research requirement; numbers of courses taught by non-nursing departments. Continued Kellogg support; improved status of administration in the National League for Nursing (NLN), American Nurses Association (ANA), and American Hospital Association (AHA); emphasis on leadership; joint nursing and health service administration programs; increasing number of master's and doctoral programs. Discovery of long-term care and home care as opportunities for nurse executives.[20]

In summary, the early leaders in nursing were administrators as well as trained nurses. They were responsible for nursing service and education and they were expected to have technical intelligence as well as executive ability. Financial knowledge and training in every detail of work as well as record keeping were essential skills. The American Society of Superintendents of Training Schools for Nursing was a major influence in supporting and establishing uniformity in the systems of instruction. It is interesting to note today that the American Organization of Nurse Executives is also the new leadership group in nursing.

CREATIVE CURRICULAR ALTERNATIVES

Various models for nursing administration curriculums abound and range from the pure nursing model with all courses taught in a school of nursing to shared models with schools of business, public health, or health services administration. Price[23] concluded that the essential components of a master's program preparing nurse administrators must include:

• administration and management
• financial management and budgeting
• organizational theory
• labor relations and human relations

- economic and political aspects of management
- research
- generalist clinical nursing knowledge

Simms, Price, and Pfoutz[24] raised the issue of preparing nurse executives for roles in acute long-term and home care settings and found comparable leadership responsibilities across settings. Lodge[20] also supports the need for preparation for executive roles in long-term care and has helped nurses rediscover the nursing home as undeveloped site for leadership in nursing practice. In her Kellogg-funded study critical needs for expert nursing care were identified.

McCloskey, Kerfoot, Molen, and Mathis[25] describe the University of Iowa experience in designing a nursing curriculum with supporting courses from the colleges of business, hospital, and health administration. Students select supporting courses in these areas to complement nursing administration courses. These courses generally include courses in organizational behavior, financial management, and legal and political issues. An administrative practicum is a key part of the curriculum. Other schools have joint- or dual-degree models all predicated on the idea that nursing cannot provide quality faculty members with administrative experience and research.

In conclusion, I believe that the time has come to move beyond current thought and recognize that nursing has become a scientific discipline with a strong research base. Nursing is a clinical discipline requiring knowledge in providing care, coordinating care, and professional skills. This means that all nurses need a strong core of knowledge in nursing, research, and leadership. The master's-prepared nurse today needs to work from a scientific base in order to exercise leadership and authority in a variety of clinical settings.

Leadership content for all graduate students needs to include:

- Organizational theory
- Role theory
- Development of professional practice models
- Innovation skills
- Technology development and utilization
- Management of human and fiscal resources
- Personal leadership development
- Ethical practice and decision making
- Gerontology
- Generalist clinical nursing knowledge

Graduate programs at the master's level should be designed to prepare clinical managers to assume leadership roles in clinical nursing, clinical teaching, or clinical management from a strong theory and practice base. The title nurse executive should be reserved for the doctorally prepared nurse who is able to conduct independent research and assume leadership roles in education, professional nursing organizations, health service systems, and other health-related enterprises. These executives will provide intellectual leadership in the conduct of nursing research and expansion of the science of nursing. They will be able to participate in health-care policy making and ethical decision making at the state and national level.

Such a curriculum promotes a research and theoretical base for study. Integrating organizational and decision-making knowledge into the required scientific base creates the environment in which doctoral study of leadership problems can occur.

Nurses are continuing to study problems related to leadership, professional practice environments, and ethical decision making and moral judgment in addition to the traditional clinical problems. More nurses in doctoral study are recognizing the need to study work environments as an important component of designing care delivery systems.

VISIONS OF THE FUTURE

The Challenge

There is unprecedented need to prepare visionary leaders who can move into uncharted waters and design and manage creative nursing systems on earth, and in space. Living and working in a permanently staffed space station is expected to become a reality by the end of the twentieth century. Nurses will work wherever people have a major responsibility for human adaptation. Resources developed by the space program will provide particular challenges for nursing.

The early pioneers in nursing moved to the Crimea, the inner city, the rural areas, and wherever care was needed. The twenty-first century demands and expects clinical coordinators who can provide leadership throughout the world and in space. They will be utilizers of enabling space-age technologies and information systems in concert with human care skills provided in various organizational environments.

The Human Resources

Instructional faculty in emerging nurse executive programs will have percentage practice appointments in and across multiple-care settings. They will play a leadership role in these settings and will be recognized as expert nurses in care provision and coordination. Students in the new nursing curriculums will come from a variety of backgrounds reflecting a liberal education in business, engineering, health science, ethics, architecture, and computer science among others. The B.S.N. will be phased out in the twenty-first century as the prerequisite for graduate study in nursing.

The first nurses were men, the Knights of St. John or Hospitalers.[26] These early monks were charged to care for the sick and defend the Holy Land. A great many of the medieval hospitals owed their origin to the Hospitalers or a similar crusading order, the Teutonic Knights.

The time has arrived for new blood, new crusaders in nursing. Nursing has arrived as a professional discipline and is ready to stand in colleagueship with other health professionals. The image of a profession transformed into a scientific discipline will attract abundant students who are seeking a challenging clinical coordination role that demands critical thinking and research skills for practice.

REFERENCES

1. Haber PA. Technology in aging. The Gerontologist 1986;26(4):350–357.
2. Roncoli M, Whitney F. The limits of medicine spell opportunities for nursing. Nursing & Health Care 1986;7(10):531–534.
3. Manson EC. Future nursing administrators: the three-piece suit image. Nursing Economics 1983; 1(2):126–128.
4. Aroskar MA. Institutional ethics committees and nursing administration. Nursing Economics 1984; 2(2):130–136.
5. National Commission on Nursing. Nursing in transition: models for successful organizational change. Chicago: The Hospital Research and Educational Trust, 1982.
6. American Nurses' Association. Nursing: a social policy statement. Kansas City: American Nurses Association, 1980.
7. American Academy of Nursing. Magnet hospitals: attraction and retention of professional nurses. Kansas City: American Nurses Association, 1983.
8. Institute of Medicine. Nursing and nursing education: public policies and private actions. Washington, DC: National Academy Press, 1983.
9. Chaska NL. The nursing profession: a time to speak. New York: McGraw-Hill, 1983.
10. Clifford J. Professional nursing practice in a hospital setting. In: Aiken LH, ed. Nursing in the 1980s. Philadelphia: JB Lippincott, 1982.
11. Stevens BJ. The role of the nurse executive. 1981; 11(2):19–23.
12. National Commission on Nursing. Summary report and recommendations. Chicago: The Hospital Research and Educational Trust, 1983.
13. Poulin MA. Future directions for nursing administration. Journal of Nursing Administration 1984; 14(3):37–41.
14. Partridge R. The decanal role: A dilemma of academic leadership. Journal of Nursing Education 1983;22(2):59–61.
15. Finneran MR. Trends in the evaluation of nursing deans. Nurs Outlook 1983;31(3):172–173.

16. Behrman JN, Levin RI. Are business schools doing their job? Harv Bus R 1984;62(1):140–147.
17. Cohen IB. Florence Nightingale. Scientific American 1984;250(3):128–137.
18. Kalisch PA, Kalisch BJ. The advance of American nursing. Boston: Little, Brown, 1986.
19. Erickson EH. The nursing service director, 1880–1980. J Nurs Adm 1980;10(4):6–13.
20. Lodge MP. Professional practice for nurse administrators/directors of nursing in long-term care facilities (phase I). Kansas City: American Nurses Foundation, Inc, 1985.
21. Erickson EH. The historical evolution of nursing administration education. Unpublished paper presented at the Council for Graduate Education for Administrators in Nursing Annual Meeting. Philadelphia, 1983.
22. Slater CH. The education and roles of nursing service administrators. Battle Creek: The WK Kellogg Foundation, 1978.
23. Price SA. Master's programs preparing nursing administrators. J Nurs Adm 1984;14(1):11–17.
24. Simms LM, Price SA, Pfoutz SK. Nurse exeuctives: functions and priorities. Nursing Economics 1985;3(4):238–244.
25. McCloskey JC, Kerfoot K, Molen M, Mathis S. Educating nurse administrators: one program's answer. Nursing & Health Care 1986;7(9):505–508.
26. Bullough VL, Bullough B. The emergence of modern nursing. 2nd ed. London: The Macmillan Co, 1969.

37

Organization and Administrative Content in Baccalaureate Nursing Programs

Barbara A. Norton

ADEQUATE preparation of professional nurses for leadership and management roles and functions has concerned nurse educators and nursing service administrators since 1893. Since Nightingale established the first nursing school, it has been generally accepted that nursing schools would assume responsibility for preparing students to function in leadership and management roles. Many nursing education programs endeavored to meet this responsibility by including content and learning experiences designed to facilitate the acquisition of the basic knowledge and skill requirements for leadership and management functions even before the league specified these competencies in the accreditation criteria in the 1950s.[1] Since that time the criteria for baccalaureate education has evolved from a statement on the development of critical thinking, decision making, and independent judgment in 1967,[1] to a criterion for the development of leadership in 1972[2] that has been expanded to include management skills for beginning professional practice in 1982.[3] Other nursing experts have also agreed that formal preparation for these roles and functions must be an integral component of the nursing curriculum.[4–10]

Nurse educators have traditionally been challenged to prepare graduates to meet changing health-care needs in changing health-care delivery systems. Complex and rapidly changing phenomenon, however, are now placing and will continue to place unusual demands on baccalaureate nurse educators to prepare graduates to practice in a highly competitive, technological and information-driven health-care world.

HISTORICAL PRESPECTIVES

The nature of the content and learning experiences selected for a curriculum depends on the particular curriculum model used and the assumptions that underly the model. Since the mid-nineteenth century, nursing education, like general education, has used five main approaches to curriculum development. These approaches are briefly described before examining how nursing education has used them. A historical review may shed some light on choices made in the past and provide some direction for future actions. Cremin noted that "The past remains present, whether we are aware of it or not. Let us work to be aware of it"[11] (p. 15).

Curriculum Development in General Education

Curriculum, usually defined as a plan for the education of learners,[12] was formally addressed by Herbart, a late-nineteenth century german philosopher whose theories about teaching and learning were widely accepted in Europe and the United States.[12–13] Recognition of the need for systematic attention to the selection and organization of subject matter, led Herbart to identify five stages for writing lesson plans and to emphasize the importance of stating the aim of instruction. Spencer initiated a broader approach to curriculum development with the proposal, in 1860, that a classification of human activities be used as the basis for designing curriculum relevant to contemporary society's needs. According to Davies,[13] Spencer's activity-analysis technique resulted in the specification of five main objectives for the school curriculum . . . "self-preservation, securing the necessities of life, rearing and discipling offspring, maintenance of proper social and political relationships, and activities that make up the leisure part of life by gratifying tastes and feelings"[13] (p. 45).

Dewey, often referred to as the father of progressive education, held that the goal of education is to maintain continued growth. He advocated organizing the curriculum to include activities that are created by the subject matter and he regarded student interest as a strong influence on the success of learning. Dewey believed that learning activities selected for the subject matter should be developed in a sequence that builds on and uses skills students already possess.[14] He stressed the importance of integrating inter-action and continuity with the longitudinal and lateral aspects of experiences to give worthwhile meaning to each experience and avoid isolated learning.[15] Dewey provided a detailed description of reflective thinking, stressed its importance as an educational aim, and held that it could serve as the means to unify the curriculum.[16]

In contrast to the humanistic and experiential philosophy of Dewey and his followers, Charters and Bobbitt designed the scientific approach to curriculum. The scientific approach, developed in the 1920s, was in response to society's demand that the curriculum become more efficient and effective.[17] Charters introduced Taylor's job analysis technique into curriculum-development theory. Job analysis, a component of industrial management principles, was a scientific method for studying a person's performance and level of achievement. Charters placed his confidence in technology as the basis for curriculum development and believed that activity analysis provided the means for developing and implementing the curricular aims and objectives.[18] Bobbitt, another curriculum theorist, used the analysis technique as the basis for creating lists of activities, which were then used to determine the specific behaviors and activities most desirable for basic educational experiences.[19] The scientific approach provided a means of delineating concrete practical activities and educational objectives for curriculum development.

Tyler's rational model for curriculum and instructional development, created in the late 1940s, incorporated the major elements of the scientific approach; Dewey's ideas on sequence, continuity, interaction, and integration; and ideas from behaviorist psychology with his own work on test construction.[20] For Tyler, the development of curriculum and instruction is based on responses to the following four basic questions, which concern the purpose, content, organization, and evaluation of educational experiences.

1. What educational purposes should the school seek to attain?
2. What educational experiences can be provided that are likely to attain these purposes?
3. How can these educational experiences be effectively organized?
4. How can we determine whether these purposes are being attained?[20] (p. 1).

These questions focus the curriculum on a linear relationship between the ends and means and place emphasis on the ends before the means. The ends, or educational objectives, provide standards used to select the subject matter, instructional methods, and methods used to evaluate student achievement. Educational objectives serve as the criteria for defining and selecting the content, materials, instructional procedures, and preparation of tests and examinations. The educational objectives are derived from analysis of the learners needs, studies of contemporary life, and subject-matter specialists. Tyler indicated that statements of objectives containing both the behavior and the content provide the specifications for further course development[20] (p. 51). Kliebard viewed Tyler's three sources of objectives as virtually meaningless because of their lack of specificity.[21] Kleibard also believed that the idea of evaluating achievement primarily by matching the behavioral objectives with the demonstrated and expected outcomes reduces the important relationship between ends and means. Use of objectives to determine achievement ignores achievement, which although delayed, may be more significant.

Curriculum Development in Nursing Education

The content and learning experiences in the Nightingale curriculum model was based on a list of duties derived from an activity analysis of nursing functions.[22] This curriculum approach was consistent with the Spencer's classification of human activities. The Nightingale model consisted of one year of formal instruction; an additional requirement of two to three years of hospital service provided time for the graduate to reinforce and apply the first year's learning. Students who demonstrated leadership potential by the end of the first year's training were assigned as charge nurses in hospital wards with responsibility to supervise and train others. Successful performance in these roles resulted in recommendation for administrative positions in hospitals and schools of nursing[22] (p. 331). A systematic course of prescribed reading and examination during an apprenticeship of two to three years provided a broader knowledge and experience base for nurses functioning in leadership and management roles. The existence of the course acknowledged the need for and importance of additional preparation for administrative and teaching responsibilities.

The Nightingale model of training nurses and preparing them for administrative and teaching roles became the dominant plan of nursing education adopted in the United States. Dissatisfaction with the quality of many nursing programs led The American Society of Superintendents of Training Schools for Nurses (the National League of Nursing Education's predecessor) to seek ways to standardize the nursing schools' curriculum and improve the quality of teaching. The problem solution rested with better preparation of nurses serving in administrative and teaching roles in nursing schools. Consequently, in 1899 the Society influenced development of a year-long course in hospital economics at Teachers College, Columbia University that offered academic preparation for leadership and management roles and functions in nursing administration[22] (p. 332).

The persistent problem of establishing acceptable standards of competence in nursing education and practice and the need to delineate clearly the scope and purpose that nursing education should have, moved the National League of Nursing Education to assume leadership by establishing committees to develop improved standards for nursing education.[23] The league's Committee on Education developed three curriculum guides that were published in 1917, 1927, and

1937.[4–6] The curriculum presented in each guide reflected integration of the major curriculum development ideas that were being assimilated into the mainstream of education in the United States. Although the curriculum presented in the first guide focused primarily on nursing tasks, the guide emphasized the need to design curriculum and plan instruction in a way that would develop students' thinking and problem-solving abilities. The scientific approach to curriculum development was used to develop the 1927 and 1937 curriculums. The latter guide included a description of progressive education ideas that were prevalent in general education. The ideas included greater emphasis on social education, developing habits of critical inquiry, greater consideration of individual differences, use of more functional experiences, greater stress on mastery of the curriculum components and building more permanent interests in the students. Nursing was defined, in 1927 and 1937 guides, as a discipline that prepares a flexible individual, capable of independent thought, problem solving, and action, able to adjust to meet the needs of a changing society, while having skill in performing the more narrowly defined activities required in providing physical care to the sick.[5–6] The definition included the holistic and pragmatic competencies required of a nurse and also represented progressive education goals.

Each version of the guide provided a total curriculum plan including course descriptions, outlines, the types of desired learning experiences and schedules for the total program. In addition to the subjects directly related to clinical practice, the first and second guides included courses in the history of nursing, psychology, principles of ethics, a survey of the scope and variety of nursing practice, and contemporary social problems. Elective courses, recommended for placement in the third year of the curriculum, focused on an introduction to institutional work, private nursing and public health nursing. The course in institutional work focused on problems and responsibilities of supervisors and head nurses; it included content on hospital organization, ward planning, personnel and head nurse roles, and functions as manager, leader, and teacher.[4]

The second and third versions of the curriculum were developed on the basis of practical objectives that identified categories of specific duties and responsibilities for the patient, the educational and service institution, the physician and medical profession, the household and friends of the patient, the social and health agencies of the community, the nursing profession, and the individual nurse.[6] (p. 558) Although the third curriculum guide did not include courses for specialized roles and functions, many courses that had been part of the previous curriculum were expanded to include more content and depth and a new two-level course for professional adjustments was added. The primary focus of the third and last curriculum guide was the professional and personal development of a graduate competent to function in any setting, use management skills for his or her own work, direct and supervise those with less experience, provide leadership to help advance the profession by participating in professional activities, and contributing new ideas to the body of nursing knowledge[6] (p. 565).

Subsequent nursing curriculum development progressed from the league's 1937 curriculum model, which incorporated the major aspects of the task-focused, objective-based scientific approach combined with some aspects of progressive education, to the adoption of Tyler's rational model. With the exception of Muse[24] and Heidgerken,[25] who applied the major tenents of progressive education in their approach to curriculum development, the majority of nurse educators have continued to use an objective-based curriculum model, deriving the objectives from an analysis of learner needs, studies of contemporary life, and subject-matter specialists.[26]

From the mid-1930s through the late 1960s the need for additional academic preparation of registered nurses to acquire the leadership and management competencies in specialized roles in nursing was met by several nondegree and specialized degree programs in nursing service, nursing education, and public health nursing. A review of Indiana University School of Nursing bulletins for this period reveals a wide variety of curriculums for each of these specialized areas with subspecialization in more narrow fields.[27] For example, the nursing administration curriculums offered specialization for head nurse, supervisor, or director of nursing service positions; nursing education curriculums offered specialization for administrators of schools of nursing, as well as for teaching fundamentals of nursing or medical specialty areas such as pediatrics and medical-surgical nursing; and public health nursing curriculums offered preparation for staff-level or supervisory positions. Depending on the registered nurse's previous experiences, it was possible for a student to take courses for credit toward a baccalaureate or master's degree.

Each of the specialized curriculums included required courses that would enhance the student's leadership and management abilities; core courses included principles of sociology, human behavior, psychology, public speaking, and principles of organization. Ward management, a senior-level course, included in the curriculum designs for both teaching and head nurse positions, included content elements pertinent to the responsibilities of the head nurse as administrator and educator. Administrative aspects focused on staffing a unit, functions and assignment, methods of supervision of personnel and orientation of personnel, delegation of responsibility, requisitioning and managing supplies and equipment, inventory and basic elements of managing the clinical unit's budget, record keeping, methods of reporting, processing medical orders, and planning time. Patient care aspects focused on planning, implementing, and supervising nursing care and discharge planning as well as specifying the elements considered important for quality nursing care. Teaching elements included identifying the learning outcomes, planning the clinical learning experiences, teaching strategies, and the use of reports.

Specialized administration curriculums designed for supervisors, directors of nursing services, and administrators of nursing schools included courses focusing on public health organization, hospital organization and administration, hospital and nursing service administration, methods and problems in administration, supervision in nursing service, principles of management, interdepartmental relationships, public relations, personnel administration, and economics. In addition to the required courses for a particular specialized curriculum, students had opportunities to enrich their educational experiences by selecting elective courses from a wide variety of courses in education, the humanities, liberal arts, and business.

Since the elimination of the specialized baccalaureate curriculums for graduate nurses in the late 1960s, all students have been expected to demonstrate knowledge and competance in the subject-matter areas included in the baccalaureate curriculum. The purpose of baccalaureate education is to prepare the graduate as a generalist who is competent to practice in any area of clinical nursing and able to assume beginning leadership functions.

CURRENT CURRICULAR ISSUES

In Tyler's curriculum model the educational objectives are derived from an analysis of learners needs, studies of contemporary life, and knowledge in the subject disciplines pertinent to the educational program. An exploration of issues and trends relevant to the contemporary life of nursing education, nursing service, and society should provide some direction for identifying subject-matter content pertinent to curriculum development for leadership and management competencies.

Studies of Contemporary Life

Observations made on the current state of society and the health-care world have stimulated nurse leaders to describe and project the demands placed on nursing and the implications of these demands for future opportunities for advancement of the professional role. Reports from experts involved in the general field of futures studies also include observations that support and elaborate on many of the issues and trends described by nursing leaders. Some of the issues directly affect nursing education, others relate to nursing practice, which of course, directly influence the curricular content.

Nursing Education

Fitzpatrick noted an increasing number of faculty who have little or no knowledge about the educational process—principles of teaching, learning, higher education, and curriculum development—knowledge that is generic to the field of education. Despite increases in the number of doctorally prepared faculty, few of them are prepared in the field of education.[28] Loss of federal financial support for baccalaureate education combined with the reduced number of qualified applicants has contributed to a decrease in the number of faculty positions.[29] Educators are also confronted with the problem of an increasing amount of knowledge that should be crammed into the traditional four-year program. Increased faculty workload decreases

faculty's ability to develop creative ways to meet the demands placed on nursing education for graduates prepared with well-developed intellectual skills and high levels of clinical competence. Rogers expressed the belief, consistent with recommendations from the National Institute of Education, that baccalaureate education in the professional fields should be extended beyond the customary four years.[30]

Fitzpatrick[28] indicated the need for nursing education to have more specific guidelines than are currently available for the National League for Nursing's accreditation criteria and the American Nurses Association's (ANA's) standards for nursing education. This position is supported by findings from some research studies of curricular patterns.

Starck suggested that the traditional nursing curricular practices used by nurse educators are not only inappropriate in today's educational environment, but that the traditional models are contributing to financial problems in schools of nursing.[31] She proposed a model that can generate an increase in revenues for schools of nursing, rather than continuing to permit other disciplines within the college or university to be the primary financial beneficiaries. Additional advantages of her model include: opportunities to enroll non-nursing students in nursing courses, a decrease in the isolation of nursing students from other students in the educational setting, reduced expense of an integrated curriculum for faculty as well as nursing students who need to repeat an entire course because of failure in one aspect of it, and earlier socialization of nursing students into the professional culture.

Starck's model involves teaching liberal arts and science course content in the context of nursing arts and nursing science courses. For example, she suggested that rather than having students take a philosophy course, that nurse faculty create a course that incorporates philosophy and bioethical issues. Nursing faculty could also negotiate with faculty in other disciplines to create science courses, such as anatomony and physiology, oriented toward clinical application. This approach would make the content more relevant to nursing practice as well as students in other health science programs. Restructuring nursing courses into smaller components taught by individual faculty, rather than faculty teams, would make more effective and efficient use of faculty and student time with the additional benefit of a cost savings. Rather than integrating concepts and content from more than one specialized body of knowledge into a single course taught by a team, individual faculty could present the specialized content in separate courses. Scheduling a seminar to follow the separate courses would facilitate integration of the content and concepts. This sequence would enhance faculty productivity while decreasing the costs for students who must repeat some aspect of the course. To reduce the delay in professional socialization incurred by having the majority of nursing courses at the upper-division level, Starck suggested permitting students to enroll in nursing electives during the lower-division period.

Quiring's survey of 53 baccalaureate curricula resulted in some insightful contributions about the state of nursing curriculum.[31] Like Starck, Quiring found nursing curricula to be mired in an outdated pattern. Many of the science course requirements are the same as those required in the diploma education model, the only difference is the amount of content included at the college level. In fact, she calculated that in the average baccalaureate program the physical and biological sciences with emphasis on chemistry, microbiology, anatomy, and physiology constituted 21% of the total program, while the behavioral sciences composed only 11% of the total program credit allocation. Science students graduating in any given field had fewer credit hours in science than the average baccalaureate nursing student. Quiring noted that the credit hours for cognate course areas represented 59% of the total program credit allocation, whereas the nursing courses represented 43%. The wide divergency in the nature of the general education courses required by the programs in the study failed to provide helpful information about the type of general education foundation on which nursing education is based. She concluded that the lower division courses in nursing curricula are a patchwork of requirements rather than a carefully planned design. This patchwork design raises questions about what the base for nursing courses should be.

Ketefian's examination of five baccalaureate programs with innovative curricula revealed that the majority of innovations could be classified into four areas related to subject matter in terms of: (1) the introduction of new content; (2) the reorganization of existing content; (3) some combination of both of those activities; and (4) the addition of two different areas of study into the curriculum[33] (p. 78). She noted that, insofar as it could be determined, knowledge specific to the nature of nursing was not used as the basis for the innovations and concluded that knowledge derived from nursing research was not being integrated into the curricula. She also noted that the changes in the curricula were not based on data from an evaluation of the previous curricula. Ketefian indicated that the use of research findings as the basis for substantive changes in nursing curricula would not be apt to occur until faculty have more respect for research findings.

Fitzpatrick believed that: (1) it is important to find ways to "regularize" nursing education curricula without losing creativity or violating the freedom of individual schools; and (2) consensus on essential points about nursing curricula facilitate progress in preparing a pool of baccalaureate-degree professional nurses with common competencies to meet future needs.[28]

Two efforts at achieving consensus have been reported recently. One is a national study conducted by the American Association of Colleges of Nursing (AACN);[34] the second is a regional project by the Midwest Alliance in Nursing (MAIN).[35]

The AACN project used a combination of regional hearings and data collected from a survey instrument to determine the essentials of education for professional nursing. The report recommends that the essential knowledge, judgments, and skills be used as a standard for evaluating curricula, graduate performance, and eventually as a base for orientation programs for new graduates. Seven values contained in the ANA's Code for Nurses are considered essential for the professional nurse; examples of personal qualities and professional behaviors are provided for each value.

Three categories of nursing roles, care provider, care coordinator, and member of the profession are used to organize statements of the essential knowledge; each cluster of these statements is followed by the associated clinical judgments and related skills used in clinical practice. Knowledge of theory and models are an integral component of the knowledge base. Providers of care are expected to have knowledge of theories and models to guide nursing practice[34] (p. 9). Coordinators of care are expected to know leadership, decision-making, motivation, and management theories; group process; and human and material resources[34] (p. 17). Members of the profession are expected to know the implications that changes in theories and technology hold for the practice of nursing[34] (p. 17). Elements of Leadership and management competencies are distributed throughout all of the roles. A list of example skills for each nursing role are labeled according to the achievement scale. The term supervision is not intended to imply a need for instruction, but is defined as a need to validate skill performance[34] (p. 20). The achievement scale consists of these three levels:

Proficient—adapts and implements clinical judgments and related nursing interventions to client and contextual variables without supervision;

Intermediate—makes clinical judgments and implements related nursing interventions with limited supervision;

Beginning—makes clinical judgments and implements related nursing interventions with supervision[34] (p. 21).

The Midwest Alliance project used a total of 29 teams, each consisting of representatives from baccalaureate nursing education, hospitals, skilled nursing-care facilities, and community-based health programs, to reach consensus on competency requirements for new baccalaureate graduates in five nursing practice areas. The competencies are clustered under the areas of teaching and collaboration, planning and evaluation, interpersonal relations and communication, leadership and two levels of critical care. Each area was rated according to whether the graduate will:

1. be effective and efficient;
2. be effective but require minimum guidance to be efficient;
3. need guidance and practice to be effective and efficient;
4. need little guidance or practice to be efficient and effective;
5. need guidance and assistance to be efficient and effective[35] (pp. 153–154).

Competencies listed under interpersonal relations and communication were rated as requiring minimum guidance to be efficient, while those under leadership were rated as needing guidance and practice to be effective and efficient.

Nursing Practice

A major issue bearing on nursing practice consists of the complex ethical conflicts and decision making in relation to quality of care and quality of life—particularly for those clients with catastrophic diseases such as AIDs and Alzheimer's, and in relation to resource allocation.[36] An increasing number of books addressing the issue of ethics in health care are being published. Bandman described research findings that revealed the significance of nurse-physician interaction and communication to the types of decision making involved in quality of care and patients' rights.[37]

The location of nurse-physician interactions is rapidly shifting away from hospitals. About 40% of registered nurses are not now working in hospitals and an increased percentage of baccalaureate graduates will continue to work in settings other than hospitals.[30] Current predictions indicate that the professional nurse will serve in a leadership role with responsibility for coordinating multidisciplinary teams. Only 25% of nurses will work in hospitals with a significant majority of patient care provided by technical nurses under the supervision of qualified professional nurses. These roles will increase nursing's accountability for quality assurance and permit greater control of practice, while requiring the professional nurse to have well-developed negotiating, collaborating, supervision, and delegation skills.[38]

Dumas indicated that nurses will need to be prepared to organize and manage work and resources effectively and efficiently, that hospitals will require nurses who are able to accept the responsibility associated with prospective payment systems, and that nurses will have opportunities to actively participate in the development of a variety of new services for consumers.[39] Multiple hospital systems, created in the private corporate sector, present new settings for nurses to demonstrate excellence in practice. Quality nursing care provided by expert clinicians is cost effective, and results in a decrease in complications and shortened length of hospitalization. Nursing practice in this environment demands expertise in the clinical and management aspects of patient care, requiring that the nurse be knowledgeable about the economics and management of health care within the suprasystem organization of this mode of health-care delivery.[40]

Marriner called attention to the current state of management in nursing by explaining the trend toward participative management. Implementation of this mode of operation has the potential for enhancing job satisfaction by providing responsibility and acknowledgment of nurses' achievements. Open verbal and written communication, problem solving, and the use of committees are some of the ways in which staff become more engaged in the management process. Marriner also addressed other issues related to cost containment and its relevance to decentralized budgeting, managers support for stress management of staff, use of power and the political process to influence forces that create the health-care world, and the importance of marketing strategies.[41]

The organizational shift to decentralized and participative management places more emphasis on the thinking, creativity, and decision-making capabilities of the individual. Individuals are viewed by organizations as capital investments who cannot be easily duplicated. Rapid decision making requiring command of information and quick analysis demands better-educated personnel. Middle managers' roles are changing in that they are becoming less concerned with supervision, with increasing emphasis on motivating others and managing projects.[42]

Cleveland viewed information as a resource that has created a new organizational environment. The increasing availability of quickly gathered information, which is rapidly analyzed and communicated, is quickly eroding the traditional hierarchal structures in which command and control have been vested.[43] The dominant mode of working in organizations during the "Third Wave" described by Toffler, is the use of information via electronic technology.[42] The new organizational environment is one of participatory decision making in which leadership is exercised primarily by persuasion, greater participation, and collective thought[43] (p. 39).

Agor indicated that persuasive and sensitive communication used in the bottom-up horizontal mode of participative management require that managers develop intuitive judgment in order to cope with rapid changes in the work environment. Intuitive skills, as well as inductive skills, are often referred to as right-brain skills. Persons with the intuitive and inductive skills are apt to prefer collegial and participatory authority structures. Persons with analytical and deductive skills, commonly known as left-brain skills, show a preference for more hierarchal organizational structures.[44] Since publication of the league's first curriculum guide in 1917, nursing educators have consistently indicated that critical thinking skills are an important attribute of a professional nurse. The 1982 National League for Nursing (NLN) accreditation criteria and the American Association of Colleges of Nursing have both reaffirmed the importance of these skills.

Broadly defined, critical thinking skills are "the mental processes, strategies, and mental representations people use to solve problems, make decisions, and learn new concepts"[45] (p. 46). A taxonomical list of critical thinking skills includes the following six classifications, each of which consists of finer discriminations of mental abilities: problem solving—10 skills; decision-making—7 skills; inferential thinking, which includes inductive and deductive thinking—11 skills; divergent thinking—6 skills; evaluative thinking—16 skills;

and philosophy and reasoning—1 skill[45] (p. 52).

Computer technology is an information resource tool that is rapidly becoming entrenched in nursing service in a variety of health-care settings. The potential this new tool has for nursing has not yet been realized, although evidence is now appearing in the literature about how programs can be designed for patient classification systems, quality assurance, nursing care plans, staffing scheduling, systems, cost control, and demographic profiles of nursing personnel.[46–48] At this time the impact of computers in nursing education appears to be limited to word processing and administrative functions because of financial limitations.[49] These limitations reduce faculty opportunities to develop competence in using computer technology to manage their teaching responsibilities and create instructional packages.[50] It is clear that nursing educators need the resources to become knowledgeable about the multiple uses of computers in nursing and opportunities to learn about the legal and ethical issues associated with its use. Grobe suggested that nursing curricula need to be designed to enable students to become computer literate as well as knowledgable about computer systems, design, implementation, and evaluation of programs.[51] Computer technology provides another avenue for professional nursing to actively demonstrate leadership and management competencies in the course of participating in the creation of programs for nursing practice.[52]

Nursing Studies in Leadership and Management

The nursing literature does not delineate clearly the leadership and management roles and functions for which the baccalaureate graduate should be prepared. Textbooks used in baccalaureate education include content consisting of multiple theories of leadership and principles of management. The content is generic for team leader, modular nurse, and primary care nurse roles as well as those of the head nurse, patient care coordinator, supervisor, and director of nursing.

An increasingly critical issue for baccalaureate nurse educators is identification of the leadership and management competencies required for a novice graduate to function adequately. A few studies address aspects of this problem. Some of the findings may provide some information that will help to give guidance to curricula developers; however, the rapid changes in the scope of responsibilities of staff in all health-care facilities could make some of the findings outdated.

Westphal found that regardless of the size or geographical location of hospitals in South Carolina, very little difference existed between the type of managerial skills needed by charge nurses and those needed by team leaders and primary care nurses. It is interesting to note that while associate degree, diploma, and baccalaureate programs in South Carolina taught basically the same managerial functions, the investigator concluded that none of the graduates were adequately prepared with the management skills required to meet the employing hospitals' needs.[53]

Brown sought to resolve the conflicting role descriptions, expectations, and real performance of recent graduates in relation to leadership and management functions.[54] She surveyed recent baccalaureate nursing graduates, baccalaureate nurse educators, and hospital nursing directors in North Carolina to: (1) validate the completeness of the list of 84 types of competencies; (2) determine agreement on the importance and relevance of 84 leadership and management competencies; and (3) determine if the new graduates felt that their educational programs had prepared them adequately to effectively function in the leadership and management roles required in their positions.

The 84 competencies were grouped into the basic management functions: planning ($N = 14$), organizing ($N = 11$), staffing ($N = 8$), directing ($N = 34$), and controlling ($N = 17$). All three groups of respondents indicated that the list of 84 competencies was complete, and they perceived most of the competencies as very important for effective practice. The rank order of the means for each competency from highest to lowest of the five functional categories was staffing, controlling, planning, directing, and organizing. The nurses, however, ranked planning competencies lower in importance than the other two groups. Planning competencies included: using multiple data-collection methods for planning patient care, effective use of interviewing skills to collect data; identifying biopsychosocial needs of individual clients; focusing on the individual patient care needs; developing patient care plans appropriate to the identified problems and goals, using nursing rounds to plan patient care; planning patient teaching; participating and conducting patient care planning conferences; using decision-making theories; making high-quality decisions in a short time period; seeking support from others for decisions, seeking cooperation from coworkers, and evaluating the effectiveness of priorities established by self and others.

Brown concluded that because 35% of the nurses believed that they had not been adequately prepared to meet the functions required for effective performance, baccalaureate preparation for leadership and management competencies could be improved. She recommended that examination of baccalaureate curriculums should focus on the particular content, and experiences related to planning functions to ensure that they are adequate.

Langer investigated the perceptions of importance placed by nurse educators and head nurses on management skills in the categories of patient care, human resources, and operations that are required for initial management positions.[55] Nurse educators' and head nurses' perceptions on the importance of selected management skills and patient care management skills did not significantly differ. Head nurses placed significantly higher importance on human resources management skills than nurse educators. Langer also found that more head nurses than nurse educators believed that the employing institution, rather than the clinical or theory faculty, should assume primary responsibility for teaching specific management skills.

Staff nurses included in the Magnet Hospital study provided information about leadership and management characteristics that provided job satisfaction.[52] Although the comments are descriptive of the values and behavior patterns demonstrated by nurse managers and administrators, consistent characteristics emerge that validate (1) the competencies required to work in a participating environment and (2) the importance of many of the competencies included in Brown's inventory.[54] Persistent themes found in the comments are that staff nurses: want to be actively engaged in a variety of shared leadership and management activities related to nursing as well as the general organization; want to have opportunities to contribute to the growth of the institution; and want to be able to demonstrate their professional competence in traditional and unique ways in a supportive environment.

Fagin reported on a study that revealed baccalaureate graduates not only underestimate their preparation for leadership but they disagreed with their supervisors' appraisal of their skills.[56] Fagin believed that part of the difficulty could be attributed to the difference in the graduates' and educators' perceptions of leadership competencies. She recommended clearer delineation of the competencies and communication of the program and course expectations to the student.

Current Leadership and Management Subject Matter

To determine the nature of content in leadership and management courses in baccalaureate nursing education Kalisz and Ryan conducted a national survey of programs accredited by the National League for Nursing.[57] The data revealed that the majority of respondents (66%) offered a leadership and management course, while 31% of the respondents indicated integration of the relevant concepts throughout the curriculum. The nature of the courses spanned a wide range of combinations. For example, some programs indicated that a required management course was taught by a school of business, while others indicated that students had the opportunity to take an elective non-nursing management course in addition to a required nursing management course. Some programs with an integrated curriculum also offered students this option.

The nature of the clinical learning experiences in 90% of the programs with separate leadership and management courses included; using team, modular, primary, or case nursing systems of nursing care delivery; designating staff for patient care; functioning as a medication nurse for a group of patients; leading team conferences; observing charge nurses, and serving as an assistant to the charge nurse[57] (p. 25). About one-half of the programs with integrated curricula indicated either placing special clinical emphasis on leadership and management concepts during the senior year or having a specific clinical learning experience. Threading of leadership and management concepts over the entire program were reported by some respondents in the integrated programs. Although the study did not collect specific data on the type of leadership and management content included in the programs, some of the topics indentified included "reality shock, assertiveness, role theory, conflict resolution, labor relations, change theory, quality assurance programs, legislative issues, and ethical issues"[57] (p. 26).

A general survey of historical and contemporary nursing literature revealed that many nurse educators have traditionally viewed courses in general education and liberal arts as critical components that provide the knowledge base of an educated person. The courses are valued with the belief that they promote development of mental and attitudinal characteristics important to personal and professional growth. The courses contribute to professional nursing's aspects of leadership and management abilities by promoting writing, reading, and thinking skills as well as contributing to the students' understanding of human nature and the physical, social, political, and economic dimensions of the world at large. These beliefs have been supported by the league's accreditation criteria and more recently by the AACN's working document on the *Essentials of College and University Education for Nursing.*[58] The importance of the biological and social sciences contribution to courses in the nursing major have also been long valued.

Program content pertinent to the development of leadership and management abilities has gradually expanded to include increased emphasis on verbal and written communication, interpersonal relations, teaching clients, and group dynamics. Within the context of these major areas, content has been added to address conflict resolution, assertiveness training, and role theory. Depending on the pattern of curriculum organization this content could be threaded vertically, horizontally, or both. Specific content and clinical learning experiences providing integration of previously achieved leadership competencies with management are traditionally taught in senior-year courses.

The major elements of management content are usually offered within the scope of a community health nursing course or a spe-

cific course focusing on management in health-care systems, or elements of the content may be portioned out in both types of courses. Content elements usually include systems theory, several leadership theories, motivational and achievement theories, change theory, principles and theories of administration and organization, and management theory. The five management functions, planning, staffing, organizing, directing, and controlling are commonly used as a framework for organizing the subject-matter content. Each functional category accommodates subsumption of content related to many aspects of nursing practice, such as quality assurance, models of nursing care delivery systems, patient classification systems, managerial tools used in nursing—reports, records, and conferences, models of staffing patterns, and human resource development. Subject-matter content pertaining to ethical, legal, legislative, and labor relations issues, may be leveled and integrated within a variety of the upper-division courses, presented in a management course or a separate course focused on multiple dimensions of the professional role.

Nursing Theory

Baccalaureate faculty interest in and knowledge about nursing models and theories has grown in the past few years as graduate education has concentrated more attention on the realm of theory development in nursing and as more information has become available through the professional literature and national programs. Nursing models, theories, or both are gradually being introduced into baccalaureate education in different ways. Some baccalaureate programs are using a single model or theory as a conceptual framework for the curriculum, while others teach students several of these. In learning nursing models and theories, students become aware of how subject-matter content from various disciplines pertinent to nursing may become organized into a body of knowledge that serves to establish the discipline of nursing.

Nursing models and theories that are known to be used in baccalaureate education include: Orem's Self-Care Deficit Theory; King's Theory of Goal Attainment; Watson's Philosophy and Science of Caring; Erickson, Tomlin, and Swain's Modeling and Role-Modeling; Roy's Adaption Model; and Neuman's Systems Model.[59] Each model is derived from different bases of nursing knowledge and theoretical sources, uses different assumptions, presents a particular frame of reference for perceiving the phenomena, and presents different foci for nursing actions. The rich variety of current models and theories provide many alternatives for faculty to examine before selecting the particular ones to use in a baccalaureate curriculum. Some models and theories, like King's, and Erickson, Tomlin, and Swain's are classified as focusing on interpersonal relationships; Watson's and Orem's are labeled humanistic; while Roy's and Neuman's are identified as systems.[59] Each model has different relevance for ill, well, or both types of client populations. With the exception of Tolbert and Gardner's description of an application of Orem's concept of leadership in the development of clinical courses,[60] there is little information available in the literature to indicate how these models and theories are used or might be used to focus on developing leadership and management capabilities.

BACCALAUREATE CURRICULUM FOR THE FUTURE

Information gleaned from observations made on the current state of nursing, the health-care world, and society combined with research and report findings provides insight into some of the major issues confronting baccalaureate nurse educators. These issues include:

1. The inadequate preparation of faculty in the process of education.
2. A need for specific guidelines to create contemporary and futuristic baccalaureate nursing curricula.
3. A need for new curricular models.
4. A need for more efficient and effective organization of all subject-matter content and learning experiences.
5. Examination of the essential knowledge and competencies required for a first-level professional graduate.
6. Increasing emphasis on the importance of leadership and management competencies.
7. Increasing importance of critical thinking skills for all aspects of nursing practice.
8. Selection of appropriate models and theories from nursing and other relevant disciplines.

Contemporary nursing practice requires most if not all of the skills traditionally used, in fact the technical skills needed continue to increase and become more complex. The essential knowledge base is also expanding. The narrow task-focused approach translated into specific objectives directing curriculum development, which has been used in the past is gradually shifting to a broader, more conceptual approach intended to be more relevant to preparing graduates to function in a larger variety of settings. This approach requires an examination of competencies required for generic situations and problems relevant to the practice realm in which the new graduate will be expected to function. If baccalaureate graduates are to be prepared with the increasing amount of knowledge and skill required for beginning leadership and management roles and functions, then faculty may find it beneficial to consider some approaches to achieve this goal.

In view of the poor preparation of faculty in the process of education, one approach would be to enlist the talents of a variety of expert nurse educators to create complete models for baccalaureate curricula similar to those developed by the NLN in the early part of this century. The model curricula could be used as a map for faculty to use as they construct their own curriculum.

It has been suggested that the Tyler objective-driven model for curriculum development has limited relevance for contemporary general education as well as nursing education. The use of behavioral objectives may serve to fragment the curriculum development and evaluation of student achievement at a time when they should becoming more unified. A reconceptualization of curriculum development focusing on some integration of liberal arts course content within the context of nursing content for both the lower- and upper-division courses can promote a more efficient and effective curriculum. Careful examination of a taxonomy of thinking skills and the finer discriminations included in each category provides considerable latitude for using critical thinking skills as a means for unifying the entire curriculum. Current knowledge about cognition and meaningful learning provide support for creating courses that meld liberal arts with nursing content and different approaches in designing the major nursing subject-matter.

Clearer delineation of the leadership and management competencies required of baccalaureate graduates is becoming more available as a result of data from recent studies and reports. Brown's complete inventory of leadership and management competencies combined with the consensus of responses from three groups of subjects about the importance of the competencies is an important contribution.[54] While replication of the study on a national level could provide additional validation of the findings, a review of the nursing literature addressing leadership and management skills lends support to the inventory and the underlying knowledge and skills included in each of the items. A content analysis of each competency in the inventory has potential for identifying the essential knowledge and experiences to be included in the curriculum.

It is clear that a major component of the essential base for leadership and management competencies consists of a large repertoire of technical skills. The number of technical skills listed in the AACN report compared to the number of skills specified for the other two roles places strong emphasis on the importance of technical skills as the base for leadership and management competencies.[34] The report provided 111 examples of technical skills listed under the provider of care role. The assigned achievement level for 36% ($N = 40$) of the skills is at the proficient level; 48% ($N = 53$) are at the intermediate level; and 16% ($N = 18$) are at the beginning level. Fourteen examples for the coordinator of care role are distributed thusly: 14% ($N = 2$) are at the proficient level; 71% ($N = 10$) are at the intermediate level; and 14% ($N = 2$) are at the beginning level. Member-of-the-profession role category contains 9 examples: 11% ($N = 1$) are at the proficiency level; 78% ($N = 7$) at the intermediate level; and 11% ($N = 1$) at the beginning level.

The MAIN project report also provided competency requirements pertinent to leadership and management with ratings of expected competency upon graduation.[35] Comparison of the AACN and the MAIN project approaches for rating competency levels reflects different philosophical orientations. The AACN rating system considers three levels of achievement that are delineated by two factors: the ability to adapt interventions in a variety of situations and the need for validation of the skill. The MAIN rating system considers four factors: the expected degree of guidance, need for assistance, and the amount of practice in relation to effectiveness of performance and the efficiency of the performance. The underlying assumptions for each approach lead to different implications for education and service. Consensus by nurse educators and nursing service personnel on a common rating system would: (1) facilitate decision making in curriculum and instructional development; (2) expedite progress toward preparing students with a common repetoire of competencies; and (3) provide direction for staff development and continuing education programs.

Use of nursing models and theories in baccalaureate education have not yet been sufficiently described to identify particular models and theories that provide optimal frameworks for leadership and management competency subject-matter content. Nurse experts with experience in working with particular nursing models and theories are in a position to guide baccalaureate faculty's efforts in the integration of leadership and management subject-matter content. Experts' experience in working with different models and theories may indicate those that are more feasible for baccalaureate education. Dissemination of descriptions of faculty experiences with curriculum development and organization and assessment of student competencies correlated with the types of specific leadership, decision-making, motivation, and management theories could facilitate decision making for curriculum and course developers. These activities could assist faculty to meet the pressing need to select pertinent subject-matter content matched with appropriate learning experiences that allows time for students to integrate the required cognitive and interpersonal learning.

Fahy noted that the demands of the future require undergraduate education to place emphasis on the use of knowledge and its sources. To meet this demand curriculum needs to be designed to provide the intellectual tools and attitudes essential for subsequent growth as a professional nurse.[61] The resources to respond to this demand are at our disposal; we need only to apply our collective leadership and management talents to resolve the issues.

REFERENCES

1. National League for Nursing. Department of baccalaureate and higher degree programs. Criteria for the appraisal of baccalaureate and higher degree programs in nursing. New York: National League for Nursing, 1967.
2. National League for Nursing. Department of baccalaureate and higher degree programs. Criteria for the appraisal of baccalaureatre and higher degree programs in nursing. 3rd ed. New York: National League for Nursing, 1972.
3. National League for Nursing. Council of baccalaureate and higher degree programs Self-study manual. Guidelines for preparation of the self-study report. New York: National League for Nursing, 1984.
4. National League of Nursing Education. Standard curriculum for schools of nursing. 4th ed. New York, 1922.
5. National League of Nursing Education. A curriculum for schools of nursing. 6th ed. New York, 1927.
6. National League of Nursing Education. A curriculum guide for schools of nursing. New York, 1937.
7. Douglass LM, Bevis EM. Nursing management and leadership in action. 4th ed. St. Louis: CV Mosby, 1983.
8. Sullivan EJ, Decker PJ. Effective management in nursing. Menlo Park, CA: Addison-Wesley, 1985.
9. Gilles DA. Nursing management: a systems approach. Philadelphia: WB Saunders, 1982.
10. Marriner A. Guide to nursing management. 2nd ed. St. Louis: CV Mosby, 1984.
11. Pinar W, ed: Curriculum theorizing. Berkeley: McCutchan, 1975.
12. Zais RS. Curriculum: principles and foundations. New York: Harper & Row, 1976.
13. Davies IK. Objectives in curriculum design. London: McGraw Hill, 1976.
14. Dewey J. Democracy and education. New York: The Free Press, 1916.
15. Dewey J. Experience and education. New York: Collier Books, 1938.
16. Dewey J. How we think. Boston: DC Health, 1910.
17. Cremin LA. The transformation of the school: progressivism in American education, 1876–1957. New York: Alfred A Knopf, 1968.
18. Charters WW. Curriculum construction. New York: Macmillan, 1924.
19. Bobbitt F. How to make a curriculum. Boston: Houghton Mifflin, 1924.
20. Tyler RW. Basic principles of curriculum and instruction. Chicago: The University of Chicago Press, 1949.
21. Kliebard HM. The Tyler rationale. School Review 1970; 78(2):259–272.
22. Stewart IM. The education of nurses: historical foundations and modern trends. New York: Macmillan, 1943.
23. Roberts MM. American nursing: history and interpretation. New York: MacMillan, 1954.
24. Muse MB. Guiding learning experience: principles

of progressive education applied to nursing education. New York: MacMillan, 1950.

25. Heidgerken LE. Teaching and learning in schools of nursing. Philadelphia: JB Lippincott, 1965.

26. Norton BA. Nursing education: evolution of curriculum development and a reconceptualized model. Indianapolis, Indiana: Unpublished paper, 1986.

27. Indiana University School of Nursing Bulletins. Indianapolis, Indiana, 1944–1968.

28. Fitzpatrick ML. Perspectives on patterns of nursing education. In: National league for Nursing. Patterns in education. The unfolding of nursing. New York: National League for Nursing, 1985.

29. Infante MS. The clinical learning experience: the evolution of the nursing work force. In: National League for Nursing. Patterns in education: the unfolding of nursing. New York: National League for Nursing, 1985.

30. Rogers ME. Nursing education: preparing for the future. In: National League for Nursing. Patterns in education: the unfolding of nursing. New York: National League for Nursing, 1985.

31. Starck P. Realism in nursing curricula. Nurs Outlook 1984;32(4):220–224.

32. Quiring JD, Gray GT. Is baccalaureate education based on a patchwork curriculum? Nurs Outlook 1979;27(11):708–713.

33. Ketefian S. Curriculum change: implications of a case study for nursing education. In: Fitzpatrick ML, ed. Present realities/future imperatives in nursing education. New York: Teachers College Press, 1977.

34. American Association of Colleges of Nursing. Essentials of college and university education for professional nursing: a final report. Washington, DC: American Association of Colleges of Nursing, 1986.

35. Stull MK. Entry skills for BSNs. Nurs Outlook 1986;34(3):138–139.

36. Nursing & Health Care editors. Ten trends to watch. Nursing & Health Care 7(1):17–19.

37. Bandman E. Ethics in health care. Interaction 1987;1(1). Indianapolis, IN: Indiana League for Nursing.

38. Maloney MM. Professionalization of nursing. Philadelphia: JB Lippincott, 1986.

39. Dumas RG. Mission for the future of nursing education. In: National League for Nursing. Patterns in education: the unfolding of nursing. New York: National League for Nursing, 1985.

40. Curran C. The corporate connection: Multihospital systems rekindle commitment. In: National League for Nursing. Patterns in education: the unfolding of nursing. New York: National League for Nursing, 1985.

41. Marriner A. Management moves. Nursing Success Today 1986;3(8):8–13.

42. Raymond HA. Management in the third wave. The Futurist 1986;20(5):15–17.

43. Cleveland H. Information as a resource. The Futurist 1982;16(6):34–39.

44. Agor WH. Tomorrow's intuitive leaders. The Futurist 1983;17(4):49–53.

45. Sternberg RJ. Critical thinking: Its nature, measurement, and improvement. In: Link FR, ed. Essays on the Intellect. Alexandria, VA: Association for Supervision and Curriculum Development, 1985c, pp. 45–65.

46. McAlindon MN, Silver CM, Edwards HK. Computer software for nursing. Computers in Nursing 1986;4(1):17–26.

47. Kline NW. Principles of computerized database management. Computers in Nursing 1986;4(2):73–81.

48. Hylton RD, Johnson JE, Moran MJ. Automating a patient classification system. Computers in Nursing 1986;4(1):27–32.

49. Walker MB. Nursing education: challenges of the computerized environment. Computers in Nursing 1986;4(4):166–171.

50. Tate J. Helping nursing faculty overcome resistance to computer use in the curriculum. Computers in Nursing 1986;4(1):5, 48.

51. Grobe SJ. The impact of computers on nursing. In: National League for Nursing. Patterns in education: the unfolding of nursing. New York: National League for Nursing, 1985.

52. American Academy of Nursing: task force on Nursing Practice in Hospitals. Magnet hospitals. Kansas City: American Nurses Association, 1983.

53. Westphal BC. Managerial aspects of the charge nurse role. Dissertation Abstracts International 1980;41(7-8):2971B.

54. Brown ST. Leadership and management competencies needed by neophyte nurses. ERIC Document, no. ED248 795.

55. Langer BE. Development of a management curricular component for baccalaureate nursing education. Dissertation Abstracts International 1985;46(9–10):2906A.

56. Fagin CM. Refocus on leadership. Nursing leadership 1979;2(4):6–13.

57. Kalisz MA, Ryan ME. Are baccalaureate students prepared to assume first-level management positions? Nursing Leadership 1982;5(3):23–27.

58. American Association of Colleges of Nursing. Essentials of college and university education for nursing: a working document. Washington, DC: American Association of Colleges of Nursing, 1986.

59. Marriner A. Nursing theorists and their work. St. Louis: CV Mosby, 1986

60. Tolbert R, Gardner K. Can you learn to be a leader? Nursing Success Today 1985;2(7):10–15.

61. Fahy ET. Baccalaureate education in nursing. In: Fitzpatrick ML, ed. Present realities/future imperatives in nursing education. New York: Teachers College Press, 1977.

38

Administration and Organization Content in Master's Programs in Nursing

Theresa L. Carroll

BEFORE any discussion of administration and organization content in master's programs in nursing can take place, it is necessary to elicit some common understanding of what is meant by the terms "administration" and "nursing administration." "Administration may be defined as all the action rationally performed . . . to fulfill a common purpose."[1] Although some authors purport to make subtle distinctions, management is a term that is frequently used synonomously with administration. For purposes of comparison, management is a generic function aimed at planning and organizing work. It involves leading workers toward accomplishment of preset goals to achieve desired results.[2] Management is intellectual work performed by people in an organizational context.[3] Management work is decision making aimed at accomplishing the goals of the organization.[4] The practice of management or administration has its theoretical underpinnings in the social and behavioral sciences. Since management work takes place in organizations, it requires an understanding of the nature, functions, characteristics, and environment of organizations that can be found in the study of organization theory.

Nursing administration is the process of setting and achieving objectives by influencing human behavior within a suitable environment. It is the job of the nurse administrator to create an environment conducive to performance of acts that will accomplish the institution's goals, as well as the goals of the participating individual.[5] The uniqueness inherent but not obvious in this definition relates to the fact that the products of any health-care organization may be patient care, education (professional, patient, and consumer), research, and community service. The employees of a nursing division in the health care organization are professional nurses and nonprofessional ancillary personnel.

In 1952 Finer, Director of a Kellogg-funded Nursing Service Administration Project, worked with 36 nursing administration leaders to determine if a science of administration was needed in the conduct of nursing service. After an analysis of the work of nursing administration, Finer concluded "It has been established beyond any doubt that modern nursing service has [a] truly pressing need of a knowledge of administration . . . . The absence of a knowledge of administration spells confused and dispersed responsibility, wasted resources, sick morale, and a defect of proper patient care."[1]

More recently, leaders in nursing administration education have agreed with Finer's conclusions and describe nursing administration as a "mediative role, requiring knowledge of the fields of both nursing and management . . . [nurse administrators use] the skills of one discipline, management, to achieve the ends of another, nursing."[6] Further, the Council of Graduate Education for Administration in Nursing recognizes that "nursing administration is an emergent discipline, evolving as a synthesis of the fields of nursing and management."[7]

The exact nature of administration and organization content that is included in any graduate nursing program is very much dependent on: (1) the faculty's philosophy regarding the importance and appropriateness of nursing administration as a valid field of study for nurses; (2) the faculty's perception of the current practice and future direction of nursing administration; and (3) the resources available both in the educational institution as well as those in the nursing and health-care community in which the graduate nursing program is located.

THE PHILOSOPHY OF THE FACULTY

The importance of the faculty philosophy about the place of nursing administration in graduate nursing programs cannot be overemphasized since their collective belief system determines the formulation of program goals, the structure of the curriculum, and, ultimately, the content of specific courses. In relation to the question of whether nursing administration is an appropriate area for graduate nursing education, a historical perspective reveals that following the Kellogg Project in 1950 to 1951; fourteen universities established nursing administration programs with financial support from the Kellogg Foundation. Subsequently, master's programs of the 1950s emphasized functional preparation in either nursing education or nursing administration. However, the 1960s saw the pendulum in graduate nursing education swing from functional preparation to

an emphasis on advanced clinical practice.[8] During this time both the National League for Nursing and the American Nurses Association issued statements that supported the preparation of clinical nurse specialists. Despite ongoing support by the Kellogg Foundation for the development of interdisciplinary graduate programs to prepare nurse administrators, the 1960s and early 1970s saw the glorification of the clinical, one-to-use bedside nursing role with stigmatization of nonclinical roles.[6] With the new focus on clinical practice, nursing administration fell into disrepute, and most schools of nursing dropped their majors and minors in the subject; some schools dropped course offerings altogether; and other schools gave nursing administration lip service. Not only was nursing administration unpopular, many in nursing, particularly those in academe, felt it an unacceptable field of study or pursuit for nurses.[9]

On the positive side, Stevens refers to this period of clinical emphasis in graduate nursing programs as the time of "professionalizing the nursing vanguard." This period resulted in an "ever-increasing number of nursing elite . . . accepting responsibilites inherent in . . . a professional practice of the discipline of nursing."[6] However, one cost of this focus on one-to-one nurse-patient care in graduate nursing programs was the lack of a cadre of well-prepared nurse administrators. Stevens goes on to point out that for the 1980s and 1990s "an exclusively clinical focus has reached the point of diminishing returns" and "the body of nursing knowledge is unlikely to develop unless systematic control of nursing practice is possible. . . . Vanguard clinicians will fail in their quest if nurse executives cannot provide a situation of inquiry where discoveries about practice can be implemented."[6]

The publication of the Institute of Medicine,[10] the National Commission on Nursing,[11] and the Magnet Hospital[12] studies reaffirmed the need for well-prepared nurse administrators to lead patient care divisions in the increasingly turbulent health-care environment of the 1980s. This evolution in health care has led many in nursing to realize that advanced clinical education may not be adequate preparation for nursing administration positions, particularly at the executive level.

What attention is given to administration and organization content, in general, and nursing administration content, in particular, in a graduate nursing program is largely dependent upon the faculty's collective beliefs about the state of nursing's evolution as a discipline and a profession. If the faculty believe that clinical nursing is the only proper field for graduate education, then the school's graduate program will focus on clinical specialization. If the faculty recognize the necessity of role development in the area of administration, they may opt for a major focus in clinical nursing and a minor one in the functional area of nursing administration. If the faculty accept nursing administration as a valid nursing specialty, then the graduate nursing program focus may take the form of a nursing administration major with an advanced generalist approach to clinical nursing content. This latter example is not a return to the 1950s in terms of functional emphasis in graduate nursing education. The question for graduate nursing education in the 1980s and beyond is not one of all or nothing—"all functional or all clinical preparation. The issue is balance."[9]

At an invitational conference titled "Nursing Administration: Directions for the Future" sponsored by Boston University in November, 1978, the balance of content between clinical nursing and administrative content in graduate nursing programs was discussed and debated. According to Stevens, the nurse administrators concluded that "there is no room for clinical nursing in a master's-level program in nursing adminis-

tration simply because there is so much administrative knowledge that must be poured into so short a time."[13] Conversely, the nurse educators concluded that "a master's-level program in nursing must contain graduate-level content in nursing; otherwise there is no justification for having such a program."[13] Stevens recognized that both sides had a valid message. She summarized the discussion by concluding that education for nursing administration must synthesize graduate-level management and graduate-level nursing. She suggested that nursing administration graduate students need to learn about the dominant models and paradigms in each area of nursing potentially represented in the institutions that they will manage. The nurse administrator's job requires a generalist approach to nursing—on a conceptual, not a practice level. Stevens concluded that the majority of the invitational conference participants probably agreed that the clinical component should use a conceptual, that is, theoretical approach as opposed to a hands-on, one-to-one patient care experience.[13]

However, this apparent accord was short lived. In 1984 Clelland wrote that the "common pattern in graduate nursing programs of having applicants elect a clinical major or a nursing administration major leaves the latter program graduates lacking significant graduate nursing content."[14] The graduate faculty in this case believed that "considerable harm has been done in nursing practice settings where nurse administrators have not been sufficiently prepared in advanced nursing to have developed a professional philosophy for guiding an interpreting nursing practice."[14] Further, Clelland pointed out that "in at least two fully accredited M.S.N. programs, the nursing faculty have not admitted graduates of their administration programs into the Ph.D. in nursing program for the reason that these graduates are not adequately grounded in nursing."[14] Based on this belief and observation, the graduate nursing curriculum that Clelland and her faculty operationalized at Wayne State University, offered students a clinical nursing major and an eight semester credit (three-course) administration minor aimed at preparing graduates academically for middle-management positions in health care settings where they had previous employment experience.[14] This is but one example of how the belief system of the faculty directly affects the amount and configuration of nursing and administration content in a graduate nursing program. However, by specifying that their program prepared graduates for middle-management positions in nursing administration, the curriculum was also reflecting the faculty's view of the state of the art of nursing administration practice.

THE FACULTY'S VIEW OF NURSING ADMINISTRATION PRACTICE: IMPACT ON CURRICULUM

In 1951 when Finer and his group of nursing leaders undertook to develop a curriculum for the preparation of nurse administrators, the initial phase of the project sought to "outline the responsibilities of directors of nursing service in modern hospitals."[15] The result of this activity is depicted in Figure 38.1. Finer proposed that this conceptualization of nursing administration could provide a model for curriculum development, that is, each component of the model could provide course content. As depicted in this model, nursing service administration has two phases. One phase is depicted by the eight functional elements, for example, budgeting, staffing, planning, and directing nursing care. The second phase is referred to as the dynamic factors, for example, human relations, communications, research, and teaching. In a later work based on the 1950–51 Kellogg project, Finer elaborated on these elements and factors and answered the question "What is the work of the executive?" by

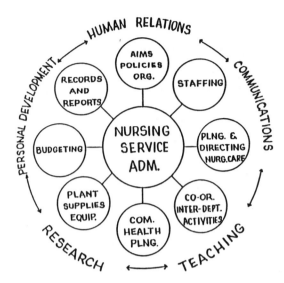

Figure 38.1   Nursing Administration as Conceptualized by the 1951 Kellogg Study. (Reprinted by permission from Finer H. Administration in nursing service. New York: The Macmillan Co., 1952.)

proposing the use of the abbreviation *A P O S D C O R B*. These letters represented Attaining (apprehension or absorption), *P*lanning, *O*rganizing, *S*taffing, *D*irecting, *C*oordinating, *R*eporting, and *B*udgeting. This is a generic definition of executive work, and Finer cautions that "it would be equal unwisdom to proceed upon the assumption that the generalizations [from other fields] can be bodily transferred without being qualified by the peculiar spirit and human elements involved in the nursing department. What is urgently needed is a marriage, on equal terms between the science of administration, as it is already known in other fields, and what is and can be known of this science from direct contemplation of nursing service."[1]

Once the work of nursing service was conceptualized, the committee on the content of nursing service administration generated seven objectives for programs in nursing service administration. These were:

1. To formulate a philosophy of nursing service consistent with a closely defined philosophy of total health services.
2. To acquire a knowledge and an understanding of health movements, including trends in nursing.
3. To develop a knowledge and an understanding of the theory of administration that will serve as a guide to administrative procedure in nursing service.
4. To develop an understanding of the need of desirable interpersonal relationships, and the techniques by which these may be achieved.
5. To recognize the importance, and learn desirable ways of utilizing and developing capacities for leadership in coworkers and members of the community.
6. To develop the ability to use research and apply findings of research in nursing practice and nursing service administration.
7. To become competent to appraise nursing care and nursing service.[15]

Nothing in the curriculum was related to clinical nursing, but throughout the project, the participants took as a given that directors of nursing would be nurses. Subsequent to this project with Kellogg support, 13 universities developed graduate programs in nursing administration. However, only objectives 3, 4, and 7 were adopted by all. Despite the lack of uniform acceptance of the objectives, some basic assumptions that seemed to be accepted by all schools were that:

1. The essential element of nursing service administration was to focus on health movements concerned with meeting the total health needs of the country.
2. Administrative style was one of skilled interpersonal relations in order to develop leadership capabilities of others.
3. Skilled administration is important.
4. Supervision and first-level management are not distinctive functions but admin-

istrative processes are inherent in every level including self-administration.
5. Sound investigative efforts are important.[16]

In terms of administration content, three themes emerge—social relations inherent in administration, the principles and practice of administration, and research and problem solving.[16] The most frequently required courses were Theory of Nursing Administration, Research Methods, Survey of Nursing, and Statistics. Courses that were less frequently required but included in some curriculums were Human Relations, Public Administration, and Principles of Hospital Administration. Little mention was made about budgeting or finance since in 1950 few hospitals operated on a predetermined budget.[15]

Following the pattern established by this Kellogg project, almost 30 years later, Stevens exhorted graduate nursing educators to "get out there" and find out what the work of nursing administration really was.[13] By observing the state of the art of nursing administration practice, nurse educators should then be able to determine what content should be included in graduate nursing administration programs.

Several nursing organizations have sought to define the work of nursing administration. Table 38.1 compares the roles and functions of the nurse administrator in an executive-level position as determined by the American Organization of Nurse Executives[17] and the Commission on Nursing Services of the American Nurses' Association (ANA).[18] The Commission on Nursing Services has identified two additional levels of nursing administration and delineated the functions of these. Table 38.2 lists the functions of middle- and first-line nursing administration positions. The ANA recognizes that "while all nurse administrators utilize common administrative processes, the emphasis and primary admin-

Table 38.1   Roles and Functions of the Nurse Executive as described by American Organization of Nurse Executives (AONE)[17] and American Nurses Association (ANA)[18]

AONE	ANA
The nurse executive is accountable for the clinical practice of nursing.	Responsibilities of the nurse executive include:
The nurse executive assesses the influence of the health-care environment on patient care and nursing practice in developing policies and programs for the nursing organization.	Participating in the administration of the total health-care agency.
	Determining clinical and administrative goals and directions of the nursing department.
The nurse executive participates in initiating and supporting organizational mechanisms and systems that ensure the provision of effective patient care.	Devising departmental functions and activities to achieve goals.
	Acquiring and allocating resources for the determined functions and activities.
The nurse executive participates in the effective management of financial, human, material, and informational resources.	Evaluating and revising the organizational goals, structures, activities, and resources of the nursing department.
The nurse executive ensures that the nursing organization has an overall plan for the development and implementation of education programs and research.	Providing leadership in problem solving.
	Providing leadership in human resources development and personnel management.
	Providing channels for consumer input into policy development.

istrative function differs among the levels."[17] In addition, the ANA has initiated a certification program to recognize proficiency in nursing service administration. One examination was developed to reflect the basic knowledge necessary to practice nursing administration at the first-line and middle levels. Another examination was developed that reflected the more advanced skill and knowledge required at the executive level. In 1982

Erickson surveyed a random sample of 300 nurses who were certified in a nursing administration (CNA) or certified in nursing administration-advanced (CNAA) to evaluate the test content in terms of their work experience.[19] An outline of the test content that was taken from Erickson's questionnaire appears in Table 38.3.

One curriculum model that reflects a concept similar to the ANA three levels of ad-

Table 38.2   Functions of Middle- and First-Line-Level Nurse Administrators as Described by Commission on Nursing Services, American Nurses Association[18]

Responsibilities of middle-administrative roles may include:	Responsibilities of first-line administrative roles typically include:
Participating in nursing policy formulation and decision making.	Providing for direct nursing care services to clients.
Problem solving and supervising the delivery of nursing care.	Evaluating nursing care given and assuring appropriate documentation, guidance, and supervision of staff members.
Evaluating care provided.	Selecting nursing personnel for hire.
Collaborating with other departments.	Evaluating staff, including disciplinary action and separation from service.
Coordinating staff activities.	Providing for teaching and staff development.
Staffing and scheduling of personnel.	Coordinating nursing care with other health services.
Arranging for equipment and supplies.	Participating in and involving staff in nursing research.
Recruiting and selecting personnel.	Providing clinical facilities and learning experiences for students.
Evaluating staff for promotions and transfers, disciplinary action, and separation of service.	
Providing orientation, training, and continuing education for staff.	
Undertaking or facilitating research activities.	
Providing and coordinating clinical learning experiences for students.	

Table 38.3 Test Content Outline From ANA Certification Examination for Nursing Administration and Nursing Administration—Advanced[19]

I. Nursing Care Delivery
   A. Philosophy of nursing care
   B. Nurse-physician relationships
   C. Relationships with other health-care professionals
   D. Quality assurance, evaluation of care delivered during audit, utilization review
   E. Changing roles in nursing
   F. Nursing care standards
   G. Creating a climate for clinical research
   H. Protection of patient's rights
   I. Patient's safety
II. Program Planning and Implementation
   A. Program planning
      1. Identification of needs
      2. Identification of program goals
      3. Determination of methods of meeting needs
      4. Determination of needed resources: human and material
      5. Relationships with relevant interacting groups, including those who will resist proposed changes
      6. Determination of criteria for evaluation
   B. Program implementation
      1. Coping with resistance to change
      2. Making and implementating a time schedule
      3. Obtaining and assigning resources: human and material
      4. Education and training of personnel
      5. Intradevelopment program evaluation and adjustment
III. Personnel Management
   A. Personnel Management
   B. Recruitment, selection, appointment, assignment, and termination
   C. Formal evaluation of personnel performance
   D. Labor relationships
   E. Orientation, staff development, training, in-service education, and continuing education
   F. Job analysis, job evaluation, and job descriptions
IV. Staffing
   A. Relationship of staffing to short- and long-term planning
   B. Staffing patterns such as team nursing and primary nursing
   C. Patient classification systems

   D. Scheduling policies and practices
   E. Utilization of staff
V. Direction and Supervision of People
   A. Motivation
   B. Establishment of an environment for favorable relations
   C. Teaching: formal and informal
   D. Conflict resolution
   E. Role modeling
   F. Integration of personal and organizational goals
   G. Counseling
   H. Recognition-rewarding
   I. Disciplining
VI. Financial Management
   A. Revenue generation
   B. Data-collection and analysis
   C. Budgeting and budget control
   D. Cost analysis
   E. Cost containment
VII. Management Styles and Techniques
   A. Leadership styles
   B. Committee use
   C. Management by objectives
   D. Communication
   E. Incident handling
   F. Operational research: systems analysis
   G. Development and implementation of policies
VIII. Community and Societal Concerns
   A. Interagency cooperative undertakings
   B. Changing patterns in delivery of health care
   C. Impact of governmental regulations
   D. Consumerism
   E. Operating constraints from court, agency, and legislative actions
   F. Impact of decisions of nursing professional organizations
IX. Executive Policies and Procedures
   A. Establishing and revising nursing department structure and functions
   B. Participating in organizational programming, goal setting, and policy development
   C. Evaluating the nursing department operation and goal attainment
   D. Long-term planning
   E. Policy development
      1. Design of policies
      2. Implementation of policies
      3. Evaluation of policies
      4. Change and revision of policies

ministrative functions has been developed at Wayne State University.[14] A conceptual model with six curricular components has been applied across four educational levels: baccalaureate, master's, continuing education certificate, and doctoral degree. The six curricular components are goals and evaluation, finance, human resources, management, nursing, and research. At the baccalaureate level students are prepared for beginning management positions. At the master's level the student is prepared for middle-management positions with a major in clinical nursing and a minor in nursing administration composed of three courses: Administrative Process in Nursing, Personnel Development, and Field Practice in Administration. Specific course content includes, organization of health services, reimbursement, group process, conflict resolution, family theories, personnel development, problems and strategies in advanced nursing, nursing practice models, and research methods.

According to the Wayne State curricular model, preparation for executive-level positions in nursing administration takes place in a postmaster's continuing education certificate program in executive administration. Content presented in the certification program includes program evaluation, financial accounting, managerial accounting; healthcare economics, labor relations, organizational change; union contract administration; executive decision-making; power, influence, and policy development; and research in the management sciences. The fourth and final level leads to the Ph.D. in nursing. Students elect a research area from any of the curriculum components of the conceptual model and develop advanced research skills using management sciences as the cognate area of study.

The need for graduate nursing administration programs to reflect the state of the art of nursing administration practice is recognized by the Council on Graduate Education for Administration in Nursing (CGEAN). However, CGEAN is less concerned about the exact structure of the curriculum than it is about the curriculum being built on a framework that includes content related to administration, clinical nursing, and research. This organization, which is composed of both nurse educators and practicing nurse administrators, recommends that the administrative component should have both a theoretical and an experiential element.[20]

In terms of the theoretical element of the administrative component CGEAN recognizes that educational programs for nursing administration have their own unique frameworks and philosophies. However, CGEAN suggests there is core content that is requisite knowledge for effective performance in nursing administration positions. These core components consist of:

1. *Organization Theory.* Nurse executives should understand how organizations are structured and behave, both formally and informally, to produce desired outcomes. Nurse executives should be able to design effective organizations and use human and material resources efficiently for the delivery of nursing care. The utilization of human resources is based on an understanding of personnel management concepts.

2. *Communication Theory.* Nurse executives should understand communication theory in order to communicate effectively with individuals and groups. They should be able to use formal and informal routes of communication in the institution and the community. Nurse executives also should be able to design and use communication systems for personnel and patient information storage and retrieval.

3. *Decision Theory.* Nurse executives should understand decision theory; they should know the mental processes in-

volved in problem solving and the techniques for improving the quality of decisions reached. They should understand principles of decision making under conditions of certainty, uncertainty, and risk. Nurse executives should be aware of the use of computer models for decision making.

4. *Nursing Theory.*   Nurse executives should have an understanding of nursing care models and theories basic to the delivery of nursing care and should be able to evaluate their appropriateness in given work situations.

5. *Health-Care Systems.*   Nurse executives should have an awareness of the nature and the impact of the health-care system on delivery of nursing care. This includes knowledge and anticipation of the effects upon the system of outside forces such as legislation, third-party payer interests, use of the medical model, health administration philosophies, consumer actions and demands, and legal requirements for health-care delivery.

6. *Management Concepts and Technologies.* In administrative practice, nurse executives should be able to utilize management techniques such as qualitative and quantitative measurement, fiscal management, information processing, and use of computers. Management concepts should be incorporated into the performance of nurse executives.

7. *Human Relations Theory.*   Nurse executives should understand and use human relations theories that explain leadership behavior, individual and group behavior, and goal achievement in organizations.

8. *Change Theory.*   Nurse executives should understand change theory and be able to use change strategies to ensure organizational development and achievement of nursing goals.[21]

A later document adopted by CGEAN suggests that this theoretical element should include specific course content such as organization theory, management science, decision making, financial management, economics, ethics, health policy, health law, strategic planning, management information systems, health-care technologies, marketing, labor relations, quality assurance, and futures.[20] Specifically, the theoretical element should prepare the student to:

1. Analyze organizational concepts and theories basic to the health-care delivery system.
2. Analyze the mission of nursing administration in the achievement of the clinical nursing goals of the system.
3. Analyze and evaluate organizational structures for the delivery of nursing care.
4. Evaluate the internal and external forces that influence the managerial processes in nursing care.
5. Assess the use of human and material resources including economic and financial aspects in the nursing care system.
6. Analyze and design information and control systems (such as staffing and patient classification) to regulate nursing care delivery.
7. Analyze the relationship of the nursing administration system to other subsystems and suprasystems of the institution, the profession, and the society.
8. Analyze the role and function of the nurse executive.

CGEAN strongly endorses an experiential element as a requisite part of the administrative component. The experiential element of the administrative component includes learning opportunities, often referred to as practicums, residencies, apprenticeships, or laboratories. The experiential element should offer the student the opportunity to:

1. Observe and analyze the performance of the nursing administrative functions by a preceptor(s)-practitioner(s).
2. Actively participate in the nursing administration of a nursing-care delivery system. An option to participate in health service administration may be offered.[20]

Further, this experience should provide the student with the opportunity to synthesize knowledge acquired in course work and to operationalize this newly acquired theory in a somewhat controlled yet realistic learning environment.

RESOURCES AVAILABLE IN THE EDUCATIONAL INSTITUTION AND THE COMMUNITY

How the administrative component with its theoretical and experiential elements is operationalized is dependent in large part on the resources available in the educational institution as well as those in the nursing and health-care community. CGEAN suggests that both core knowledge and specific content can be offered in interdisciplinary courses as well as in courses specific to nursing.

Kelley at the University of Alabama-Birmingham supports an interdisciplinary approach to graduate study in nursing administration stating that "no longer is it possible for one health discipline to practice isolated from the talents and contributions of other members of professions and related fields of study. Health schools need to foster closer relationships and facilitate an interchange of technology and human resources with other fields such as business administration so that a vast fund of relevant knowledge may be tapped and used in the delivery of quality health care."[22] Kelley goes on to describe the process of bringing faculty from the School of Nursing, School of Community and Allied Health Resources, and the School of Business together to develop a master's-level program of studies for the preparation of nurse adminstrators. A collaborative and productive working relationship had existed among faculty as a result of collaboration between nursing and business in developing courses in Human Relations and Organization Behavior that were meaningful to both businessmen and health-care professionals.[22] This spirit of acceptance and professional respect is the basis for any interdisciplinary effort, whether the effort involves one course or an entire curriculum. Kelley cautions that the interdisciplinary approach to curriculum planning and implementation is "more appropriate to the university medical center where a multiplicity of facilities, resources, and services are available rather than to nursing programs located in small colleges and universities without health centers. The initial investment of faculty effort in bringing the interdisciplinary philosophy to life is expensive in terms of the time and compromises required, but the benefits and the end product . . . are well worth the price."[22]

While leaders in nursing administration education support an interdisciplinary approach to the presentation of content in graduate nursing programs, interdisciplinary efforts need to be approached with some caution. Nursing administration melds two disciplines: nursing and management.

However, the nature of nursing and its unique setting makes it necessary to adapt, rather than to adopt, managerial science. For example, unlike most management situations, nursing management: (1) is labor-intensive rather than machine-intensive; (2) relies primarily on knowledge workers rather than semi- or unskilled workers; (3) requires continual and significant decision making at low hierarchic levels of the organization, for example, by the staff nurse at the bedside; (4) has a nonstandardized consumer (the patient) and a unique product (despite shared goals for groups of similar patients); (5) calls for frequent individual adaptations of worker behaviors, even where standard operating procedure exist; and (6) takes place in the ongoing present, for 24-hours a day, every day, where the nine-to-five workday mentality of the industrial management discipline cannot be applied. These and other differences in the practice environment make it counterproductive merely to superimpose the science of management on nursing.[6]

Therefore, courses and learning experiences that offer the student the opportunity to debate, synthesize, and apply administrative and organization theory to the practice of nursing administration are absolutely essential.

The effectiveness of these application courses is very much dependent upon the knowledge, educational background, and experience of the faculty who plan and teach these courses. There is an ongoing urgent need for doctorally prepared nurse educators who have both a knowledge base in organization and administration and experience in nursing administration. The curriculum and course offerings in a graduate program will only be as good as the effectiveness of the faculty in planning, teaching, and selecting meaningful content and learning experiences.

The availability of meaningful learning experiences in the nursing and health-care communities is another factor that affects the experiential element of the administrative component. CGEAN recommends that practicums or residencies be planned after analyzing: "(1) the student's professional goals and experiences; (2) the program's content and goals; (3) the academic preparation, administrative goals, and experiences of the potential preceptors; and (4) the commitment of the care organization to work cojointly with the students toward goal attainment."[20]

In summary, nursing administration is a mediated role that involves the use of one discipline—management—to accomplish the goals of another discipline—nursing.[6] Both

the quantity and exact nature of administration and organization content that is included in any graduate nursing program is dependent upon: (1) the faculty's philosophy regarding the importance and appropriateness of nursing administration as a valid field of study for nursing; (2) the faculty's view of nursing administration practice; and (3) the resources available in the educational institution as well as in the nursing and health-care community. The administrative component in a graduate nursing program should have both theoretical and experiential elements. Core knowledge and content in administration and organization have been identified by the Council on Graduate Education for Administration in Nursing. CGEAN further recommends that each nursing administration graduate program offer the student the opportunity to synthesize and operationalize theory through a planned field-experience such as a practicum or a residency.

REFERENCES

1. Finer H. Administration in nursing service. New York: Macmillan Co, 1952.
2. Stevens WF. Management and leadership in nursing. New York: McGraw-Hill Book Co, 1978.
3. Kast FE, Rosenzweig JE. Organization and management: a systems and contingency approach. 4th ed. New York: McGraw-Hill Book Co, 1985.
4. Charns M, Schaefer M. Health care organizations: a model for management. Englewood Cliff, NJ: Prentice-Hall Inc, 1983.
5. Arndt C, Huckabay L. Nursing administration: theory for practice with a systems approach. 2nd ed. St. Louis: CV Mosby, 1980.
6. Stevens BJ. Administration of nursing services: a platform for practice. In: Nursing administration: present and future. New York: National League for Nursing, 1978.
7. Council on Graduate Education for Administration in Nursing. Guidelines for development and evaluation of graduate programs in nursing administration, 1979.
8. Poulin M. Education for nursing administrators: an epilogue. NAQ, 1979;3:45–51.
9. Freund C. Director of nursing effectiveness DON and CEO perspectives and implications for education. JONA 1985;15(6):25–30.
10. Institute of Medicine. Nursing and nursing educa-

tion: public policies and private action. Washington, DC: National Academy Press, 1983.

11. National Commission on Nursing. Initial report and preliminary recommendations. Chicago: The Hospital Research and Education Trust, 1981.

12. American Academy of Nursing Task Force on Nursing Practice in Hospitals. Magnet hospitals: attraction and retention of professional nurses. Kansas City: American Nurses Association, 1983.

13. Stevens BJ. The clinical component: what are the issues? NAQ 1979;3:62–64.

14. Clelland V. An articulated model for preparing nursing administrators. JONA 1984;14:23–31.

15. Mullane MK. Education for nursing service administration. Battle Creek: Kellogg Foundation, 1959.

16. Erickson E. The historical evolution of nursing administration education, unpublished paper presented to the Council on Graduate Education for Administration in Nursing. Philadelphia: May 31, 1983.

17. American Organization of Nurse Executives. Guidelines: role and functions of the hospital nurse executive. Chicago: American Hospital Association, 1985.

18. Commission on Nursing Services. Roles, responsibilities and qualifications for nurse administrators. Kansas City: American Nurses Association, 1978.

19. Erickson E. Characteristics of nurses certified in nursing administration and nursing administration-advanced and their evaluation of test content and outline. Unpublished paper prepared for American Nurses Association Commissions on Nursing Services Certification Board for Nursing Administration, April 1982.

20. Council on Graduate Education for Administration in Nursing. Guidelines for educational preparation in nursing administration, 1986.

21. Council on Graduate Education for Administration in Nursing. Position statement on the administrative component of graduate education for administration in nursing, 1977.

22. Kelley J. An interdisciplinary curriculum approach to the preparation of nursing service administrators. Paper presented to the Council on Graduate Education for Administration in Nursing, 1976.

39

Organization and Administration Content in Doctoral Nursing Programs

Enrica Kinchen Singleton

PROGRAMS in nursing service administration at the doctoral level are designed to prepare nurse executives. They generally include a synthesis of theoretical knowledge from the disciplines of nursing and management.

THE ENVIRONMENT FOR PRACTICE

In designing such programs, it is important to look at the environment in which the role will be implemented. In the health-care delivery system today, a number of issues are receiving major attention. These include institutional cost containment and prospective payment; competition in overbedded communities, which is causing extensive efforts by the hospitals to attract and maintain health-care providers; marketing the equality, or supremacy of health-care technology and services in institutions; catering to informed consumers; diversifying hospital services to include home care, same-day surgery centers, ambulatory care facilities, and satellite clinics; restructuring the organization to facilitate management of increasingly complex entities; and installing computer systems to facilitate the flow of information. There is competition among the increasing numbers of private for-profit corporations and the traditional nonprofit health-care entities. All of this activity is taking place in a nation with a less than ideal employment rate, a new poor

among health-care consumers, and a market where health-care expenditures comprise 10% of the gross national product.

In this environment, there is increasing competition among health professionals for primacy in the delivery of services that many nurses consider to belong to the preeminent domain of nursing (e.g., discharge planning, patient education, rendering oral medications, supporting the dying patients and their relatives, etc.). In the same milieu, the nursing profession is taking an increasingly hard line on requiring a baccalaureate degree for entry into professional practice. Yet graduates from practical nursing, associate degree, diploma, baccalaureate, and masters' and doctoral programs often work in the same organization, and their roles and functions require periodic differentiation and refinement. Additionally, nurse shortages persist in certain geographical areas, in institutions, especially on night and evening shifts, and in intensive care and speciality units.[1] Hospitalized patients today are more acutely ill, and the geriatric population service needs are increasing.

There is an increasing need to develop interdisciplinary relationships among hospital administrators, nursing personnel, physicians, social workers, nutritionists, accountants, pharmacists, lawyers, marketers, and other professionals who are responsible for direct and indirect patient services. All these professionals will seek to protect their vested interests as they compete for control of limited resources. Consider, for example, that the nursing budget formerly constituted 60% to 80% of an institution's total budget.[2] A 1986 survey of nurse executives found that the nursing budget constituted approximately 33% of the average hospital budget.[3] Certainly, increasing emphasis on areas like legal and marketing departments and restrictive payment mechanisms has meant a redistribution of income.

Even so, the health-care business must be administered within a framework of valuing sick or well patients and clients in a variety of settings who require measures for health promotion, disease prevention, cure, or comfort while dying, and who have significant others who need attention.

Other forces that influence health services include government, as a policy maker and third party payer; private insurers, who are competing for clients, packaging health services to appeal to the market, and promoting growth of their organizations; and private industries or corporations, who are looking for ways to cut costs so their business can compete effectively in the marketplace. Indeed, the health-care industry is in a period of change and uncertainty and it is a challenge to strategic planners.

During the same period, nursing is increasing its research emphasis, its scientific knowledge base, and its interest in competing and complementary nursing theories, and all of these considerations need to be examined in a practice setting. Nurse leaders in complex organizations are called on to be responsive to changing demands in their institutions and to contribute to the leadership in a complex emerging discipline.

The ideas expressed here are only a representation of the factors that influence the discipline and, ultimately, curricula for doctoral programs in nursing service administration. According to Grace, the Nursing Division of Health Education and Welfare (HEW) proposed that all directors of nursing in health science centers and coordinators of research in these settings become doctorally prepared. Further, in speaking to the need for doctorally prepared nurses, Grace states, "administrators of nursing services in complex health science settings need a sound base in research as well as the substantive content related to their specialization."[4] A 1983 survey of nursing service representatives indicated there would be a need for 176 doctorally prepared nurse administrators in major centers by 1988.[5]

THE TYPES OF DOCTORAL PROGRAMS

Essentially, the Ph.D. is the academic degree focusing on research and knowledge development; the D.N.S., D.S.N., D.N.Sc., and the Ed.D. are the professional nursing doctorates. Though there is a theoretical distinction between the Ph.D. and the professional doctorates, Grace states that program models across the country "are remarkably the same"[6] and states, "while there are differentiations between the degree offered at varying schools throughout the country, the objects are not clearly differentiated nor the end product clearly distinguished."[7] Similar views on degrees were presented by Jamann in the proceedings of a conference on doctoral programs in nursing sponsored by the American Association of Colleges of Nursing (AACN) and the Division of Nursing, Department of Health and Human Services (DHHS). Attendees agreed:

1. Some programs have not clarified their focuses; thus, some doctor of nursing science programs seem more like doctor of philosophy programs, and vice versa.
2. The purpose of doctoral education in nursing is the development of nursing knowledge.

3. The primary emphasis of the doctor of philosophy is on research and creative scholarship.
4. The professional degree emphasizes advanced clinical experience for the integration of research and practice to improve patient care.[8]

In addition, Jamann quotes Elliot, who states that nursing is a practice field and "the goals of all doctoral programs in nursing are service education and research."[9] Snyder-Halpern found more similarities than differences in doctoral programs in nursing. In studying eight programs, four Ph.D. and four D.N.S. or D.N.Sc., she found that both types were geared toward preparation of educators and applied researchers. However, Ph.D. programs were "more oriented toward preparation of pure researchers" and D.N.S. or D.N.Sc. programs "felt that the communication of research findings relevant to nursing practice was a primary consideration." The D.N.S. or D.N.Sc. programs "considered themselves more flexible in program organizational structure and less traditional in terms of types of instructional strategies."[10]

From another perspective, the nature of the program of study and the degree offered depends on the setting. According to McPheeters:

Some nursing programs will be located in universities where the majority of other doctoral programs are basic research programs featuring the Ph.D., while others will be located in health science centers where the other schools offer professional degrees and where there are more opportunities for interprofessional collaboration. In the first case, the Ph.D. might be the more appropriate degree. . . . In the latter situation the D.N.S. might be more appropriate.[11]

Also, the type of degree a program offers might be influenced by the position of the Association of Graduate Schools in the Association of American Universities and the Council of Graduate Schools in the United States. They consider the degree of doctor of philosophy "the mark of the highest achievement in preparation for creative scholarship and research" and state that "the Doctor's degree in a professional field is the highest university award given in that field in recognition of the completion of academic *preparation for practice* and other professional activities."[12] Authorities in the discipline state, "It seems clear . . . that the Ph.D. in nursing is most highly valued, allowing its achievers to gain a wide range of employment opportunities within varied settings."[13]

In terms of providing an appropriate degree, McPheeters's needs assessment of nurses who plan to obtain their doctorates indicates that most plan a career in teaching or administration rather than research. He indicates that since they need to know enough about teaching and evaluation skills to evaluate clinical and program outcomes, the D.N.S. would seem to be the appropriate degree.[14] In support of this view Brimmer and associates, in their study of nurses holding doctoral degrees in May 1980, showed that 67% were employed in baccalaureate or higher-degree programs; 3% were in hospital inservice or administration; and only 6% to 8% reported their primary function as research, though a number of nurses who were hired primarily for another role were conducting research.[15] Though Leininger contends that both types of degrees have value, she also notes that some nursing leaders argue that the research-oriented Ph.D. is essential to support nursing and should be the primary focus, while others view the clinical-based degree as invaluable to determine the areas of nursing empirically, i.e., from experience and observation; and the identification of clinical nursing problems.[16]

According to Shores, "no research studies are available to attest to the value of either type of doctoral preparation for nurses." Her 1983 study of 25 schools with doctoral programs that offered preparation for administrators and clinical specialists showed that

57% of the respondents from professional programs indicated that "some group outside of the school of nursing determined that the school would be allowed to offer only one specific type of doctoral program." This was true of only 8% of the respondents from Ph.D. programs.[17]

SELECTED ASPECTS OF EXISTING DOCTORAL PROGRAMS

According to Brodie, the doctoral curriculum should provide a framework that examines the tasks of nursing, its intellectual suppositions, and its philosophical implications. It should also provide opportunities to explore knowledge of other disciplines so students will "encounter new paradigms and metaphors that might be brought to bear in developing new knowledge."[18]

For the purpose of this paper, the blurred distinction between doctoral programs in nursing, regardless of the degree offered; the importance of research for the development of the discipline; and the need for nursing and management content in doctoral programs in nursing service administration are acknowledged. However, there will be no attempt to distinguish the difference in administrative content based on the intent of the degree.

Bulletins were requested from all programs clearly offering nursing service administration or research in nursing service administration as a major area of study according to a 1983–1984 listing of doctoral programs in nursing.[19] Of the bulletins received, eight programs offered the Ph.D., one offered the Ph.D. and the Master of Business Administration, two offered the D.N.S., one offered the D.N.Sc., and one offered the D.S.N. The bulletins of these 13 programs were examined to determine, from a broad perspective, admission requirements, program objectives or characteristics of the graduate, course offerings, content, concepts, and theories or organizing themes in course descriptions. Bulletins from all colleges and universities do not adhere to the same format, so all areas were not covered in every bulletin. However, the assumption was that all bulletins reflected the primary information that an informed career-oriented nurse needed when a decision about selecting a doctoral program in nursing service administration was imminent.

ADMISSION REQUIREMENTS

Graduation from National League for Nursing (NLN)-accredited baccalaureate and masters' programs was a requirement for admission to most programs. In two instances, graduation from either an NLN accredited masters or baccalaureate program was acceptable. One school would accept applicants who had graduated from an NLN-accredited program or its equivalent with admission to the Ph.D. program pending demonstration of advanced knowledge and skills in a nursing speciality area. One school stated that the master's must be equivalent to the one offered at that university. In another instance, a school was acceptable if a student graduated from a nonaccredited program that later achieved accreditation under the student's curriculum.

Quantitative Requirements

Eleven programs required applicants to submit their Graduate Record Examination (GRE) scores; six programs required satisfactory scores on the verbal and quantitative components; and five programs wanted satisfactory scores on the verbal, analytical, and quantitative components. One of these programs indicated that, ordinarily, verbal and quantitative scores below 500 were not acceptable. In one instance the student could either have had 1000 on the verbal and quantitative components, or 1500 on the verbal, quantitative, and analytical components.

In one program a score of less than 350 in either area was unacceptable. Of schools listing scores, the range was 900 to 1100 on the verbal and quantitative components of the GRE. Also, one program required satisfactory scores on the GRE and Graduate Management Admissions Test (GMAT); another required satisfactory scores on either the GRE or Miller Analogy. Two programs indicated that the GRE must have been taken within the last five years. Five programs also indicated that foreign students must submit a minimum score of 550 on the Test of English as a Foreign Language (TOEFL). One school indicated that 600 was preferred.

Nine programs specified grade point averages (GPAs) in masters' programs in their criteria. On a four-point scale, eight programs required a GPA within a 3 to 3.5 range, and one program required a GPA of 4 on a 5-point scale.

Licensure

Most schools indicated that a license to practice nursing in a state in the United States was acceptable, with one program specifying a license in the state in which the school was located. Four schools addressed admission of foreign graduates; requirements included licensure in the country of origin, evidence of certification by the Commission on Graduates of Foreign Nursing Schools, and state licensure prior to the first clinical course.

Prerequisite Courses

Two programs stated that a basic statistics course was a prerequisite, though in one instance students could satisfy that deficit by taking one of the courses offered at the university. One program required an inferential statistics course with a grade of B or better, one required a graduate-level statistics course, and one program required either an introductory or a higher-level statistics course that had been taken within the last five years.

Prerequisites that were specific to the nurse executive focus included three graduate semester-hours in management theory with a grade of B or above for one program and one course in organizational studies for another.

Goals and Personal Interview

Seven programs indicated that they required written statements of students' goals or objectives for doctoral study or their career or professional goals. One program obtained this information at the time of interview. One program looked specifically at congruence of applicant goals, program goals, and the resources of the university; two programs specified that statements should contain research interests. One program also asked for a statement of the strengths the applicant would bring to the program and for views on contemporary issues.

The personal interview was addressed by twelve programs. Nine of these programs stated that a personal interview was required, two said a personal interview was highly recommended, and one program said the interview was optional.

Experience

In addressing experience, one program required three years of experience with at least one year of postbaccalaureate experience in nursing service, one required two years' experience as a registered professional nurse, one required one year of experience in an area of specialization, and another required one year of experience for citizens and two years of experience for foreign applicants. One program required an unspecified amount of work experience in nursing education or nursing services, one required appropriate practice for proposed research specialization. One program required information on professional and academic experience, and another required a curriculum vitae containing such information.

Other Requirements

Five programs listed criteria regarding professional scholarship, research, or both, asking for such things as evidence of advanced scholarship; a sample of writing and research scholarship; evidence of oral communication skills; or a master's thesis or the equivalent.

Three programs addressed the need for professional liability insurance. One program said this was necessary when the student was in clinical courses.

LENGTH OF PROGRAM OF STUDY

Time required to obtain the doctoral degree differed according to program designs. One program required three years to complete course work plus time required for the dissertation; one required two academic years, one summer, plus time required to complete the dissertation; another required three to four years; one required three years of full-time study.

In terms of maximum time allowed for completion of the degree, one program allowed a total of 10 years with a five-year maximum for completing the dissertation and the final oral examination after advancing to candidacy; one allowed seven years from the time of the first graduate course following admission; two programs allowed six years postmaster's; one allowed five years to become a candidate plus three years to complete and defend the dissertation; one allowed five consecutive calendar years after advancing to candidacy.

Residency requirements were addressed by only two programs. One program required two consecutive semesters, excluding summers, in continuous registration. The other required one academic year of full-time study or two consecutive summers with one intervening regular semester. However, several programs required continuous matriculation from the time course work was completed until graduation.

All schools would accept transfer credits; twelve semester credit-hours beyond the master's degree for acceptable graduate courses in which the student had earned a grade of B or above was the maximum number cited.

COMMITTEES AND EXAMINATIONS

As students advanced through the various programs, dissertation committees were appointed. These committees consisted of a three, four, or five persons, including the chair. Some programs limited the committee to five persons. Usually, one of these persons was a member of the graduate faculty or a doctorally prepared person from a school outside of nursing. In one instance, a person outside of the university faculty could be added.

The examination sequence varied. All programs required a final examination, either a defense of the dissertation or an examination that included the defense of the dissertation. Examples of examination sequences include a preliminary examination, a qualifying examination, and a final examination or defense of dissertation; a preliminary, comprehensive, and a defense of dissertation or final examination; a qualifying, comprehensive, and final examination; a comprehensive examination and a defense of dissertation; an oral and written candidacy examination and a defense of dissertation; and a proposal examination and a defense of dissertation. In addition to three other examinations, one program required two written tool examinations. These included written proficiency in a computer language; either proficiency in a computer language or proficiency in multivariate statistics; or reading proficiently in a modern language. Other requirements by various programs included second-year proficiency in a foreign language in one program; tool requirements of a computer analysis or computer science sequence instead of a foreign language in one program; and computer

Table 39.1 Nursing Administration Objectives Reflected in Selected Progams

Nursing Administration Objectives	Number of Programs
Graduates should be able to:	
1. Assume leadership roles	
a. in a top-level executive-administrative position in a health-care setting or a complex organization.	6
b. in the profession.	2
2. Synthesize research knowledge; design and conduct independent investigations that are (a) critical to the advancement of nursing administration or nursing science or (b) focus on the design, support, management, and evaluation of health-care delivery systems.	3
3. Formulate problems, design investigations, analyze and interpret findings, judge the merits of research for its application to and incorporation into nursing knowledge, or advance theory and research to develop the scientific base of the profession.	4
4 Exercise leadership in the formation and implementation of public policy in health care.	1
5. Analyze strategies for program planning, health-care delivery, and program evaluation.	1

science and statistics courses prior to candidacy in another program.

PROGRAM OBJECTIVES AND CHARACTERISTICS OF THE GRADUATES

In looking at the separate listings of objectives or characteristics of the graduates of doctoral programs in nursing service administration, or at administration-oriented objectives included in overall program objectives, several ideas were evident (see Table 39.1).

COURSE WORK

The number of post-master's credit hours required to complete course work ranged from 40 prescribed graduate credits plus a noncredit dissertation to 75 semester credit hours. All programs required core courses in nursing theory and research, including courses in theory development; theory testing and conceptual models, or concept analysis; and some combination of design and measurement, data analysis, principles and qualitative and quantitative methods, hypothesis testing, research projects, an advanced empirical research seminar, and research in nursing administration. Core courses in some programs included advanced statistics, organization and development of nursing knowledge, nursing science, philosophy of science, and advanced nursing trends, problems, and issues. The types of nursing administration, cognate, or supporting courses include those shown in Table 39.2. Courses were selected by the student and advisor in keeping with the student's goals, the dissertation, and the program of study.

No attempt will be made to list the wide range of electives that are available in the various programs. However, required business courses specific to the combined degree were accounting, business administration, microeconomics, macroeconomics, statistics, marketing, management, and social systems sciences.

In addition to identifying course titles, course descriptions were perused to get more detailed information about course content. Some of the titles in certain programs appeared as content in others. Content that was not clearly reflected in the titles previously listed included the role and function of a nurse executive, including control, responsibility, accountability, delegation, fiscal planning, and effectiveness evaluation. Other content reflected in course descriptions included examining (a) research-based theories underlying nursing care delivery in complex organizations, (b) intraorganizational structure and process, (c) interorganizational and environmental relationships among health-care organizations and the nursing care de-

Table 39.2 Types of Administrations, Cognate, or Support Courses Offered by Selected Programs

Type of Course	Programs Requiring
Financial management	7
Organization policy	1
Public policy and health or nursing practice or health policy	8
Health-care delivery or financing and delivery systems	2
Environmental health-care systems	1
Human resource management in nursing	5
Theories in nursing service administration or administration and organization theory	4
Legal issues relevant to nursing administration	1
Ethics	1
Nursing administration (course or seminar)	3
Contemporary nursing issues or professional nursing	4
Program or nursing planning	2
Nursing administration management systems	1
Patient care management systems	1
Computers or computer analysis or computer science statistical software packages for health-care professionals	6
Decision theory	1
Organization, administration, and governance or negotiation process or labor relations	3
Organization analysis in nursing	1
Economics in nursing administration or health economics	2
Residency or practicum or internship in nursing service administration	5
Independent study in nursing service administration	1
Nursing science integration seminar	1
Psychometrics	1
Evaluation or organizational structures and outcomes in nursing	4
Development of leadership skills or administrative processes	2
Dissertation	13
Foreign language (no credit)	1

livery system, and (d) assessment of organizational development, structures, and outcomes within theoretical frameworks. Course content also included strategies for determining goals and resources to promote delivery of progressive nursing services, education, and research.

Attention was given to developing interpersonal skills and competence, and to the relationship between the administrator's personal style and organizational role; societal and other underlying forces impinging on nursing; financing health-care; political forces affecting legislation and the legislative process; health systems planning and evaluation; credentialing of health-care personnel; and consumerism and quality assurance.

Practicums, internships, clinical laboratories, or field experiences with an administrative nurse preceptor included observing or participating in the following functions within an organization: departmental organization, budgeting, staffing, the communication process, directing personnel, evaluating observed events by an administrative model, personnel and employee relations, evaluation of personnel services, staff development, continuing education, performance appraisal, job evaluation and payment scales, staff procurement, employee organizations, employment contracts, rewards, discipline, and promotion. Students also received experience in planning, organization, managing a division of nursing service, responsibility for supervisory evaluation of outcomes, designing strategies for effecting change, utilizing management principles and process, and developing patterns of nursing care. Further, students examined the facilitative process used by managers and the use of managerial tools and techniques. Synthesis of previous learning in nursing service administration was promoted through discussing selected problems and alternative managerial approaches to their solution. Clearly this content does not specify all that is available in all programs, nor what is expected in every nursing administrative role. It does imply that mastery is expected for most of this content and reiterates the position that nursing and management are major components of the administrative role.

Curriculum Research Findings

Beare, Gray, and Ptak conducted a survey of twenty doctoral programs in universities with NLN-accredited baccalaureate and master's programs. Using responses from 12 programs, they reported on ideal and actual content of doctoral curricula that could be identified as a common core of theories, processes, and concepts in the cognitive domain that would fulfill the requirements for a doctoral degree in nursing, regardless of clinical area of concentration or functional component. In part, their findings showed that the actual and ideal content listed by all respondents included nursing theory, theory development, concept formulation, and quantitative analysis. Other content areas that 50% or more of the respondents identified as actually being taught and ideal included experimental testing, research, ethics in health, legislative issues, trends and issues, nursing ethics, publishing, political issues, and grantsmanship. Fifty percent or more of the schools believed that ideally the following content should be taught: computer instruction, health care delivery, role theory, accountability, change theory, resource planning, health, wellness, systems theory, stress theory, leadership theory, role socialization, and quality assurance. None of the respondents identified financial management, teaching learning theory, or teaching learning process as actual curriculum content. Beare and associates indicate that doctoral programs in nursing do not seem to prepare nurses for the discipline's priority needs, which include "outstanding and strong nurse leaders and administrators."[20]

Beare and associates identified the same core and many of the same areas listed in the catalogs of programs offering doctoral preparation in nursing service administration. Unlike the findings of Beare and associates regarding doctoral programs financial management was listed by all programs. Though

knowledge of the teaching learning process was not listed per se, staff development and continuing education, which require such knowledge, were listed by some programs.

Since nursing service administration is a synthesis of nursing and management, the findings of Miner are important. Miner used Lewin's statement "nothing is as practical as a good theory" as a testable hypothesis. "Practical" was understood to mean "useful in an applied setting to achieve some goal" and "good theory" referred to "theory that produces valid knowledge (understanding, prediction)." Miner looked at established theories in the management field using the nominations of 35 knowledgeable scholars in the field. At least 110 distinct theories were nominated, and 24 of these theories were selected as established because they received 10 or more nominations. These theories were:

1. Contingency theory of organization
2. Expectancy theories
3. Contingency theory of leadership
4. Decision making concepts and conducts
5. Need hierarchy theory
6. Psychological open systems theory
7. Technological determinism
8. Job characteristics theory
9. Behavior modification and operant learning
10. Path-goal theory
11. Sociological open systems theory
12. Equity theory
13. Theory of system 4 and 4T
14. Motivation-hygiene theory
15. Technology in a comparative framework
16. Goal congruence theory
17. Goal setting theory
18. Achievement motivation theory
19. Sociotechnical systems theory
20. Mechanistic and organic systems theory

21. Theory X and Theory Y
22. Decision tree theory of participative leadership
23. Theory of bureaucracy
24. Theory of bureaucratic demise

Other less frequently nominated theories included:

25. Classical management theory
26. Control theory
27. Theory of strategy and structure
28. Role-motivation theory
29. Vertical dyad linkage theory
30. Group-focused systems theory
31. Influence-power continuum theory
32. Leadership pattern choice theory

Miner categorized these theories as being "one of four types—motivation, leadership-supervision, organization development, and structuring. The first two are of micro-organizational behavior nature; the latter two of a macro nature." In looking at validity and usefulness of these theories, those rating "high on *both* validity and usefulness in application are motivation theories." Specifically, these are job characteristics theory, goal setting theory, achievement motivation theory, and role-motivation theories. Miner states that available data are insufficient to say why the theories nominated are considered important if the knowledge is not valid and useful. The possibilities presented are concerned with the congruence with pre-existing nonscientific values, amount of related publication, and the size of the interpersonal network around them. He states that the theories that are high in validity and usefulness "occupy limited, rather, circumscribed domain," within the area of motivation and are successful "within their specialized, focal areas."[21]

In view of Miner's findings, if preparation for nursing service administration is preparation for the practice role, then doctoral programs should give priority attention to the useful and valid motivation theories. This does not mean others should be excluded, but when they are used, their estimated usefulness in application should be noted. For example, Maslow's need hierarchy theory—also a motivation theory, and Tannenbaum and Schmidt's leadership pattern choice theory—a leadership and supervision theory, were both low in scientific validity and low in usefulness in application. These theories appear frequently in the nursing literature. Certainly, information about the current limitations of these theories can be very useful to students as they begin to prepare for their dissertations or to seek models for theory construction.

Concepts, Theories, and Models

Meleis, in her discussion of nursing theory and scholarliness in doctoral programs, makes certain assumptions. Two of these are, "nursing is still a developing science" and the "the discipline of nursing does not have a single tradition guiding its scientific work."[22] Likewise, the framework for preparing persons whose career goal is nursing service administration in a complex organization is also developing.

Chaska, in looking at the nursing component of nursing service administration, states "nurse administrators are the significant representatives and translators of nursing at the highest level of administration in an organization." She also says the nurse executive "must be able to assess, analyze, and evaluate the appropriateness of a partial or complete nursing theory or conceptual model for utilization by clinicians given the organizational setting, characteristics, and mode of care provided."

To be sure, the curriculum for the nurse executive should provide familiarity with several nurse theorists and their models. This could include Roy's adaptation model and its four modes—physiologic needs, self-concept, role function, and interdependence; and

Neuman's health-care systems model, which was derived from the theories of gestalt, field systems, and Selye's stress adaptation model.[24] Other nurse theorists that might be included are Orem, who discusses self-care; King, who discusses the operation of people in social systems through communication; and Johnson, who speaks of the human being as a behavioral system.[25] Attention might be given to Watson, who proposes a "philosophy and science of care," and Peplau, Travelbee, Orlando, Wiedenbach, Riehl-Sisca, Erickson, Tomlin and Swan, and Bernard, who address interpersonal relationships.[26] According to Riehl and Roy, "Nursing theoreticians have focused predominately on developmental, systems and interaction models"[27] and the curricula will probably have a similar focus. Also, King states that disengagement, consistency, systems theory, communication theory, self-actualization theory, and grief and loss theory are theories from other disciplines that are currently used in nursing research,[28] so this content should be considered. Faculty developing curricula in nursing service administration can be selective about the extensiveness of the theory component, but they need to be fully aware that staff nurses will bring a knowledge of nursing theory to the organization, and the nurse executive must be able to relate to their views.

Chaska discusses developing integrated models for nursing administration and the need to identify the "essential elements and concepts of management thought, administrative, and organization theory; nursing concepts, nursing theory; and/or nursing conceptual models, that might be critical to the management role of a nurse administrator." According to Chaska, certain behavioral processes are evident in some of the conceptual-theoretical formulations in management, sociology, and nursing. She lists many of the concepts previously mentioned and adds conflict, power, conflict interaction, and self-actualization. She also suggests examining the management processes of planning, organizing, controlling, and evaluating as concepts.[29] From another perspective, Chaska cites Hall who addresses the categorization of traditional and contemporary organizational theories that include structural, group, individual, technological, economic, and contingency theories.[30]

According to Chaska, "any one concept, [or] categories of concepts, from nursing, management, administrative, and organizational theory might be employed to construct an integrated model." However, the model must be "logically consistent in using the concepts to ensure compatibility with the organization structure and design where the model may be tested and implemented." She suggests "integrating multiple nursing concepts or partial theories for compatibility with multiple management concepts employed in complex organizations." Also, in implementing the integrated model, the critical variables are the "personality and administrative style of the nurse administrator, the setting and the environment itself, the mode of care provided, the professional level of the nursing staff, [and] the needs of the consumer client."[31]

Curricula must be designed to help students select theoretical models for use in practice. Stevens warns that structures need to be modified to reinforce (or require) use of a theoretical model. For example, she states that staffing will reflect theory if only professional staff are used in nursing positions or if a diverse staff, one that is "interchangeable" with professional nurses, is used. Further, care must be exercised to see that different elements of theory do not provide conflicting messages. For example, requiring problem-oriented charting and the use of the Kardex version of the nursing process will cause nurses "to have to think in two diverse thought patterns at the same time."[32] Nurses and administrators must be prepared to consider factors like these when they choose their philosophical stance and the concepts they value to incorporate in their professional practice or in nursing practice in the organization.

Many of the concepts presented earlier can be considered components of traditional organization theories. Ouchi discusses the contemporary Theory Z. Using his perspective, the curriculum should address (1) trust and subtlety (e.g., pinpointing personalities and putting together work teams), thus yielding greater productivity through more effective coordination, (2) intimacy (caring, unselfishness), close, personal relationships in the work organization and elsewhere, long-term employment, and concern for the self-esteem of employees, and (3) "management by walking around," conveying the necessity of hands-on, direct participation of managers (not to be equated with direct patient care). In this design, management is dedicated to "setting objectives that permit every individual to satisfy their own interest while simultaneously serving the corporate interest." Also, it is imperative that organizations "change their internal social structure in a manner which simultaneously satisfies competitive needs for a new, more fully integrated form, and the needs of individual employees."[33]

Indeed, in this highly competitive health-care environment, nurse executives must rethink their management philosophy as they become involved in the organization's quest for survival as it competes for consumers and providers of service. They need to be ready to embrace appropriate new concepts and to prepare staff to implement newer modalities.

The work of Peters and Waterman is also important. After studying several organizational forms in successful companies, they proposed a hybrid alternative to all these forms and presented a "structure of the eighties." This was based on three pillars: a stability pillar to respond to the need for efficiency, an entrepreneurial pillar to respond to the need for regular innovation, and a "habit breaking" pillar to avoid calcification. The stability pillar is tangible and honest and is based on "maintaining a simple, consistent, underlying form, and on developing and maintaining broad yet flexible enduring values." They say "the old, simple, divisionalized organizational structure is probably the best form around now and for the future." The entrepreneurial pillar views smallness as a requisite for continual adaptiveness. Organizations can stay small by removing new or expanded activities and placing them in new divisions with simpler systems. The "habit breaking" pillar encompasses a "willingness to reorganize regularly, and to reorganize on a 'temporary basis' to attack specific thrusts." Among other things this means "a willingness to take the top talent and bring it together on project teams aimed at solving a few central organizational problems or at executing a central organizational thrust." These three pillars represent a "theoretical" response to the issues that emerged in the matrix structure.[34] Certainly, understanding these pillars is important to the nurse as he or she prepares to participate on the top management team in the health-care organization. It is particularly important to master the "habit breaking" pillar because employees frequently counter ideas for change by saying, "but we have always done it this way."

The concepts set forth by Peters and Austin advance a model for excellence that includes (1) care of customers via superior service and superior quality, (2) constant innovation (in resource exploration technique and market development), (3) turned-on people—which involves listening and displaying trust and respect for the dignity and creative potential of each person in the organization, (4) leadership—"vision, cheerleading, enthusiasm, love, trust, verve, passion, obsession, consistency, the use of symbols, paying attention . . . , creating heroes, coaching, effectively wandering around. . . ." According to Peters and Austin, the prices of excellence are time, energy, attention, and focus. They say achieving excellence is not easy but acting on a passion for excellence will provide a sense of purpose, of making a difference, and a sense of self-respect. In this model, leadership must be present at all levels in the organization.[35] These concepts seem to deserve attention in doctoral curricula.

Certainly, curricula in doctoral programs cannot provide the student with all the knowledge that is available or all of the new or reorganized concepts that will facilitate the administrative function. The curriculum must offer a framework of theories and concepts that give attention to the learner's baseline knowledge, to the knowledge needed in the field, and to providing experiences that use that knowledge in a wide range of health-care management activities. Certainly, the content needs to be relevant now and later, allow one to postulate and recombine old forms, and consider new knowledge related to patients, management, and nursing.

Given these ideas, the graduate of a doctoral program in nursing service administration should be prepared for the nurse executive's role from core courses related to nursing theory and nursing research, specialization courses in administration, and electives and cognate courses. The names of courses and areas of emphasis will vary, depending on the nature of the university and the goals of the program. However, any program in nursing service administration should create an awareness of the interface of the nursing component within the larger system. This relationship is reflected in Figure 39.1.

An administrative clinical experience, practicum, internship, or residency in nursing service administration should be a curriculum requirement. Administering or problem solving from a theory base in a real-world organization is very different than reading

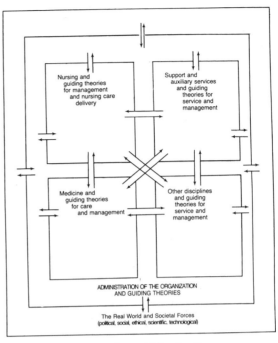

Figure 39.1. Nursing within the Systems Framework of a Health-Care Organization. The lined areas and the arrows represent areas of overlap and exchange.

about or discussing how to administer. The clinical laboratory helps the student see action-oriented administration.

THE FUTURE

Is it more important for nursing's doctorally prepared members to obtain what is generally considered the prestigious academic degree or the professional degree? Ideally, programs would offer the professional degree to emphasize preparation for administrative practice and evaluative research and to provide a clinical mentorship to facilitate the required practice and research process. Programs would offer the academic degree to emphasize a more intensive research focus and the acquisition of research skills that would address nursing administration and related clinical problems, and also organizational political problems related to nursing. Concurrent theory development would be expected of candidates for this degree.

In looking at the future of the D.N.S., D.S.N., D.N.Sc. degrees, the findings of the Mayhew and Ford must be kept in mind. They state that at Syracuse University, when recipients of the Doctor of Social Science Degree, "a well contrived program producing people generally in demand as college teachers" were offered an opportunity "to exchange their degrees for the Ph.D. . . . almost 90% jumped at the opportunity." Also, the history of the Doctor of Education degree, which "was conceived as equal in rigor but different in substance from the Ph.D. degree," shows one or two developments: "either the Doctor of Education has been consistently regarded as a second-class degree with less rigorous requirements—for example, no language requirements—or the demands have been so modifiedd that there is no perceptible difference between the Ed.D. and Ph.D. degrees." Given this situation, the question arises: "If there is no difference, why not concentrate on the more prestigious degree?[36] Perhaps in nursing, the trend toward the Ph.D. is already being established. Anderson and associates report that of doctoral programs planned in the next five years by respondents to their survey, 36 were proposing a Ph.D. program and seven were proposing the Doctor of Nursing Science program.[37] In 1984, of the 30 doctoral nursing programs in place, seven offered the D.N.S., D.N.Sc., or D.S.N., one offered the Ed.D., and 22 offered the Ph.D.[38]

Even with current and projected programs, the future demand for doctorally prepared nurses will be difficult to meet. Just how difficult is clear from the data of Anderson and associates. The 232 schools responding to the survey projected that 3,489 full-time doctorally prepared faculty would be needed by 1988. As of February 1983, 1790 nurses held the doctorate. The 116 schools respond-

ing to their survey indicated that 200 faculty members were enrolled in programs in nursing and 346 were pursuing degrees in other fields. Also, the projected need for nurses in service agencies by 1988 totaled 482.[39] Certainly, institutional constraints and resources, prestige, and appropriateness of the degree for the program of study are important factors in the types of degrees programs offer. However, many nurses will select programs because of their accessibility. Schools will compete for prospective students and will recruit from the available doctorally prepared faculty. Faculty will often seek positions based on attractiveness and availability regardless of their degree or the organization's primary focus.

Just as distinguishing preparation required for doctoral degrees is important, it is also important to concentrate on preparing a nurse executive who can administer the department; explain, interpret, and promote the nursing agenda related to patient care, nursing research, and nursing theory; and develop systems that are efficient and effective for agenda implementation. Also, the executive needs to be able to work to achieve the goals of the organization as a member of the top management team. Essential values include efficiency and innovation to reduce cost; responding to the needs of an increasingly aging population; attention to needs for speciality care, regular curative care, disease prevention, palliative treatment, and family involvement; and assisting patients toward a peaceful death. A bilingual education (nursing and management) is vital to success in the nurse executive role. Doctorally prepared nurses in the multidisciplinary health environment need to be able to control nursing service and gain greater influence in the larger organization. If the product of the doctoral program is ineffective in the complex environment, nursing administration will lose some of its position power, and by the time differences about the appropriateness of a particular degree have been settled, nursing will have to fight to recover its influence, prestige, and territory.

However, the lack of congruence within the discipline cannot be overlooked. Brodie states that "nursing administrators, many currently functioning with a bachelor's degree, favor master's degrees in either nursing administration or business administration" and "nursing educators tend to argue for a doctorally prepared director."[40] If doctoral preparation in nursing is important, then there must be dialogue between these parties in both areas to share views, discuss the difference in perception, and make reasonable adjustments to achieve an acceptable program. Perhaps there should be shared efforts to predict the nature of the complex organizations of the future and the types of nurses needed to function therein. Both groups should desire nurse executives who are abreast of management and nursing needs in an increasingly dynamic health-care delivery system. Surely, doctoral-level management content can be appropriately organized to prepare nurse executives for complex organizations.

REFERENCES

1. Institute of Medicine. Nursing and nursing education public policies, private actions, Washington, DC: The Academy Press, 1983, pp. 60, 76.
2. Stevens BJ. The nurse as executive. Wakefield MA: Nursing Resources, Inc, 1980, pp. 236.
3. Survey profiles nurse executives of the '80s. The Nurse Executive, 1987; 14–17.
4. Grace HK. Doctoral education in nursing: dilemmas and directions. In: Chaska NL, ed. The nursing profession: a time to speak. New York: McGraw-Hill Book, 1983, p. 150.
5. Anderson E, Roth C, Plamer IS. A national survey of the need for doctorally prepared nurses in academic settings and health service agencies. Journal of Professional Nursing 1985;1(1):23–33.
6. Grace HK. 1983, p. 148.
7. Grace HK. The development of doctoral education in nursing: in historical perspective. Journal of Nursing Education 1978;17(4):24.
8. Jamann JS, ed: Proceeding of doctoral programs in nursing: consensus for quality. Journal of Professional Nursing 1985;1(2):118, 119.
9. Elliot JE. In: Jamann JS, ed. Proceedings of doctoral programs in nursing, 120.
10. Snyder-Halpern R. Doctoral programs in nursing: an examination of curriculum similarities and differences. Journal of Nursing Education 1986;25(9):364.
11. McPheeters HL. Planning for doctoral education in the South (Draft report). Commission on Health and Human Services, Southern Regional Education Board, Atlanta, 1984.
12. Liston MF. Graduate education in nursing: preparation for functional roles. In: National League for Nursing, extending the boundaries of nursing education—the preparation and roles of the functional specialist. New York: National League for Nursing, 1970, No. 15-1397, p. 2.
13. Gorney-Fadiman MJ. A student's perspective on the doctoral dilemma. Nurs Outlook 1981;29(11):654.
14. McPheeters HL. 1984, p. 27.
15. Brimmer PF, Skoner MM, Pender NJ, Williams CA, Fleming JW, Werley HH. Nurses with doctoral degrees: education and employment characteristics. Research in Nursing and Health 1983;6(4):157–165.
16. Leininger M. Doctoral programs for nurses: trends, questions, and projected plans. Nursing Research 1976;25(3):201–210.
17. Shores LS. Analysis of decisions to initiate doctoral programs in nursing. Nurse Educator 1986;11(1):27.
18. Brodie B. Impact of doctoral programs on nursing education. Journal of Professional Nursing 1986;2(6):355.
19. Council of baccalaureate and higher degree programs. Doctoral programs in nursing 1984–1985. New York: National League for Nursing, 1985.
20. Beare PG, Gray CJ, Ptak HT. Doctoral curricula in nursing. Nurs Outlook 1981;29(5):315.
21. Miner JB. The validity and usefulness of theories in an emerging organizational science. Academy of Management Review 1984;9(2);296–306.
22. Meleis AI, May K. Nursing theory and scholarliness in the doctoral program. Advances in Nursing Science 1981;4(1):32.
23. Chaska NL. Theories of nursing and organizations: generating integrated models for administrative practice. In: Chaska NL, ed. The nursing profession: a time to speak. New York: McGraw-Hill Book Co, 1983, pp. 722, 723.
24. Chaska NL. 1983, p. 724.
25. King TE. Scholarly pursuit of excellence: doctoral education in nursing. Nursing Papers 1981;13(4):41–46.
26. Marriner A. Introduction to analysis of nursing theories. In: Marriner A, ed., Nursing theorists and their work. St. Louis: CV Mosby Co, 1986, p. 9.
27. Chaska NL. 1983, p. 724.
28. King TE. 1981, p. 44.
29. Chaska NL. 1983, p. 724.
30. Hall RH. Organizations: Structure and process. 1982. See note 23.
31. Chaska NL. 1983, pp. 724, 727.

32. Stevens BJ. Applying nursing theory in nursing administration. In: Chaska NL, ed. The nursing profession: a time to speak. New York: McGraw Hill Book Co, 1983, 713.

33. Ouchi WG. Theory z: how American business can meet the Japanese challenge. New York: Avon Books, 1981, p. 177.

34. Peters TJ, Waterman RH Jr. In search of excellence: lessons from America's best-run companies. New York: Harper & Row, 1982, pp. 315–317.

35. Peters T, Austin N. A passion for excellence. New York: Random House, Inc, 1985, pp. 4–6.

36. Mayhew LB, Ford PF. Reform in graduate and professional education. San Francisco: Jossey-Bass Publishers, 1974, 163.

37. Anderson E, Roth C, Plamer IS. 1985, p. 28.

38. Andreoli KG. Specialization and graduate curricula: finding the fit. Nursing and Health Care 1987;8(2): 65–69.

39. Anderson E, Roth C, Plamer IS. 1985, pp. 26, 27, 29.

40. Brodie B. 1986, p. 354.

40

Professional Issues Facing the Field of Administration of Nursing Services

Loucine M. D. Huckabay

TRENDS affecting health care and nursing are of vital importance to the welfare of society; the existence and well-being of both health care and nursing depends on a variety of interacting factors including trends in society, in human values, and in economic conditions. What role registered nurses will play in the future of health-care delivery is an issue of interest and consequence not only to nursing professionals, but to other health professionals, policy makers, the media, and the public. Preparation for that role, according to Andrioli and Musser (1985), is the main responsibility of nursing, and can only be achieved with full recognition of and planning for those factors that will change health-care delivery and modify nursing practice.[1]

The main purpose of this chapter is to present some of the major issues affecting health care and nursing, as well as implications of these issues to the nursing director's role and educational preparation, and to nursing research. The five major issues presented are nursing practice issues, cost-containment, nursing education issues, collegiality issues between nursing service and education, and ethical issues. The basis for this selection is a national-level survey study on nursing issues conducted by Urquhart, Wooding, Budinger, and Henry (1986);[2] these issues constituted 90% of the responses of the nurse executives and faculty.

MEGATRENDS IN HEALTH CARE AFFECTING NURSING

When we look at the megatrends occurring at the national level we see there are five major ones that will have the greatest impact on nursing's role in both the near and distant future. These are increased technology, oversupply of physicians, emphasis in self-care and health promotion, escalating health-care costs, and the substantial increase in the number of people over the age of 65. Nursing's growth and even the survival for some nurse specialists, according to Andrioli and Musser (1985), depend on understanding these trends, predicting their potential impact over time, and developing skills to adopt to an ever-changing marketplace.[2]

And the megatrend of growing biomedical technology has already affected health care. Computers are now being used to manage patient records, perform diagnostic tests, and regulate medications. Computers are being used to forecast staffing requirements months in advance. In some situations this is cutting down the need for nurses. Computers are being used in patient assessment at admission and analysis of tests and diagnosis. The expanded technology will require more technological skills among nurses in expanded nursing roles. We have seen the effect of this trend in the care of critical care patients and in tripling of critical care beds since 1978.[3] In order to benefit from the technological advances, nurses must learn the necessary technological skills and also provide personalized care in a depersonalized environment.

Oversupply of physicians is the second trend that will affect health care and nursing. It is estimated that by the year 2000 more than 700,000 physicians will be practicing in the United States. This is a 54% increase from 1980.[4] As the number of physicians increases in the cities, more and more physicians will be attracted to serving the underserved rural and inner-city areas. They will also provide services that are currently being done by nurses and other health professionals, such as patient teaching, inhalation therapy, counseling, and charge for them. This may cause lower demand for nurses in doctors' offices. The nurse practitioners who are now working in expanded roles will be displaced, if the health-care system can bear the increased cost. Physicians will also adversely affect legislation expanding nurses' role and oppose direct reimbursement for nurses and nurse practitioners.

The third megatrend that will affect health care and nursing as Naisbitt (1982) predicted is a shift from institutional help to self-help.[5] Health care is being reconceptualized from a sickness orientation to wellness orientation, from short term to long term. This will mean that individuals will take more responsibility for their own health habits, environment, and life-style. The emphasis will be on prevention and wellness, holistic care over the old model of illness, drugs, surgery, and treatment of symptoms. Naisbitt also points out that the shift toward self-help is a move toward greater participation in decision making at all levels of society. Nursing already embodies the essence of the self-care trend.[6] The American Nurses' Association (ANA) Social Policy Statement defines nursing as the diagnosis and treatment of human responses to actual and potential problems.[7] Even though nursing is atuned toward this trend, unfortu-

nately, insurance providers do not reimburse health promotion or education programs unless they are prescribed by a physician. Patients want these services and nurses have special opportunities to bring their skills into homes, schools, and work sites. For instance, school nurse practitioners have provided this role in school settings. Also health promotion and disease prevention have become increasingly important in work settings. With an estimated 101 million Americans on the job every day, the workplace is an ideal setting for health screening, education, promotion, and follow-up care for chronic diseases.[8] Nurses have already established control in corporate settings. There are nine times as many occupational nurses as occupational physicians; and according to a survey, 73% of corporate benefits officers and 78% of insurance executives concerned with employee productivity and absenteeism said that they would accept a health-care system that encourages the use of nurse practitioners, midwives, and physician assistants rather than physicians.[1]

Escalating medical costs is another major trend that is having a tremendous impact on health-care delivery systems and nursing. According to Naisbitt (1982),[5] Chrysler has paid 34 cents per hour for health care in 1975; today they pay $3.30 of each hourly wage. Nurses must let the society and business community know the extent of the services they can offer, that their services are less expensive compared to physicians, and that prevention is more cost-effective than intervention. Also in 1985, as the government was trying to reduce Medicare costs to reduce the federal deficit by $200 billion dollars, scrutiny of productivity and hospital operation started taking place and the prospective payment system based on diagnostic related groups (DRGs) took effect. To control hospital costs and to increase revenues, the trend to modify services will continue. Hospitals plan to add home health services, health promotion, and outpatient diagnostic services. As more highly technical services are needed in the home to assist patients with chronic diseases, the trend to noninstitutional-based nursing practice will be more prevalent. Also, legislation mandating direct insurance reimbursement for nurses will take place.[2]

The last megatrend that will affect health care and nursing is the increasing proportion of older people. It is estimated that by the year 2030 Americans over the age of 65 will make up 20% of the total U.S. population. The elderly, with high incidence of chronic illness, currently use one-half of all acute-care hospital beds. As the number of older people increases they will use not only more hospital beds but will need care in nursing homes and other long-term care facilities in the home and community agencies, such as adult day-care centers, community mental health, and day-treatment facilities.[9] The principal providers of care in these facilities will be nurses. The geriatric nurse practitioners of the future will be indispensable members of the health-care team. They will act in the role of clinicians, administrators, planners, coordinators, negotiators, and consultants to provide quality care.

It is extremely important that the resource-conscious nurse executive be very aware of the current events. He or she should be able to see the broad picture to be able to prioritize which issues to address and which direction to take. In the context of these megatrends affecting health care, the five major issues facing nursing that were identified by the selected nurse executives and faculty across the nation will be presented in the next section.

NURSING PRACTICE ISSUES

Nursing practice issues were described most frequently. Review of the literature also revealed the following to be the most notable concerns under nursing practice issues: control over practice, entry into practice, changing demographics of the patient population, emphasis on self-care and health promotion, and other forces in the practice setting leading toward collective bargaining. Each of these will be briefly described with implications to the role of the nurse executive.

In outlining characteristics of a profession, Kast and Rosenzweig (1974) state that the professional has an authority based upon superior knowledge that is recognized by his or her clientele. This authority is highly specialized and is related only to the professional's sphere of competence. They also point out that society recognizes and expects a professional to be an authority in a specialized field to serve its needs. This authority is legitimized through a superior knowledge base.[10]

Other occupations in the United States have given the prestigious title of profession only to those who have the bachelor's degree as a minimum prerequisite for practice. Professional nursing continues to rely overwhelmingly on the services of persons who have not received a college education. As Mauksch (1983) points out, only nursing allows a nurse's aide to give care to a patient, and chart this care as though it were the equivalent of the care given by a professional nurse. The professional nurse, on the other hand carries out tasks that are also performed by physicians, while only the physician receives either the financial or professional credit. Why has nursing done the reverse? asks Mauksch.[11]

When there was shortage of nurses, nurses aides performed definitive nursing care. Nurses supervised the care and those things the aides couldn't do, they did. Thus, nursing allowed the requirements of a professional presence to become expandable because there was a nursing shortage. This was compounded by the fact that hospital administrators used their prerogatives to intensify this replicability. Administrators also encouraged directors of nursing to continue this practice and staffing pattern under the guise of its economic benefits, although studies pointed out that the fewer the nonprofessional care providers, the better the nursing care and the most cost effective the overall running of the nursing departments.[11] Mauksch also states that for a long time we have operated on the misconception that supervising someone who is not professionally trained results in care equal to professional service. This type of service is technical at best, and the accountability for it, while assumed by a supervising nurse, cannot truly be assumed because actions and interventions that are already performed cannot be eliminated, nor can deficiencies be met.

Patients have been confused by the great variability of the quality and the range of services offered, having assumed that it was all nursing care. The sooner the nurses face the professional imperative that only they deliver nursing care and establish appropriate levels of quality care, the sooner the public's confusion will be eliminated, and nurses can assume control over their practice.[11] Nursing directors should support this stand and require the baccalaureate degree to be the minimum requirement for entry into practice. Some nurse executives have already taken a stand and implemented primary nursing with only professional nurses giving nursing care.

Another contributing factor that is directly related to control over one's practice is the economic status of the nurses. Because nurses traditionally have been women, and are in an occupation of employees, the improvement of their economic status has been difficult. Mauksch (1983) questions why nurse executives and those in managerial decision-making roles have been uninterested, if not actually counterproductive, in supporting the economic progress of the profession. Rather than promoting better salaries and benefits for nurses in their employ, nursing directors

seem to identify with hospital management and look at patient-care cost from their perspective. Because they have no contact with their employees, they are vulnerable as advocates for their employees. Most nursing directors also have the problem of identity, and they have not resolved their perceived dilemma of being part of management or part of a professional practice group. Mauksch[11] does not perceive this to be a dilemma. She states that "professional leadership roles can espouse a nursing identity and combine it with directing professional providers."[6]

Improving the economic status of nurses also requires a basic change in the attitudes of nurses toward economic competitiveness. It is not enough to do a job well; we need to place an economic value on it. The nurse has no visibility as a service deliverer, but is considered part of the room charge. This certainly contributed to nursing's low self-esteem, which in turn made nurses refrain from demanding better working conditions and better salaries. Mauksch recommends that the best economic hope for nursing's future lies in abandoning the status of employee. There are more nurses now who are becoming individual entrepreneurs or forming groups to provide care on a contractual basis. If this trend continues, nurses will contract their services for an equitable fee to hospitals, not as an employee of another agency, but by being their own contractors[11] (p. 7).

There is another possibility to enhance the economic plight of nursing. It is through pricing the nursing care requirements of each DRG patient. We have already developed patient classification systems based on unit values given to each nursing activity, and each unit is equivalent to three minutes of nursing care. Once the minutes of care are accumulated for the 24 hours, it can then be multiplied by the professional nurse's hourly wages. Stanford University Medical Center's Nursing Department have already started pricing about six DRGs.[12] The nurse executives have the primary responsibility for initiating and implementing such a project in their health-care institutions. Nurse researchers also need to investigate and validate the nursing care requirements of each DRG patient.

To summarize at this point, therefore, nursing executives together with their nursing staff need to understand and subsequently eliminate nursing's replicability, require the baccalaureate degree as the minimum for entry into practice, and justify and place a dollar value on nursing services. All these factors bear a direct relationship to nursing's ability to control its practice.

Two other major areas of concern affecting nursing practice are legislative and court challenges to nursing practice and challenges to the social and economic welfare of nurses.

Because of the broad spectrum of services provided by nurses, and because of the budgetary cuts, nursing is very vulnerable to attempts to limit its activities. As Curtin[13] (1983) points out, court challenges to the scope of practice initiated by physicians and various technicians to pass legislation to restrict certain practices to their domain are increasing. It is important that nurses collectively take action against such moves. In order to do that effectively, nurses need to strengthen their public image, especially among elected officials who have antiquated concepts about nursing but are in positions to make important decisions about nursing practice. Curtin also stresses the urgency of establishing a national legal fund to finance the defense of nursing practice and to protect one another. This type of legal fund needs to be sponsored by all of our major nursing organizations. Nursing directors need to take an active role in getting their nurses to see the importance of defending our practice and participate in improving the public image of nursing. As Dugan[14] (1985) quotes, "Public policy follows public opinion. We have to stop talking to ourselves and get out front and talk to the American public" (p. 30).

Challenges to the social and economic welfare of nurses will also have tremendous impact on nursing practice. Current trends indicate that nurses' job security cannot be taken for granted. For the generalist nurse, the shortage of the mid-1970s has been replaced by the supply and demand equilibrium.[15] According to the survey conducted by Muller, Byre, and Whitehead (1983),[16] more than 40% of U.S. hospitals reported no vacancies in 1983. This balance is expected to continue throughout the decade according to Institute of Medicine (1983). Curtin[13] also points out that nurses' jobs have already been threatened, and some nurses have been laid off because of organizational changes, budget cutbacks, and ambiguity about nursing's area of expertise. Already some institutions have replaced nurses with technicians in certain areas of the hospital. There will be more pressure in the near future to reduce nurses' salaries and fringe benefits.

Nurses need to take collective action to protect themselves and their practice. When in an institution there is a strong nursing administration who directs the nursing department, nurses need to support and rally behind the administrator as he or she protects and adjusts the practice of nursing to meet the changing needs. If an institution has a poor nursing administration, nurses will surely form collective bargaining units to achieve their goals. According to Spitzer,[17] vice-president of Nursing Services at Cedars-Sinai Medical Center in Los Angeles, union activity grows in an atmosphere where fiscal restraints prevail and when there is weak administration. Speaking at an Annual meeting of the American Society for Nursing Service Administrators of the American Hospital Association in Chicago, she said that unions are avoidable if nurse executives are responsive to concerns raised by their nursing staffs. Survey conducted at Cedars-Sinai

Medical Center has revealed that factors causing dissatisfaction among nurses were lack of meaningful participation in policy-making communication and feeling of distrust of management among employees. Spitzer recommends that nurse executives have open and prompt communication established between themselves and their staff. Hospitals need to have good management systems and procedures to ensure that employees have an opportunity to grow and advance in their jobs. In the area of benefits and incentives, nurse executives should take steps to ensure that they are competitive with other neighboring facilities and they should ensure that employees have equal employment and advancement opportunities. Responsiveness to the nurses' work environment is also key. Spitzer[17] states, "unions are only necessary if a company makes them necessary" (p. 60). She also recommends that nurse executives be very knowledgeable about labor laws and keep abreast of union issues related to nursing.

The concluding comments of Curtin[13] regarding the challenges to the social and economic welfare of nurses are that "the profession's future depends [on] how clearly nursing leaders see the problems, how effectively they articulate nursing's positions, how efficiently they build coalitions inside and outside the profession, how rapidly they implement nursing's responses to the problems, and to what degree nurses as a group are prepared to grasp opportunities" (p. 9–10).

Curtin feels that decisions made by 1993 will determine the course of events for nursing in the coming decade. She states what the nursing profession needs in the nineties is a decade of unity under pressure—unity of purpose, direction, and action.

COST-CONTAINMENT ISSUES

Cost containment of the health-care industry and costs of the nursing services were the second most frequently mentioned issue facing nursing by the Urquhart and associates (1986) study.[2]

In 1981, Americans spent $287 billion on health care, which is equal to 10% of our country's gross national product (GNP). In 1985, health expenditures reached $438 billion or 10.5% of the GNP.[6] Hospital care accounts for 41% of our nation's health-care expenses. No wonder hospitals have been the largest of recent cost-containment measures. Because of the high cost of health care, approximately 33 million Americans have no medical insurance coverage, and 15 million have inadequate coverage.[18]

Accelerating costs have also affected providers, insurance carriers, and the federal government. Health care is now the fourth largest item in the federal budget. Medicare costs have doubled every four years, and it is predicted that by 1990 the Medicare system will collapse.[19] As of 1985 Medicare costs are rising 60% higher than payroll taxes.[1,20] The federal government is retreating from guaranteeing health care and is restricting its financial outlays. The federal retrenchment in health care represents a shift away from the concept that government should ensure equal access to health care for all. This change was marked most prominently by the shift of Medicare hospital reimbursement from a per-diem cost basis to the DRG-based prospective payment system. Hospitals are paid a set amount of money according to the patient's DRG category at discharge, irrespective of the costs incurred. If treatment costs fall below the reimbursement rate, the hospital will profit. If treatment costs exceed payment rates, the hospital will lose money. No longer will it be cost effective to keep patients hospitalized providing care on a fee for service basis. Instead, shorter patient stays will be favored to cut total costs per patient. More recently, the program has authorized "HMO vouchers" whereby Medicare will pay for all or a share of the premium for enrollees to join prepaid plans. The usual fees used in setting physician reimbursement rates have been frozen.[21] These changing health imperatives will cause a shift from the use of hospitals for a broad range of services to the development of a variety of community facilities. This emphasis on cost containment and Medicare's DRG prospective payment system will influence both health-care delivery and the types of professionals who will dominate the marketplace. Also as the population ages, insurers will be hard-pressed to meet spiraling costs. Medicare will have to expand to meet the needs of a growing elderly population as the size of the population contributing to the system will be shrinking. U.S. Census Bureaus predict that more than one-fourth of our nation's population will be over the age of 65 by 1990.[22]

Changes in the focus of the nursing practice will take the form of a shift from inpatient to outpatient services, with the accompanying trend leaning toward more acutely ill patients in hospitals, and the need for coordinated community and home services.[2] By the year 2000, there will be a need for a 66% increase in the number of registered nurses. The greatest needs will not be in hospital nursing, but where the largest increase will be—in nursing homes. It is predicted that nursing homes will experience a 223% increase in patient load, and community health nursing will increase by 90%.[23] This change of focus from acute care to preventive and chronic care follows the movement of patients from hospital settings to outpatient clinics, continuing care facilities, and home care. Acuity levels in hospital have increased as admissions are limited and patients are discharged earlier.[24]

With respect to the influence of these changes in the type of professionals who will dominate the marketplace, there will be competition among providers and new roles for nurses will emerge. Studies show that in many situations nurses can provide care comparable to physician care at lower total cost.[25] According to Andrioli and Musser[1] if nurse's care can be substituted for physician's care without risk to the patient, hospital and health agency administrators may choose nurses to assume some of the clinical responsibilities of physicians, causing an increased demand for nurse anesthetists, certified nurse-midwives, clinical nurse specialists in hospitals, and nurse practitioners in public health clinics and other agency-administered ambulatory health-care centers. Also as sicker patients get discharged earlier from the hospitals, they will need nurses for high-technology home care services such as intravenous therapy, chemotherapy, and hyperalimentation.[26]

The Role of Nursing in Cost Containment

The nursing literature in administration has ample citations about means of controlling health-care costs, but very few of the suggestions are backed with supporting evidence. In this next section each of these suggestions will be reviewed, the role of the nursing director will be identified, and implications for further research and education of nursing director and managers will be made.

In reference to cost containment by the nursing department, Stevens (1985)[27] proposed that belief in comprehensive care may be a real threat to the survival of nursing in its present form. She states that nursing has only one alternative: the abolishment of a goal-driven model for care. This model is similar to management by objectives approach whereby one sets goals, finds the necessary resources, implements the intervention, and evaluates the outcome. In this model, the sequence of events is from goal to resources to product. On the other hand, the new model's sequence of events is from resource to goal to product. It asks what nursing measures are possible with available resources. The new model conflicts with the patient's health bill of rights, which states that health care is the right of a patient not a privilege. Under the new model, if the patient cannot afford the necessary but expensive care or testing, the patient will either have to do without it entirely or settle for something less than what is needed. The challenge to nursing through research is to find economic ways of giving the best care, which the patient deserves. We also submit to testing and research the validity and the practicality of the new model proposed by Stevens. In reference to the new model, Lancaster[9] (1986) raises another big question—will hospitals recognize that patients will have fewer complications if they employ a sufficient number of well-prepared nurses, or will they seek the least expensive providers? This last question raises two researchable questions that have not been answered convincingly. One is, will patients recover faster, have fewer complications, and spend fewer days in hospital when care is given by a professional registered nurse than if care is given by technical registered nurses and other less-qualified nursing personnel? The second researchable question is, when patients are given a choice between care given by professional registered nurses and technical registered nurses or other less-qualified personnel, and the price associated with each option, which alternative will the patient select? Answers to these two questions will provide the necessary data to determine if Steven's new model of "resource of goal to product" will be acceptable to patients. Nurse executives need to engage in research providing answers to these and similar questions before substituting unqualified, cheaper care providers for qualified professional nursing personnel.

The second major role of nursing and probably the most important one at this time is for nursing to accurately determine its worth. Curtin[28] (1986) and Kuhn[22] (1985) state that total nursing costs average less than 30% of a hospital's operating budget, although 90% of patient care is delivered by nurses. Curtin[28] writes, "any department which produces 90% of the product while consuming less than 30% of the budget is a profit center—a revenue producer, an asset par excellence" (p. 7). Both of these authors, however, do not cite data to back their statements.

It is very important that nurses develop methods to determine exactly how much their services cost for each category of patient under each DRG, and to determine precisely what they do and what outcome they seek to produce. For instance, when nurses say they teach the patient or provide psychological or emotional support to the patient, what exactly do they do? What outcomes can be expected? How should these outcomes be measured, and how much should it cost? According to American Nurses' Association[7] (1980), patients have a limited understanding of nurses' educational preparation, the scope and range of their services, or their ability to make effective decisions.

Research in pricing of nursing services has already started in several health centers. In an interview, Walker, former nurse executive at Stanford Medical Center in California[12] says that at Stanford they have determined the cost of the care for six DRGs. They have kept track of the hours of care for every shift and totaled them for the hospitalization. What they have found was that 10% of the patients' hospital bill was attributable to direct nursing care costs. They are in the process of revalidating their evaluations. They are using their patient classification system in predicting the nursing care requirements. They will put their direct nursing care costs on patient's bills in all areas. According to Walker, the preparation of the nurse is very important to cost containment, and he sees the need for more geriatric nurse practitioners in the long-term care facility. He also states that when hospital administration talks about cost containment, the first place they look is at nursing. He states that cost containment is never going to be effective until we have a way to put a lid on the doctor's reimbursement. There are no disincentives to the escalation of costs in physician services or other services that are controlled by physicians. Also, in teaching hospitals there are no incentives for doctors to limit the duplication of tests, which is part of their teaching philosophy.

Madsen and Harper[29] (1985) are also determining the cost of nursing by using the acuity coordinator. With a patient classification system matching staffing, budget requirements and patient acuity in place, they are using the acuity coordinator to match the patient case-mix on a given unit with different levels of nursing personnel. This is accomplished by analyzing the specific types of nursing tasks required at various acuity levels for specific diagnostic categories of patients, which will enable one to track the impact of nursing costs per DRG. They will then use this information to justify an all-R.N. staff in specialty units such as neonatal intensive care unit.

DRGs are also having tremendous impact on community health nursing. They need to develop partnership approaches with both acute and long-term facilites. More and more patients are having their preadmission work-ups done at home, and assessment for discharge planning are also being done by the public health nurses. Research is urgently needed in the areas of how to reduce hospital stays, assure quality, and prevent readmission. The nurse executives of both the acute care settings and the public health—home health care—agencies need to take an active role in these investigations. Two other very important areas for research are (1) determining the cost of home health-care for each specific DRG in the home health-care situations and (2) developing a methodology to separate the actual cost of nursing services in

the long-term care facilities from the extraneous costs that are usually included in the nursing budget.

Several other suggestions are cited in the literature to curtail cost of nursing services both in acute care settings and in occupational health. All these suggestions also await further testing.

The first suggestion is negotiating non-nursing task redistribution to other departments. According to Haw, Claus, Lafferty, and Iverson,[30] the key in-house groups to target for task reduction and redistribution are the medical staff, radiology, laboratory, pharmacy, and nonprofessional support service departments of housekeeping, clerical, dietary, and so forth. In meeting with these groups, nursing must be prepared with data in hand, to identify all the non-nursing and low priority tasks that are currently being performed by the nursing staff and the cost to the organization in terms of actual dollars, as well as the effect on quality of nursing care if nurses are to continue to do so. The authors suggest that an assertive stance on the part of nursing will be needed to preclude the delegation of additional tasks as departments and support services are further reduced at a time when patient acuity is expected to increase. Among the identified tasks that nurses do for other professional service departments are taking messages for the doctors, preparing unit doses, and filling requisition slips for laboratory and radiology. For the nonprofessional service departments nursing staff perform such functions as meal service tasks, such as distributing and removing meal trays; transport service tasks, such as taking patients from one unit to another, clerical tasks, such as answering the phone, relaying messages, and making up patient charts; housekeeping tasks, such as cleaning up the utility room, removing trash, restocking shelves with cleaning supplies, and so on.[30–32] In negotiating task delegation with the other service departments, especially the nonprofessional service departments, an aim should be to reduce the nurses' non-nursing tasks away from the patient's bedside that are time-consuming and could be performed by less-costly personnel.

The second suggestion for cost containment in the hospital setting was to have an admitting professional registered nurse. Hartman[33] recommends that having a professional nurse in the admitting department makes it easier to screen the diagnosis of the patient for appropriateness prior to admitting them to the nursing units. The nurse can recommend to the physician preadmission testing, which will cut down on the length of stay in the hospital or rule out a diagnosis for which the hospital may not be reimbursed, or screens out those patients who, due to abnormal test results, are not able to have surgery at the chosen time. She states that once the patient is in the hospital unit and has on the hospital attire these alternatives to care cannot be discussed without either the hospital or the doctor losing face. Hartman also suggests that having a nurse in the admitting department, enables discharge planning to be initiated even before the patient arrives on the nursing unit. The earlier the social services or home health-care agencies are notified of potential problems, the better chance there is of containing cost by cutting down the length of stay. Hartman has also found out that having an admitting nurse in the hospital has reduced significantly the transfer of patients between units or between beds on the same unit. She states, "what a rude awakening it was to find that each time a patient is transferred, it costs the hospital (not the patient) anywhere from $120 to $200."[33] (p. 33). This concept of having an admitting nurse is very appealing, but again, it awaits further testing and verification.

Reduction of nurse absenteeism and turnover is another worthwhile cost-containment suggestion proposed by Aiken.[34] The Institute of Medicine and the National Commission on Nursing have agreed that the major responsibility for improving the retention and satisfaction of nurses lies with the employers. Both these groups have proposed the following recommendations for employers to initiate in their institutions:

1. Provide opportunities for career advancement in clinical nursing and administration.
2. Give salary differentials for nurses with advanced educational preparation, experience, and merit.
3. Raise nurse salaries for times when it is difficult to recruit, such as evenings, nights, or weekends.
4. Have the nurse be a part of decision making in areas dealing with patient care, unit management, and hospital governance.
5. Have the fringe-benefit packages adapt to the special needs of the nurses, such as having child-care arrangements or educational programs in lieu of traditional benefits that may duplicate already existing coverage or be inappropriate.[34]

Research is definitely needed to test the effectiveness of each of these suggestions in reducing absenteeism and turnover.

Establishing an organizational climate conducive to cost containment is another suggestion proposed by Madsen and Harper.[29] The authors have implemented a specific strategy starting at the head-nurse level to create the climate receptive to cost-containment changes. They believe it is important that such an effort be directed at supporting the head nurses who are the first-line managers and critical to the success of any planned changed. In examining the roles, organizational problem-solving opportunities, and communication lines of first-line managers in their institution they have found that many of the units were decentralized and functioning autonomously. The nurse managers had a fairly narrow organizational perspective, and certain available resources were underutilized. On the basis of this data they have initiated a series of strategic retreats and management programs designed to broaden the role of the nurse manager, strengthen unit-level problem solving, encourage creative use of existing resources, and develop administration and supervisory skills. These retreats are conducted by the nursing director once every 6 weeks for the 11 associate and assistant nursing directors and twice a year for the head nurse and nurse executives combined. During these sessions, they are asked to formulate yearly and five-year goals, draft position papers, plan the implementation of divisionwide programs, and brainstorm special projects that require uninterrupted blocks of time. At these sessions future directions and trends are presented, yearly goals developed by the executive group are reviewed, and the head nurses are invited to give their feedback, suggest changes, or make additions. As part of their management development, Madsen and Harper (1985) also point out that the head nurses are introduced to the quantitative methodologies to better equip them to deal with the business aspect of the hospital. They learn not only Maslow's and McGregor's theories, but also to deal with critical path methods, Gaant charts, and cost account. One of the side benefits observed of having the director of nursing conduct or facilitate these sessions was that the nurse managers have an opportunity to learn the director's philosophy and have a forum to share their concerns. This strategy also has initiated a better team spirit and fostered a commitment to organizational goals. And access to the director has created an awareness of the complexities of his or her role in the hospital administration hierarchy. Consequently, nurse managers have become more knowledgeable about what kind of information the director requires to fulfill his or her nursing advocacy

role. Similarly, the director has developed awareness of the day-to-day issues at the grass-roots level. As a result of these management-development series, the authors point out that middle managers are engaged in more creative problem solving. It has created a supportive environment for risk taking and has enabled nurse managers to be more persuasive in dealing with other health-care professionals such as hospital administrators, facilities planner, and computer analysts.[29]

The development of creating a climate conducive for cost containment and at the same time making this opportunity a learning experience for all involved is a worthy challenge for all directors of nursing. More of these types of undertaking need to be done, and consequences in terms of money saved and job satisfaction of nurse-managers and staff need to be tested and validated.

U.S. corporations are another influencing source in containing health-care costs. As providers of health-care benefits for many Americans, corporations have identified strategies to reduce health-care related expenditures. Employees are paying a greater percentage of the health-care costs from their own pockets. To reduce hospitalization costs, they are encouraging their employees to seek outpatient treatment, second opinions, and preadmission certification. If hospitalization is required, reimbursement is designed to reduce length of stay. Employees are encouraged to check their hospital bills for overcharges. Some states require hospitals to provide patients with hospital bills. Maine is the first state to require that the hospital bill specify the cost of nursing services.[24,25]

Corporations are also opting for health maintenance organizations (HMOs) and preferred provider organizations (PPOs) to provide health-care coverage for their employees. This is an area where nurse practitioners have found that their skills are needed. They can provide the same quality care as those provided by physicians at much reduced cost.

Nurse practitioners are also making inroads in the occupational and industrial settings. They are doing physical examinations for initial employments, patient teaching for employees with chronic illnesses, and so forth. This trend will increase as long as health-care costs are increasing and nurse practitioners are doing a good job of providing satisfactory care to the employees of corporations.

Research is also needed here to determine: (1) the savings in dollars and cents when care is given by a nurse practitioner versus a physician in occupational health-care settings; (2) amount of patient teaching done to employees, (3) reduction in absenteeism due to illness; (4) the effect of nurse practitioners performing preventive care and teaching health promotion on reduction in illnesses and accident prevention in the work setting.

The curricular implications of cost-containment issues on the educational preparation of the nurse executive is of great importance. Urquhart and associates[2] point out that the intense, price sensitive, comprehensive environment of 1986 and the foreseeable future have changed activities of nurse administrators and have quieted the disagreements among nursing faculty about the place of health economics and finance in nursing curricula. Justifying nurse costs relative to patients' severity of illness and classification is now an essential and critical activity.[36]

Price-driven decisions that compete with professional values, and competition for traditional markets, generate unavoidable issues for professional nurses, nurse executives, and education working with both. As questions are raised about capital shortages and profit declines as well as nurse productivity and cost effectiveness, there is demand for nurse executives to find creative methods to solve complex problems.[37]

In order to meet the economic challenges of today and tomorrow the nurse executive needs to have formal educational preparation in such subject areas as accounting, health economics, marketing, budgeting issues effecting labor relations, personnel psychology, fiscal responsibility, and policy making. The role of federal, state, and local governments in health economics, creative problem solving, computers, and advanced research methodology need to be included in the educational preparation of the nurse executive. The trends affecting health care will have a profound effect on the practice of nursing. If we are to foster a successful transition for nursing from the challenges of today to the promise of tomorrow, the nurse executive needs to have appropriate educational preparation to meet these challenges in a creative and resourceful manner.

NURSING EDUCATION ISSUES

Nursing education issues range from the need for a consistent core curricula, to decline in student enrollments in nursing schools, to the appropriate educational preparation of the director of nursing. All these issues affect the practice of nursing.

McFarlane[38] in *The Proper Study of a Nurse* states that the unique function of the nurse is to give nursing care. To this function both nursing management and nursing education are in a service relationship. Their excellence can only be judged by the excellence of the nursing care they enable. According to Jarvis,[39] the profession is not the end product of professional education, the recruitment to the profession and the practice that they undertake as a result of their education are its end products. Glick[40] further points out that the purpose and meaning of nursing as a profession have been defined by society. Society both recognizes and expects a professional to be an authority in a specialized field and this authority is legitimized through a superior knowledge base. This concept of superior knowledge has been historically determined to be the bachelor's degree as the minimum prerequisite for professional practice.

Agreement on a coherent educational base for nursing practice is essential if we are to defend nursing practice before a legislature or a court of law. As Bartkowsky and associates[6] point out generic programs must offer a consistent core curriculum, with emphasis on preparing a generalist rather than a specialist. In a world of unprecedented diversity, those with a generalist education will have the advantage. They agree with Naisbitt's[5] warning that individuals who overspecialize do so at the risk of their specialty becoming obsolete in the long run. Americans will also witness greater ethnic diversity, and will have to be fluent in at least one second language—not to mention the computer's language. In reference to the future of nursing, Lancaster[9] comments that to gain entry into the profession of nursing, practitioners must possess specialized knowledge and skills based on a formal program of education that reflects considerable difficulty and is consistent with the health-care trends. For example, with the "graying of America" both baccalaureate and master's degree programs must address the needs of the elderly. In light of a knowledge and technologic explosion, students will need to be computer literate. In an era of cost containment and competition among providers, students should be exposed to content on health economics and the marketing of services.

Agreement on a coherent educational base for nursing practice is essential Curtin[13] states. It is important that generic programs provide a consistent core curriculum, that graduate programs identify the knowledge necessary for advanced practice, and that credentialing agencies develop consistent standards for certifying excellence in practice. She also states the necessity for what nurses do and can do being based on an identifiable core of knowledge; we cannot develop methods for determining the cost of our services until we can define those services and base our claims to expertise on a coherent educational foundation.

Another important educational issue that awaits further testing and investigating is the importance of adding to nursing's scientific knowledge base, and continuing to communicate unique health-care contributions of nursing to fellow health professionals, policy makers, the public, and the media.[1]

Declining enrollment of generic students in our nursing programs is another challenge facing nursing educators. Already the shortage of nurses in the practice setting is being felt. Unless urgent measures are taken to correct this recruitment problem, the shortage is going to be even more severe in the next five years. Admissions to nursing schools have declined by as much as 45%, and the number of college-age persons will drop from 8.5 million in 1975 to 6.5 million in 1995.[41] Lay offs and strikes may be disillusioning young people about the field. Nurses have done an effective job telling the media and the public that nurses work hard, go through years of education, are underpaid, and poorly appreciated. This image dissuades some of our potential applicants, especially the more mature, leadership-oriented persons who also would like to be financially successful. Even college freshmen are aware of these factors. The more altruistic applicant who wants to enter nursing is likely to seek the shortest, least expensive educational program when faced with rising tuition costs. Another factor that has contributed to this shortage is the women's movement, which has provided the freedom for young women to enter other disciplines. The bright and capable women are entering high-ranking professions formerly occupied almost exclusively by men. Figures also show that only 2% of registered nurses are men.[42] A major recruitment strategy would be for our profession to change nursing's image from feminine, passive, and helpless to more analytical, compassionate, sensitive, assertive, autonomous, and leadership-oriented. Then we might see changes in recruitment statistics. More men and more leadership-oriented female nurses would enroll in our nursing programs. Holtzclaw[42] (1983) recommends other recruitment suggestions. For example, when portraying the profession to college-bound freshmen, it may be helpful to give them the average salary figure that they would expect to earn upon graduation and licensure and compare it to the salary and job availability of those graduating in other majors such as English, psychology, history, social sciences, and so on; nursing will look very attractive to them. Also, instead of leaving our image-building to chance, she states that we should actively seek a variety of forums in which to publicize the accomplishments of our leaders in nursing education, research, practice, and administration of schools of nursing and hospitals.

Educational Preparation of Nurse Managers and Directors

With respect to the educational preparation of the nurse executives, supervisors, and middle managers, they all need different levels of formal educational preparation to implement management principles. Management in itself is a job requiring knowledge of management science. The nurse managers and superiors need to synthesize two types of sciences—nursing and management.[43] As recognized by business, management is critical to achievement of objectives, and it is making serious attempts to strengthen management skills at all levels. An article in the *Wall Street Journal*[44] demonstrates the commitment of business industry to management development. Some of the facts presented were: (1) approximately 500,000 managers take some form of management education at least once a year; (2) there has been a six-fold jump since 1974 in the number of applicants

to University of Pennsylvania Wharton School minicourses for executives—the number has soared to 7800 applicants per year; and (3) American Telephone and Telegraph company enrolls 14,000 of its managers in in-house management seminars per year.

It is, therefore, extremely important that nurse executives and nurse managers at different levels not only have management science in their formal educational preparation but keep up their knowledge of management principles on a continuing basis, to keep abreast of issues in this area. The question is raised as to where these leadership-oriented nurses should get this information. Should they get the management principles from a nursing school, or should they enroll in schools of management or administration? Urquhart and associates[2] point out that if entrepreneurship and participation in policy making are trends, then they predict an increasing number of leadership-oriented nurses will seek graduate degrees outside of nursing, unless educational programs in nursing administration are available and provide pertinent courses on marketing, finance, policy, and other related subject areas. The authors recommend that the curriculum task for nurse educators and researchers be the identification of how nursing, marketing, finance, and policy can best be integrated, investigated, and contribute to nursing theory.

COLLEAGIALITY ISSUES IN NURSING

Issues related to colleagueship were described fourth most frequently by nursing leaders in the national-level survey study conducted by Urquhart and associates.[2] The two major areas that need special attention are: (1) the development of better relationships between nurses and physicians and health care professionals in other disciplines, where they can work together cooperatively, collectively, and collaboratively; and (2) the establishment of a closer relationship between nursing service and nursing education.

Few members of the health-care team have become noteworthy due to their efforts at cooperation, collaboration, and collegiality according to Lancaster.[9] She raises a very pertinent question and makes several recommendations for establishing collegiality between nursing, medicine, and other health-care professionals. She asks, "When will we stop defining ourselves in terms of who we are against?" (p. 37). To be for nursing, she states, does not mean that we have to be against our colleagues in medicine, hospital administration, or other sciences. She recommends that nursing cultivate and nurture collegial relationships with people or groups of people who are willing and able to exert their influence to improve our image. There are many doctors, hospital administrators, and educators who are not threatened if nurses gain respect or stature. She states that we should avoid stereotyping them as "bad guys" and seek their help in making policy decisions that will affect the nursing profession.

Mauksch[11] has already observed a trend toward an improved relationship between nursing and medicine. She states that more recently nurses are taking more responsibility in making their own decisions. The impetus to change in the nurse-doctor relationship occurred concurrently with two other significant events. In the society at large, the women's liberation movement became real. Within nursing, the nurse-practitioner role emerged. This new role of the nurse mirrored the characteristics of liberated women, which are: accountability, assertiveness, autonomy, and self-direction. As doctors recognized the nurse practitioner's competence as competitive, and as they encountered heretofore unexpressed demands for colleagiality, the rearrangement of their relationship called for mutual respect and greater knowledge of each other's competencies.

Mauksch has also observed the emerging of a different division of labor both in the ambulatory care settings and in the hospital. Increasingly, nurses and physicians are assessing the patient-care needs together and then deciding on the what needs to be done and by whom. Doctors and nurses are doing much more sharing in the areas of patient information, teaching, and communication. These changes are resulting in the delivery of better quality patient care. This new relationship will enhance the self-worth of the nurse and decrease the stress and accountability requirements of the doctor; but the greatest beneficiary is the patient who is being cared for by the nurse-doctor team working together toward the same goal and respecting each other's competence.[11]

With respect to the collaboration issues between nursing service and nursing education, major efforts to unite the two branches of the nursing profession are contributing to the evolution of nursing as a profession and the actualization of the full professional role. According to Baker,[45] the declining quality of nursing care and the lack of role models for students provide impetus to the reconciliation effort. She also points out that nursing is compromised because of the lack of consensus between education and practice on the goals for the profession, on the direction of nursing practice and education, and on the scope of research necessary for practice and education.

In her recommendations for an improved relationship and better collaboration between nursing service and nursing education Baker[45] states that recognition of the interdependency of nursing education, practice, and research is the first step toward creating models to facilitate collaboration. Increasingly, nursing leaders are realizing that relevant practice requires relevant education, and both must be grounded in research. As each branch of nursing continues to mature, the interdependence of these components become even more apparent. In citing the advantages of a better relationship between nursing practice and education, Baker points out that collaboration enables both practice and education to benefit qualitatively by associating with each other and economically by allocating scarce resources to nursing's needs. This process may be threatening to some institutional administrators if they perceive it as threatening their power and destroying their autonomy. Baker recommends that these administrators take a broader view and reformulate their goals to be consistent with the profession's needs.

Baker recommends three strategies to improve the state of collaboration between nursing service and nursing education. The first strategy is to have joint appointments. The success of a collaborative movement is dependent on the capabilities of faculty and the effective use of nurse leaders and consultants. She states that nursing faculty have the knowledge base and the educational perspective and that the nursing service directors need to recognize if useful changes are to occur. When nursing education, practice, and research overlap it creates a professional academic position and policies need to be revised and negotiated to make legitimate time for practice, to ensure proper reimbursement for professional services, and to engage in academic and professional activities to meet promotion and tenure requirements. In this regard she also recommends for those faculty involved in collaboration efforts, that the academic administration put a temporary moratorium on tenure decisions and reduction in committee assignments and salary supplements.[45]

The second strategy to promote collaboration between nursing service and education is to increase the financial status of both branches of nursing. Baker (1983) points out that collaboration projects have not attracted much foundation support, the Kellogg Foundation being the exception. The need for collaboration is so critical that federal, state, and foundation supports are essential to experimental and innovative approaches to collaboration, with added monetary incentives for those institutions who demonstrate solid outcomes.[45]

The third strategy recommended by Baker[45] and Sharp,[46] to promote collaboration between nursing service and education is for the accrediting body, such as the National League for Nursing and the Joint Commission on Accreditation of Hospitals, to endorse the need for collaboration and establish guidelines for implementation. This will have a definite impact. Sharp (1978) further recommends that if future licensure and credentialing required that nurse educators demonstrate currency and excellence in nursing practice, it might challenge nursing leaders futher.

The issues of collaboration between nursing service and education are age-old. They have existed as long as both branches of the nursing profession have existed. Sometimes the gap between the two widens, and when the profession is in crisis the gap narrows and the forces for collaboration are renewed. The recommendations to enhance collaboration between nursing service and education and colleagiality between nursing and medicine and other disciplines are excellent, however, hard-core data and research is necessary to document their benefits and measure the outcomes and the advantages of these to each discipline and to each branch of nursing.

ETHICAL MORAL ISSUES IN NURSING

Ethical moral issues related to health care of patients and the management of nursing services have received more attention during the past five years than previously. As technology increases and the need for cost containment becomes more acute nurses and nursing executives are finding themselves confronted with ethical dilemmas that require moral sensitivity and a sense of justice. Two categories of ethical issues are presented in this next section as well as what the role of the nurse-executive should be in offering support to these nurses. Then, the moral dimensions of decisions that nurse executives currently face are presented.

In a recent study[47] (Applegate 1984), practicing nurses were asked to identify ethical-moral issues they encountered in their clinical setting that required them to make moral decisions. Nurses identified six categories of ethical-moral issues that required some form of moral decision. The first category was those issues related to "standards of care." Thirty percent of the responses fell into this category. They cited 18 instances of clients receiving poor-quality care as a result of nurse, physician, and system lowering of standards. In 14 situations, doctors rendered poor care because of lack of communication, lack of assessment, overt class bias toward indigent patients, ordering contraindicated medications, medical mismanagement leading to patients' death, and inappropriate orders. In two situations nurses rendered poor care by ignoring the patient, resulting in the patients' death.

The second category of ethical-moral issues were related to patients with "terminal illnesses." Twenty-eight percent of the responses were in this category. There were 17 situations cited that dealt with artificial life-support systems and requests for euthanasia. In five situations nurses were asked to "code" the patient so that family members could arrive to the hospital. In one instance "coding" was done because doctors couldn't agree. In four situations patients had requested not to be coded, but the nurse was ordered to code. In four situations nurses were asked to "pull the plug" on respirators by the doctor or family members, and three times the nurses were asked to overdose the patient by giving morphine sulfate as an active euthanasia.

The third category of ethical-moral issues faced by the practicing nurses was "relationship" issues. Fifteen percent of the responses were in this category. For example, conflict between nurses and doctors was reflected in two situations (1) where the doctor refused to pronounce the patient dead, and (2) where blame was projected on a nurse in an emergency problem involving a nurse-patient relationship when there was a threat to trust and spreading of rumors about patients. Four instances of patient-doctor relationship problems were reported such as: lack of honesty, nonprofessional relationship, verbal and physical abuse, and passing of verbal judgment on a patient. There was one situation of a nurse-nurse problem involving a manipulative power struggle.

The fourth category of ethical issues were those related to "rights" issues. Fifteen percent of responses were in this group. Nine situations were reported where nurses experienced conflict when giving experimental medications and placebos to psychiatric patients, and in practices where pediatric psychiatric patients were placed in solitary confinement. Three situations were also reported where nurses were ordered to obtain informed consent from patients where the patients were either uninformed or confused. There was also one case of police brutality of a prisoner in an emergency room setting, and one other case where a decision had to be made as to whether the mother or the fetus was going to live. Finally, a nurse who objected to abortions was assigned to assist the doctor in an abortion case.

The fifth type of ethical issues faced by practicing nurses dealt with the care of babies with "congenital anomalies." Seven percent of the responses fell in this category. The nurses encountered mixed feelings of sustaining the life of a newborn that had anomalies incompatible with life, or those infants who would survive but lead a "vegetable" life.

The sixth category of ethical issues encountered by the nurses dealt with "setting priorities." Five percent of the responses were in this group. There were three problems reported in health-care priority. One dealt with utilization of staff in the operating room during combined emergency-nonemergency situations. The other two situations dealt with inadequate staffing in the neonatal unit and the problem of bed utilization in intensive care units.

In reviewing the findings of this study, Applegate[47] points out that 66% of the situations cited involved both physicians and nurses. She also raises the question, What is the role of the nursing director in providing support to the practicing nurses confronted with ethical issues requiring moral decision-making? She makes the following recommendations:

1. Offer special programs in bioethics and ethical decision-making to the staff by the staff-development department.
2. The director of nursing should keep him- or herself and the staff informed about the legal and regulatory requirements related to the above-mentioned issues.
3. Foster accountability and collaboration between nurses and doctors.
4. Establish nursing policies that provide guidance for situations with ethical overtones and ensure that all nursing personnel adhere to these policies.
5. Provide adequate resources to nurses so that at least minimal nursing standards of care are upheld.

Many institutions are convening ethics committees to find innovative ways to help their nurses with ethical dilemmas. These committees establish policies and also discuss the specific issues at hand. The authority of the committee ranges from consultation to decision-making power.

The moral dimensions of decisions that nurse executives make entails the allocation of nursing services, the quality of care, and values involved in these decisions.[48] Since 1980, the need for cost containment in health care has thrust nursing and the cost of nursing services into the limelight of health-care economics. With the advent of DRGs, nursing services must now authoritatively justify and defend nursing cost and the nursing care component of each DRG. Accompanying this new opportunity for nursing is the obligation to articulate the moral dimensions of and to be morally accountable for nursing services in health-care relationships.

The allocation of nursing services and the quality of care have been singled out by Frankena[49] and Fry[50] as having moral dimensions because they involve a balancing of moral values essential for health-care practices. Fry[48] (1986) points out that allocation of nursing services involves the identification of criteria for determining how resources should be allocated. For example, relevant criteria might include patient needs, ability to pay, prestige of the patient, age, prognosis, or in the case of DRGs, quick recovery and return to the community. The selection of one criteria over another entails normative assessment of the benefits obtained and norms averted as the basis for decision making. Also, values considered important for humanistic nursing need to be balanced against values deemed important for cost containment. The way in which these values are balanced determines how resources will be allocated; thus it is an ethical decision.

The criteria for quality of care also reflects the balancing of benefits and harms, and helps establish standards against which quality is measured. Selecting criteria to measure quality of care is an ethical decision. According to Fry,[48] "it involves the normative assessment of what constitutes benefit and what constitutes harm in terms of nursing services, often in response to moral principles fundamental to human interaction" (p. 161).

With respect to values in ethical decisions,

the values of equity, self-determination, and well-being are involved in the balancing of nursing services' potential benefits and harms.[51] According to Fry,[48] decision making for the value of equity means the fair and impartial consideration of individuals in terms of access to health. The value of self-determination in decision making entails giving the individual the freedom of making choices without outside interference. Decision making about the value of well-being deals with provision of human-welfare interests as determined by consumers or others.

The ethical issues discussed above have immense implications to the educational preparation of the nurse executive and for further research. In order for the director of nursing to make ethical decisions about allocation of nursing resources and quality of care, he or she must resort to a knowledge base in values and how they are balanced in terms of benefits and harms. Such a knowledge base is not found in the educational preparation of most nurse executives. Some may have obtained aspects of this knowledge base from business management courses. Some may have acquired it through the socialization process of their management role. Others may have learned it through common sense, insight, or trial and error.[48] There is no research that indicates which method of acquisition of knowledge in the area of value formation and decision making is preferable. Most existing research on ethical decision-making has been on the types of decisions that clinical nurses make when faced with a moral dilemma.[52–54] Research is needed in determining how nurse executives weigh their personal, professional, and institutional values in making decisions about allocation of resources to different aspects of nursing services and about quality of care. Knowledge from these research studies can determine the critical cognitive behaviors for moral-ethical decision-making that can then be in-

stituted in the educational preparation of the nurse executive.

In conclusion, as of 1988, when issues in health and nursing abound, this is a time of opportunity and change for nursing to take advantage of. We need to be creators of, not reactors to change. Knowing our destination and developing plans to meet our goals requires each of us to be active participants in promoting a positive public image of nursing, agreeing on the baccalaureate degree as the minimum requirement for entry into professional practice, promoting public accountability and professional autonomy, improving the economic status of nurses, justifying our costs—especially at a time when there is increased competition and stringent cost-containment measures. Nurses need to establish better colleagial relationships with physicians and hospital administrators working with them; nurses should negotiate policies that provide for just and fair decision-making, autonomy, improved staffing, and adequate resources. When this relationship is established nursing will have a better chance of controlling its practice and clinical research. This control can be further enhanced when there are colleagial relationships between nursing service and nursing education. In order to reach our destination, nurses need to possess the skills of political savvy and effectiveness. Nurses need to learn how to influence the political machinery; become politically assertive; and influence, develop, and implement health policy. Our professional nursing organizations must encourage and help members to lobby at the local, state, and national levels. Andrioli and Musser[1] also recommend that "as an organized, educated, and cohesive force, nurses must identify, rank, and confront political issues that affect them" (p. 49).

The current and projected health-care trends require that nursing establish through research and documentation its unique contribution to the future of health care and document the effectiveness of nursing practice. By so doing, it will also enhance the profession's image and reputation in scholarship and research. Andrioli and Musser[1] recommend four areas of timely research in response to the current trends. These are studies of (1) the impact of nursing on health care of the elderly; (2) cost effectiveness of nursing services; (3) effectiveness of the nurse in health promotion and education programs; (4) the impact of biomedical technology in nursing practice.

Finally, the role of the nurse executive in response to these health-care trends requires that he or she possess the knowledge base necessary to act appropriately and lead the nursing department in achieving its objectives. The knowledge base necessary includes an understanding of and skill in management sciences, marketing, finance, policy making, labor relations and negotiations, ethical-moral issues, the politics of health-care and health policy formulation, research methodology, human relations, personnel psychology, and knowledge of current trends in health care and how they effect nursing. This list (by no means exhaustive) covers some of the essential cognitive skills that a nursing director should have. The extent to which the nurse executive possesses these and related areas of knowledge and is articulate in presenting the contributions of nursing to the health-care delivery system, is the extent to which nursing will find its worthy place alongside other health professions, and meet the challenges of tomorrow.

REFERENCES

1. Andrioli KG, Musser LA. Trends that may affect nursing's future. Nursing and Health Care 1985: 6(1):47–51.
2. Urquhart AL, Wooding G, Budinger KM, Henry BM. Perspectives on nursing issues and health care trends. J Nurs Admin 1986;16(1):17–23.
3. Fagin C. The national shortage of nurses: a nursing perspective. In: Aiken LH, ed: Nursing in the 1980s: crises, opportunities, challenges. Philadelphia: JB Lippincott Co, 1982.
4. White D. HRSA predicts health professions balance by 2000. Washington actions on health. July 23, 1983.
5. Naisbitt J. Megatrends: ten new directions transforming our lives. New York: Warner Books, 1982.
6. Bartkowski JJ, Swandby JM. Charting nursing's course through megatrends. Nursing and Health Care 1985;6(7):375–377.
7. American Nurses' Association. Nursing: a social policy statement. Kansas City: ANA, 1980.
8. Bureau of Labor Statistics. Employment and earnings—April 1983. Washington, DC: U.S. Government Printing Office, 1979.
9. Lancaster J. 1986 and beyond: nursing's future. J Nurs Admin 1986;16:(3):31–37.
10. Kast FE, Rosenzweig JE. Organization and management: a systems approach. 2nd ed. New York: McGraw Hill, 1974, p. 44.
11. Mauksch I. An analysis of some critical contemporary issues in nursing. J Cont Educ 1983;14(1):4–8.
12. Foster LB, Walker DD, Bernadette M, Schraff SH. Nursing service in transition: four perspectives. Nursing and Health Care 1984;5(3):312–316.
13. Curtin L. Editorial opinion, the decade ahead: five major issues. Nurs Manage 1983;14(10):9–10.
14. Dugan AB. Expanding nursing's practice terrain: imperatives for future availability. Public Health Nursing 1985;2(1):23–32.
15. Institute of Medicine, Division of Health Services. Nursing and nursing education, public policies and private actions. Washington, DC: National Academy Press, 1983.
16. Muller R. Byre CS, Whitehead SF. Hospital nursing vacancies. Am J Nursing 1983;83(40):547.
17. Job security seen as main issue in unionization drives. Hospitals 1984;58(23):59–60.
18. Fuchs V. Current factors affecting society's willingness to pay. Protecting and advancing health in an era of constrained resources. Presented at the Institute of Medicine's annual meeting, October 10, 1984.
19. Medicare may go broke by '90, experts say. Houston Post, Sept. 8, 1983.
20. Reeves R. Mondale knows, but won't say. Houston Post October 14, 1984.
21. Little A. The health care system in the mid 1990's. A study conducted for the Health Insurance Association of America by Arthur Little Inc, 1985.
22. HMO enrollment to 19 million. Health Care Report 1985;14(9):9.
23. American Nurses' Association. Environmental assessment: factors affecting long range planning for nursing and health care. Kansas City: ANA, 1985.
24. Kuhn R. Creativity: survival in turbulent times. Heart and Lung 1985;15(3):21A–30A.
25. Gortner SR. Commentary. In: Aiken LH, ed. Nursing in the 1980s: crises, opportunities, challenges. Philadelphia: JB Lippincott Co, 1982.
26. Kleinfield NR. The home health care boom. New York Times. June 30, 1983, 29–30.

27. Stevens B. Tackling a changing society head on. Nursing and Health Care 1985;6(1):27–31.
28. Curtin L. Who says "lean must be mean?" Nurs Manage 1986;17(1):7–8.
29. Madsen NL, Harper RW. Improving the nursing climate. J Nurs Adm 1985;15(3):11–16.
30. Haw MA, Claus EC, Lafferty ED, Iverson SM. Improving morale in a climate of cost containment. Part 2, program planning. J Nurs Adm 1984;14(11):10–15.
31. Byrnes MA. Non-nursing functions: the nurses state their case. Am J Nursing 1982;82(7):1089–1093.
32. National Commission on Nursing. Initial report and recommendations. Chicago: Hospital Research and Foundation Trust, 1981.
33. Hartman P. Frontdoor cost containment. Nursing Success Today 1985;2(10):32–38.
34. Aiken LH. Nursing's future: public policies, private actions. Am J Nursing 1983;83(10):1440–1444.
35. Maine's 42 Hospitals, obeying a unique law, begin to charge their patients for nursing care. Am J Nursing 1985;85(10):1166–1167,1190–1192.
36. Bermas N, Vanslyck A. Patient classification systems and the nursing department. Hospitals 1984;58(22):99–100.
37. Harju M, Sabatino F. Productivity efforts on the rise. Hospitals 1984;58(22):89–90.
38. McFarlane JK. The proper study of the nurse. London: Royal College of Nursing, 1970.
39. Jarvis P. Professional education. London: Croom Helm, 1983.
40. Glick MS. Educational entry level in to nursing practice. J Cont Educ Nursing 1985;16(6):185–188.
41. Glick MS. Schools alarmed by downturn in applications: "pool is down in quantity and quality," some say. Am J Nursing 1985;85(11):1292, 1299–1300.
42. Holtzclaw BJ. Crisis: changing student applicant pool. Nursing and Health Care 1983;4(8):450–454.
43. Stevens B. Improving nurses' managerial skills. Nursing Outlook 1979;27(12):774–777.
44. Ricleft R. Back to school, more executives take work related courses to keep up advance. Wall Street J, 3 March, 1980.
45. Baker CM. Moving toward interdependence: strategies for collaboration. J Nurs Adm 1983;12(4):34–39.
46. Sharp E. The coming crisis for nursing faculty: joint appointments in a practice discipline. In: Licensure and Credentialling. New York: National League for Nursing, 1978, no. 52-1706, 12–31.
47. Applegate M. Capsule: does your staff need help? J Nurs Adm 1984;14(6):14–15, 27, 41.
48. Fry St. Moral-values and ethical decisions in a constrained economic environment. Nurs Economics 1986;4(4):161–164.
49. Frankena WK. Ethics. Englewood Cliffs, NJ: Prentice-Hall, 1973.
50. Fry St. Ethical issues: politics, power and change. In: Talbott S, Mason D, eds. Political action: a handbook for nurses. Reading, MA: Addison-Wesley, 1985, pp. 133–140.
51. President's Commission for the Study of Ethical Problems in Medicine and Biomedical and Behavioral Research. Securing access to health care. Volume 1: report. Washington DC: U.S. Government Printing Office, 1983.
52. Ketefian S. Moral reasoning and moral behavior among selected groups of practicing nurses. Nurs Res 1981;30(3):171–176.
53. Ketefian S. Professional and bureaucratic role conceptions and moral behavior among nurses. Nurs Res 1985;34(4):248–253.
54. Murphy CC. Levels of moral reasoning in a selected group of nursing practitioners. Unpublished doctoral dissertation. Teachers College, Columbia University, New York, 1976.

41

Issues of Academic Administration

Doris Froebe

MORE than two decades of growth and substantial disciplinary accomplishments have placed schools of nursing in the United States as established entities in the university community. Integration into the university affords nurse educators recognition as a national educational disciplinary force. Although today's schools of nursing will be destined to show less growth in the future, they will still be essential to the university structure and to the health-care community at large. In this context, administration of schools of nursing can continue to grow in stature in the university and the nursing discipline.

Problems facing the administration of schools of nursing during the 1980s are legion. The reason is clear. Nursing's unique disciplinary problems are combined with higher education's more general set of problems. Lowering enrollments, aging faculties, short-falls in funding, and increasing external controls are examples of problems that cross most of the disciplines in the university. After nurse administrators cope with these problems, they must address problems of knowledge explosion and technological advance unique to nursing, the matter of being a largely female work force in a male milieu, and the need to further integrate the practice and profession of nursing into the academic community. Today's nurse is recognized for his or her contribution to health care. With this recognition nursing emerges with increased eminence, and alumni, donors, ac-crediting bodies, government funding agencies, allied health collaborators, and unions expect to exact influence over nursing education and do so.

Administrators of nursing units could function in more propitious times using looser administrative and organizational structures. Propitious times could be labeled as times of fiscal affluence, and prominence for pursuing higher educational autonomy. As conditions change, so must academic management techniques. The use of administrative concepts in day-to-day management should be considered by academic administrators if they are to operate effectively in complex and changing times.

Concepts of administration that hold significance for academic administration parallel those used by nurse administrators. Several concepts are selected for limited interpretation.

GOVERNANCE

University governance is complex. Nurses in faculty and administrative roles in the university find themselves facing at least three sources of authority and control. One source of authority comes from the university's charter. In this case, faculty hold certain rights that do not extend into the administrative ranks. An example of such faculty authority rests with curriculum generation and implementation. Another source of authority comes from the university's bureaucratic structure. From this source, administrators in nursing have authority over staffing and budgets. Both of these sources of authority are internal to the university. As faculty move to structure and implement curriculum policy, the authority of the dean to budget and staff meets point-counterpoint with curriculum authority of faculty. A structure needs to be considered to handle these two essential tracks of authority. In no other realm of nursing does a subordinate group hold authority granted by charter. This makes a structure delineating dual authority essential. Usually the administration's executive group operates to formalize policy. Faculty committees suggest and appeal policy.

Nurses are also members of a profession. One form of the profession's control comes through the profession's accreditation process.

The accreditation process exerts an external influence. Professional associations are responsible for enforcement of standards of educational performance in secondary schools, colleges, and universities. "In performing this function they have long expressed substantial influence, or even control, particularly over the newer and marginal colleges and universities. That influence has been enlarged as federal aid of higher education has grown and federal aid has generally been made available only to accredited institutions."[1] (p. 27) Accreditation activities such as self-studies, adequate library volumes, established faculty-student ratios, preparation of faculty, physical plant properties, and curriculum implementation place external demands on administration.

Where unions exist, another form of external authority and control needs to be considered. Unionization of faculty makes establishing administrative policy even more tenuous. Unions want to protect economic interests primarily. Union agreements affect management's policy making.

STRUCTURE

The primary product line in schools of nursing is student education. Research and service follow as secondary product lines. The organizational structure and processes that prevail to maintain product lines in schools of nursing are patterned after the structure of business. The organization of the school follows bureaucratic lines with the dean at the apex of the organization.

Authority for maintaining the organization flows from higher university administration to the dean of the school of nursing. This authority ultimately converges at the faculty level where teaching occurs. Where there are no intermediate levels of faculty or staff between the dean and faculty, we see a decentralized organization. In other words, decentralization means that the dean interacts directly with the faculty to administer the school. The more the dean can interact with the faculty, the closer the dean operates to the school's product line—the students.

In most large- or medium-size schools of nursing the dean administers the school with the help of others. These deans have assistants, associates, or directors who form an executive group or cabinet to advise the dean. The scope of the program, the size of the school, and use of regional school sites have required the move from total decentralization to an organization with more hierarchic levels. Assistants to the dean extend the intent of the dean through the organization.

For example, assistants may direct product lines such as associate, baccalaureate or graduate student educational units. Product lines may also be formulated for regional campuses. The extension of teaching to multiple campuses separates the dean from faculty and students by hierarchic level and geographic distance.

Whether continuing education is defined as a product line varies among schools, although it is usually not a major product line.

Splintering of personnel, student, finance, research, and administrative tasks to other than the product-line assistant deans further compounds the delegation patterns. These persons render help in their given areas of expertise, and in doing so tend to move the dean further from faculty in decision making. None the less, today's larger schools require enough highly specialized personnel to initiate the placement of a number of support staff and administrators in the school of nursing structure.

Executive and faculty groups function in a parallel fashion. Neither group holds pre-emptive authority over the other, with the exception of authority dealing with staffing and budget issues generating from the dean's position power, and authority dealing with curriculum issues generating from faculty-position power. A typical faculty organization meets at least quarterly, and its committees meet monthly. Committees constitute the actual bodies that frame potential policy for consideration by the dean. The dean's assistants meet at least once a month. Faculty proposals and administrative logistics are handled. Minutes of both groups' meetings and the generated directive statements comprise the formal mechanisms used to link the dean and faculty bodies.

Assistant deans, associate deans, and directors work directly with faculty and directly under the dean. As such, these individuals serve as human linking mechanisms to resolve conflict in academic settings. In selected instances, task forces composed of individuals from both faculty and executive groups serve as links to formulate issues and resolve conflicts. Staff personnel holding high expertise in a given area also serve as linking mechanisms between faculty and executive groups. An example of this is an expert in student services.

Some nurse academicians question the suitability of a hierachic bureaucratic structure for schools of nursing that exist in settings of higher learning. They hold the premise that the school of nursing's faculty is a corps of highly specialized, competent individuals who hold equal and often similar preparation to the preparation and competence of their administration. Hage[2] (p. 58) has stated that "occupational or other interest groups want the same rank in power, prestige, pay, and privileges as they have in training and skill." This becomes a substantive issue today with school of nursing faculties becoming largely doctorally prepared. It would seem that organizations with fewer hierarchic levels will emerge. Meanwhile, matrix organizations may be juxtaposed over the existing bureaucratic structure. Matrix organizations are found useful as interim organizations.

COMMUNICATION TECHNOLOGY

There can be little doubt that the use of existing data in and between schools of nursing can be improved. Today's technology offers refined computer programs that can exchange information on academic problems, fiscal applications, staffing-student imbalances, and a score of related issues. Departments in a school can be ascertained by a statistical look at the current student population.

The investment in a management information system to deal with these problems is a significant one. Mayhew[3] (p. 100) cites the conditions whereby such an expenditure should prevail. Conditions are reinterpreted here for the dean's level in the organization as follows: the dean should understand and want the system; resources for purchase and maintenance of the system can be handled on university monies; there are personnel on board to operate the system; subordinate administrators are also trained to use the system; faculty morale is high enough to withstand careful performance screening; and the organization has demonstrated that it can sustain change.

COORDINATION

The hierarchic bureaucratic organization, with the dean at the apex and levels of personnel functioning below, provides a format for the process of coordination existing in the school. Linkages by individuals and groups were noted under the section describing structure. These linkages, to a large extent, become the major source of coordination of faculty and administration. Electronic data controls in a few organizations augment the coordination processes in a school of nursing.

Coordination weaknesses can occur from the limitations that the external environment places upon the dean. For example, today's research funding mechanisms often place individual faculty outside the fiscal control of department chairs and dean. This may result in unequal work expectations across faculty. A rise of external regulations relating to research and affirmative action brought controls from newly appointed directors of university research, sponsored programs, and affirmative action to bear on product-line management. Staff, faculty, and administrative-line personnel all must coordinate their authority and functions for the school to succeed. Successful modification of the process of coordination becomes important as schools grow in size, complexity, and become instruments of change.

CONCERNS IN THE 1980s

A discussion of governance, structure, use of data, and coordination provide a base for examining trends in the 1980s. Continued growth of schools of nursing appears unsupportable without a realistic plan for student enrollment, personnel, and finance. Assistance in using the planning process in the school can be drafted from outside organizational planners, schools of business, and committees of selected administrative personnel working in the school. Regardless of who is

involved in planning, the planning parameters need to be defined. Planning periods of one year become more realistic in times of change. One-year plans can be structured to fit into three- to five-year organizational strategic frameworks.

Personnel

Education and experience backgrounds of academic leaders assume increasing importance as positions are opened through resignation or retirement. Movement from teaching to administrative positions still occurs, but evidence of increments of management education, training, and experience is now critically reviewed by search and screen bodies. A few programs exist that prepare academic administrators for nursing programs. Sources of knowledge concerning programs that prepare leaders in academic nursing administration can be secured from the National League of Nursing.

Applying management theory in practice, the dean must work through faculty and staff to locate and utilize scarce human and material resources. The placement of personnel in the form of assistants, consultants, task forces, and faculty into strategic positions in the organization at the right time demands a sense of timing, fiscal aptitude, and management expertise. Along with this, the dean "must cultivate the professions they serve, derive financial support from them, and maintain an independence from them."[1] (p. 257) This alone requires adept leadership skills.

The bureaucratic structure of the school of nursing will undoubtedly remain intact for purposes of overall personnel organization and control. Nevertheless, the working distance of the dean to the faculty needs to be bridged to keep an increasing number of doctorally prepared faculty creative and functional in the organization. A shortened working distance is not meant to imply that more controls, such as closer supervision, are needed. It is intended to mean that as a manager increases the number of staff for whom they are responsible, they support goals but give less direct supervision. More decentralized decision making will be demanded by a highly prepared faculty work force.

The issue of dealing with an aging faculty population in the school of nursing will need to be considered in the 1980s. An aging faculty needs to address potential content deficiencies. In a parallel vein, the administrator dealing with the aging faculty needs to address the issue of having the majority of the faculty hold tenure. Deficiency in faculty expertise can result in curricular problems. A high percentage of faculty holding tenure can create recruitment problems. It must be recognized in the academic arena that years of practice in teaching a subject cannot be equated with teaching competency any longer.

The majority of tenured faculty were educationally prepared in a period before computer technologies were widely used in education. Resources are now being directed to faculty populations expected to meet changing educational needs with changing technologies. Resources are directed by way of course reimbursement, released study time, or retirement benefits phased in at an earlier age. It will take a wide variety of approaches to keep faculty expertise in line with educational needs through the 1990s. The need for knowledge updates can become a costly faculty development initiative. In the early 1980s we experienced the costs related to merely bringing a majority of faculty into computer literacy. Other technologic systems will require other faculty developmental expenditures.

The issue of nursing as a largely female work force has been of concern to schools of nursing for a long time. Significant wage differentials between male and female fac-

ulty, lower promotion rates to the few professor levels for women in the university, and fewer opportunities for promotion into administrative ranks in the university for women are representative problems facing the female nursing workforce. Federal assistance for adjusting workplace equality appears to be vanishing. While there are no pat answers, women in nursing who continue to raise consciousness levels will help. Advances for the educated woman working in the academic arena will undoubtedly be slower and advances will be the result of local activities by women.

Enrollment

Recruitment of students demands a significantly higher expenditure of money and effort if the school of nursing is to obtain its market share. Brochures will become more attractive, and more expensive. Markets will be targeted and segmented to include more recruitment of R.N.s and L.P.N.s into mobility programs. Visits by faculty to other school's recruitment days, to hospitals, and to public schools will be tested for efficiency and effectiveness. Data sources will be more complete using computers. Therefore, statistical studies on which mechanism brings students into enrollment will be used to help administrators allocate funds. An often forgotten source of undergraduate recruitment is the graduate program. Reputable graduate programs attract promising students. Selective interpretation by recruiters of long-range opportunities in nursing will become important.

Fiscal Impact

A shortfall in fiscal resources faces nearly all programs and cannot be ignored. A number of mechanisms will be attempted in the 1980s to protect programs and faculties. Some will succeed and others fail. In all cases, a knowledge of the budget process will be needed.

The need for careful scrunity of every expenditure will prevail over the 1980s and possibly thereafter. Searches for funding in the form of grants, endowments, and subsidies will be concentrated.

Larger schools will seek the professional help of fund-raisers. Fiscal needs will be translated into larger faculty-to-student ratios, fewer support services, and less-institutionally financed faculty development in the form of travel to scholarly events. Deans will aggressively seek donor funding. Name chairs will become more visible. Since the majority of the donors in nursing are not highly paid, deans will need to be creative in looking to a number of donors for one chair. Partial funding for a chair may be considered. A topper chair is an example of a partially funded chair. For example, a smaller sum of money may fund only the topper chair faculty's research.

Data generated from computer sources will help to examine expenditures allocated to marketing the program. Linear models can be plotted to determine which recruitment expenditures were effective in bringing students into nursing. The expenditure levels to be experienced in pursuing marketing will be new to nursing administration.

A typical school of nursing of the 1980s is housed in a structure built in the 1960s and 1970s. These physical plants will need to be modernized to accommodate the technologies available to faculty and teaching. Programming for such modernization will require planning, coordinating, and data-processing skills of faculty and deans.

External Forces

External forces will continue to influence all of the health community. The school of nursing will probably experience less government control due to lowered government nurse-education subsidies. On the other hand, nurse administrators will probably experience more controls as diagnosis related groups (DRGs), catastrophic health insurance, and home-care subsidies affect patient-care arenas and in turn affect nursing education.

Accrediting bodies exact significant staffing and fiscal controls on the educational program today. If the costs generated in pursuing the accredition process and its policies are not modified, university administrators may alter their position on accreditation. Accreditation costs are not limited to fiscal imperatives, but include pressures that appear to result in less organizational creativity. For example, pressures for relatively explicit faculty-student teaching ratios exist, despite newer available teaching technologies. If only four or five of the larger institutions moved away from the accreditation process as we know it, the impact of the accreditation status on other schools' programs would be modified. For example, if graduate programs accepted students from other than accredited program, the accreditation process would be weakened. This could end in a decrease in the quality of educational programs in the future.

Unionism will continue to be an external condition to be considered. The extent to which unions will influence the teaching programs in nursing is uncertain. Turnover of nursing faculty in higher education is much lower than in recent decades. Decreasing mobility by faculty has decreased job opportunities. This could positively or negatively influence unionism.

In summary, administrative processes in the school of nursing combine middle management and executive authority. In conceptualizing the school, today's deans and faculties hold specific positional power and responsibility. Structure and governance are instituted to accommodate this dual authority. Internal and external issues of the day were noted to impinge on both function and organization. Issues relating to lack of funds, an aging faculty population, and lowering enrollments were specifically addressed. The peculiarities of the academic setting and forces impinging on the dean and faculty have been addressed in order that the dean and faculty might consider, and possibly create, a more productive milieu.

REFERENCES

1. Corson J. The governance of colleges and universities. New York: McGraw-Hill Book Co, 1975.
2. Hage J. Theories of organizations: form, process, and transformation. New York: John Wiley & Sons, 1980.
3. Mayhew L. Surviving the eighties. San Francisco: Jossey-Bass Publishers, 1980.

42

Emerging Paradigms of Nursing Administration Education

Mary Jane Reinhart

EVEN though the title of this chapter evokes expectations of a crystal-ball discussion of things to come, the intent is not to be a horoscope of future nursing administration paradigms. The purpose of this chapter is to provide a body of information to nursing practitioners, educators, and students so that they may build a common understanding of paradigms and theories, apply this understanding to past and present organizational paradigms, and predict and plan for future paradigms. The chapter begins by considering the nature of paradigms and theories.

PARADIGMS AND THEORIES

The world in which we live is a dynamic arena of changes. Time passes, water evaporates, rocks and soil erode, and continents shift. Changes in the world's phenomena require new explanations if we are to understand the way the world works. Reliable new explanations aggregate in an orderly fashion with related established explanations into clusters that broaden the scope of understanding in a synergistic manner. When large clusters of explanations become a common body of beliefs, they are called paradigms. If paradigms are widely accepted and utilized over time to guide beliefs and practices, they join with related paradigms to become traditions. Traditions and their component paradigms serve as norms or standards by which people bring order to their thinking and behavior.

Like other phenomena in the world, paradigms change. However, they do not change by simply accumulating new explanatory theories. Rather, paradigms are subtly shifted or transformed in a somewhat revolutionary manner when component explanations of the paradigm are replaced by new explanations that are perceived as important enough to entice a lasting body of believers away from previously held beliefs. Individual explanations found in paradigms are actually theories, each theory explaining a segment of the paradigm. Theories that have been replaced become past history and are eliminated from the paradigm. Kuhn suggested that these eliminated or outdated beliefs become myths.[1] This tantalizing idea that myths were once thought to be scientific theories leads one to imagine a line of historical nursing research in which the origins and disposal of nursing myths could be explored. It is also possible that mythical beliefs have not been eliminated from nursing's paradigms as they should have been when new theories took rightful places in the schema of nursing practice.

The importance of educationally establishing a common understanding of paradigms and their nature cannot be overstressed. Ask 10 people what a paradigm is and there are likely to be 10 different definitions. Kuhn, in relating the term "paradigm" with actual scientific practice, noted that "The study of paradigms . . . is what mainly prepares the student for membership in the particular scientific community in which he will later practice"[1] (p. 226). How can nurses who are being educated as administrators and leaders be expected to sense the emergence of new paradigms that will guide future nursing practices if there is no solid understanding of what constitutes a "basic" paradigm? A further discussion of the characteristics and makeup of paradigms is warranted.

A jigsaw-puzzle is a good analogy of a paradigm in the making. The completed product projects the image of a whole situation through the mosaic union of parts. Like many large jigsaw puzzles, paradigms are usually missing a number of component parts, leaving the paradigm sufficiently open to redefinition of the composite image. A paradigm differs from a jigsaw puzzle in that individual paradigm parts are subject to challenge and replacement when more appropriate parts are discovered and accepted. In this manner, a paradigm's large picture is flexible enough to take on a new image. When one remembers that the component parts of a paradigm are theories, the paradigm's missing parts may be thought of as unexplained areas that give rise to a wealth of opportunities for research leading to a more refined understanding of the workings of the phenomenon in question. A paradigm is not merely an image, but acts as a guiding schema; a grand plan; an explanatory overview of a complex naturalistic phenomenon. Kuhn defined a paradigm as a "universally recognized scientific achievement that for a time provides model problems and solutions to a community of practitioners"[2] (p. 21).

There is an implied hierarchy in the process of explaining how the world works. Questions or problems that occur at the base of the hierarchy lead to concepts that interrelate under the situation of the phenomenon in question. As explanations to the questions and problems are formulated, these inter-related concepts become integral parts of theories—the next rung on the hierarchic ladder. When the theories inter-relate or enhance one another, they unite on the hierarchy to form a paradigm. Related paradigms that exist over time ultimately become traditions.

"Theory" is a commonly misused, misunderstood, and therefore an often-disdained term. However, a well-constructed and well-researched theory is not an object of scorn, but is the best explanation we have of how a small segment of the world works. There are certain criteria that are essential in theory construction. Not meeting criteria has been the main cause of the disdain that pseudo-theories have suffered, blighting whole attitudes toward the subject of theories. A true theory should stand up to analysis in much the same way that it was once popular to break down and diagram grammatical construction of sentences. Gale[3] described a theory as the basis for a scientific conceptual system, a "fairly structured entity which includes at least two elements: the set of observation correlations, and the metaphysical hypothesis which is linked to the correlations" (pp. 73–74). One should be able to study a purported theory and break it down into Gale's two basic elements for further analysis. A metaphysical hypothesis is an abstract explanation about a real-life phenomenon. The abstraction must represent something that happens in nature, but cannot be directly observed. The abstraction cannot represent a supernatural explanation. "Thor, the God of Thunder, is the reason for the noise following lightning" would not be a metaphysical hypothesis. "Gravity is the reason things fall to the earth" would be a metaphysical hypothesis, albeit oversimplified. The observation correlates in a theory are composed of a set of inter-related objects or concepts that provide a supportive and definitive milieu for the metaphysical hypothesis. The collective nature and behavior of individual concepts must be sufficient to logically cause the observed correlations. It is important to remember that for every set of observed correlated concepts there are undoubtedly at least two, and perhaps a whole range of naturalistic explanations that are possible.[3] Since it is often difficult for a number of scientists to reach a consensus among a variety of alternative explanations, theories become vulnerable to testing and possible later replacement with explanations that seem to fit the observed correlations more appropriately. In this manner, new theories replace old theories, old theories become myths, and a new quality emerges in the paradigm. Therefore, when one wishes to watch for paradigm shifts, one first develops a sensitivity to shifts and alterations in component theories. It is causal vulnerability that leads many scientists to hesitate proposing theory hypotheses in the first place. Thus, golden opportunities for inquiry may be missed, and a portion of the world's workings goes unexplained awhile longer.

Gale noted two goals of science: (1) prediction and control, and (2) explanation and understanding. Studying correlations among observed concepts may lead to making predictions about the chance of future occurrences of the phenomenon, and imply control through manipulation of variables. However, it is the riskier development and testing of hypotheses that ultimately satisfy the human mind's higher need to explain and understand nature's phenomena.[3] A distinction between predictive and prescriptive theory must be addressed. While studying observation correlations may allow prediction of future variable correlations, widespread prescription of actions and behaviors is precluded because there is no basis of explanation, no causality shown by correlations. When one remembers that theories may have whole ranges of explanations, that paradigms contain myriad theories, that the nature of the world is to change, and that environmen-

tal influences may confound situations, then it follows that prescription of specific beliefs and behaviors based on theories that have not been repeatedly tested is inappropriate. Indeed, existence of prescriptive theory at all is questionable—a point to be taken into consideration when nurses set out to develop one theory to direct all nursing curricula or practices in a given program or practice setting. When searching for unique prescriptive nursing theories, nurses have often eschewed theories from other fields or disciplines. When one remembers that a theory is simply an explanation about how a segment of the world works and that no one lives in isolation from the world, it becomes obvious that a theory cannot be "borrowed" since it does not "belong" to a specific person or group, but belongs to all inhabitants of the world. For example, the theory of gravity works for you and me just as well as it did for Newton. Thus, nurses would be well advised to seek the best explanations possible, whatever the sources, for problems facing the profession. It is the specific mixture of theories and their synergistic nature that give a paradigm its unique quality, not that each theory is especially formulated for one discipline or situation.

The preceding discussion of paradigms and theories was not meant to be a sophisticated all-inclusive philosophic or scientific presentation, but rather a basic discussion designed to build a common understanding to be used as a foundation for the ensuing discussion of specific organizational-administrative paradigms.

ORGANIZATIONS AND PARADIGMS

Organizations are good examples of paradigms in action. An organization's paradigms are what direct policies and technology, set standards of practice and behavior, and establish shared meaning. Evidence that a paradigm is present may be witnessed when an employee says, "That's the way we do things here." Most, if not all, nurses practice within the boundaries of some type of organization. An important assumption for this chapter is that nursing administration is related to, and is an integral part of generic organizational administration. According to Pfeffer,[4] "one of the critical administrative tasks involves the articulation of the organization's paradigm" (p. 228). Therefore, administrative changes and trends resulting from organizational paradigm shifts will affect the practices of nurse administrators. Nursing administration educators need to assume a reconnaissance position to detect common changes across organizations if the educators are to maintain relevant curriculum content and prepare students for the future. Reciprocal networks among nurse administrators and nursing administration educators can be resource reservoirs, and are essential for optimum functioning of both roles.

Paradigms that are serving an organization in a satisfactory manner (at least in the eyes of top administrators) tend to gel into the self-protective nature of a closed system with resistance to changes. Pfeffer noted, "if paradigms are the glue binding the organization together and differentiating it from its environment and other organizations, paradigm shifts are traumatic and fundamental events"[4] (p. 228). Reluctance to initiate traumatic and unsettling changes in organizational paradigms is one explanation of why nurses have experienced relatively powerless roles in health-care organizations for so long.

When organizational paradigms change, the shift is likely to be from one of two mechanisms.[4] A profound change may come when fundamental assumptions of the paradigm are challenged following acquisition of consistent information indicating that the organization's technology is ineffective, inefficient, or is outdated. A second mechanism of change that doesn't start out to be quite so profound begins subtly when the paradigm's

individual theories undergo corrections. As more and more theories are replaced by new theories, a positive feedback loop is established, chipping away at the paradigm's structure until the paradigm takes on a whole new composite personality. The first-type change is likely to occur because of external environmental influences, often with economics as chief catalyst. Profound changes in the paradigms of health-care organizations because of initiation of Medicare's Diagnosis Related Groups (DRG) prospective payment system is an example of how the first change mechanism works. A combination of external and internal influences such as increased technology and initiation of the baccalaureate degree as entry into professional nursing practice may bring about the second-type paradigm change. As the concentration of college-educated nurses increases to meet the needs of more complex technology, theories of efficiency through rote obedience will presumably be altered as nurses take rightful professional organizational positions. These two mechanisms of paradigm change afford nurses a fertile field for reflection and research.

If we are to gain a sense-making picture of how paradigm shifts have occurred, an overview of organizational paradigms across time must now be considered. Evidence that dominant organizational paradigms have had direct influence on nursing practice will be presented.

Orthodox Organizational Paradigms

Up until around the end of the 1930s, few people raised serious theoretical questions about organizations. The period might be referred to as a time of unchallenged classicism; a time when the emphasis was on structure and profit for the employer with little or no regard for the people who worked in the organization. The "Protestant work ethic" was in full force. It was considered "good" to

Table 42.1 Orthodox Organizational Paradigms

Time Frame of Popularity: 1940s to 1960s.

Sample of Theories:
1. Weber:[5] ideal bureaucracy; formal authority structures.
2. Taylor:[6] scientific management movement.
3. Fayol:[7] Formula for management: "POCCC" (Planning-Organizing-Command-Coordination-Control).

Characteristics:
- Mechanical; task orientation.
- Emphasis on efficiency and productivity.
- Quantity rather than quality.
- Strong bureaucratic authority structures; power concentrated at top of organization.
- Control of workers by rules and regulations; close supervision to enforce rules.

Evidence of Paradigm Effects on Nursing:
- Hospital administrators and physicians established policies and rules and retained high-status roles.
- Nurse administrators enforced rules and policies established by hospital administrators and physicians.
- Nurse administrators directed supervisors; supervisors supervised head nurses; head nurses supervised staff nurses.
- Close adherence to rules and policies.
- Staff nurses received assignments and practiced functional nursing.
- Salary, prestige, and privileges became progressively less down the chain of command.

---

work and "evil" to be idle. Indeed, if one did not work, one stood a good chance of starving. Working conditions were likely to be deplorable, with pay matching the conditions. World War II served to marshal a need for order in the schema of organizational paradigms. People who had never been in the work force joined in the production of goods and services that were major contributions to winning the war. Out of this time period, Weber[5] emerged with his rationalization of bureaucracy, establishing the basis for orthodox organizational theories. Although Weber's studies and writings began before World War II, it was not until 1947 that his writings were translated into English, spawning a persistent interest in organizational theory. With his quest to describe an ideal bureaucracy, Weber developed a theory whereby authority structures accounted for efficiency in productivity. Weber's theory of bureaucratic organizations is important to note since the theory has produced the underlying assumptions that we carry with us into the workplace. Weber's bare-bones theory was that the authority structures of centralization—where policies and rules are made—stratification—where rewards are divided—and formaliza-

tion—where workers are controlled by rules—account for the degree of efficiency in production. The higher the degree of authority structures, the higher the degree of efficient productivity. Degree of efficiency in production was another way of saying degree of profit for the organization's owner or top management. Efficient production was accomplished through a scalar principle with authority and supervision flowing downward. Even in the late twentieth century, most organizations are a variation on this mechanistic theme, despite modifications that have occurred over time. Table 42.1 illustrates the major characteristics of the period of orthodox organizational paradigms and its effects on nursing. Nurses who practiced in the 1950s and 1960s can readily recognize the paradigms of the period.

Neo-Orthodox Organizational Paradigms

The crack in the orthodox period occurred when people began to question why consideration of the individual wasn't part of the schema, and how one methodology could possibly cover all the situations arising in an increasingly complex world. The questioning

Table 42.2   Neo-Orthodox Organizational Paradigms

Time Frame of Popularity: 1950s to present.

Sample of Theories:
1. Mayo:[8] Hawthorne investigations; importance of human element as a variable rather than a constant.
2. Barnard:[9] interactions of people and activities within organizations.
3. McGregor:[10] Theory X and Theory Y.
4. Hage:[11] Effects of increased complexity on bureaucratic structures.
5. Drucker:[12] Management by objectives.

Characteristics:
- Emergence of human relations movement superimposed on mechanistic task orientation.
- Task (primary) plus people (secondary) orientation.
- Modified bureaucratic authority structures; increased decentralization; role redefinitions.
- Increased complexity of technology and specialists.
- Emphasis on quality as well as quantity, but quality may be sacrificed for increased efficiency and productivity.

Evidence of Paradigm Effects on Nursing:
- Changing job descriptions and role titles: director of nurses becomes vice-president for nursing; head nurses become coordinators; frequent elimination of supervisor position.
- Trend away from functional nursing to primary nursing care.
- Primary care nurses formulate own care plans, assume responsibility for own practitioner actions.
- Nurses recognize need for carrying own liability insurance.
- Coordinators participate in operational decision-making committees and budget preparation.
- Nursing administrators participate in making policy decisions.
- Many hospitals revert to more mechanistic team or functional nursing practices on evening and night shifts.
- Some increase in nurses' salaries; still large gap between hospital-administrators' and nurse-administrators' salaries and prestige.

in the system ushered in the human relations movement characterized by a whole generation of neo-orthodox humanist theorists who tried to fit people into bureaucratic organizational structures by using reconstructed logic. Table 42.2 illustrates an overview of paradigms and their effects during the Neo-Orthodox period, which is still in evidence. The majority of nurses in the late 1980s still practice in hospitals that are some variety of modified bureaucracy. Although nurses have made progress in participating in policy decisions (decentralization), have gained new titles and diversified positions, make more money, and have more autonomy of practice, the underlying bureaucratic assumptions are still present. We still search for ideal organizational methodology; profit and productivity are still dictators, nurses are still constrained by many rules, and there are still dining rooms exclusively for top hospital administrators and physicians. Care must be taken that nurses who move up in organizational administration are sensitive to the dif-

ference in making progress as full colleagues in health care versus simply being thrown crumbs or tokens of appeasement. For example, one might question whether decentralization is truly a step toward progress in administration, or whether nurses are simply being exploited in a new fashion. Where is the body of research that supports one view or the other? It is possible that decentralization is just another way of delegating troublesome operational tasks to lower status members of the organization; an easier way to ensure profit and productivity? This is an area worthy of attention by nurse administrators, nursing administration educators, and graduate nursing students who are seeking research topics.

Emerging Nonorthodox Organizational Paradigms

While there is continued emphasis on the importance of the individual in the organization, several other forces are operating in the emergence of nonorthodox organizational paradigms. The women's movement has been a catalyst prompting women nurses to take risks their older sisters would not have attempted. The women's movement has also had the effect of raising the percentage of women in medicine, a phenomenon that bears watching. Medicare's prospective payment system (DRGs) has exerted gigantic external pressure to change the system of health care, necessitating rapid development of new paradigms. When the DRG system spreads to other third-party payment systems, the effect will be even more profound. Changing economic systems have forced all types of organizations to reformulate their paradigms, and health-care agencies are no exception. The concept of profit has come out of the health-care closet with many hospitals becoming acknowledged for-profit institutions. Profit has become a goal in seeking institutional survival. One strategy for profit that has emerged is the methodology called diversification, a method where health-care agencies develop diversified services, or product lines, in an effort to increase revenue. Nursing administration educators would do well to prepare their students to capitalize on the opportunities afforded by diversification.

In the field of electronics, the development and endemic dissemination of computers, both personal and large organizational mainframes, have had major impact on organizations. In Weber's ideal bureaucracy, information by communication flowed upward so that top administrators could formulate rules and policies that then flowed downward. In late twentieth-century organizations, data from computers are rampant with communication flowing every which way. The immense increase in information flow caused Naisbitt to call the late twentieth era a virtual information society.[19] Horizontal flow of information has opened up the field of matrix management whereby projects are conducted across departments, eliminating duplication of tasks

and optimizing use of personnel. If nurses expect to thrive as well as survive in tomorrow's health-care field, it is imperative that nurses, especially nurse administrators, have user-knowledge of computer capabilities as well as knowledge of innovative applications for using increased communications.

A further event that has tremendous potential for nursing's professional growth and resultant paradigm changes in health care is the movement to establish the baccalaureate degree as an entry level requirement for professional nursing practice. According to Kanter,[14] as more and more workers become college educated, they attain higher degrees of knowledge, and "new attitudes about dignity, entitlement, and using their skills." Further, "Education creates another pressure for autonomy, flexibility, and freedom." The overall effect is to reduce the authority structures of top administrators as the workers become " 'knowledge workers' who cannot be closely supervised and controlled, because the organization counts on their knowledge and internal commitment to get the work done" (p. 56).

Table 42.3 suggests some of the emerging organizational paradigms of this complex age we live in. Tables included in this chapter are not meant to be exhaustive outlines of organizational paradigms, but are designed to offer the reader a flavor of how paradigms shift and affect both people and organizations. It is hoped that the figures will stimulate the reader, whether administrator, student, or educator to engage in further analyses of the dynamic nature of paradigms.

IMPLICATIONS FOR NURSING ADMINISTRATION EDUCATION

Nursing administration educators assume a great responsibility in preparing tomorrow's nurse administrators. Administration curriculum must include both the paradigms of the past and present for application to and ap-

Table 42.3 Emerging Nonorthodox Organizational Paradigms

Time Frame of Popularity: 1970s to future.

Sample of Theories:
1. Herzberg:[13] job satisfaction.
2. Kanter:[14] innovation through corporate entrepreneurs.
3. Weick:[15] organizational sense-making; coupling systems.
4. Matrix Management:[16] multiple-command system with overlapping roles.
5. Clark:[17] Alternative perspectives in administration.
6. Guba:[18] Context of emergent paradigm research.
7. Naisbitt:[19] Onset of the information age; the computer attack on established paradigms.

Characteristics:
- People (primary) plus Task (secondary) orientation.
- Further modification of bureaucratic structures.
- Overt challenge of orthodox paradigms; consideration of alternatives in decision making.
- Further emergence of new organizational roles.
- Tasks designed to benefit both worker and consumer.
- Increased awareness of environmental-economic impact.
- Emergence of the intra-organization entrepreneur.
- Reliance of quality to ensure profitability of organization.
- Overlapping of roles; networking and project cooperation across departments.
- Increased emphasis on organizational complexity.
- Increased communication from increased computer data.

Evidence of Emerging Paradigm Effects on Nursing:
- Nurse administrators are expected to develop new services to meet environmental needs.
- Nurses assume roles in product-line management.
- Nurses participate in marketing of services; primary nursing care proves to be profitable as well as beneficial.
- Increasing numbers of nurses complete higher-education degrees to qualify for complex practitioner roles; there is increased emphasis on professionalism.
- Increasing numbers of nurses are becoming self-employed.
- Salaries of nurses rise, particularly for top nurse-administrators.
- Clinical ladders afford upward mobility.
- Voice of nurses becomes stronger through nursing research.
- Increasing numbers of nurses are becoming computer users.

preciation of today's circumstances. Of greater importance, however, is the need to include curriculum content that addresses long-range projections of administrative activities and responsibilities. Although future administrators cannot be experts in all the complex technologies and theories, they need to have a working knowledge of as many potential aspects as possible if they are to participate actively in the moving and shaking of events. Educators are truly reconnaissance scouts and long-range crystal-ball gazers when planning administration curriculum. Table 42.4 presents a sample of curricular areas that need particular emphasis in order to address emerging paradigms of nursing administration.

In conclusion, if you are to be left with a few final words about organizational paradigms, let them be this: Look critically at the paradigms you have accepted in your professional life. It is entirely possible that the focus has been on the wrong side of the coin. Always consider alternatives; perhaps alternatives offer better explanations of the way the world works. For example, are we managing by objectives, or do our objectives manage us and limit our creativity? Another example, if the nonorthodox theorists are right, then organizations are simply places where a set of people come together to conduct their work in the most satisfying and self-actualizing manner possible. According to this alternative, the focus is on the worker, not the client or product. Our present-day nursing paradigms lead us to believe that organiza-

Table 42.4 Implications for Educational Emphasis

Source of Implications: Emerging Nonorthodox Organizational Paradigms.

Assumption: Paradigms that affect organizational administration also affect nursing administration.

Implicated Areas for Emphasis:
- Critical analysis of past and present theories and paradigms of organizational administration.
- Increased awareness of how paradigms shift.
- Change theories: effects of change theories on organizations; strategies to bring about desired changes.
- Power: attitudes toward power; acquisition of power; management of power; propensity to risk using power.
- Organizational Development.
- Critical analysis of environmental concerns that have potential impact on health care.
- Matrix management: what it is, and how it might be applied to nursing practice situations.
- Research concerning effects of organizational paradigms on nursing: inquiry into all organizational areas where questions might be raised concerning nursing's position or participation.
- Communication: strategies for improving interpersonal communication, networking, and diplomatic negotiation.
- Computer usage: minimum of an introductory course on word processing; encouragement of computer use through increased availability of computers in department.
- Budget analysis and preparation: health-care economics.
- Innovation: techniques and applications.
- Marketing: product-line management; improved techniques of recruitment and retention of nurses.
- Long-range planning: techniques and implementation.
- Decision-making techniques: emphasis on choosing quality (effectiveness alternative) over quantity (efficiency alternative).
- Development of theories that explain how nursing may grow as a viable power component within the health-care field.

tions should be client-centered, student-centered, and/or product-centered. So strong is this socialization that the suggested alternative will be shocking to some. But, think about it. What if the goal of nurse administrators or nursing administration educators was to create a facilitating environment where workers could aspire to self-actualization, to reaching their highest potentials? Would the client or student be the loser? Hardly, since workers who are professional nurses, whether practitioners, administrators, or educators, all share a mission of providing excellence in their practices in the field of health care. The client, student, product, or service would be an essential recipient of excellence in the worker's quest for self-actualization. Emerging paradigms can be winners. Think about it. The changes are up to us.

REFERENCES

1. Kuhn TS. Science does not develop by accumulation. In: Mosedale FE, ed. Philosophy and science: the wide range of interaction. Englewood Cliffs: Prentice-Hall Inc, 1979.
2. Coughlin EK. Thomas Kuhn's ideas about science: 20 years after the revolution. The Chronicle of Higher Education 1982,22:21–23.
3. Gale G. Theory of science: an introduction to the history, logic, and philosophy of science. New York: McGraw-Hill Book Co, 1979.
4. Pfeffer J. Organizations and organization theory. Boston: Pitman, 1982.
5. Weber M. The theory of social and economic organization. New York: Free Press, 1947.
6. Taylor FW. Scientific management. New York: Harper & Row, 1947.
7. Fayol H. General and industrial management (Storrs C, Trans). London: Pitman, 1949.
8. Mayo E. The human problems of an industrial civilization. New York: Macmillan, 1933.
9. Barnard CI. Organization and management. Boston: Harvard University Press, 1948.
10. McGregor D. The human side of enterprise. New York: McGraw-Hill, 1960.
11. Hage J. Theories of organizations: form, process, and transformation. New York: John Wiley & Sons, 1980.
12. Drucker PF. The practice of management. New York: Harper & Row, 1954.
13. Herzberg F. Work and the nature of man. New York: World Publishing Co, 1966.
14. Kanter RM. The change masters: innovation and

entrepreneurship in the American corporation. New York: Simon & Schuster, 1983.

15. Weick K. The social psychology of organizing. Reading, MA: Addison-Wesley, 1979.

16. Davis SM, Lawrence PR. Matrix. Reading, MA: Addison-Wesley, 1977.

17. Clark DL. Emerging paradigms in organizational theory and research. In: Lincoln YS, ed. Organizational theory and inquiry. Beverly Hills: Sage Publications, 1985.

18. Guba EG. The context of emergent paradigm research. In Lincoln YS, ed. Organizational theory and inquiry. Beverly Hills: Sage Publications, 1985.

19. Naisbitt J. Megatrends: ten new directions transforming our lives. New York: Warner Books, 1982.

43

A Practicum Experience: Use of the Charns and Schaefer Model for the Managerial Assessment of a Nursing Unit

Arlene Lowenstein

THE PROCESS of nursing management has been described as paralleling that of the nursing process.[1] Both nurses and nurse administrators assess, plan, implement, evaluate, reassess, and replan. Obtaining a patient history and performing a physical assessment is the first step in assessing for patient care. Nurses are taught a systematic method to carry out the assessment and obtain data to be used in the development of patient care plans. Planning for a nursing department or unit also requires a systematic approach to assessment. A nurse administrator should be able to take an organizational history, perform an organizational exam, and use that data to develop a managerial care plan.

Educators often use the case study method and practicum experiences to assist nursing administration students learn organizational assessment skills. The case study method allows the student to gain analysis skills, given specific data. The practicum allows the nursing administration student to observe and work with a practicing nurse administrator in an actual health-care setting. Analysis in the actual setting is more difficult than case study analysis, because the information needed for analysis must be selected by the student. In

the real-world conditions change over time, new information is constantly entering the system, and interpersonal dynamics change as people enter or leave and new coalitions are formed.

An organizing framework can be helpful in assisting students in a practicum experience to analyze the organization to which they are assigned. Charns and Schaefer[2] have defined and systematized the elements in an organization that can be assessed for both operational, or short-term, and strategic, or long-term, planning and decision making. In the same manner that the nurse assesses the cardiovascular system or gastrointestinal system of a patient and makes a nursing diagnosis, a nurse manager or student using the elements identified by the Charns and Schaefer model, can assess organizational systems such as the external environments, mission, purpose and goals, and the work of an organization, to develop an organizational diagnosis. While the taxonomy for nursing diagnosis exists, there is no accepted taxonomy for organizational diagnosis currently available. Although there may be no specific diagnostic term available, the model can still be useful in categorizing problem areas.

The model is geared toward a macroanalysis of health-care organizations, but adaptations can be made for microanalysis at the unit or departmental level of many types of organizations, since the model is based on universal management concepts. This needs to be done with some caution, however, recognizing that this is an adaptation, and concepts may not fully translate from macroanalysis to microanalysis. The model elements and theoretical constructs have been used effectively by students in practicum experiences in nursing service departments and educational settings at the divisional, departmental, and unit levels.

The Charns and Schaefer model for health-care organizations is based on contingency theory, which holds that managerial decisions are contingent on situational factors, therefore single prescriptive actions cannot be universally appropriate. However, there are guidelines that an administrator may use to gather information, and strategies that may be chosen once an assessment has been made. Students can use the model to become aware of areas to analyze and questions to ask. The model incorporates many organizational theories. Students can also use the model to become more familiar with organization theory and terminology, and can refer back to the original theorists and their writings when developing managerial strategies.

The Charns and Schaefer model is based on the following premises:

1. Organizations are open systems that exist in and interact with their environments.
2. Organizations exist to do work.
3. Requirements for organizations depend on the characteristics of work. (p. 26)

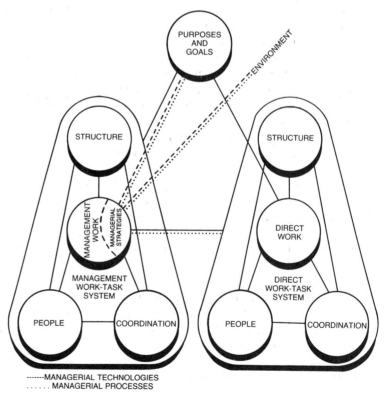

Figure 43.1. A Contingency Model for Organization and Management. (Adapted by permission from Charns MP, Schaefer MJ. Health care organizations: A Model for Management. Englewood Cliffs, New Jersey: Prentice-Hall, Inc, 1983, p. 285)

Table 43.1 Organizational Management Decision Making

	Time Dimension	
Decision-Making Categories	Operational	Strategic
I. Interface of the Organization with its external environment		
1. external environment		
2. mission, purposes, and goals		
II. Organizational Design		
1. work		
2. structure		
3. coordination		
4. people		
III. Managerial Strategies (tools and techniques)		
1. technologies		
2. process		

Sources (unpublished): Schaefer MJ, University of Pittsburgh.

Eight major elements have been identified for assessment (see Figure 43.1). Each element can be further broken down by use of key words to identify situational factors, potential problem areas, and strategies to be considered.

The major elements include:

- External Environment
- Mission, Purpose, and Goals
- Work—direct, management, and indirect or support work
- Structure
- Coordination
- People—individuals and groups
- Management Technologies
- Managerial Processes

Schaefer[3] placed the model elements into three major decision-making categories that can be examined over two time frames. The time dimension consists of both operational decision making and strategic decision making. The operational dimension refers to the current period of time and short range planning, while the strategic dimension refers to the future and long range planning. The first category—interface of the organization with its external environment—contains two elements, external environment and mission, and purpose and goals. The second category—organizational design—includes the elements of work, structure, coordination, and people. The final category is that of managerial strategies—or tools and techniques—and includes the elements of managerial technologies and managerial processes (see Table 43.1).

There are no right or wrong answers in using this model. Each choice is an individual one, based on the unit of analysis and the individual organization. Although the model is set up in categories, those categories often have fuzzy edges, and may change or overlap. It is important to be flexible and view the model as a guide. The model provides a framework to use to identify important areas for assessment, to increase observational skills, and to develop conscious planning efforts instead of spur-of-the-moment or impulsive planning.

Examination of each element has been modified to include both a physical assessment of the conditions in the element and a strategy assessment to identify dynamics and current strategies in use. Each model can be assessed to recognize areas of strength that can be utilized and reinforced, and to identify problems that need to be addressed.

INTERFACE OF THE DEPARTMENT WITH ITS EXTERNAL ENVIRONMENT

The first two elements, external environment and mission, purpose and goals, deal with the interface of the department with its external environment. The first step in the analysis is to identify the departmental boundaries, thereby separating the internal from the external environment. In the clinical setting, this means identifying the people who directly contribute to the work of the department. This is not as simple as it sounds. In one student assessment, the internal nursing unit consisted of nursing staff, including registered and practical nurses, nursing assistants, plus two unit clerks. Although the clerks were not structurally under the nursing department, two specific individuals were designated to the nursing unit and contributed regularly to the work of the department; therefore, they were considered internal to the unit. In the same manner, specific resident physicians were considered internal because they regularly contributed to the unit. Other residents who covered patients sporadically were considered external. In some settings, certain physicians who consistently admit patients to the unit and physicians designated as unit medical directors could be considered internal, even though those physicians are not employed by the hospital. The unit boundaries are established by including those persons falling under the criteria of regularly contributing to the work of the unit, and not by administrative structural design.

External Environment

The physical assessment of the external environment requires identification of categories of people and organizations that relate to the department. These categories include customers, suppliers, competitors, regulators, and other stakeholders (people who have an interest in the department but are not part of it). By identifying patients as customers, marketing techniques and strategies can be selected to work with specific market segments, depending on the desired clientele, and can be used to identify group needs. In many of the student assessments, physicians were also considered customers, since they were responsible for patient admissions. In some cases nursing administration and hospital administration were considered customers when a unit had developed a specific project it wanted funded. Recognizing these groups as customers helps in the selection of strategies for working with them.

Assessment of each of the other categories, looking at strengths and problem areas, can increase awareness of relationships and dependency on the external environment. Hospital and nursing administration were recognized as regulators but also as suppliers of resources. Nursing units compete with each other for a share of those resources. Similar units in other hospitals may also be classed as competitors for both customers and for human resources. Students analyzing intensive care units needed to be aware of the competition with other local hospitals for attracting and keeping intensive care nurses. Recognition of major competitors within and outside of the health care setting encourages conscious competitive strategy formation.

The next part of the physical assessment of the external environment consists of looking at the environmental characteristics. The environment is assessed in relation to stability, complexity, population dynamics, hostility, market diversity, and legitimacy, or the acceptance of departmental services. One student found that legitimacy was the major problem in a program of pulmonary rehabilitation. Even though the nurse clinical specialist was well respected and the role and program was supported by administration, the physicians and staff nurses did not refer patients for the program, although they did consult with her in other areas. Assessment pointed out that different strategies were required to demonstrate the need for the service and positive patient outcomes to physicians, staff nurses, patients, and the community at large. In addition, it was found that mechanisms for self-referral by patients and families were needed and possible once the community was aware of the need for the service.

Students assessing population dynamics looked at both the potential patient population, the physician population, and the labor pool. For some settings this was a critical problem, while other settings were found to be comparatively stable at the unit level. Potential changes in physician population were found to have a major effect in long-range planning for an obstetric unit in a community hospital. Community physicians were aging and many were reducing obstetric practice but continuing to care for gynecologic (GYN) patients. Unit survival in the organization could depend on the ability to attract new physicians interested in obstetric practice, or the decision could be made to decrease obstetric beds and increase GYN beds. Even though the actual decision to change the bed ratio may be made by hospital administration, nursing is influenced by that decision, and should be involved in strategy formation and in the decision-making process.

The strategy assessment includes identifying strategies that are being used to decrease organizational dependency on the external environment, protecting the core technology, reacting to competition, and identifying and participating in political activity. Recognizing and using these strategies allows the nursing manager to manage the external environment for the benefit of the nursing unit. Reducing organizational dependency is important in reducing uncertainty, conflict, and the frustration that can occur when the influences of the external environment override the perceived needs of the unit. Examples of strategies to decrease organizational dependency include cooptation, coalition formation, contracting, vertical integration, and public relations. Students can assess if these strategies are being used and if they are

effective or needed. Developing coalitions with consumers was found to be an important strategy in establishing and encouraging the role of the nurse practitioner in an ambulatory setting. Vertical integration, or control over unit resources, was demonstrated in one setting by the establishment of a distinct staffing pool specifically for one unit, thereby reducing the need to depend on a centralized staffing pool in which many units competed for resources.

Protecting the core technology could mean buffering, smoothing, anticipation or forecasting, and rationing. Overhiring unit nursing staff when nursing school graduations occur is an example of both buffering and forecasting. In one assessment, turnover was usual in July and September due to the nature of the community in which a medical center was a major employer. By overhiring when a supply of nurses was available, orientations and state boards were completed when the turnover materialized.

Mission, Purpose, and Goals

The second major element for assessment is mission, purpose, and goals. Categories for assessment in this element are identification of domain, task system, formal and informal goals, and distinctive competence. The departmental domain includes the product and services offered, customers, technology utilized (including professional services), and the location where the work is performed. The task system is identification of the major missions of multipurpose organizations, including an understanding of priority standings of those missions. This is particularly important in teaching hospitals and research universities, since priority of mission may indicate how resources will be allocated. Even though patient care may be most important to the unit, it may not be most important to the organization.

Along with identification of formal and

written goals, it is also important to assess the informal goals, which may be very different from the formal goals. In one unit, the student found that the major written goal was care of the psychiatric patient, but the unit was also used for overflow for medical-surgical patients. The unwritten purpose of providing care to other than psychiatric patients created a significant amount of uncertainty in the work of the unit and demonstrated a lack of control in the unit's internal environment.

Distinctive competence includes understanding what the unit can do best and how this differs from the competition. Competition may include similar units in other health care settings, or other units in the same organization that compete for resources. Recognition of distinctive competence can assist in promoting the unit and in the development of competitive strategies.

Strategy assessment in this category includes identifying dominant coalitions that set formal goals, informal goals, or both. It is important to assess nursing's position in those coalitions. Is nursing a part of those decisions, or are those decisions made elsewhere and is nursing left to react? Formal goals can be set by one coalition, but the staff may form a coalition to set informal goals if they are not in agreement with the formal goals. Efficiency is compromised in that instance, and conscious or unconscious sabotage may occur.

It is important to identify the information base and understand how information can be obtained for both external and internal goal monitoring. Students were able to examine quality assurance programs in this area. In some instances it may be necessary to develop an additional information base, such as patient satisfaction questionnaires. It is also important to understand the unit's role and participation in the institutional strategic planning process, and how information is transmitted for planning purposes.

ORGANIZATIONAL DESIGN

The model elements of work, structure, coordination, and people are internal to the unit of analysis and influence decision making about organizational design. The element of work is critical to the model. The analysis is geared to understanding what the work of the organization is or should be. Charns and Schaefer call work "the link between what the environment presents as opportunities, constraints, and demands—from which are developed the organization's purposes—and the structure, coordination, and people required to meet those purposes." (p. 81) There are different types of work. Direct work is directly related to the organization's purpose and is done to reach an organizational goal. Management work is another form of work required by the organization and requires different skills. Managerial work includes decision making authority and responsibility. Support work, or indirect work, provides support for direct work and for management work. It does not directly affect the organization's goals, but is needed to promote efficient direct work and management work.

Direct Work Analysis

The analysis of the direct work element includes the identification of the components of work. It is important to distinguish work from working. Working deals with the people who do the work and those who affect how the work is carried out. Separating out what is currently being done and what needs to be done, regardless of the worker, allows a more objective view. The two concepts of work and working come back together in the analysis of the people element. Management work, support work for direct work, and support work for management work can also be analyzed using the same categories discussed below.

The components of work include an analysis of individual pieces of the work that need to be done to carry out the goals and objectives of the unit. It was emphasized to students that the assessment needs to take into consideration work that needed to be done, even though it was not being done at that point in time. Breaking the work into component parts allows identification of areas of interconnectedness and uncertainty. These are important concepts in deciding structure and coordination, and in identifying areas of potential conflict. The direct work of patient care includes more than nursing, although nursing is, of course, a major component. Students were able to focus on total care for patients for the assessment. Analysis of the pieces of work and the complexity of the work required provides information necessary to make decisions on the personnel qualifications most appropriate for the job. It was also important to separate ritual from the real work need.

Identification of time boundaries for work is important in resource allocation. This explores the differences in the required work—daily and over time. Patient acuity changes over time in the units, and different tasks are required at different times of the day. In some surgical units patient care needs increased in the evening or on specific days due to operating room scheduling. Weekends were found to be light on some units because of patient discharges, while on other units work was particularly heavy on Sunday afternoons because of patient admissions. In assessing ambulatory care settings, it was important to consider patient needs when clinics were not normally in session. It was also important to consider where the work was done. For the surgical patient, part of the work of patient care is done off the unit, in the operating room and recovery room. Patients may also leave the unit for X Ray and physical therapy. This analysis becomes important in looking at coordinating the work.

There are also technological boundaries to work. In this analysis technology is considered to be more than hardware, but also includes skills and training requirements, interpersonal requirements, and practice differences. Various professions and services have defined their work. Students were requested to look at this broadly, analyzing the skills needed to carry out the work before making personnel decisions. Professional boundaries do change as new technology comes in. Nurses function very differently today than in the past, even the recent past. Nurse practitioners and clinical specialists provide patient care that not so long ago was considered medical practice, rather than nursing practice. In the same vein, in some settings respiratory therapists or physical therapists provide some patient care during the day, but nurses pick up those treatments during evenings, nights, and weekends. This may or may not be appropriate, depending on the work required. The rate of technologic change was also found to be important. In some facilities students found frequent changes in technology, but others were slower to incorporate those changes.

Students were able to assess the interconnectedness of the required work. Some elements of work can be performed independently; others can be performed sequentially or simultaneously. In the delivery room simultaneous attention needs to be given to both mother, baby, and in some instances the father. Recognition of this element provided information for personnel decisions and coordination strategies. Along with interconnectedness, students also assessed task uncertainty. The more uncertain the task, the more professional judgment is needed. Different pieces of work may require different skill levels. In complex settings more professional nurses will be needed than in simpler, more programmable settings where licensed practical nurses or nurse assistants may be used. There is always an element of uncertainty in health-care work, but in some settings prior experience and familiarity with the work allow for different levels of staff to be chosen.

Task uncertainty is also affected by the environmental influences previously mentioned—stability, complexity, diversity, and hostility. The age and size of the organization and the unit of analysis also influences task uncertainty.

The impact of power strategies on the work was also assessed by students. Organizational ownership affects the work and the level of uncertainty. Government-owned hospitals and clinics function differently than for-profit corporations, even at the unit level. The ability to respond to change and environmental pressures differs from setting to setting. Fashion also influences work. New techniques and technologies may be brought into the setting because someone influential likes them, or they are the current trend. Trends can change quickly, however, and something that works in one setting may not effectively translate to another.

Also included in the work analysis is identification of resource requirements needed to carry out the work. These include human resources—based on job requirements, financial resources, information, equipment and supplies, space, and the need for support work. Work controls also need assessment. This includes an analysis of how feedback is given to direct workers and identification of work controls in use or needed. In all settings students assess if the work needs control the schedules or if the schedules control the work to be done.

Structure and Coordination

The analysis of the elements of structure and coordination are related. It entails examination and identification of the basic structure of the unit that allows the work to be accomplished, and a look at strengths and problem areas found in both the structure and coordinating the work of the unit. In addition it is important to identify collateral organizations and overlays to the basic structure, such as committees and task forces. Students are

asked to examine the formal and informal organizational structure to assess where decisions are actually made. Points of similarity, differences, and interconnectedness in work and the work group are important to assess. These points demonstrate the potential for conflict and the dynamics that are being used formally and informally in dealing with conflict.

The health-care arena has been changing rapidly. With the implementation of Diagnosis Related Groups (DRGs) into a prospective payment system for hospitals, many hospital organizations are restructuring to provide product- or service-line management, using DRGs to define "products." In some cases nurses are becoming service-line managers, but physicians or other administrators are taking on that role in other organizations.

For many units a functional structure exists, with nurses reporting to a department of nursing. But all nurses in the organization are not necessarily included in that organizational structure. Nurses may be employed in the outpatient area, emergency services, X-Ray department, or operating room, but the formal organization does not include them in the nursing department. At the same time, policies and procedures developed for the nursing department may also apply to those nurses. Service-line management and program structures may actually create matrix structures, where there is accountability in more than one area. The establishment of mechanisms for communication and input into decision making through collateral organizations, committees, and coordinators may be needed to address this issue.

These are complex issues for students to assess. Students are asked to examine the functional and dysfunctional characteristics of groupings for work. This includes identifying the work group, looking at the impact of specialist groups, and identifying geographic groupings. At the same time students assess groups that address interconnections in the work required. This is the area where centralization versus decentralization issues are explored. It is often difficult to focus on the internal unit and not get into complications regarding the interface with the external environment. A major purpose of this assessment is to recognize points of potential conflict, increase work efficiency, and clarify responsibilities. Organizational structural design always involves trade-offs.

Assessment of the coordination element involves identifying where resources need to be shared, identifying the existence and effectiveness of vertical information systems, noting rules and regulations developed to increase clarity of expectations, and observing the dynamics of conflict resolution currently occurring in the organization. Students look for conflict behaviors that may include avoiding, smoothing, unilateral-decision making, forcing, confronting, and bargaining. Some of these behaviors may show up again in the areas of people and managerial processes.

People

This is the area that addresses working. Analysis includes people as individuals and people as part of groups. In looking at individual workers, students assess individual perceptions of the work that needs to be done as well as values, skills, and abilities of the workers internal to the department. Recognition of cognitive dissonance can help in understanding readiness for change. An assessment of the organizational fit between the work and the worker should be carried out. Assessment of turnover can provide information about organizational fit. Understanding unit expectations is important in recruitment and retention of new staff. Students found that when there was clarity and agreement by staff with the goals and objectives of the unit, job expectations could be clarified and accepted. Feedback could be accepted in a constructive manner when it was related to goals and objectives and clear job expectations.

Reward systems and motivation strategies can have both positive and negative effects on individuals. Students assessed the existence and effect of extrinsic and intrinsic rewards. In particular, they looked at staff expectations of the results of their behavior and behaviors that were actually rewarded in the system. Some people are rewarded for good work by being given more work because they can do it so well. This is not always perceived as a reward. Individuals differ in their needs for power and achievement.

Assessment of job design is an integral part of this model. Job design includes more than addressing the work needed. It also addresses the needs of the worker. Areas of skill variety, task significance, autonomy, and feedback are pieces of job design that can be assessed. Appropriate and regular feedback is important to job performance. Feedback provides information to the worker about job performance and comes from many different sources. Besides supervisors, feedback was found to come from patients, physicians, and peers. Informal feedback can be valued and may not be the same as formal feedback. Differences between informal and formal feedback may lead to worker confusion and resentment or hostility. Feedback given sporadically, only in the form of criticism, or both can be destructive to job performance.

Assessment of people as groups entails identification of both formal and informal groups, and formal and informal group leaders. Types of groups identified were work groups, committees, task forces, teams, and informal liaisons. Some groups span the boundaries of the internal and external environments. Boundary spanners need to be recognized and can be utilized in strategy formation.

People make different decisions as individuals than they do as part of groups, and it is important to understand the effect of the group and of the dynamics occurring. Groups develop norms that need to be consciously understood. Group norms were found to be both functional and dysfunctional. Socialization and acceptance needs of individuals influence group formation and efficiency.

Groups also perform differently depending on their size, age, and composition. Team nursing may be used as one method for delivering patient care, but teams will function differently if they are kept constant over a period of time, or established each day by head nurse assignment.

Two types of group leadership were assessed by students, task leaders, and socioemotional leaders. Task leadership behaviors were geared toward getting the work done, while socioemotional leadership behaviors were oriented toward the interpersonal relationships in the group and how group members worked with each other. These behaviors can be found in both formal and informal group leaders and may surface at different times in the group process. The amount of emphasis needed in each area may depend on the purpose and composition of the group. Group process may be time-consuming, but may also be advantageous in expanding thought processes. However, even though a group consensus can ostensibly be reached, all members may not agree or be invested in the decisions, and group decisions may not be effectively implemented in the work setting. Recognition of group dynamics assisted students in recommending when tasks could be performed more efficiently by a group or an individual. Assessment of the effectiveness of group leadership strategies assisted in further strategy development.

MANAGERIAL STRATEGIES

The elements of "managerial technologies" and "managerial processes" are the tools and techniques that assist in the development of managerial strategies. The Charns and Schaefer model describes the technology as both hardware—such as computer systems,

and other or nonhardware based—such as rules and regulations, policies, and so on. The process strategy is an interpersonal one. Students have found major problems in these areas. Policies do not always effectively address the problems for which they were formulated. Some policies are ignored and others may be followed too strictly, prohibiting flexibility when needed. Budget information systems may not be current enough to provide effective monitoring. Communications are often viewed as a problem between administration and staff. Change strategies may create discomfort and hostility. But there are also strengths to these elements. The technology assists in reducing uncertainty and the process compliments the technology with the human element and can motivate and increase productivity. Even though change or conflict may be uncomfortable, it is necessary to continued efficiency and development of an organization. Understanding barriers and dynamics can assist in developing more effective strategies. Managerial strategy assessment can be carried on simultaneously with the other model elements.

Managerial Technologies

The managerial technologies element includes examination of management information systems, budgets, rules, regulations, policies, and procedures to determine impact and effectiveness. Managerial technologies are tools to assist in decision making. They are used to program work—to make it simpler to accomplish—and to facilitate information-gathering, thereby reducing uncertainty. Students assess both potential positive and negative effects of these technologies. Technologies can be developed and used proactively as well as reactively. Students can examine the effectiveness of current information systems, but also identify superfluous information and needs not addressed by the system. Students may not need to examine every unit policy and procedure, but they should recognize consistent infractions or confusion.

Managerial technology assessment can be accomplished systematically by categorizing policies according to the other model elements, although many technologies are used in more than one area. Examples of technologies that may affect the environment are accreditation and reporting requirements; examples of those that may affect purpose and goals are information systems and standards and formal goal-planning systems. Direct work technologies may include patient care procedures and policies. Structure and coordination technologies are reflected in organization charts, job descriptions, staffing systems, patient acuity systems, and general and specific policies and rules. People technologies may include personnel evaluation, staff education systems, and reward and compensation systems. Financial systems and planning systems assist management work.

Managerial Processes

Managerial processes are interpersonal processes and strategies used in the organization. The processes of communication and change come into play in this element. Students can perform a power and influence analysis to know who makes decisions, and who needs to make them. Nurse administrators need to recognize which decisions need to be influenced; students can explore the impact of decisions to identify potential problems. Actors may change with new or different decisions, so that analysis needs to be ongoing. The element calls for analysis of leadership styles and recognition of informal leaders. Governance issues and communication systems are important here. Both overt and covert conflict situations and strategies need to be recognized and assessed.

PRIORITY SETTING

Assessment of the model elements is the first step in diagnosing the unit or organization. When areas of strength and weakness have been identified, strategies can be formulated to utilize and reinforce the strengths and deal with the problems. Systematic assessment provides the student with information needed to move on to the next step, prioritizing those problems and developing an administrative action plan. Even the simplest of organizations is complex and will have many areas of strengths and weaknesses. Only certain areas can be selected for action plans. The assessment model provides the student with a systematic way to consider the vast amount of information in a practicum setting and can be used to validate the selection of priority areas and actions.

Systematic assessment can be time-consuming for students during the learning process, in the same way that it takes time for the nurse to learn health assessment to develop patient care plans. In the beginning, students found it helpful to use a work book that incorporated the model elements. After they used the model a few times it became easier to consolidate areas and concentrate on specific sections. They began to recognize how to categorize staff comments to focus in on specific problem areas or identify strengths. In patient care the initial history and physical assessment provides a base to continue monitoring health-care status. An in-depth organizational analysis provides base-line information for students to continue monitoring organizational health and the effect of managerial strategies.

REFERENCES

1. Gillies D. Nursing management: a systems approach. Philadelphia: WB Saunders, 1982.
2. Charns M, Schaefer MJ. Health care organizations: a model for management. Englewood Cliffs, NJ: Prentice-Hall, Inc, 1983.
3. Schaefer MJ. Unpublished classroom discussions, University of Pittsburgh, 1985.

V

Introduction: The Practice of Nursing Administration

Marie Di Vincenti

NURSING administration is part and parcel of health care in the United States. It influences and is influenced by prevailing policies, science, and culture. Commitments to theory, research, education, and practice form a tradition in nursing that must be comprehended for nursing administration.

The practice of nursing administration and its symbiotic relationship to theory and inquiry has been a recurring theme in this book. Theory in nursing administration—its development, testing, and use—is an idea that is coming of age. Nurse administrators increasingly use theoretical knowledge, viewing such knowledge as an extension of scientific principles and perceiving it as useful for guiding everyday actions and making sound decisions. Theories are analytic tools for nurse administrators who wish to sharpen and focus their perspectives on the problems they face. The use of theory enables nurse administrators to make clearer sense of complex situations and to formulate the best possible strategies for rational action. Without a strong grounding in the finest knowledge, we run the risk of floundering aimlessly at work in a random tide of events.

Nursing administration is a full-fledged professional endeavor responsible for doing basic and applied research, which builds knowledge by testing existing theories and formulating new ones. Nurse administrators, who are concerned with nursing care and the effective administration of nursing services,

attend both to the art and science of nursing and management, and they support the scientific approach to research and education. This approach rests on the identification and articulation of suppositions, principles, and hypotheses about the *why* of events in the workplace with respect to the provision of nursing care and to the management of health care services.

Strong educational programs and sound research are inextricably tied to the development of knowledge and to the practice of effective nursing administration. Theoretical knowledge orders empirical observations and serves to stimulate the generation of new knowledge through research. Theory based on research findings applied to individual action is transformed, tested, and refined in practice. Nurse administrators are in a pivotal position to determine the important problems that need to be studied to generate new, useful knowledge addressing the dilemmas found in health care organizations.

There is an abundance of critical questions in need of answers in the field related to the costs of services, quality of care, productivity, and much more. Both educators and practitioners are reflecting, therefore, on practical as well as existential questions about the purpose and meaning of decisions and actions in a complex technological society and in large complex organizations. Many ways of thinking and numerous methods of analysis are being probed to educate future nurse administrators to function in a world of nearly constant transformation and flux.

Planned collaborative efforts to facilitate progress and adaptation are needed on the part of educators and administrators. Nurses in education and service can pave the way for students who must learn to deal with uncertainty, rapid transition, and a nearly endless stream of paradoxes. Both faculty and administrators have unique positions in the communities they serve and can set the scene for new innovative educational programs in universities and health care agencies. By strengthening the relationship and lessening the gap between nursing education and nursing service, both consumers and students profit.

Nursing administration is changing both in private and public institutions. To retain a capacity for responding imaginatively to the current dynamic social environment, educators and administrators are encouraged to take a leadership role in identifying and incorporating educational and scientific advances into newly designed training and academic curriculums. Seeking a shared sense of purpose and vision, which is grounded in the realities of the present, nurses in both capacities can lead in the development of sound, sensible scientific programs.

One of our goals must be the conceptualization and organization of a system of education for the future. Such a model may well include participative curriculum planning and flexible, alternative teaching strategies. In addition, an educational agenda needs to be promoted that encourages a fundamental concern for high standards of effective practice, quality care, and intelligent empirical observations. The formation of partnerships and other cooperative arrangements between higher education and health service institutions can expand the resources available to both groups, and contribute to each group's goal to elevate nursing beyond the level of apprentice training to a professional discipline.

The future for nurse administrators and nurse educators can be bright. But we are our main limitation: The question is whether we have the vision, faith, and zeal to rise to the challenge and successfully meet it. There has never been a time when there has been a greater demand for improved, high-quality health care. Both academicians and providers of services can transform the meaning of education for the practice of nursing administration by transmitting understanding of the past, preparing for the present, and creating a new, brighter future.

The majority of the chapters in this section represent collaborative efforts by managers and educators to understand one another and to compose in writing central ideas about problems they encounter and ways they consider reasonable for solving those problems given existing knowledge.

Departments of nursing and health care organizations vary widely in size, age, history, and level of maturity. Modes of departmental governance also vary, as do the personalities of nurse administrators, and the approaches to decision making and to accomplishing the tasks relative to the work that needs to be done. To develop a set of absolute prescriptions that would provide every administrator with solutions to each and every problem would be an impossible task and certainly beyond the scope of any single volume.

This section of the book, however, describes a number of problems relevant to contemporary practice, and provides insights about how some dilemmas can be addressed. The selected problem-solving models contributed by the authors—nurse educators and administrators and consultants, often writing in teams—encourage creativity and foster a determination to explore different views. Our goal in this section is to present readers with substantive, practical, and theoretical knowledge about developments in the fields of nursing and management, including fresh concepts and current research.

In the opening chapter "From the Transition Stage to the Transformed Organization," Fine suggests that major forces and changes occurring in society call for a restructuring of health care organizations. An understanding of the basic changes occurring during transitions in a health care setting can be valuable to nurse administrators. The need to manage transformations successfully is paramount to survival. Fine provides a theoretical framework that can be helpful to members of any organization.

Chapter 45, entitled "Value Conflicts in Nursing Administration," is written by Scalzi of the University of Texas at Austin, and by Nazarey, a nurse administrator at Harbor-UCLA Medical Center. Their concern is about promoting an awareness of personal, professional, and organizational values, and improving understanding of the role these values play in decision making and leadership. The authors discuss the nature of valuing, the consequences for interpersonal relationships, and the conflicts that can result.

Comparable worth is an idea that Swansburg and Barnett believe is important to nurses and deserves to be understood from several perspectives: the dissatisfaction of professionals in organizations, societal values with respect to the work of women, occupational segregation, and free markets and fair wages. Personal change and crowding theory are also discussed by the authors.

"Labor Relations: Theory, Research, and Strategies" is the title of Chapter 47, by Throckmorton and Kerfoot. These authors provide an overview of the dimensions of labor relations and discuss strategies used by employees when they perceive that management is arbitrary or working conditions are substandard. Although nurses use traditional modes of collective bargaining, their concerns center on achieving professional autonomy and control over standards of practice. A choice of routes for action that emphasizes avoidance of collective bargaining and tradi-

tional union representation is described. Supporting research related to the reasons nurses are dissatisfied and thus support collective action or leave their jobs provides knowledge for guiding administrative action. The authors also discuss how faculty attitudes toward collective action affect students' perceptions of unions and unionization.

The importance of collaboration when conducting nursing research is described in Chapter 48 by Kelley and Patterson of the University of Alabama in Birmingham. The essential dimensions of cooperative research endeavors are identified, followed by a description of the collaborative model developed by the authors. The usefulness of the model, the research studies which have been done, and the team work at various levels of administration and education demonstrate how the valuing of research has been translated into practice and how this translation has changed education.

In Chapter 49, Snowden, academic coordinator of the community health nursing program at Louisiana State University, and Steedley, a nurse administrator in a home health care agency address the changing role of administrators in home health care in the context of historical and legislative perspectives. Although nurse administrators encounter many critical problems, defining the nature and boundaries of home care is one of the most critical. Nurses in home health care organizations find themselves juggling resources trying desperately to maintain an economically viable position. Two theoretical perspectives—change and marketing—can serve as a basis for making decisions about the problems encountered. The care of clients in their homes is a fertile ground for nursing research and the generation of new knowledge to deal with very real and extremely complex problems.

Chapter 50 by Barbara Stevens Barnum is entitled "Contributions of Nursing Administration to the Development of Nursing as a

Discipline." This soliloquy on the contributions of nursing administration to the development of nursing as a discipline is thought provoking. The author expresses the view that nursing administration is a scapegoat and discusses her concerns about the relationship of administration to professional practice, the existing realities and images of nursing administration, and the need to differentiate between nursing practice and nursing as a discipline.

"Quality Care" by Donaho addresses the quality of nursing and nursing administration from the perspective of the nurse executive at work in a large, multisystem corporation. Assuming the nurse executive position in many health agencies requires an understanding of the nature of multi-institutional arrangements and the implications of these kinds of organizational structures for administrative and clinical practice. Donaho begins with a description of the characteristics, growth, and complexities of multi-institutional arrangements. She identifies seven functions or roles corporate nurses assume and offers substantive pointers for how to effectively assure quality services.

"Nursing Administration in Long-Term Care" is the title of Chapter 52 by Bahr, a nurse educator, and McConnell, administrator of a nursing home. The major problem the authors focus on is the unavailability of professional nurses interested in employment in long-term care facilities. The problem of too few professional nurses is viewed historically and within the context of today's educational system, and in terms of the image and practice of nurses employed in nursing homes. A model of the critical issues is provided accompanied by suggested mechanisms and strategies to alleviate some of the problems nurse administrators in these agencies face.

Malkemes and Wisener, authors of Chapter 53, entitled "Consultation and the Nurse Executive," are practicing health care consultants. Malkemes holds a position as an independent technical advisor to a large international consulting firm and Wisener is in a principal administrative position with this same firm. Their work focuses on the various modes of consultation, the roles of consultants, and the benefits to nurse executives of using consultants. They suggest that both process and technical consultation can be extremely helpful and supportive to practicing executive nurses.

"Executive Succession" is the chapter written by Fuszard, on faculty at the Medical College of Georgia, and by Tilby, a practicing nurse administrator. The replacement of a nurse executive in a health care setting commands considerable attention in most instances. The primary question is: Does replacement come from within the organization or from outside? Theory and research addressing this question are explored and the implications are discussed in some detail. The authors also describe various models for studying managerial success as well as the existing research relevant to the varying dimensions of executive succession, which they caution is in its infancy. The nursing literature offers little on the topic and yet the turnover rate among nurse administrators is high. The information in this chapter begins to fill a gap in our understanding of who succeeds whom and why.

Poteet and Goddard contribute Chapter 55, entitled "Issues in Financial Management." The financing mechanisms in health care are of major concern to nurse administrators and require the meticulous attention of governmental leaders, health care administrators, consumers, and communities at large. Health care finance is of particular concern to nurse administrators who are currently striving to do more with proportionately fewer and fewer resources. Selected social forces affecting the economics of nursing are described with a focus on population demographics, ethnic diversity, technological change, and economic status.

"Application of Neuman's Model in Nursing Administration and Practice," by Raborn, a director of nursing, and Hinton, a nurse educator, provides a description of how one health care organization used the Neuman model as a basis for both nursing administration and clinical nursing practice. In this final chapter, the rationale and criteria for selecting Neuman's model are discussed. Administrative problems inherent in the application of the model requiring future research are identified.

44

From the Transition Stage to the Transformed Organization

Ruth Barney Fine

HEALTH-CARE organizations today face turbulent environments and organizational instability. The advent of prospective reimbursement in October 1983, caused the health-care system to experience more uncertainty than at any other time in the last 30 years. Some observers have termed this a time of revolution in health care.[1] Major forces exerting pressures on the health-care system are: changing health economy; increasing use of high and low technology; aging of the population; and expanding shortage of registered nurses.

ECONOMY

Evidence of revolutionary changes can be seen in the recession of the hospital economy in the United States. It is predicted that this recession will continue until the year 2000.[2] Patient days in short-stay hospitals declined 5 to 15% between 1983 and 1985, with an associated decrease in length of hospital stay. In 1983, 7.6 days was the average length of stay. This decreased to a national average of 6.7 days in 1985, and is anticipated to decline by another 8% by 1995.[3]

Changes in the health-care economy have brought about turbulence in the environment in which health-care organizations exist. Market competition has become intense, new markets and clientele are being sought, and joint ventures and corporate restructuring are appearing to facilitate a more competitive position in the market place. The outcome of such restructuring are megasystems that drastically change the internal relationships among institutional members such as hospitals, as well as change the mission and the interaction with external bodies.

TECHNOLOGY

The need to shorten the patient's hospital stay has increased the application of high technology in hospital patient care. The use of computer-aided diagnosis and computer-assisted medicine will decrease the length of the patient's stay. The use of laser technology, angioplasty, CT (computed tomographic) scanning, ultrasound, organ transplantation, and artificial organ implantation are all predicted to improve the quality of health care for hospitalized patients, offering earlier diagnosis and hope of improved quality of life, and at times of life itself.[4] But this use of high technology will also profoundly change the character of the organizational structure and vitality. Associated with use of high technology in hospitals is the expanded use of low technology in ambulatory situations and home care. These shifts have created a need for new modes of delivery systems in both hospital and ambulatory care environments.

POPULATION CHANGES

Another major force is the changing composition of the population. In the first quarter of the twenty-first century there will be 60 million Americans over 65 years of age.[5] Forecasts suggest that by 2010 there will be nearly 5 million people 65 years or older in the work force. This represents an increase from 21% to 26% in their participation in the work force.[6] The continuation of the older worker will also have a direct impact on organizations and will add to uncertainty in the organization. In addition, the rapidly increasing elderly population and their associated health problems will add to the complexity of ethical and religious issues faced by health-care institutions.

SHORTAGES OF REGISTERED NURSES

Shifts in the national economy as well as expanding opportunities for women in the work force are adversely affecting the nursing work force, resulting in a shortage of registered nurses and decreased enrollment in schools of nursing. Such shortages bring an increasing need to examine organizational structure, values, and culture and the need to improve the quality of work life and offer positive incentives for the recruitment and retention of registered nurses.

THE STAGE OF TRANSITION

The wide-ranging economic changes, increasing regulation, external competition, rapid technological changes, changing composition of the work force, and the general population call for a restructuring of health-care organizations. Nurse administrators enmeshed in this revolution often find themselves between two worlds, that which has been and that which will be—a period of transition, uncertainty, and adaptation to expanding service demands such as new markets and decreasing demands in other service

areas. Often the nurse administrator's immediate reaction to ambiguous demands is to respond with vagueness regarding long-range goals and to reduce the length of time to achieve those goals. Uncertainty often leads to a feeling of powerlessness. There is a need, therefore, to understand the transitional state so the feeling of powerlessness can be managed and change can be viewed in a positive manner.

The transitional state may be likened to a bridge—it is neither the old organizational world nor the transformed organizational world, it is rather the bridge that leads from the old to the new. The transitional state is a time of disengagement and re-engagement, a time when organizational personnel step from one shore onto the bridge (the transition stage) that will lead to the other shore where individuals will find their vision of a transformed organization.

The transition state is neither the old organization nor the new but the link that leads from one to the other. As the bridge is different from each shore, so is the transition state different from the old, traditional and the new, transformed organization.

Transition is different from change.[7] Change has a beginning and an end. Transition, however, begins with an ending. Transition requires that those wishing to progress to other organizational arrangements must let go of the past, disengage from the former patterns, and move into a "twilight zone" in which thoughts and actions are geared toward new situations not yet fully defined. The disengagement from the old order causes a fundamental difference in individual and collective thinking, and often produces a crisis in individual and group concepts.

Change starts with a beginning whereby the participants may go straight from what was to what is. It is often abrupt and clearly defined. In contrast, the transition stage may extend over time and require separate structures that differ from the old and may or may not differ from the new structures and structuring that will emerge. Some bridges are longer than others; some have guard rails or special regulations such as "no passing on the bridge." The major emphasis in this "bridging" stage is that the individuals, organizational groups, or both begin to act in new ways in order to undertake a successful journey.

Thus, the transition stage is a period of awakening, instability, unfreezing, restructuring, and changing of values. It is a time of reorganization and rebirth, and of building new cultures.

MANAGING IN THE TRANSITION STATE

Vision

The first step in the transition state is creating a vision. Nurse executive and nurses must have a vision of the future state. Nurses on each unit should ask where they want their organization to be in five years. What should the preferred future for this unit be? What should be the philosophy of patient care? of leadership? and of management? How do we wish to be treated, and how do we plan to treat patients, coworkers, and others? As nurses, executives, and staff begin to envision the future state, they identify hopes and expectations for an excellent organization. These statements of vision can be expressed as a philosophy. They are an essential part of the transition process.

It is important that each employee participate in building this vision. Personnel in each division or unit should be asked to contribute their visionary thoughts. Statements that express idealism should be encouraged to identify the kind of organization to be created. Organizational structures and structuring that best fit the desire for individual and organizational growth, development, and autonomy should be identified. Block lists in his book three criteria to achieve a great vision:

1. It comes from one's innermost being.
2. It is personal.
3. It is forceful and fundamental.[8]

Views of desirable states can be collected through nominal group technique; zeroing-in technique, derived from the nominal group technique; or another more elaborate process, such as the Delphi process.

The delphic technique is a tool for short-term forecasting. It consists of approximately three rounds of questionnaires given to a panel of experts and asks their expert opinions or judgments about a specific topic of interest. Feedback is given to the members of the expert panel by summarizing each round of questionnaires and returning to the experts a new questionnaire. Thus, a process of response–analysis–feedback–response is repeated (usually three times) until a general consensus is obtained.

As the vision of the future is articulated, a sense of accountability is established. Each member of the organization should hold themselves accountable for actions that are consistent with the vision. The creation of a vision is essential for the transition stage to be successful in helping individuals to disengage from the past and engage in the preferred future. The expression of a vision tells others where the organization is going and opens dialogue with others. But expression of a vision may also cause conflict since not all members will agree with it.

Block believes that the expression of a vision creates a feeling of autonomy among members, which may lead to conflict among participants.[9] Autonomy is defined as the attitude that one has choice and can make meaningful decisions. When organizational personnel contribute to the vision of a future they are declaring their stake in that organization. Further, they are demonstrating that they believe their views count and that their desires make them feel in charge of what is happening. The development of the feelings of autonomy moves the organization beyond participation to a more democratic workplace. Such changes may be resisted by present power holders.

Since visions are highly idealistic and therefore usually difficult to negotiate, there is an inherent risk of conflict when they are made visible.

Temporary Management Structures

During the transition period, temporary management structures need to be established. The establishment of temporary task forces or other intervention strategies should be put into place. When organizations collectively and individually disengage from the past, there is a need for the formation of new groups to assist the unfreezing process: new relationships can be started and trust can be established among group members. These mechanisms decrease conflict that may center around the vision statement.

A transitional manager or leader should be named to monitor, plan, and direct the movement through this stage. The transition manager should have attributes such as:

1. credibility and respect of those in leadership positions.
2. a reputation for wisdom and fairness.
3. ability to work with others.
4. creativity and flexibility.

The transitional leaders should be selected from those who have high right-brain activity, that is, those who can fantasize, dream, and be creative about the future. They should accept the vision of the future as a cause. The problem in selecting such leaders is that often they are not seen as credible by those left-brained, logical, analytic people in the organization. However, in the transition phase creativity, vision, and innovation are essential. Once the organization has moved into the new organizational mode, different

leadership can be put into place. But, during the transitional stage, it is important to keep the processes from falling into standardized routine; hence, the need for creative, innovative leadership.

The management structure devised for guidance through the transition stage should be manifestly different from the old structures, since those structures may or may not be the same ones desired for the new organization. During the transition a mission statement for the transformed organization should be developed. The mission statement should answer the following questions:

1. What does the organization (division or unit) see as its specific social function?
2. What levels of care and service should be provided?
3. What population groups and geographic area does the organization wish to serve?
4. What is expected of personnel who will provide this service?
5. How will personnel maintain the quality of their productivity?
6. What type of relationships does the organization wish to have with external groups, including competitors (cooperative, competitive, or antagonistic)?

Gaining Commitment

During the transition stage it is necessary to gain commitment to the vision and the mission for the transformed organization. Garnering this commitment and building a winning coalition is a political process and requires political skills.

To develop a political strategy one must first determine:

1. What people or groups are needed for the issue to succeed?
2. Further, are these people or groups for, against, or neutral toward the issue?

3. What is the power of the individual or group? Can they obstruct, aid, or otherwise influence the decision?
4. How important is the issue to the individual or group?[10]

Political Analysis through the Prince System, by Coplin and O'Leary, is useful for answering the above questions.[11]

Block, in *The Empowered Manager,* proposes developing a matrix that uses the dimensions of agreement and trust to place those who are seen to have influence on decision making. The categorizing of those individuals needed to further the aims of the transition movement is the first step in the political process of gaining commitment. Block suggests that individuals can be categorized as "bedfellows," "fence sitters," "allies," "adversaries," and "opponents."

The next step is to identify those who are in agreement with the issue and can be trusted. These people are called "allies" and can be further identified as exhibiting high or low levels of trustworthiness and agreement.

The same procedure can be followed for those falling into the groups of "adversary," "fence sitters," "bedfellows," and "opponents." Following the classification of the various actors, Block advocates giving special attention to "allies" to increase their support and to seek other allies. Attention should also be given to the opponents, those in whom a high level of trust is placed but who disagree with the purpose and direction of the vision, mission, and goals.

"Opponents" serve a useful purpose in the transition phase since their conflicting views help those who are formulating the vision to examine their arguments and plans and use their negative comments to refute and solidify a positive approach.

"Bedfellows" are those who agree with the vision, but are classified as deserving a low to moderate amount of trust. These individuals,

groups, or both are treated with caution in sharing information since their loyalty may be questionable. However, a continued relationship is necessary to maintain agreement.

The "fence sitters" do not deserve much attention since they tend to vacillate with each passing issue.

"Adversaries" are those people or groups who are not open to negotiating either trust or agreement. It is best to dismiss a relationship with them after making them aware that their viewpoints have been recorded and understood.

The process of negotiating with those who have influence and power to further or inhibit the vision for the transformed organization is designed to increase trust and agreement. The value of developing the matrix and classification of those involved is in its ability to assist in setting priorities for individuals and groups that deserve the most effort and attention.

One of the major differences between the two systems described above is that the *Political Analysis through the Prince System* furnishes a method to quantify the positions, interest, and power individuals or groups may have for or against an issue, while Block does not offer such a quantification method.[12]

Culture

In the transition stage attention must be given to the organization culture in which the old organization is embedded. Schein defines organization culture as:

a pattern of basic assumptions—invented, discovered, or developed by a given group as it learns to cope with its problems of external adaptations and internal integration—that has worked well enough to be considered valid and, therefore, to be taught to new members as the correct way to perceive, think, and feel in relation to these problems.[13]

Just as organizations are composed of many subsystems, each subsystem may have a different subculture. During the transition stage, a decision must be made as to which features of the old culture and what subsystem's cultures should be studied regarding its fit or nonfit for the transformed organization.

Allen and Kraft advocate a systematic culture approach.[14] In this approach members of the organization participate in the analysis; this participation is thought to increase a feeling of awareness, control, and ownership of the cultural changes.

The normative model advocated by Allen and Kraft for transforming organizational culture involves four stages.[15] The first stage involves all participants in defining the culture in which they work. In this analysis stage various instruments can be administered to determine the cultural norms that are deeply buried within the organization.

During the second stage, all participants are involved in workshops or retreats to examine the cultural norms found in the first stage. At such retreats new cultural norms are discussed and tied to the vision of the transformed organization.

Stage three introduces the implementation of the change. This stage might be called the stage of development of personnel. Attention is given to the behavioral changes necessary for the new organizational arrangements being envisaged. For instance, if an entrepreneurial culture is in the vision, then open discussions of risk taking and innovation should be offered with attention to the discovery of the early innovators in the organization—those who accepted reasonable risks and were capable of living with situations of high ambiguity. It is in this stage that the members begin to put into practice new behaviors that fit the vision of the transformed organizations. Appropriate mentoring systems should be established to reinforce and sustain the behavioral changes.

The last stage in the normative model is the assessment stage. Evaluation mechanisms are established whereby members can continue to examine their behavior in light of the new cultural norms. This stage should extend throughout the transition stage. Individuals need to receive frequent feedback and support during a time when their beliefs are being challenged and new behaviors are being developed.

Nelson and Burns use a "high performance programming model" to diagnose how the organization's past performance operated and how to plan future cultural changes.[16] In this model, organizations are classified into reactive, responsive, proactive, and high-performing organizations. Here again, as in the normative model, an assessment of the organization is advocated. Once the assessment of the present culture is determined, definitions of the future culture need is often made clear.

Certain values are selected as being critical to achieving the vision, and appropriate strategies are developed with the goal to develop a responsive, proactive, or high-performance organization. The emphasis is on the selection of appropriate cultural changes to fit the vision of the transformed organization. For instance, if the organization chooses a responsive culture, the frame of reference appropriate for this culture would be a focus on goals, problem solving, team building, and use of situational leadership theory. The environment would encourage team work in which members support and encourage each other in working toward mutually developed goals. The leader's style would be based on the maturity of the employees for the task at hand, with the leader acting in different roles—director, coach, or counselor—according to the situation. On the other hand, if the high-performance organization is chosen, the culture would include beliefs in autonomous democratic work arrangements, networking for individual and group support, empowering of individuals, and feed-forward and feedback communication channels. In this organization the culture would support the continued development of the individual in the workplace.

Schein proposes that cultural changes in the organization are dependent on the developmental stages of the organization and the extent to which the organization is unfrozen.[17] Further, he predicts that those influences that cause organizations to be receptive to cultural changes differ according to the developmental phases of the organization. The growth stages of organizations are depicted as "birth and early growth," "organizational midlife," and "organizational maturity."[18]

Different mechanisms for change and cultural functions are proposed for each stage. If the organization were in the midlife stage of growth such as hospital *A,* which is faced with severe external regulatory pressures, declining patient days, severe competition, and price discounting, and if hospital *A* were also faced with a staff that was resistant to change, liked the status quo, and otherwise showed lack of innovation, the culture would be diagnosed as deeply embedded. Schien is pessimistic about making people aware of their culture unless there are forces, crises, or other problems that effect the organization in a major way.[19] These forces cause unfreezing to occur and, during the unfreezing phase, enable an examination of the culture.

Unfreezing forces for hospital *A,* which is in midlife growth, will probably come from external forces. Economic pressures on hospitals are the most common cause of unfreezing. In many hospitals, survival is at stake. Survival pressures provide strong impetus for evaluation of the culture to determine its compatibility with the vision of a new organization.

Schein proposes three change mechanisms for the midlife organization: coercive persuasion, turnaround, and reorganization and rebirth.[20] If the transition manager and the task forces managing the transition select the strategy of coercive persuasion, then the tactics would be to retain key essential administrators and managers, while offering rewards and support for change in cultural beliefs.

If the turnaround option were chosen, many of the strategies already outlined in the transition stage would apply. These are: a turnaround transitional manager is selected, a vision about the organization's future is verbalized, and a systematic cultural-change model is developed. In addition power is given to implement these strategies.

The third change strategy advocated by Schein is "reorganization and rebirth." While Schein states there is little known about this process, it can be suggested that it is similar to the transition stage, which is comparable to the cycle of death and birth. In the transition stage old, nonfitting cultures are relinquished and new cultures are accepted to fit the vision of the transformed organization.

Attention to culture is essential in the transition stage. Unless cultural changes are made that fit the vision of the new organization, organizational members will continue to strategize and act on assumptions from the old culture, and changes will be blocked. Attention to culture is increasingly paramount in health-care organizations as mergers of different organizations become increasingly common. Such mergers bring together groups with many different cultures and necessitate mechanisms to mesh these diverse values.

Goals and Objectives

As personnel in the transition stage begin to see more clearly the new transformed organization, goals and objectives become necessary. When the basic components of the new organization have been established, the articulated vision furnishes the basic foundation. The mission statement adds specificity, and political processes identify the commitment of organizational members to the vision. The basic culture of the organization has been examined, and strategies for change have been outlined. It is now necessary to begin the freezing or solidification of these ideas so that the members of the organization are not seduced into journeys into secondary visions at this time.

Setting goals consistent with the vision enables the left-brained leaders to begin to focus their energies on anchoring the vision in specific organizational realities. Goal setting has the effect of speeding up the transition process. The presence of visionary, appealing strategic and innovative goals contributes to the feeling of progress and prepares organizational members for the transformed organization.

Goals are defined as descriptions of aspirations and the fruition of the ideas established through a systematic, cultural approach. Goals may be stated in broad general terms, but are designed to focus the possible direction in which to move.

Through a participatory process goals are generated throughout the organization and are then matched with the vision statement for congruence. Goals with the greatest possible concurrence among organizational members are identified as ends to be accomplished. Goals with special appeal to certain groups or units in the organization may be claimed as theirs to monitor, guide, and implement. This process generates a feeling of ownership, commitment, and accountability.

Groups, units, or individuals who hold or own these goals may then proceed to develop the objectives to achieve them. Objectives are defined as specific end points established for the transformed organization. These objectives define goals in terms of time, place, quantity and mode of impact for program efforts. In other words, the objectives turn the goals into reality.

It is equally important for the objectives to have ownership. Who will be responsible for carrying out the objectives? Usually those who hold ownership in a specific goal are assigned responsibility, resources, and time to complete objectives that bring the goal into reality.

TRANSITION AND TRANSFORMED ORGANIZATIONS

Revolutionary changes are occurring in health-care institutions. Such changes generate transition stages in organizations. Organizational members need to understand the basic processes inherent in the transition stage or stages in order to manage effectively during this unique period.

Throughout the transition stage the organization is moving toward a new vision. Again, the transition stage is the bridge between the ending of one phase and the beginning of another. This bridge provides the vehicle that carries the organization through to a metamorphosis of organizational life more in keeping with societal changes.

Each organization will have a different view of the transformed organization. In general, a new perspective of organizational life is being proposed—a reformation into a new, exciting, and more responsive institutional life.

Effective institutional life for employees may be difficult to achieve given the present trends toward health-care mergers leading to megasystems. Smith and Mitry found consistent relationships maintained according to hospital size.[21] Nurses demonstrated increased tensions, fewer opportunities for self-actualization, and lowered feelings of self-esteem, all related to increased size and complexity of the hospital. However, counteracting the evils of size and complexity is the need to establish an entrepreneurial spirit in the organization in order to be competitive and survive.

The emergence of the idea that health-care institutions must adopt an entrepreneurial spirit will force the traditional organizations into a transitional stage leading to a transformed organization. Such entrepreneurial organizations will need to have structures and cultures in which new ideas are nurtured into successful ventures. These organizations will be quite different from the traditional health-care institution. The need for openness in the environment in order to encourage innovative ideas places emphasis on individualism, independence, moderate risk taking, and creativeness—characteristics quite different from those found in traditional health-care agencies.

The encouragement of individual growth in the entrepreneurial agency should lead to greater democratization in the workplace. Ewing makes a very strong argument for "Americanizing" the workplace.[22] He stresses the differences between the political environments outside and inside organizations. Americans have many more rights outside of organizations than inside them. Such civil rights as freedom of speech, due process of law, and fairness in the work environment may not exist in all organizations. Elimination of the two standards, one inside the organization and the other outside, would encourage a wholeness in our society.

The movement toward a whole society with equal civil rights inside and outside the workplace could transform the authority structures of organizations, leading to self-managed, more democratic structures. Research, while not conclusive, suggests that democratic organizational structures provide socialization of workers toward a more active, fully democratic citizenry.[23] Certainly this is a worthwhile societal goal, given that in the presidential election year of 1980 only 59.2% of those of voting age reported voting, and in 1984 59.9% reported voting.[24]

In conclusion, we live in interesting, exciting, and stimulating times, but organizational life is complex and at times confusing. We have the opportunity to restructure organizations, and are being required to do so. Restructuring, if done properly, can benefit organizations, individuals in the workplace, and the society as a whole. But such transfor-mations of organizations cannot be successfully achieved unless the transition period is managed with great expertise.

REFERENCES

1. Califiano J. A revolution looms in American health. New York Times, 25 March, 1986.
2. Coile RC Jr. Health care industry outlook: macro-trends for 1990. Paper delivered at annual meeting of Oregon League for Nursing, Portland, Oregon, 25 April, 1986.
3. Ibid.
4. The American College of Hospital Administrators. Health care in the 1990s: trends and strategies. Chicago: Anderson and Co, 1984.
5. Coile RC Jr. Health care industry outlook. Paper delivered at annual meeting of Oregon League for Nursing, Portland, Oregon, 25 April, 1986.
6. Bezold C, Carlson RJ, Peck JC. The future of work and health. Dover, MA: Auburn House Publishing Company, 1986.
7. Bridges W. How to manage organizational transition. Training 1982;19(9):28–32.
8. Block P. The empowered manager. San Francisco: Jossey-Bass Publishers, 1985.
9. Ibid.
10. Coplin WD, O'Leary MK. Political analysis through the Prince system. Croton-on-Hudson, NY: Public Affairs Program, Syracuse University, 1983.
11. Ibid.
12. Coplin WD. Political analysis through the Prince system. Croton-on-Hudson, NY: Public Affairs Program, Syracuse University, 1983.
13. Schein EH. Organizational cultures and leadership. San Francisco: Jossey-Bass Publishers, 1985.
14. Allen RE, Kraft C. Transformations that last: a cultural approach. In: Adams JD, ed. Transforming work. Alexandria, VA: Mills River Press, 1984.
15. Ibid.
16. Nelson L, Burns L. High performance programming: a framework for transforming organizations. In: Adams JD, ed. Transforming work. Alexandria, VA: Mills River Press, 1984.
17. Schien EH. Organizational cultures and leadership. San Francisco: Jossey-Bass Publishers, 1985.
18. Ibid.
19. Ibid.
20. Ibid.
21. Smith HL. Quality of working life. Nursing Management 1983;14(1):14–18.
22. Ewing DW. Freedom inside the organization. New York: EP Dutton, 1977, p. 237.
23. Elden JM. Political efficacy at work: the connection between more autonomous forms of workplace organization and a more participatory politics. American Political Science Review 1981;75(1):43–58.
24. Bureau of the Census. National data book and guide to sources. Statistical abstracts of the United States 1986. Washington, DC: Bureau of the Census, 1986, p. 256.

45

Value Conflicts in Nursing Administration

Cynthia C. Scalzi
Peggy Nazarey

CHANGING values are shaping new directions for the future of the health-care industry. Since 1980 economic constraints have had a greater influence on the health-care environment than in the previous 50 years. Hospitals are undergoing tremendous changes to adjust to decreased resources, increased demands, and advances in technology. Humanistic values that have been inherent in the service-oriented health-care industry must now be balanced with cost effective, product-oriented values. This change from service to product brings with it a shift in the basic value framework of the industry. The provision of hospital services historically has been based on values that are very different from those typically associated with competitive free-market processes.[1] This change in value framework demands clarification by all key decision-makers functioning in the health-care arena. The nurse executive, as a vital participant in the planning and delivery of health care, needs to be able to positively and productively respond to the changing environment.

The primary purpose of this chapter is to increase the awareness of personal, professional, and organizational values and the role they play in decision-making and leadership behavior. In addition, we identify several common value conflicts experienced by nurse executives and discuss some ways to manage them. We conclude by raising further questions and implications for nursing practice, education, and research.

THEORETICAL BACKGROUND

Philosophers place the study of valuing in the field of ethics, and apply the term "axiologists" to those who concern themselves with the nature of valuing.[2] Axiology is a relatively new and emerging branch of inquiry with only a short history of professional concern.[2-4] Simmons discusses three types of literature on values: works that present models for the structure of value system content (Spranger, Kluckhohn and Strodtbeck, Rokeach), models for value fulfillment (Cantril, Frankl, Maslow), and methods to measure valuing competency (Hartman, Dewey, Kohlberg).

A selective review is given here to provide the theoretical background necessary for a discussion of value conflicts experienced by nurse executives. This review covers the definitions of values, value systems, value sets, and the distinctions between values and value indicators.

Value Definitions

The concept of "value" has been defined somewhat differently by various theorists. However, there are four significant elements that are essential to the definition of a value and can serve to organize the similarities of the definitions identified by most of the major theorists. These elements are awareness, selection, desirability, and behavioral guidance.[5]

According to Rokeach, values deal with modes of conduct and end states of existence.[6] To say that a person "has a value" is to say he or she has an enduring belief that a specific mode of conduct or end state of existence is personally and socially preferable to alternative modes. Once a value is internalized it becomes, consciously or unconsciously, a standard or criterion for guiding action, developing and maintaining attitudes toward relevant objects and situations, morally judging the self and others, and comparing the self with others.

Smith, in contrast, defines values as simply conceptions of the desirable—a belief in what is right and what should be attained at the ideal level.[7] Raths, Simon, and Harmin use the term "value" to denote "those beliefs, purposes, and attitudes that are chosen freely and thoughtfully, prized, and acted upon."[8] Values are not seen as static; rather, they change as the individual matures and changes. However, Raths and associates are less concerned with the particular values one chooses than with the process one uses to obtain them.

Value Indicators and Valuing Process

Value indicators include goals, attitudes, interests, feelings, convictions, and beliefs. Value indicators are potential values, and are important because they indicate expressions that approach values. However, they are not considered values because they do not meet all the steps of the valuing process that define or describe a value. According to Raths, a belief, attitude, goal, or feeling becomes a value only when all seven steps of the valuing process described below are satisfied.[8]

When one values something, one "chooses" (freely; from among alternatives; after care-

fully considering the consequences of each alternative); "prizes" (is proud of and happy with the choice; is willing to affirm and share the choice in a public manner); and "acts" (the choice is reflected in behavior; the choice is a consistent pattern of behavior).

The first step assumes the individual is consciously choosing to take on a belief as a personal principle. Steps two and three suggest that one reviews all options before deciding on a course of action, and considers the consequences of the alternative selected. The fourth step implies that for a belief to be a value it must be something the person is proud of; the fifth step is sharing in some public way what is of value. The fourth and fifth steps together suggest that if a belief is really of value, one feels good about it and is committed enough to the view to share it. The sixth step requires that the individual act on the value. The seventh and final step in the valuing process is that a value is reflected in one's behavior in a consistent, repetitive fashion. Steps six and seven suggest that there must be a shift from insight about one's belief to a behavioral change based on this value.

Clarifying values does not imply that all of our values are fixed. Except for a precious few, most of our values are in a process of development—being repeatedly tested, altered, and reapplied.[9]

Value Systems

Human beings are unique in their reliance on a value system that enables them to resolve conflicts and make decisions. Values serve to maintain self-esteem by assisting the individual in adapting to society and by protecting his or her identity. Although humans have a relatively small number of values, there are unlimited numbers of variations in value systems. The closer individuals are in culture, experience, and needs, the more their value systems will be related.

Values are clearly for the most part cultural products. Children learn values from their contact with society and significant others. Over time, values are given priorities in order of importance in relation to other values. When a value is activated it will be selected based on the importance it has in relation to other values. In other words, all values do not hold equal importance, and under pressure a person will select the value with the highest priority.[10]

Values are organized into hierarchic structures. This ordering of values is a rational plan. The emerging value system has a rank ordering of values along a continuum that reflects their relative importance; therefore, each value relates to a series of higher values.

Value Sets

Value systems of individual professionals can be thought of as being composed of three distinct value sets—personal, professional, and organizational. These value sets have considerable overlap, and their boundaries are not sharply delineated (see Figure 45.1). These value sets are described here primarily

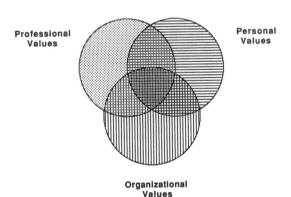

Figure 45.1 Individual's Value Sets. The three circles represent the personal, professional, and organizational value sets of an individual. Presence of both unique areas and areas of overlap of two or three sets indicate that the boundaries of the value sets are not always distinct; values may be included in more than one set.

from the viewpoint of the nurse executive as an individual, a professional, and a member of an organization.

Personal Value Set

An individual's values are hierarchic and developmental, in that they change as the individual grows and matures. Maslow identifies values with needs, and categorizes subsets of values based on his well-known hierarchy of needs: safety, security, love, self-esteem, and self-actualization.[11] He believes there are hierarchies of basic needs, and that a person's values are controlled by his or her dominant need-level beginning with the lowest one. When one level of needs is met, consciousness is then opened to a higher need. The ultimate personal value is self-actualization, which means becoming fully human or everything a person can become. Maslow defines some good values as serenity, love, kindness, courage, knowledge, honesty, and goodness.

Individuals enter the profession of nursing with values or value indicators that guide personal actions. Steele and Harmon state it is unlikely that anyone can completely separate personal and professional values, and that professional values are ultimately an expansion and reflection of one's personal values.[12] Some of the personal values that influence the selection of nursing as a career might include: serving others, respect, caring, autonomy, financial security, tradition, health, responsibility, and marriage.

Professional Value Set

All groups of people who call themselves professionals function within a code of ethics based on the values of the profession. Professional values include a claim to competence, a socially valued goal, and autonomy.[13]

Belonging to a profession places demands on its members. The professional group sets high standards based on beliefs about the profession and the role that it plays in society. When persons select a profession, they are not always aware of the values of the professional group. As a result, the values of the profession can be in conflict with personal values. Identifying values that guide one's personal life and professional role offers an opportunity to assess how personal and professional values relate to one another, although it is unlikely that anyone can completely separate personal and professional values.

The socialization process into the profession is structured to pass values of the professional group on to a new member. In a profession, such as nursing, that is predominately female, contemporary issues that relate to women have a substantial influence on it. Gilligan's research suggests that men and women speak different languages that they assume are the same.[14] Fry also states that moral values in a predominately female profession may need to be assessed differently.[15] Women value cooperation and care in relationships and responsibilities, whereas men value rights, justice, and equality.[14]

Organizational Values

This term is not used here to describe values *of* a particular organization, but rather to describe those values that an individual holds *for or about* organizations. These values may or may not be consistent with the values expressed by a given organization's policies.

Peters and Waterman describe the dominant values of excellent companies, which are a reflection of the organizational value sets of the leaders of those companies.[16] The values are:

1. a belief in being the best.
2. a belief in the importance of the details of execution, the nuts and bolts of doing the job well.
3. a belief in the importance of people as individuals.

4. a belief in superior quality and service.
5. a belief that most members of the organization should be innovators, and its corollary, the willingness to accept failure.
6. a belief in the importance of informality to enhance communication.
7. an explicit belief in and recognition of the importance of economic growth and profits.

It is still unclear how nurse executives acquire organizational values, and how they might differ depending on educational and experience backgrounds.

Internal Value Conflicts

Conflict originating from within an individual's value system causes internal discomfort that can have three sources. First, persons can be forced into behavior that is inconsistent with their present value system. Second, persons can be exposed to new information that calls into question part of their value system. Third, persons can be made aware of inconsistencies that already exist in their value system. Persons can tolerate some inconsistent values unless the inconsistency threatens their self-concept. Before a value can be changed, the person needs to bring the value into his or her awareness for examination and evaluation.[6] The process of examination and evaluation must be a part of any professional socialization; otherwise, the individual may experience discomfort and confusion.

Unless value systems are consciously examined, it is possible to have inconsistencies that are not immediately obvious. When two values become inconsistent, they must be reassessed. The reassessment may merely result in an acknowledgment that, under certain circumstances, some values that are held by the individual can be inconsistent with other values. In other circumstances, it may be wise to change values that are so inconsistent that they interfere with determining alternative courses of action. This may involve reordering ones's hierarchy of values.

RELATIONSHIPS OF VALUE SETS AND DYNAMICS OF VALUE CONFLICTS

This section of the chapter describes value conflict as it directly relates to nurse executives. We give specific examples of conflicts between value sets, both internal and external. In addition, we describe the various dynamics of value conflicts involving individuals and groups, with examples of combinations that the nurse executive might experience.

The nurse executive needs to examine and clarify values because of their relevance to role performance. Some of the ways that values influence managerial functioning are:

1. decisions are ultimately based on the decision maker's value system—values are significant determinants of action at each state of the decision-making process;[17]
2. an individual's values can cloud perception and ultimately eliminate or limit alternatives;
3. values determine style of leadership and managerial actions;
4. values and value systems of individual leaders direct and determine the vision, mission, and strategies of an organization;
5. values influence decisions on resource allocation;
6. clearly understood values may increase productivity and decrease turnover; and
7. conflicts are frequently rooted in value differences.

Conflict is an inevitable part of everyday life. Conflict of some type exists when two or more parties differ with regard to facts, opinions, beliefs, feelings, or values. The resolution of any of these conflicts requires knowledge of the basic ideological differences

underlying them. On the other hand, failure to understand ideological differences often leads to conflict. Our specific focus here is on conflict arising from differences in values.

Value Sets of Individuals as Sources of Possible Conflicts

The three value sets that the nurse executive needs to be aware of are personal, professional, and organizational (see Figure 45.1). Balancing these three is not easy, and requires frequent re-examination and clarification. Balancing also requires that the nurse executive be flexible in looking at the changing environment and in allowing his or her value systems to expand.

A value conflict for the nurse executive may arise from differences involving any or all value sets. For example, many women experience a value conflict in meeting the time demands of a professional career as well as the time demands of a family. This conflict can be represented as internal conflict between an individual's personal and professional value sets (illustrated by line *a* in Figure 45.2). Value conflicts between individuals can also involve a variety of value sets. A conflict

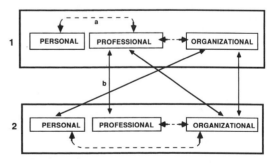

Figure 45.2 Value Set Conflicts. Two individuals (1 and 2) are represented by the rectangles, each with their own personal, professional, and organizational value sets. The arrows depict common value conflicts, with dotted lines showing conflicts between a given individual's value sets (internal) and solid lines showing conflicts of value sets between individuals (external).

between the nurse executive and the chief executive officer (CEO) over resource allocation might arise from differences in their professional value sets, (illustrated by line *b* in Figure 45.2).

Value Conflict Dynamics

Value conflict exists for every nurse executive. The dynamics of value conflicts can be divided into four major categories according to who is experiencing the conflict: intrapersonal, interpersonal, intergroup, and intragroup (see Figure 45.3). Value conflicts do not necessarily occur in isolation. At any given time a nurse executive may be faced with one or more value conflicts in all four dynamics categories.

"Intrapersonal conflict" is conflict that occurs in a person in response to a value difference, either between that individual's values and an external value system or between two values of the individual. For example, the professional value of "management by walking around and being visible to staff" is frequently at odds with the professional value of keeping up with administrative paperwork. Intrapersonal value conflicts are frequently not expressed, and can result in a great deal of personal stress.

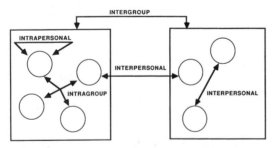

Figure 45.3 Value Conflict Dynamics. Types of conflict that can arise from value differences are categorized by the person(s) experiencing conflict. Two professional groups are shown by the rectangles, and individuals in the groups are represented by circles. Arrows show the possibility for types of conflict.

"Interpersonal conflict" is conflict that involves two or more individuals, either in the same or different professional groups. An example of this is conflict between the nurse executive and the finance director arising from professional value differences concerning the span of control the nurse executive should have in budget planning. This occurs when the finance director believes that the nurse executive's input regarding resource allocation should be limited to the nursing department, whereas the nurse executive believes that as a top administrator he or she should help determine the resource allocation in ancillary departments.

"Intragroup conflict" is conflict that occurs in a group arising from value differences among individuals of the group. The "group" can range from a work group of four or five people to an entire profession. For example, a nurse executive's professional value may dictate that nurses in the institution be accountable for their practice outcomes. All nurses in that organization, however, may not believe accountability should be an expectation of practice. This results in intragroup conflict because of differences between professional values sets.

"Intergroup value conflict" is conflict that occurs between two or more groups. This usually occurs along with other kinds of conflict dynamics. Some examples of intergroup conflict are included in the next section.

"Multiple dynamics of conflict" can arise from a single situation, leading to very complex relationships among both value sets and individuals in conflict. To examine the dynamics of conflicts that can stem from value sets in opposition, consider the issue of quality care versus cost restrictions. The nurse executive's personal and professional value sets include valuing quality care. However, the hospital CEO's professional values are reflected by primary interest in the bottom-line costs. Thus, the CEO's expectation is that hospital beds will remain open, whereas the nurse executive may believe that beds should be closed if there are not adequate numbers of nurses to provide safe, quality care. Several dynamics are involved in this conflict of values. An interpersonal conflict clearly exists between the CEO and the nurse executive. Conflict may become intergroup to the extent that the entire nursing organization is in conflict with all of hospital administration. The nurse executive can also experience intrapersonal conflict, depending on the degree to which the nurse executive's professional values about quality care conflict with his or her own organizational values that may be similar to the CEO's.

As another example of multiple dynamics of conflict arising from one situation, consider a nurse executive whose professional values dictate that nurses be involved in research and publishing. An interpersonal value conflict occurs with a CEO who does not value these professional activities in nursing and does not support the nurse executive in taking time to engage in these activities. An intragroup value conflict in the nursing department results if there is one group that includes the nurse executive and other staff who value these activities, and another group of nurses who do not. In addition, intergroup conflict exists between physicians who do not feel nurses should be involved in these activities and the group of nurses who give high priority to nursing research and professional writing.

Conflict Resolution

Instances of inadequate sharing of values and conflicting values are numerous. Health-care organizations are complex, in part due to the presence of many groups of professionals and a high degree of technological sophistication. This complexity results in diversity of value systems.[18] Analysis of value conflict and values clarification is vital to effective functioning in the nurse executive's role. Little attention, however, is given to this area during the educational process. Traditionally, nurse executives have not been educated to consider the importance of values explicitly in decision making or conflict management. Before any resolution of value conflicts can take place in practice, nurse executives must examine their attitudes and understanding of values. Each individual can then develop his or her own approach to resolving value conflict. It is important to remember value differences do not necessarily imply value conflict; values that are different are not necessarily incompatible.

When serious conflict does exist, the ability to effectively identify what values are in conflict is critical to successful conflict management. Value differences need to be carefully assessed and analyzed. Priorities given to values by individuals can fluctuate according to the situation. Individual nurse executives must decide what, if any, flexibility exists in their values and determine their positions in conflict resolution accordingly. Resolution of a value conflict does not require one value winning over the other, but rather an understanding and appreciation of the value differences and a willingness to develop shared goals.

IMPLICATIONS

Education and practice

An examination of values and value clarification should be a part of the education of the nursing professional. It is essential that a clear understanding be developed during initial socialization into the profession of the relevance of personal, professional, and organizational values. Without this value clarification, future value conflicts will be more difficult to recognize and resolve. Nursing students need to develop realistic professional and organizational values that will be compatible with today's health-care industry; the development of idealistic values that are impossible to achieve is likely to lead to frustration and unresolvable conflict. Role models with sound value systems are needed to help guide the students' development and testing of values.

The professional value systems of nurse executives in the 1970s were for the most part developed in a stable health-care environment that is not fully relevant to a changing industry of the 1990s. There could be harm in rooting value judgments in the past when such rapid value shifts are occurring. Nurse executives must examine their values carefully in relation to the changing environment and decide whether or not they are still realistic and appropriate. The danger exists that values that should be retained are let go, and that those that should be expanded in new directions are left as they are. Nurse executives need to learn to promote and protect personal, professional, and organizational values if excellence is to be achieved and maintained.

It is important that change be analyzed in relation to potential value conflicts. Open communications regarding value differences should be encouraged. Nurse executives could be more aware of the influence that values have on leadership and management actions.

All nursing professionals need to examine the values of organizations and their people before deciding to work in a particular environment if potential for future conflict is to be reduced. Nurse executives must be prepared to collaborate with other health-care professionals in shaping industry values. Finally, the values of our patients need to be considered carefully in the delivery of nursing care.

FUTURE RESEARCH

Although theories exist, there is little empirical work concerning values, particularly the professional and organizational value sets.

This is probably due to the difficulties in measuring the attributes in question as well as due to limitations of the perspective usually used to study values. Gilligan's research implies that women's moral development is different from men's; new descriptive studies are called for that focus on better understanding of these differences and their implications for a predominantly female profession such as nursing.[14]

Although it is generally accepted that educational experience influences development of values, possible mechanisms and stages of this process remain unknown. The rapid changes and shifts in the health services industry imply changes in the roles of the nurse executive and nursing staffs. Studies are needed to identify inconsistencies that exist or might arise between the values instilled through educational preparation and those encountered in practice. Also, questions remain regarding how nurse executives' professional and organizational value sets might differ with graduate preparation of a master's in nursing versus an M.B.A.

Hall and Allen have described a controversy in the nursing profession regarding a split in those professional values that relate to health and disease.[19] Different values arise depending on which of the two perspectives on nursing are accepted—one focusing on the illness state and the other on the health state. With the development of nursing frameworks, it became clear that nursing education was moving from the disease model to the health model. However, much of the health service industry reflects an illness-based orientation. What are the implications for the nurse executive who has a health-based professional value set but works in an illness-based acute care medical center? The assumption that greater value differences leads to greater potential for conflict needs to be supported or modified by research on this issue.

Similarly, an implicit assumption in discussions of values and value conflicts is that clarification of values and anticipation of value-conflict situations can help to reduce or manage conflict. However, research that might support this assumption has not yet been done.

According to Fry, decisions regarding the allocation of nursing resources and the quality of care are drawn from the nurse executive's values.[15] As of 1987 there is little research on the type of moral decisions made by nurse executives. Thus, we have little information about how nurses in executive roles learn to balance values, integrate moral and other values, or make value centered decisions. Decisions will be based on each individual's value system—a value system in which important personal, professional, and organizational values are arranged in a hierarchy of relative importance to the decision maker. We need to learn more about mechanisms that nurse executives use to balance competing values in the organizational and policy-making structures in which they function and make decisions.

ACKNOWLEDGMENT

The authors wish to acknowledge the assistance of Sondra T. Perdue, Dr.P.H., in helping to clarify the concepts of value sets and value dynamics by translating them into schematic diagrams.

REFERENCES

1. Peters J, Wacker R. Strategic Planning. Hospitals 1982;56:90–92.
2. Simmons DD. Personal valuing. Chicago: Nelson-Hall, 1982.
3. Hartman R. The science of valuing. In: Maslow A, ed. New knowledge in human values. New York: Harper & Brothers, 1959.
4. Findlay J. Axiological ethics. London: Macmillan and Co, 1970.
5. Kluckhohn F, Strodtbeck F. Variations in value orientations. Evanston, IL: Row, Peterson, 1961.
6. Rokeach M. The nature of human values. New York: Free Press, 1973.
7. Smith H. How hospitals can respond to changing values. Hosp Topc 1984;1:13–17.
8. Raths L, Harmin M, Simon S. Values and teaching. Columbus, OH: Merrill, 1966.
9. Uustal D. Values and ethics in nursing: From theory to practice. East Greenwich, RI: Education Resources in Nursing & Holistic Health, 1985.
10. Rokeach M. Beliefs, attitudes, and values: a theory of organization and change. San Francisco: Jossey-Bass, Inc, 1975.
11. Maslow A. Toward a psychology of being. 2nd ed. New York: Van Nostrand, 1968.
12. Steele S, Harmon V. Values clarification in nursing. 2nd ed. Norwalk, CN: Appleton-Century-Crofts, 1983.
13. Hinshaw AS. Socialization and resocialization of nurses for professional nursing practice. New York: National League for Nursing, 1977, no. 15-1659.
14. Gilligan C. In a different voice. Cambridge, MA: Harvard University Press, 1982.
15. Fry S. Moral values and ethical decisions in a constrained economic environment. Nurs Econ 1986;4 (2):160–164.
16. Peters T, Waterman R. In search of excellence: lessons from America's best-run companies. New York: A Warner Communications Company, 1982.
17. Gibson JL, Ivaniwich JM, Donnelly JH. Organizations: structure processes behavior. Revised ed. Dallas: Business Publications, Inc, 1976.
18. Binder J. Value conflicts in health care organizations. Nurs Econ 1983;1(5).
19. Hall B, Allen J. Sharpening nursing's focus by focusing on health. Nurs and Health Care 1986;2: 315–320.

46

Comparable Worth

Russell Swansburg
Kathryn Barnett

THROUGHOUT the United States women are concentrated in the lower-paying jobs. Nursing is one of these lower-paying occupations in which approximately 96% of the nation's 1,531,000 nurses are women.[1] These women run the gamut in terms of intellect, ingenuity, innovation, creativity, knowledge, skill, and talent. In any one of these traits there are nurses to match the male captains of business and industry. Job segregation by gender has been perpetuated by traditional wage-setting practices that pay more for male-dominated occupations and less for female-dominated occupations.[2]

Some nurses believe they are "members of an occupation that has historically been victimized by sex-linked job classification and salary systems."[3] The nursing job-market is gender-segregated by the nursing profession, within the health-care industry. To a large extent the mobility of nurses is tied to hospitals.[4]

In 1982 women earned 59 cents of every dollar earned by men as compared with 64 cents in 1955.[3] In 26 years they have lost comparable pay by five cents per dollar earned. This has been reported to have improved by 1986 when fully employed women earned an average of 69 cents for every dollar earned by fully employed men.[5]

Women are still held back from corporate promotions causing continued narrow career ladders. They have been historically and deliberately hired into certain types of jobs. It is not feasible to attempt to increase salaries of women by recruiting men into traditionally female occupations. Men won't go. In the past 40 years only between 2% and 4% of nurses have been male.[6]

Although wage discrimination is largely basic to women minorities and their families, disparities in earnings continue to be greater between men and women than between minorities such as blacks and whites. While disparities in the latter have improved in recent years, the disparities between men and women have gotten worse.[7] During the past 30 years, the number of women entering the labor force increased only 25%.[3] To add insult to this disparity, women are frequent targets of demeaning forms of workplace harassment. These include making the coffee, running personal errands, and social and sexual propositions.

IMPORT TO NURSE ADMINISTRATORS

With few exceptions the last four decades have been marked by acute shortages of nurses. There is little evidence that the dissatisfactions stated by nurses, and reported in descriptive studies, surveys, and reports, have been remedied. These dissatisfactions focus on problem factors of inadequate salaries and fringe benefits; staffing—philosophy, clerical work, floating and rotating shifts; professionalism—physician-nurse relationships, autonomy, and public relations; staff development; and, administration support.[31] Women students are entering other professional schools and occupations such as medicine, dentistry, veterinary medicine, engineering, and accounting in large numbers. Enrollment in schools of nursing are down. Unless the dissatisfactions of nurses are addressed by nurse administrators, the nursing profession will not recruit its share of the best women students nor increase the number of men students.

Nurse administrators can promote the establishment of strong programs to decrease job dissatisfactions of professional clinical nurses. This will require aggressive salary improvement programs, career development programs, and programs to enhance participation of professional clinical nurses in decision making at all levels in the organization.

Before the industrial revolution, men and women shared work and child-rearing responsibilities. With urbanization of society and the industrial revolution men went to work in factories and women became homemakers for husbands and children. Women's work opportunities were limited to being nurses, clerks, secretaries, schoolteachers, and waitresses. In factories men were paid more for their work than women were for theirs; therefore, men's work became more important.[8]

While their paychecks belie their value, nurses are respected by the public. When their intellect, education, and competencies are compared with male occupations people know that nurses are equal to engineers, accountants, and others; however, they are paid less than semiskilled or unskilled workers, such as garbage collectors. Their education does not equate with their earnings.[8] Pay inequities run the gamut of occupations, industries, and geographical areas for nurses within the health-care industry. To quote the Texas Nurses' Association "the issue is comparable worth, the problem is gender-based wage discrimination, and the goal is pay equity."[9]

VALUE BY SOCIETY

It is a public viewpoint that women work to supplement the family income, and they are secondary wage earners. The fact is that 85% of women can expect to be self-supporting in their lifetime.[10] They will be single-parent heads of households, married heads of households, or single heads of households. Their marital status should have nothing to do with the pay they receive for doing their jobs.

Society does not pay for occupations that serve, nurture, and demonstrate concern for people. This could mean that people don't value such occupations, despite the lip service they give to the life-saving work of nurses. Society rewards what it values, and women's occupations are undervalued. Historically, jobs held by men have had higher status than those held by women.[10-11]

Many women like the profession of nursing and do not want to leave it—or any occupation that is satisfying to them. They enter traditionally female occupations voluntarily and therefore voluntarily do the kinds of work for which they are paid 40% less on the average than men. While male-dominated occupations are open to women, many nurses do not want to change occupations to achieve equity.[10-11]

Society views some jobs as "women's jobs"—a mindset that has begun in elementary schools, continued into high schools, and solidified in college. Employers value these jobs less and seldom consider that women work because of economic need—the need to support themselves and their families.[4] When they do consider the economic needs of nurses, employers do so negatively saying, "She won't quit! She has to have a paycheck!"

Silver refers to the fact that there is job segregation in occupations that are predominately male. Physician specialists do not get comparable pay for comparable work. This applies to both fees and salaries for such specialists as pediatricians versus obstetricians, or internists versus clinical laboratory specialists, and radiologists. Physicians are not satisfied with these inequities and although a "relative value scale" is used to determine specialists' fees and salaries, Silver predicts that there will be many court cases by physicians. There are cultural and economic factors involved. Silver states, "We pride ourselves on our advanced levels of education and modern concern for equality and social justice. Yet it is clear that we are a male-oriented culture, male-dominated, and despite our understanding of social justice theorems, indistinguishable in these matters from older and (in our view) less advanced societies."[12]

Eighty percent of employed women work in undervalued service or support organizations. The service sector of the economy is expanding with more jobs in the service industries that are traditionally filled by women. It is the secondary segment of the labor market. Nursing is part of this secondary segment in which the "characteristics of jobs in the secondary segment include relatively low wages, generalized skills that can be used in several job situations, acquisition of skills usually paid for by the worker, short career ladder for advancement, and high turnover.[13]

When professions switch from being dominated by males, they become less valued; or when men enter them they create valued titles. This occurred when women became bookkeepers—men then created the Certified Public Accountant; and when men came to be librarians they called themselves library scientists. In the Soviet Union, general medical practitioners are 90% women, and men are specialists who are better rewarded. In society in general, cheap labor is designated by gender and race.[14]

According to Steinem, counting women into the gross national product (GNP) for their housework would cause it to rise 25%.

Not counting this work undervalues the contributions of women's work and worth to society. Human work should be valued according to its true contribution to the community. In the struggle to equate women's work to that of men Steinem concludes "But every day gives us a bit of our own full identity and makes us see what we could be and what we as individuals will be. And we will begin to have societies into which, at least, no one is ever again born into an inferior role because of sex or race or class, and we each have a chance to be the full, unique human being we could be."[14]

Among the evidence of devalued worth in nursing is the fact of requiring nurses to rotate shifts. This would not be necessary if nurse administrators all worked to provide incentives, including adequate financial differentials and child-care facilities. Not only would these incentives solve the shift problems, they would contribute to recruitment of people into nursing and to retention once employed. Nurses have poor compensation programs related to retirement; only 18% to 20% of R.N.s reported ever having received retirement benefits. Although some worked 20 to 30 years in one hospital, they only received $80 to $120 a month.[15] Nurse administrators can correct this dissatisfaction by pressing for a sound retirement system or providing personal financial counseling.

When great shortages of nurses occur they turn to registries for higher wages, preferred hours and units, and control of their practice. The health-care industry has recruited foreign nurses to keep profits up and wages down. Nurses from the United Kingdom and the Philippines have been recruited, ostensibly because of acute shortages. Higher salaries and increased fringe benefits would have increased the supply of U.S.-educated nurses. The salary range is a major reason the nursing profession cannot recruit and retain adequate numbers of nurses. Among hourly wage rates of eight occupations studied in

Table 46.1 Hourly Wage Rates of Selected Occupations in California

Registered nurse	$10.20
Truck driver	$13.07
Cannery worker	$11.87
Typist	$11.55
Tire changer	$13.00
Pharmacist	$15.87
Biomedical electronics technician	$13.62

Adapted from Absalom KC. Collective Bargaining: Comparable Worth. Calif Nurse 1982;17(9):7,13.

California, the registered nurse was lowest (see Table 46.1). Other than the pharmacist, the R.N. probably required the highest level of education and skills.[15]

Women want to be valued in work according to the same set of rules applied to men. This value should be related to the work and not the gender of the person doing it. Administrators of health care, including nurses, can improve the public image of nursing in society, thereby increasing its value by society. They can portray nursing as an occupation for both men and women; publicize the technological knowledge and skills required of and used by nurses; improve the incentives for working mothers, for shift demands; and improve salaries, pension plans, and other benefits. Nurse administrators can be mentors, sponsors, or leaders of these nurses. Other values placed on the work of women versus men are listed in Table 46.2.

OCCUPATIONAL SEGREGATION

Occupational segregation is defined as any occupation in which 70% or more of the employees are all men or all women.[16] Eighty percent of women workers are concentrated into between 10 and 25 out of 427 defined occupations with lower pay and fewer advancement opportunities than male-dominated jobs. Only 19% of the professions are constituted by women and yet over 50% of them are concentrated in jobs such as librarians, schoolteachers, and registered nurses.[3]

Table 46.2 Values Placed on the Work of Women Versus Men

- Pay rates discriminate in all sectors of the economy for men versus women.

	Men vs.	Women
Overall	$1.00	$0.59
State and local government	$1.00	$0.71
Federal government	$1.00	$0.63
Private sector	$1.00	$0.56[2]

- There is a 20% to 40% pay difference between men and women in comparable jobs.[18]
- During the first quarter of 1985, full-time male workers in the United States had a median weekly paycheck of $404, while female workers' median weekly paycheck was $268, or 66% of what men earned.[19]
- Craftwomen earn 67% craftmen's earnings.[3]
- Female accountants earn 72% of male accountants' earnings.[3]
- Female salespersons earn 52% of male salesperson's earnings.[3]
- A nurse with 14 years of education earns 6% less than a deliveryman.[4]
- Male college teachers are paid $5,000 (23%) more annually than female college teachers.[20]

Women are segregated into female occupations where wages have been discriminantly depressed. In 1960 only 12% of professional-technical employees were women.[17]

As occupations have become feminized they have dropped in status and pay. As obstetricians replaced midwives and anesthesiologists replaced nurse anesthetists, the status and pay increased. As this situation is reversed due to liability costs to physicians, it will be interesting to see whether costs come down. State laws frequently protect the male-dominated medical profession requiring nurse practitioners to be supervised by them.[10] One could argue that the M.D. degree is required for the justification in increased pay and status, however the level of selective work performed by nurse midwives is the same as for physicians in these same specialties. Nurse administrators can help in identifying the knowledge and skills of graduate-level preparation and credentialing of these nurse specialists. The suboccupations must continue to require this and provide standards for employment and practice. Nurse anesthetists demand higher salaries and more fringe benefits than do other equally or better-prepared nurse specialists. This fact is sometimes criticized by the other nurses, a criticism antithetical to the goals of comparable worth.

It remains to be seen whether increased numbers of women graduates of medical schools will bring about comparable worth. Will a female obstetrician, anesthesiologist, surgeon, orthopedist, or other specialist be paid as much as her male counterpart?

Other predominantly female occupations include seamstresses, private household workers, food service workers, dental assistants, and bank tellers. It is a fact that employers make money from gender-based occupational segregation. Job segregation also exists on the basis of race, ethnicity, and similar criteria.[4]

Aldrich and Buchele estimate that occupational sex segregation explains only approximately 15% of the female-male wage gap. Their econometric model contrasts male and female wages in many occupations. It is their contention that a percentage of female workers must be included in each occupational group as a component of this mold. When this is done and the concept of comparable worth adopted, women would have a net gain in their aggregate earnings of about 10%.[21]

WHAT DO MARKET FORCES DO?

Although the free labor market is reputedly operated to the advantage of scarce occupations, it has not determined fair wage rates for nurses. Lower wages are supposed to increase hiring and decrease the number of people entering these occupations or professions, thereby creating shortages that increase salaries and wages. Higher wages decrease hiring but cause more people to enter occupations or professions, thus creating surpluses and lowering wages and salaries.

Nurse shortages have not improved wages to any great extent.[11] There have been occasions when employers paid fees for nurses to interview, bonuses or special deals such as automobiles for initial employment, and moving expenses. However, these have seldom been given to nurses already employed in an organization. One wonders if nurses are adept at negotiating meaningful salaries and employment benefits from a long-range perspective. The time to do this is prior to employment; and it should include a signed contract that spells out amounts and frequency of wages, and fringe benefits six-months after employment (or the probationary period) and at annual intervals thereafter. The nurse administrator can take the initiative to do this.

Some persons view the free-market system as another bias. Employers frequently use it as an excuse for not raising nurses' wages. They say they pay salaries competitive to other local health-care institutions.[10]

Disch and Feldstein describe three theories for women entering occupations:

1. Human Capital Theory. Women invest less time and money in their careers than men do, and so get less in return. This is because they are more interested in homemaking and child rearing. Women choose to enter female-dominated fields for other than economic reasons if they know the wages are lower than male-dominated fields requiring equal education and experience. Otherwise they are not informed about the equality of these characteristics. (This theory has some of the strong characteristics of a myth.)
2. Personal Change Theory. Choice of entry into an occupation is based on lower-economic losses from intermittent absences. Women enter male-dominated fields if they do not anticipate absences. Research indicates no difference in

wages, so there is no financial advantage to choosing a female-dominated career field because of anticipated intermittent absences.

3. Crowding Theory. Large numbers of women in female-dominated occupations decrease entry by others, thereby increasing wages. This theory is not supported by facts.[11]

The market system is not working to the economic advantage of women and nurses. Nurses and other advocates of comparable worth do not accept market approaches to wage discrimination. They want jobs that are comparable in value to be rewarded equally.

Youngkin echoes the perceptions of others that there is wage discrimination; that performance appraisal is unfair, that promotion and tenure systems are unfair, that occupational opportunities are unfair, that legal avenues for recourse are unfair, and that there have been no economic gains for women in 60 years. She also perceives that there are other causes of the problem than gender discrimination, education, experience, personal choice, and supply and demand. With regard to the market, wage surveys are seldom standardized, the going rate may not be acceptable to the employer, and survey results may be invalid or unreliable. Hospitals have had a monopoly over nurses leading to job channeling, job crowding, and weak salary-negotiating power.[17]

The free-market system is manipulated in agriculture, steelmaking, automobile manufacturing, and other industries and businesses. The short supply of nurses did not raise nurses' salaries spectacularly.[22] Employers use multiple pay plans for different categories of jobs. Sometimes these work to the advantage of nurses when there are true career ladders that pay meaningful differentials and provide other incentives in the form of work assignments that challenge intellect

and ability. Brennan indicates that there is little validity to use of "marketplace" factors for paying women less.[23] These factors are ignored if employers don't want to use them. "The same economic arguments that were used to oppose the emancipation of slaves are now raised to oppose pay equity for women."[23] Employers of nurses won't go broke and there will not be an economic disaster. Cost is not a valid defense against comparable worth. "Employers fought the costs of the Pregnancy Determination Act, the Minimum Wage Act, the National Labor Relations Act, safe workplace legislation, and more, all on the basis that it would cost too much and hurt the economy."[24]

Many factors are considered in determining wages and salaries including union pressure, internal equity, relative importance of job, financial constraints, and value systems. Market surveys, are again inconsistent and invalid. Companies usually deviate from them. If the deviation is for men but not women, they are considered fair. Pay rates in the same organization should not be related to gender but should follow valid and consistent internal pay practices.[23]

Research Selection for Jobs

It is illegal to discriminate on the basis of gender, race, or age, so employers often turn to psychological testing to assist them in decision making. Stewart and Stewart report the findings from a survey of a large manufacturing company that showed the application form, the interview, and the grapevine were used to make decisions about promotions. Psychological tests and performance appraisals were seldom used. Personality tests have indicated profiles for certain jobs or environments but have also been proved invalid as predictors of success in job performance. Appraisal is often based on traits rather than performance. Analysis of 236 appraisal forms from eight companies showed only 7% of cases had concise statements of strengths or effective behaviors. There was one study, by Ramsden, of nonverbal behavior as an appraisal factor. Developing techniques for selection of people for employment in the right job is a time-consuming and comprehensive effort.[25]

Noncompetitive Markets

Some professions and occupations have had restricted entry into the market. One of these is medicine, the excuse being maintenance of quality in education and training of physicians. Their tasks have been restricted by law as "the practice of medicine." Until recently they have been restricted from advertising, and consumers of their services have been loath to ask for and compare their fees, thereby curtailing competition for their services or products. This has caused a lack of cost restraint even with Medicare's prospective payment system. This noncompetitive market has raised and maintained the income of physicians. Only in recent years have women had equal access to some medical schools.

Licensing has restricted entry into other occupations, not always to the individual's financial benefit. Unions have also restricted entry into occupations by gender, although this is slowly changing. This has resulted in predominantly male occupations such as stevedoring, truck driving, carpentry, plumbing, electrical work, and many others.

In the health-care industry the illegal monopoly or restraint of trade by employers acting together to set wages has been subtly circumvented. Hospital administrators discuss prevailing wage rates for nurses among themselves. This activity can be forestalled by nurse administrators developing more planned career ladders with pay equity relative to comparable jobs in the organization. This will include input by the practicing nurses and performance evaluation that is

objective and includes self-evaluation, peer evaluation, and supervisor evaluation.

THE CONCEPT OF COMPARABLE WORTH

There exists in the United States a significant disparity between earnings for men and for women. This disparity cannot be explained by unequal pay for the same work, such as two staff nurses with equal education, experience, and ability to care for patients. They are protected under the Equal Pay Act of 1963 in which pay equity relates to the goal of equal pay for equal work. Job segregation by gender exists because of salary differences between men's work and women's work. National women's groups consider comparable worth the most important women's issue of this era.[2,13]

The issue is, "what is paid to women for the work they do, and what is paid to men for comparable work, but not the same work, that they do." "Comparable worth is a theory which holds that employers should provide equal pay for jobs that are of comparable value even though they aren't identical."[4] If jobs require comparable education, skill, effort (physical and mental demands), responsibility, and working conditions those performing them should be equally compensated, whether male or female. Jobs are dissimilar in nature but equal in value.[2]

In the process of determining comparable worth, the goal is to place a value on the work performed for an employer without consideration of whether the worker is a man or a woman. An equitable pay policy is based on the value of the job to an employer, and not the value of that job to other community employers. It is important to note that comparable worth does not always compare jobs in the community.[6] The concept is "that jobs which are equal in value to an organization ought to be equally compensated whether or not the work content of those jobs is similar."[9]

As an example of jobs that have been equated for comparable worth, in Massachusetts, R.N.s were compared to Accountants III, Personnel Directors I, Chemists III, and Engineers II in projecting inflation factors for nurses. None of these occupations was more than 24% female and all averaged $8,000 to $10,000 more in annual salaries.[3] Questions remain about what jobs can be equated or compared. Since plumbers learn by apprenticeship and do not work on people, can nurses be compared to plumbers as performing work of equal value? Is the comparison true if plumbers are paid more than nurses, or nurses more than the plumbers? It is if both jobs require comparable but not identical education, skills, demands, and responsibilities. If the value of the nurses's work equals the value of the plumber's work, they should be paid equally. That plumbers are mostly men and nurses are mostly women does not mean nurses should be paid less.

The United States Supreme Court defined comparable worth as "increased compensation on the basis of a comparison of the intrinsic worth or difficulty of their job with that of other jobs in the same organization or community."[7] Obviously, if the tenets of comparable worth are settled in court, they will apply beyond one employer. Organization and community will have to be further defined as to whether they relate to a town, city, government, or a whole field such as the health care community.

Employers argue that the comparable pay concept has many problems including:

1. Job measurement systems are judgmental and subjective. They can give relative degrees of weight to working conditions and make male jobs worth more.
2. It transcends job market conditions of supply and demand. This could hurt those nurses who have received higher wages due to shortages.
3. It could cause economic disruptions in

the United States if salaries of predominantly women's jobs were all raised. The Federal Court ruled against the Denver nurses saying that the suit was "pregnant with the possibility of disrupting the entire economic system of the United States of America."[4,23]

Comparable worth is the concept that has emerged to remedy the situation in which unequal pay is a primary function of sex-based occupational segregation. Arguments against it summarized by Youngkin include the concepts that: comparable worth rejects free-market notions of supply and demand; it could be a disaster leading to lost dollars, myriad regulations, and the end of collective bargaining; all salaries would be linked to one so only one would need negotiation; equal pay would eliminate competition, and personnel policies would be less responsive; higher pay could eliminate some positions to pay for it; and comparable worth is a women's rights issue and so is an emotional one.[17]

Quoting Chi, definitions of comparable worth share two assumptions: "(1) jobs that are dissimilar in content and demand on the worker may nonetheless be compared by objective criteria to determine their relative value to the employer, and (2) jobs that are of the same value or worth should be paid equally."[2]

THE COURTS AND COMPARABLE WORTH

During World War II the U.S. War Labor Board was created by Executive Order 9017. It created a system for examining jobs to see if women were paid according to requirements of the positions they held and not by gender. Inequities were corrected by this executive order. After the war ended in 1945, a bill embodying the concept of comparable worth was introduced in every Congress.[7]

The Equal Pay Act

The Equal Pay Act was passed in 1963, to establish the standard of equal pay for equal worth. This bill is restricted to equal pay for the same work. It did not provide real benefits for women who are segregated into occupations such as nursing. The law is not enforced because too few people challenge it. Discrimination by gender is often subtle. This federal law and most state laws require that men and women be paid equally for equal work requiring equal skill, effort, and responsibility, performed under similar working conditions. These laws apply to male nurses versus female nurses but not to female nurses versus female pharmacists. The Equal Pay Act has been interpreted to mean that women must perform work that is identical to men's work. A female supervisor of 20 nurses does not equal a male supervisor of 20 respiratory therapy employees even though the work is of equal importance to the organization and is of equal difficulty, responsibility, and value to the company.[8,18]

The Equal Pay Act allows occupational segregation of jobs by gender. It allows wage differentials between men and women to be produced by a seniority system, a merit system, a productivity system, or a differential system other than a gender-based one. There must be evidence of intent to discriminate in wage rates by gender, and this is difficult to prove. Other evidential factors include a sequence of events that depart from normal procedures or statements by the decision-making body. It must be proved that the employer treated an employee less favorably because of race, color, religion, gender, or national origin. Also, employers cannot defend salary or fringe benefits based on actuarial distinction or higher employer costs.[16,26] When employers were taken to court, women have had to prove that their jobs were identical and they were paid less than men.

An example of litigation under the Equal Pay Act is that of *Hodgson* v. *Robert Hall Clothes, Inc.* Male employees of the men's department were paid higher wages than women employees of the women's department. The plaintiff asserted that the women did the the same work (equal work) as men and were entitled to equal pay. The women employees lost. The U.S. Circuit Court held for the employer. The men's department was more profitable than the women's department; therefore, the men could be paid more than the women.[26]

The Civil Rights Act

Under Title VII of the Civil Rights Act of 1964, as amended, women in an occupation cannot be paid less than men who perform the same job. The legal term used is gender-based wage discrimination. Persons performing identical responsibilities under the same conditions must be paid the same. It has been interpreted that differences in pay are legal if based on seniority, merit, differences in productivity, or factors other than gender. This could be interpreted to mean that an R.N. who can care for only two patients should be paid less than one who can care for six patients with the same acuity. The difference is justified on the basis of productivity.[7,11]

A number of suits have been brought to court under the Civil Rights Act. Few suits have been filed against the federal government. Most have been filed against municipal governments. This does not indicate that comparable worth is only an issue of municipal governments.

JOB EVALUATION

Job evaluation serves the purpose of ordering jobs hierarchically on the basis of objective criteria of relative skills, knowledge, effort, working conditions, and responsibility among other factors. They are then grouped on this basis for payment purposes. Job evaluation

Table 46.3 Disparity in Annual Salaries for Comparable City Jobs in Favor of Predominantly Male Classifications, City of San Jose, California*

Predominantly Male Workers		Predominantly Female Workers		Annual Salary Difference
Custodian	$15,210	Library page	$11,154	$4,056
Park ranger	$18,304	Senior typist clerk	$15,600	$2,704
Equipment operator	$18,304	Police records clerk	$15,600	$2,704
Gardener	$19,292	Secretary	$17,784	$1,508
Civil engineer	$21,528	Neighborhood recreation supervisor	$18,460	$3,068
Plumber	$26,260	Programmer analyst	$21,398	$4,862
Assistant master fire mechanic	$27,648	Employee health nurse†	$18,528	$9,120

* Selections are random in comparable-city job categories.
† An Employee Health Nurse would not have the comparable worth of a hospital-based nurse.
From: How to establish the comparable worth of a job—or one way to compare apples and oranges. Calif Nurse 1982;17(9):10–11. Used with permission.

does not consider market factors, although the courts do. Under the concept of comparable worth, the process of job analysis is used to compare different jobs of equal or identical worth.

Job evaluation systems rate jobs in a given agency according to knowledge, skills, abilities, and responsibilities necessary for job performance by assignment of points for each factor. Weights are used for the various job factors measured. Factors can be weighted to discriminate for men and against women. Job structure can be segregated by gender, race, or ethnicity. Job-analysis evaluation systems choose weight factors biased against women. Four systems are used to evaluate jobs: the classification ranking system, the point rating system, the factor comparison or benchmark ranking system, and whole job ranking in which all jobs are ranked by relation to top position. The system and the process can both discriminate.[7,9,17]

Table 46.3 shows annual salaries for comparable city jobs in the city of San Jose, California, 1981.

Problems with Job Evaluation

There are many flaws in job evaluation. A Westinghouse plant in New Jersey was sued by female employees because they were paid less than male employees for jobs rated comparably by the company's job-evaluation system. The female employees won.[27]

All current pay systems are considered inadequate: hourly, output, job contract, supply and demand, and everyone-paid-the-same. They could be improved if employers and employees agreed on critical factors and values assigned.[18] Since no good job-evaluation system is reported to exist, job evaluation is not done in 80% of organizations across the country even though job evaluation systems have been developed for two-thirds of the labor force. They contain gender and race factors that need to be eliminated.[28] Nurse administrators should press for development of a job evaluation in their organizations. It is one of the most objective activities for establishing pay equity, regardless of its lack of widespread application.

Career Development and Job Evaluation

Career development and job evaluation can be combined as major objectives of nurse administrators. Nurse job-applicants should be apprised of career opportunities at the time they apply for jobs. These should be strategic objectives once nurses are hired. The clinical nurse should be entered into a career-development program in which job evaluation has established promotional opportunities based on credentials, require-ments, and productivity. The promotion pro-gram will have financial and titular rewards.

PROGRESS

Despite claims that pay equity for women has not made gains for the past 2000 years, there are actions that have and can be taken to make progress. Pay equity only became an issue after 1945. These actions include:

- Political action will cause legislators to change laws on municipal, state, and fed-eral levels. Bruntland is prime minister of Norway for a second six-year term. She has appointed eight women to her cabinet. Forty percent of the Norwegian civil service are women and 34% of 157 parliament seats are occupied by women. Voters support Bruntland.[29] If women in the United States acted in concert po-litically they could accomplish similar results. Nurses can influence politicians to support comparable worth for state employees, particularly during election campaigns and legislative sessions.
- In 1984 the City Council of Seattle estab-lished a reserve account for comparable worth.[8]
- Individual nurse administrators can im-plement a bias-free job-evaluation system.[8]
- States implementing comparable worth studies or bills include Maine, Minne-sota, New York, Nebraska, Connecticut, Idaho, New Mexico, Louisiana, and Washington. Approximately 13 other states are collecting data and evaluating job-equity concerns.[30]
- Nurses could establish a model bias-free job-evaluation system through their pro-fessional associations.

The question remains: Will the best bet for comparable worth be employers, the courts, or both? Nurses should use job-evaluation studies, re-evaluation studies of wage scales,

political organizing, collective bargaining, legislation, lobbying efforts, and public edu-cation. The National Science Foundation's position is that a nonbiased job-classification system is possible. Laws do exist and can be enforced. Society must value the people who perform its services, and nurses are a major group among these people.[4,10]

Change is slow in reducing occupational channeling and crowding. The system will adapt with gradual change. Collective bar-gaining will increase in some areas not af-fected by comparable worth. Comparable worth will be achieved through legislation and at the collective-bargaining table. Policy follows politics, and nurses must be involved in both.

In summary nurses, being predominantly women, are party to the concept of compara-ble worth, a concept that asks to be remedied by correcting salary inequities based on job segregation by gender. While some headway has been made in the decade of the '80s, it has been made by women entering predomi-nantly male occupations. This does little to correct the inequity in the value or worth of nursing as a profession. While society has given lip service to a high worth for nurses, occupational segregation in nursing makes it a predominantly female profession with lower salaries and wages than comparable male professions and occupations.

Market forces are touted by economists as a remedy that will bring about comparable worth. Nurse shortages have reached crisis proportions, yet there have been no signifi-cant pay increases. Court decisions on com-parable worth center around the Equal Pay Act and the Civil Rights Act. They have not advanced the cause of comparable worth. While job evaluation has as its purpose scien-tific analysis of jobs based on objective criteria of relative skills, knowledge, effort, working conditions, and responsibility, it has had rel-atively minor application. Unions have achieved only modest results.

Nurses, and women in other sex-segregated occupations, need to proceed with the quest in the courts, in job evaluation efforts within professional organizations, in the political arena, and with the collective-bargaining process. They should intensify their efforts in all areas if nursing is ever to be valued by society and to continue to attract intelligent and able women and men into its ranks.

If mutual trust is to be established between the clinical nurse and the nurse administrator, the latter must act decisively and promptly. This will include addressing all the issues of comparable worth—issues crucial to ending the dissatisfactions of professional nurses, and subsequently to ending the shortage of nurses.

REFERENCES

1. U.S. Bureau of the Census. Statistical Abstract of the United States, 108th Ed. Washington, DC: U.S. Government Printing Office, 1988.
2. King L. Comparable worth: economic issue of the '80s—in Kansas? Kans Nurse 1985;60(7):1–2.
3. Finnin M. Finnin testimony. Mass Nurse 1983;52(4):8–9.
4. Pollard S. Comparable worth. Mass Nurse 1981;50(11):5.
5. Waintroob A. Comparable worth issue: the employer's side. Hosp. Manager 1985;15(4):6–7, Women's Pay. Advisor 1987; 14(3):4.
6. Curran P. Comparable worth study shows state classification system discriminated. Mich Nurs 1982;55(6):4, 23.
7. Thomas C. Pay equity and comparable worth. Labor Law Journal 1983;34(1):3–12.
8. Bedell J. Another look at comparable worth. Wash Nurse 1984;14(8):3, 10.
9. TNA's Professional Services Committee. Nurses & the comparable worth concept. Tex Nurs 1985;59(4):12–16.
10. Felmley J. Comparable pay for comparable worth. JNY State Nurses Assoc 1981;12(4):12–16.
11. Disch JM, Feldstein PJ. An economic analysis of comparable worth. J Nurs Adm 1986;16(6):24–32.
12. Silver G. Comparable worth. Lancet 1984;3(8408):917.
13. Weingard M. Establishing comparable worth through job evaluation. Nurs Outlook 1984;32(2):110–113.
14. Steinem G. Let us revalue work. Calif Nurse 1982;17(9):7–9.
15. Absalom KC. Collective bargaining: comparable worth. Calif Nurse 1982;17(9):7, 13.
16. Stober RP. Comparable worth: part I: the basis of the controversy. Penn Nurse 1983;38(4):1–2.
17. Youngkin EQ. Comparable worth: alternatives to litigation and legislation. Nurs Econ 1985;3(1):38–43.
18. Esquire CC. Comparable worth: a brief explanation. Florida Nurse 1985;33(9):7.
19. Pay equity/comparable worth: an update of public sector activities. Penn Nurse 1985;40(9):4, 10.
20. Stober RP. Women are paid less than men. Solution? Comparable worth. Weather Vane 1984;53(3):3–5.
21. Aldrich M, Buchele R. The economics of comparable worth. Cambridge, MA: Ballinger, 1986.
22. Pennsylvania nurses file bias lawsuit. Mobile Press Register 1986;173(216):15D.
23. Brennan EJ. Sex discrimination and comparable worth. Personnel Journal 1984;63(10):56,58–59.
24. Robinson B. Robinson testimony. Mass Nurse 1983;52(4):9.
25. Stewart A, Stewart V. Selection and appraisal: the pick of recent research. Personnel Management 1976;8(1):20–24.
26. Wisniewski SC. Achieving equal pay for comparable worth through arbitration. Employee Relations Law Journal 1982;8(2):236–255.
27. Carter MF. Comparable worth: an idea whose time has come. Personnel Journal 1981;60(10):792–794.
28. Anderson D. A hospital administrator responds: comparable worth is not the issue. J Christ Nurs 1984;1(1):9–10.
29. Shearer L. Even break for women. Parade Magazine 1986, p. 18.
30. Washington Women United—Comparable Worth Project. The issue is comparable worth. Wash Nurse 1984;14(5):6–7.

BIBLIOGRAPHY

Wandelt MA: et al. Why nurses leave nursing and what can be done about it. Am J Nursing 1981;8(1):72–77.
Report from the Task Force to Study Nurse Shortage Situation in State of Alabama. Montgomery: Alabama Hospital Association, December, 1981.
National Commission on Nursing. Summary of the Public Hearings. Chicago: American Hospital Association, Hospital Research and Educational Trust, and American Hospital Supply Corporation, 1981.
American Academy of Nursing Task Force on Nursing Practice in Hospitals. Magnet Hospitals: Attraction and Retention of Professional Nurses. Kansas City: American Nurses' Association, 1983.
Alabama Hospital Association. The Alabama Nurse Study: A Survey of Registered Nurses' Attitudes About Their Profession. Montgomery, Alabama, 1983.
Committee on Nursing and Nursing Education, Institute of Medicine. Recommendations: Meeting Current and Future Needs for Nurses. Washington, DC.

47

Labor Relations: Theory, Research, and Strategies

Terry Throckmorton
Karlene Kerfoot

NURSES who function as executives in health-care institutions control the largest number of employees in the institution. If they also have responsibility for ancillary services such as housekeeping and dietary, the volume of employees becomes even more significant. Whether these administrators are responsible for nursing staff alone or for nursing and ancillary service staff, the mix of personnel provides them with a challenge in terms of personnel management and labor relations.

Employees enter the work force for many different reasons and are motivated in different ways. Administrators who are interested in the satisfaction and retention of employees as well as their productivity, will apply management theories and historical perspectives in assessing: (1) factors that motivate employees to join or remain in the work force, (2) factors that lead to dissatisfaction, and (3) needs that employees see as unmet.

The foundation for the current composition and context of nursing as well as for the approaches of nurses as a group to work satisfaction was laid in the period between 1860 and 1930, when nursing first emerged as a distinct profession. Nurses, in the earliest period of their history, functioned relatively independently in homes and in public health settings. However, nursing, a predominantly female profession, developed in a male-dominated society and its functions naturally grew to be defined in terms of the feminine role in society. These functions included the nurturing of children and the sick, housekeeping, and assistance in ancillary tasks.[1] In keeping with this concept, the education of nurses was relegated to hospital systems which, according to Sleeper, enforced severe discipline and instructed nurses in passive subordination to physicians.[2] Their security in the work force depended upon the goodwill of physicians and hospital managers, and their status as professionals remained vague. The relationship of employers toward nurses was paternalistic with rewards provided as deemed appropriate by the employer rather than by the employee and with encouragement of individual rather than collective bargaining.[3] Nurses responded to dissatisfaction with the work environment through turnover, absenteeism, and exit from employment, a pattern that has continued into the 1980s.

Loss of nurses from the work force and frequent turnover among nurses who remained actively employed created significant increases in staffing costs, forcing managers to focus on the volume of nurses exiting from the work force and on the factors related to that behavior. Although some nursing directors viewed turnover as an insoluble problem resulting from the unavoidable family obligations of nurses, analysts indicated a variety of causes and potential for resolution.[4] Fournet, Distefano, and Pryor found that turnover related to unavoidable family obligations accounted for only 36% of all turnover, and that 64% was voluntary and possibly preventable.[5] The responses of nurse managers to the high turnover among nurses took the form of requests for nursing input through innumerable surveys assessing satisfaction. Many of these surveys were based on the theoretical premises presented by Maslow, Herzberg, and Vroom as approaches to management.

Benton and White assessed the responses of 565 registered nurses regarding 16 job factors categorized into Maslow's need hierarchy (excluding physiologic). Respondents ranked the categories in order of importance as follows: safety and security, social, esteem, self-actualization, and nonspecific (salary and benefit needs). Specific factors listed as deficient in the work environments were: adequate personnel (safety), management recognition (esteem), promotion opportunities, inservice training programs (self-actualization), pay differential for education and experience and written job descriptions (nonspecific). The value and level of deficiency assigned to each factor by administrative nurses varied considerably from that assigned by staff nurses.[6]

Ullrich compared results from his study on the work motivation of nurses with studies by Herzberg, using Herzberg's two-factor theory of motivation.[7] Herzberg postulated that factors intrinsic to the work itself, such as achievement, responsibility, and recognition could serve as sources of motivation, whereas factors extrinsic to the work, such as working conditions, administration, and personnel policies, would more likely be sources of dissatisfaction. He therefore attributed turnover among workers to extrinsic job factors.

However, Ullrich, in his survey of 40 nurses, found that 44% of the factors cited by nurses as reasons for leaving the job were intrinsic to the work. Although Ullrich's sample was a small, systematically chosen one, his findings were similar to those of other nursing investigators.

Brief, as well as Seybolt, Pavett, and Walker, assessed turnover among nurses using models based on Vroom's expectancy theory and the modifications made by Porter and Lawler. Vroom theorized that behavior was determined by the individual's motivation in the job situation. He defined motivation as a combination of the individual's perceived value of the outcomes of work and the organization (valence), perception of a connection between performance and outcome (instrumentality), and the actual value of performance (valence of performance). If individuals valued the outcomes of work and perceived a connection between performance and outcomes, they would have a high valence of performance. Vroom defined expectancy as individuals' perceptions of whether their efforts would lead to high-level performance.[9] Porter and Lawler added ability and role perceptions to motivation as determinants of performance leading to a result perceived as satisfying or dissatisfying. They also postulated that the perceived equity of the outcome affected the level of satisfaction.[10]

Brief surveyed available research on turnover in nursing and applied Vroom's expectancy theory in analysis of the data.[11] Seybolt and associates surveyed 212 nurses (20% L.V.N.s; 80% R.N.s) regarding the importance of work issues and followed one year later with an assessment of turnover in the group.[12] Data from both surveys supported the concept of turnover among nurses due to failure of the job to meet their expectations for autonomy, growth, and development.

More complex and comprehensive assessments of motivation and turnover among nursing employees were based on causal models that were focused on multivariate correlates of turnover and the psychology of the withdrawal process in order to better predict turnover. March and Simon developed one of the earliest integrative models of employee turnover, the Decision to Participate Model, which served as a stimulus for the development of subsequent models. The model has two distinct, but interrelated elements applied to employee participation: perceived desirability of movement from the organization and perceived ease of movement from the organization. It was the first model to include integration of the economic-labor market and individual turnover behavior and was based on a large volume of research.[13]

Subsequent models have again been based on extensive literature reviews and deal with the same variables consistently identified in these reviews. These variables include: individual differences, job satisfaction, probability of finding alternatives, withdrawal cognitions individual values, and affective responses. Individual differences frequently include: age; sex; education; personality factors such as achievement, aggression, independence and self-confidence; vocational interests, aptitude, and ability; source of job referral; tenure in the organization; professionalism; performance; and absenteeism. Job satisfaction usually covers personal, institutional, and job related characteristics (e.g., pay, promotion, job content, coworkers, supervision and working conditions) and is usually measured using a Likert (e.g., strongly agree, agree neutral, disagree, strongly disagree) or a ranking scale. The probability of finding alternatives refers to the ease with which an employee can find a job of equal or better value to them. Withdrawal cognitions are defined as the employee's thoughts about leaving the job or actual intent to quit the job. Individual values include variables such as religious beliefs, emphasis on work or nonwork activities, philosophy of life, and service- versus self-orientation. Affective responses are defined as the emotional reactions of employees usually in relation to stress, treatment by managers, treatment by peers, and ability to live up to personal standards in the work setting.

The variables included in each of the mod-els are usually placed in sequence according to the process by which they affect turnover. An example of the sequencing in these models can be seen in the model developed by Mobley, Griffeth, Hand and Meglino in which Individual Values influence Affective Responses that lead to Intention to Search and Intention to Quit (simultaneously) that result in Turnover. In this model, economic and market condition variables are included as determinants of the intention to search and quit. In other words, the employee who observes an abundance of jobs and the ability to obtain equal or better salary and benefits through the available jobs will be more likely to search and leave the current job.[14]

The model by Mobley and associates has been tested with employees in various occupations and professions, including nursing. Each time the model has been tested, decisions have been made regarding revision of the model in order to more accurately predict turnover. The key to the successful use of any model of turnover is continued testing with the employee group of interest and continued refining of the model to achieve a better fit of the model with the behavior of the employees.[14]

Although nurse executives usually do not have control over all of the variables presented in these surveys and models of turnover behavior, they can make recommendations to those who do have control over these factors and they can create a supportive environment for employees, making the setting as convenient as possible for the achievement of both employee and institutional goals. This type of management is the best method for the prevention of dissatisfaction, and the resulting absenteeism, turnover, and unionization.

EMPLOYEE RESPONSE TO MANAGEMENT

In the absence of satisfactory management and working conditions, employees will select a way to make their dissatisfaction known. Employees relate to and negotiate with management according to their individual circumstances and backgrounds. The existence among nurses and ancillary staff of different ideologies (Nightingalism, employeeism, and professional collectivism), educational levels (diploma, associate degree, and baccalaureate), occupational levels, and reasons for working results in different responses to management. The ideologies most prevalent among nurses correlate with the historical development of nursing. In Nightingalism, the service ideal is stressed with greater emphasis on helping society than on personal gain and relates back to the service-oriented image portrayed by Nightingale. Employeeism is based on the belief that the employer has the best interest of the employees in mind, and will therefore provide for them. The survival of this attitude may be due to the authoritarian system of hospital schools in which many nurses have been educated. Professional collectivism developed as a result of the failure of the first two ideologies to meet nursing needs and to permit the provision of quality care. In professional collectivism, the responsibility for maintaining high standards of service was placed with the individual as well as with the group of professionals.[15]

Underlying this division of nurses according to philosophical belief is the problem of multiple routes for entry into practice. Inferred in the views of Habenstein and Christ is the premise that the varying types of educational preparation for nurses direct them toward one of the three ideologies. They seemed to indicate that those nurses who espouse professional collectivism tend to be more recent graduates of collegiate programs, whereas proponents of Nightingalism tend to be older nurses who graduated from hospital programs, and proponents of employeeism tend to be graduates from shorter programs designed to provide skills to make a living.[16]

The varying occupational levels or career directions of nurses also contribute to the differences in their responses to management and to dissatisfaction with their jobs. Throckmorton, in her survey of 445 Texas nurses found that staff nurses with heavy work loads as well as middle managers favored collective action and strikes in dealing with unsatisfactory working conditions, whereas nurses isolated in doctor's offices and in float pools favored sanctions such as letters and newspaper articles.[17]

According to Udy and Hirschman, employees as individuals with unique characteristics may select exit or voice behaviors and may respond individually or as a group.[18–19] Exit behavior represents individual or group response in the form of tardiness, absenteeism, or turnover. As already discussed, exit behavior seems to represent a pattern among nurse employee groups. Voice behavior may include individual complaints to administration or group protest through such actions as demonstration, strike, and collective negotiation. Health-care workers have been associated with many of the conditions that generally result in the use of exit behaviors. These conditions include low wage in comparison to peers with equal or less education, availability of alternative employment with increased benefits, wages and better working conditions, and subscription to middle-class values and mores.[20] In recent years, conditions that foster the use of voice option have also begun to exist for health-care workers. These conditions include changes in the economy making jobs less plentiful, concern with the quality of work and of the care provided, and the availability of assistance from traditional unions or the professional association. Health-care employees represent one of the last large industries to be organized by traditional unions. As such, they have been targeted for extensive and comprehensive campaigns, making collective bargaining more obviously available and perhaps more appealing.

In addition to understanding the satisfaction level of employees, nursing managers require an understanding of the views of nurses as a professional group toward collective bargaining. Historically, nurses as a group have been ambivalent about the concept of unionization and remain divided on the issues related to unionization. Those nurses who oppose the use of collective bargaining primarily refer to the effect of the process on the professional status of nursing, the separation of nurses in bargaining units, the conflict of interest question in representation by state nurses' associations and the adversary relationship created between staff nurses and managers. Because nursing is a service-oriented profession composed of both staff and managerial employees who belong to the same professional association, opponents of collective negotiation view it as disruptive to the unification of nurses and to achievement of the primary goals of nursing.[21]

Proponents of collective bargaining for nurses present a view of a new type of professional practicing within a bureaucracy and adopting the collective tactics traditionally used in bureaucratic organizations to achieve autonomy and control over standards of practice. They see the process of collective negotiation as the same for all employees and stress that the issues for professionals center around control over professional practice, thus making it a clear expression of professionalism.[22] According to Wilensky, collective negotiation for nurses provides a means by which they can bargain for and enforce standards of professional practice in a written contract.[23] He added that collective negotiation for professionals results in a hybrid-type professional association that combines the element of professional practice with that of collective negotiation.

Nurses usually function in health-care institutions such as hospitals or community agencies. The setting is therefore an important factor in the decision of whether or not to organize as a collective bargaining group. In some settings, collective bargaining is a very strong force, while in others it is not recognized as useful to the nursing staff. Unions have not been as ingrained in the nursing culture as in that of other work groups. The nursing profession has cyclicly experienced either an oversupply or an undersupply of nurses. This cycle has resulted in a very inconsistent and staggering progress toward unionization. In times in which the supply of nurses is plentiful, when nurses are facing layoffs, it is difficult to organize nurses into unions. When there is a shortage of nurses and the available nurses have more power because they are a scarce resource, unionization is easier. There are many more issues around which nurses can coalesce during staff shortages.

The key to the formation of unions in nursing is the ability of the union to define issues that those in power are not able or willing to address satisfactorily. The structure of nursing in institutions has come from a background of extreme centralization of authority and hierachic decision making with power and responsibility centered at the top of the organization. The military and religious influences on nursing have contributed greatly to this heritage. Consequently, nursing organizations in institutions often have traditional hierachic organizational forms. Many young nurses are not satisfied with this model. Younger generations of nurses desire autonomy, independence, control, input into the workplace and work rules, and job satisfaction and autonomy that previous generations did not expect. Nursing administration in institutions has been slow to reorganize and respond to these needs. The groundwork for conflict is often laid in organizations when this expectation of the current generation is not recognized.

The lack of recognition of nurses can also be a contributing factor leading to unionization. This lack of recognition can come from the institution, but it can also come from the nurse leaders. As nurses climb the corporate ladders of hospitals and become nurse executives, it is common for their roles and identities to become blurred. The nurse executive can be perceived by the nursing staff as no longer identified with nursing and supportive of the institution, not of nursing colleagues. A result of this perception is the "labor-management split" that can precipitate and support unionization. Once this split occurs, open communication, problem solving, and negotiation are no longer plausive conflict-resolution tools.

Lack of respect for individual rights is another powerful factor in causing an institution to be at high risk for unionization. Respect and recognition are demonstrated not only through deeds such as logical salary adjustments, fair promotion procedures, and other employment practices, but also through the culture developed in the institution. If administrators are unavailable, distant, aloof, and set themselves aside as "better than everyone else," resentment and anger will build. Protecting and respecting the rights of the employees should be standard operating procedure for people in administration.

There are many forms of management available to solicit and recognize input from nurses. The Japanese bottom-up type approach, quality circles, participative management, and shared governance are all key words to the organization of departments of nursing. If one truly does establish a participative management model, the need for a union decreases. However, if the model exists on paper only and not in actual practice, the institution immediately places itself in a situation of high risk for someone coming in from the outside.

Unions need a cause to exist. It is virtually impossible to organize a satisfied, happy group of people. It would not make sense to these people to spend extra money in union

dues to obtain problem resolution they may have without paying the additional fees. Job satisfaction is integral to the decision to form or not to form a union. Therefore, the administrator who pays close attention to job satisfaction and is perceived as being genuinely concerned about job satisfaction of the nursing staff will not have to contend with a group's decision to unionize. Unions become necessary when the principles of open communication, participative management, respect, and fairness are perceived as absent. Institutions that are not able to actualize these concepts are at high risk for unionization.

Organizations that are not at high risk for unionization have some common characteristics. The administrators of these organizations respect the employees and show recognition for their contributions to the organization. The administrators have established upward- as well as downward-communication channels for employees and acknowledge and use their information and decisions. Finally, they have a very discretely defined and effective grievance procedure; the nurses believe that the procedure is fair, meets their needs, and is administered logically.

It is also important to consider the role of the nurse educator in the attitudes that people develop toward unions. Nurse educators are powerful figures in the inculcation of nursing students and have a far-reaching effect on their views of nursing and hospitals. If a nurse educator voices a preference for unions and is able to support this view, the nursing student often learns that unionization is a viable option for the future of the nursing profession. On the other hand, if an instructor does not believe that unions are appropriate, the student will often develop a similar view. In a survey of senior students in baccalaureate schools of nursing, information was solicited about their perceptions of the faculty members' view of unions. Overwhelmingly, the senior students reported that their faculty members supported unions for the profession and the faculty members' views correlated positively with the individual student's view of this matter.[24]

As more nurses have obtained educational degrees in two- or four-year colleges, they have been exposed to an academic culture that varies dramatically from the culture of the hospital diploma school. Academic freedom, student access to committees by membership, and the concept of sharing the governance of the academic institution becomes part of the nurses' awareness. If this atmosphere is not available in a service setting, the lack of ability to participate in decision making and to collaboratively work with people becomes rich fuel for unionization.

LABOR LAW

The availability of union or other collective-negotiation group assistance to health-care workers has been primarily influenced by three federal labor laws: the Wagner Act or National Labor Relations Act (1935), the Taft-Hartley or Labor-Management Relations Act (1947), and Public Law 93-360 or the Taft-Hartley Amendments (1974). The Wagner Act was designed to govern labor relations in industry and included the rights of employees to organize, defined unfair labor practices for employers, and established the National Labor Relations Board (NLRB). The NLRB was formed to administer the basic law under the Wagner Act with authority to seek enforcement through the courts. Some of its responsibilities included overseeing the elections of union representatives, investigating charges of unfair labor practices by employers and employees, hearing appeals and making decisions about possible violations of the National Labor-Relations Act. The law included under its jurisdiction both private and nonprofit hospitals.

The Wagner Act prohibited employers from:

1. Interfering in employees' right to organize and bargain collectively,
2. Discriminating against employees considering collective bargaining in hiring, tenure, or treatment during employment,
3. Interfering with or contributing to the formation or management of labor organizations,
4. Refusing to bargain collectively with the employees' selected representative, and
5. Discriminating or discharging employees who file charges or give testimony under the Taft-Hartley Act.

The act also defined the election procedure for selection of a bargaining representative by employees.[25]

The Taft-Hartley Act of 1974 (Labor-Management Relations Act) amended the Wagner Act to exclude government-owned corporations, voluntary, nonprofit hospitals, and government-owned hospitals. The Taft-Hartley Act also recognized state "Right to Work" laws that prevented the requirement of union membership as a condition of employment. The act prohibited unions from:

1. Restraining or coercing employees to join their membership or select a specific representative to deal with the union,
2. Causing employers to discriminate against employees because of union membership,
3. Refusing to bargain in good faith for employees who have selected the union as a representative,
4. Initiating obstructve procedures to force an employer to discontinue doing business with any other union,
5. Encouraging employees to stop work in order to force an employer to deal with a union when another union has already been certified as the bargaining agent,
6. Initiating a strike to force an employer

to assign work to members of one union over those of another union,

7. Charging excessive membership fees, and

8. Causing an employer to pay fees for work that had not or would not be performed (featherbedding).

The Taft-Hartley Act also permitted only one election per year for a particular bargaining unit.[26]

Four amendments to the Taft-Hartley Act were passed in subsequent years. In 1962, federal legislation was passed allowing employees of federal health-care institutions to engage in collective bargaining. Legislation passed in 1967 included employees of investor-owned hospitals and nursing homes under collective bargaining legislation. In 1970, nonprofit nursing-home employees were also included under the law, and in 1974, the major amendment affecting the health-care industry was passed.

The Taft-Hartley Amendments of 1974 re-established legal support for collective negotiations for nongovernment health-care facilities. The definition of a health-care institution was expanded to include: hospitals, convalescent hospitals, health maintenance organizations, health clinics, nursing homes, extended care facilities, or other institutions devoted to the care of sick, infirm, or aged persons.[28] The amendments mandated a 90-day notice of termination or expiration of existing union contracts to the employer and to the Federal Mediation and Conciliation Service and a 10-day note of intent to picket or strike in order to allow administrators to plan for continued patient services.[20] The amendment included provisions that no strike or lockout could occur during the 90-day notice period. It also included a requirement for mediation by the Federal Mediation and Conciliation Service and the possible use of a Board of Inquiry to settle disputes. The

amendment allowed for employee refusal to join or support a union for religious reasons.

REPRESENTATION

Professional workers who seek a voice in factors related to employment have a choice of routes for action, including avoidance of collective action, professional association representation, and traditional union representation. Avoidance of collective action and a focus on individual bargaining or on exit from the work setting as methods for dealing with work issues has been well documented as a persistent trait among nurses.[28] However, increasing numbers of nurses are finding these methods unsatisfactory and are turning to group action through formal representation. The choice of a representational group is based upon a variety of factors including: perceived professionalism and ethical standards, the behavior of management, perception of the success of the representative, understanding of the process of collective negotiation, and immediate goals.

Nurses historically have opted for both traditional and professional representation. In 1980, Beletz found that nurses who valued professional membership and dominance, understanding of nursing, and concern for the public interest tended to choose professional association representation. Those nurses whose interests were primarily oriented toward economic gains tended to consider representation by traditional unions, although actual use of these groups remains controversial.[29] In 1983, Throckmorton found that nurses in Texas ($n = 450$) agreed with both professional association representation (390) and union representation (107). Only 15 of the 450 nurses disagreed with collective negotiations for nurses. She also found that there were no significant differences between the choices made according to whether or not the nurses belonged to the American Nurses' Association.[17]

DIFFERENCES IN COLLECTIVE BARGAINING AGENTS

A union by definition is an organized group of employees that uses formal procedures to negotiate with an employer to determine the conditions under which the employees perform their jobs. Divisions of professional associations or autonomous state professional associations that serve as collective bargaining agents fulfill the criteria for the title union. The structure of the American Nurses' Association (ANA) for collective bargaining purposes is composed of local units (core groups of nurses in individual hospitals), district units that facilitate communication between local and state units, state units that function as autonomous agents representing local units to the employer, and the national organization that acts as an advisor. The distribution of nurses in the state and district units frequently correlates with that of employing organizations with supervisors, directors, and educators in governing positions, although the configuration varies from unit to unit.[30] The conflict of interest that arises as a result of a membership composed of staff nurses and nurse managers is avoided by ANA through separation of the national association from autonomous state associations. State associations are still faced with the conflict of interest issue in some instances because of dominance by nurse managers and educators. As a result, there has been a trend toward decertification of these state associations as well as separation of nurse managers and educators from control over this function in the associations.[31]

The structure of traditional unions is similar to that of ANA with the national, state, and local units. However, multiple national traditional unions exist each with state and local units and most linked together in a federation. The membership of traditional unions differs significantly from that of ANA with only nonmanagement personnel eligi-ble, and in some instances including nonprofessional employees (L.V.N.s or L.P.N.s and aides) as well as professionals.

Traditional unions have several advantages over the professional association in competing for contracts in terms of focus and availability of resources. The membership of ANA is small in proportion to the number of nurses represented by it; as a result funding and staffing may be restricted. In addition, nurses as a group exhibit a lack of knowledge about collective bargaining. As a professional association, ANA has many other functions besides collective bargaining.[31] The traditional union in contrast, has a single orientation, years of experience, and a better source of funding since in many states they can either require all workers in a unionized institution to join the union (union shop), or require them to pay dues (agency shop).

THE ORGANIZING PROCESS

Selection of an organization as a target for union organizing efforts can occur in several ways. The initial contact with the union may be made by dissatisfied employees who wish union representation, or the union organizer may select organizations for an organizing campaign. The organizer's selection may be based on the vulnerability of an institution to union organizing efforts, its position as a key institution in an area, or simply the convenience of an organization for the union.

The union may use a top-down approach in which representatives try to convince management that the union has employee support and demand recognition. Since the employer may not legally recognize the union unless it actually does have the support of over half of the employees, most employers refuse to accept the union organizer's word alone as evidence of employee support. This approach is therefore the least successful one used.

The bottom-up approach is most frequently used and involves contacting employees and convincing them to sign authorization cards and vote for union representation. The union organizers are usually interested in specific employees in the organization who have essentially the same interests and demands. These employees form a bargaining unit.

The next step after selection of the targeted institution is a detailed survey of its resources and workings to gain as much information as possible about it. Information is obtained from employees and other sources in the community regarding the work force, services, working conditions, shift hours, personal and occupational characteristics of the employees, salaries, benefits, supervision, management, and financial status of the organization. Employees are approached in public places, their homes, the organization's parking lot, and other nonwork areas and are asked for their opinions, ideas, and needs or wants. As the organizers become familiar with the employee perspective, they begin to present their campaign to help employees negotiate with management.

Key employees are selected to serve as leaders and to provide information about problems and complaints of employees. These leaders usually represent each of the factions in the employee group such as women, men, or racial minority groups. The leaders collect and deliver union authorization cards to the organizers. The cards indicate the employees' authorization of the union to act as their bargaining agent. The union must receive cards or a signed petition from 30% of the employees in order to file with the National Labor Relations Board for a secret ballot election.[32] Unions usually try to obtain the support of 50% or more employees before they petition the NLRB for an election. Once the petition for the election has been granted, the union organizers devote their efforts to convincing employees to actually vote for union representation.

PREPARATION FOR NEGOTIATIONS

Negotiation of a collective bargaining agreement requires extensive preparation and knowledge. If the nurse managers and administrators are not already familiar with labor law and the collective negotiation process, the first step should be to educate all managers with this basic information. In many institutions, managers are required to attend formal didactic courses on collective negotiation preparation and strategies. Along with this information, managers will require a clear understanding of the NLRB certification. They should be aware of which employees are legally represented in the bargaining unit and the short- and long-term implications of placement of these job classifications in the unit.[33] It is also necessary to decide who among the employee groups should be classified as supervisor under the NLRB definition.

In Section 2.11 of the National Labor Relations Act, Supervisor is defined as:

> any individual having authority, in the interest of the employer, to hire, transfer, suspend, lay off, recall, promote, discharge, assign, reward, or discipline other employees, or responsibly direct them, or to adjust their grievances, or effectively to recommend such action, if in connection with the foregoing the exercise of such authority is of not a merely routine or clerical nature, but requires the use of independent judgment.[34]

Employees who are classified as supervisors are important for two reasons. First, they are needed to represent management to organized employees on a day-to-day basis. Second, they are needed to cover for absent employees during a strike so that patient care is not interrupted. Who is to have supervisor status must be decided on prior to the union election.

Selection of the negotiation team is the next step. Membership on the team is based on the areas of expertise required for the negotiation, usually including personnel management or labor relations, finance, nursing, and general administration. The membership should not include top-level managers in any of the areas. Absence of the main decision makers from the team permits more time for decisions since the negotiating team must check with administration before making any agreements. Preliminary planning with top management provides goals and basic parameters for the team's negotiations. A main spokesperson should be appointed from the committee members so that negotiations will be organized.

Once the team is selected, data covering all areas of potential negotiation should be collected and made available to team members. Areas to be covered include: internal cost data (current job rates), wage history for at least five years, fringe benefit costs and upgrade costs, employee data (seniority rights and demographic data), external wage and fringe benefit data (industry survey), environmental survey (availability of jobs, contracts, and availability of replacement personnel), and existing data on employee factions and complaints. Information about the union should also be obtained. This search should include: the constitution and bylaws of the union; names and biographical data of the union officials; and demographic, professional, and employment background of the union negotiators.

The third type of data to be collected is a list of potential union demands and the estimated cost of each item. These data are usually obtained from known areas of dissatisfaction among employees and from contracts negotiated throughout the United States by the respective union. A useful format is to place current wages, benefits, rights, and costs in a column parallel to predicted values for easy visual comparison during negotiations. The same procedure can be used for clauses from previous and predicted contracts.

When all data have been collected, management objectives and proposals are developed and placed in a written format that includes the rationale and supportive data for each item. A useful approach is to prepare three levels for each item: the highest- and lowest-acceptable levels and the actual predicted level. The same format can be used to outline projected union demands. These data plus all supporting data should be organized into books according to the negotiation agenda or previous contract clauses.

The last item in preparing for the negotiations is to select the place and time for the initial meeting. Issues to be considered include: location at or away from the organization, and timing during or outside of working hours and with or without pay for team members. During the first meeting, the participants exchange proposals. The length of the proposals, the number of demands, and the degree of differences between the groups will be the basis for determining the number and length of meetings. Decisions regarding placement of the meetings and payment of members are usually based on previous practices or the current practices of others in the region.

THE NEGOTIATION PROCESS

Meetings are divided into four types: the first meeting for exchange of proposals and the setting of meeting times, the second meeting for responses to the proposals, middle meetings of two to four hours at one- to two-day intervals for preliminary negotiating and the final meetings, usually longer, for actual contract agreement. Usually the union's first demands are high and management's offers low. During the negotiation process, demands and offers gradually approximate each other until an agreement is reached, or remain disparate until mediation is requested or a strike or lockout is called.[34]

The negotiation process usually includes four types of bargaining: distributive, integrative, attitude structuring, and intraorganizational.[35] Distributive bargaining involves attempts to obtain the largest portion of fixed benefits. Gains by one side are reflected in losses on the other side. Integrative bargaining is based on achieving mutual benefit with both sides gaining from the final agreement. Attitude structuring involves efforts to change the attitudes of the opposing negotiators. Union and management representatives attempt to affect each other's attitudes about specific items in the contract. Intraorganizational bargaining occurs among the members of each side in an attempt to negotiate acceptance of necessary compromises among their own memberships. All four types of bargaining usually occur during the process of negotiating a contract.

NEGOTIATION DEADLOCKS

In the event that the negotiating parties fail to reach an agreement in the designated time limits, or if it becomes apparent that neither side is willing to make concessions, essentially four procedures are available for resolving the dispute. These procedures include mediation, fact-finding, arbitration, and strike or lockout. Mediation involves assistance from an outside source—either federal, state, or private—in resolving the conflict. The mediator can explore the options and offer advice, but has no authority to dictate terms. Fact finders are also obtained through federal, state, and private sources to collect data from both sides and make recommendations. Again, there is no authority to dictate terms. In interest arbitration, the third option, responsibility for establishing the terms of the contract is delegated to a third party. The third party makes final decisions without participation of the parties other than the supplying of information. Although riskier than mediation or fact-finding, arbitration can be an alternative to strike or lockout. Mediation, arbitration, and fact-finding services can be obtained through the American Arbitration

Association (AAA) or the Federal Mediation and Conciliation Service (FMCS).

A strike by the union or lockout of union employees by management both involve the cessation of work by union employees until some resolution can be reached. A strike is a cessation of work by employees in order to achieve contract demands or to protest unfair labor practices. A lockout involves closure of an organization in order to make employees agree to terms. Strike and lockout are the ultimate weapons for each side and as such incur the greatest negative public sentiment and impose the greatest hardship on the opposing parties. In health-care industry contracts, it is not uncommon to see the elimination of the strike and lockout weapons as special clauses. This strategy is used to eliminate the use of tactics that are unpopular with the consumer group and to apply pressure toward the resolution of disputes.[25]

CONTRACT ADMINISTRATION

Once a contract has been ratified, the issue then becomes how to deal most effectively with the union so that the needs of the nursing staff and of the patients can be simultaneously met. Working with the union means working with the right mind-set. It is necessary for those involved to believe that there can and must be collaboration and negotiation. It is imperative that each problem be approached with the thought that the relationship between the union and the management will be stronger because of this positive interaction. Extreme polarization between union and management means the end of effective negotiation.

Unions can potentially make the job of the administrator easier. There are definite work rules, clear expectations and guidelines, and little latitude allowed on the part of the administrator and the nursing staff. The structure of many interactions is spelled out by the union contract, which results in less ambiguity.

The administrator needs to appeal to the rationality of members of the union and the management staff. If nurse administrators are willing to listen to the issues and make changes based on the recognition of real problems, the respect for them and their authority will grow and the power of the union will lessen. The members of the union need to feel that the nurse executive is committed to their welfare.

Unions grow and mature in the face of inadequate, poor leadership. Their greatest impetus for growth exists when they are placed in a position in which they deal with people in management who are naive and uninformed and with whom it is difficult to relate. Unions in these situations are perceived as a vehicle to obtain results when the management staff are unable to do so. Poor management often gives unions their best excuse to exist.

Knowing the techniques of contract administration is particularly important for the smooth running of a unionized institution. Knowledge of these techniques means literally memorizing the contract and becoming fully aware of interpretations. Orientation of everyone to the contract will result in effective administration of the contract and efficiency in the organization.

PREPARATION FOR A STRIKE

Survival of a strike by employees in any significant number requires extensive planning on the part of both the union and management. Considerations for both sides include: current and future costs, ability to meet financial obligations during a strike, effect on the employees and clients, the potential effectiveness of the strike, whether employees will remain loyal to the union or to management, and public opinion regarding union and management behavior. The decision of a union to strike, or of an administrator to allow an impass to result in a strike or a lockout, is made only after serious review of these considerations and consideration of the resulting cost-benefit data.

Planning by management should occur well in advance of the strike date. Typical decisions include: which, if any units to close; which services to discontinue or reduce; who will be available to provide continued services and how should they be scheduled; what role physicians will play; what other groups or suppliers will honor the strike; and what, if any, services will be offered by striking employees. Once decisions are made in each of these areas, a formal plan can be developed so that there are few interruptions in patient care or in communication with union representatives.

Although effective planning by either or both parties can result in an orderly strike or lockout, the chances for negative results are great. The cost of a strike in terms of strike benefits for employees, loss of wages by employees, and loss of business by the employer is extensive. An end to the strike may be forced by either or both sides with or without an agreement as a result of inability to sustain additional losses. Because of the cost of strikes and the negative public opinion toward strikes by health-care employees, the option of a no strike/lockout clause in union-management contracts has become fairly common.

In conclusion, the future of nursing depends on the development of a strong profession, a profession that is united on many issues, and a profession that does in fact work together to better patient care. If this goal is to be achieved, excellent working conditions must exist in institutions with and without union contracts. The key to the success of nursing in an institution is not whether the nursing staff is or is not unionized. The real survival issue rests with the ability of the nursing staff and the management to work together in a way that provides great job satisfaction for the nursing staff and excellence in nursing care for the patients. Whether an institution does or does not have a union is not really the issue. The real crux of the matter is how successful the nursing staff and managers have been in developing an organizational structure and a communication system that leads to positive job satisfaction for all concerned.

REFERENCES

1. Devereux G, Weiner F. The occupational status of nurses. American Sociological Review 1950;15(5): 628–634.
2. Sleeper R. The two inseparables—nursing service and nursing education. Am J Nurs 1948;48:678–691.
3. Sheppard H, Sheppard A. Paternalism in employer-employee relationships. Am J Nurs 1951;51(1):10–14.
4. Beyers M, Mullner R, Byre C, Whitehead S. Results of the nursing survey, Part 2: RN vacancies and turnover. J Nurs Admin 1983;83(5):26–31.
5. Fournet G, Distefano M, Pryor M. Job satisfaction: issues and problems. Pers Mgmt 1966;19(2):165–183.
6. Benton D, White H. Satisfaction of job factors for registered nurses. J Nurs Admin 1972;2(6):55–63.
7. Ullrich R. Herzberg revisited: factors in job dissatisfaction. J Nurs Admin 1978;8(10):20–24.
8. Herzberg F. The motivation to work. New York: John Wiley & Sons, 1959.
9. Vroom V. Work and motivation. New York: John Wiley & Sons, 1964.
10. Porter L, Lawler E. Managerial attitudes and performance. Homewood, Ill: Richard D Irwin, Inc, 1968.
11. Brief A. Turnover among nurses: a suggested model. J Nurs Adm 1976;6(8):55–58.
12. Seybolt J, Pavett C, Walker D. Turnover among nurses: it can be managed. J Nurs Adm 1978;8(9):4–9.
13. March J, Simon H. Organizations. New York: John Wiley & Sons, 1958.
14. Mobley W, Griffeth R, Hand H, Meglino B. Review and conceptual analysis of the employee turnover process. Psych Bull 1979;86:493–522.
15. Grand N. Nightingalism, employeeism, and professional collectivism. Nurs Forum 1971;10(3):289–299.
16. Habenstein R, Christ E. Professionalizer, traditiona-

lizer, and utilizer. Columbia, MO: University of Missouri, 1955.
17. Throckmorton T. Attitudes of registered nurses in Texas relative to collective negotiation (Dissertation). College Station, Texas: Texas A & M University, 1983. p. 180.
18. Udy S. The comparative analysis of organizations. In: March J, ed. Handbook of organizations. Chicago: Rand McNally, 1965, pp. 678–709.
19. Hirschman A. Exit, voice and loyalty: responses to declines in firms, organizations and states. Cambridge, MA: Harvard University Press, 1970.
20. Miller M, Dodson L. Work stoppage among nurses. J Nurs Adm 1976;6(12):41–45.
21. Rotkovich R. Do labor union activities decrease professionalism? Sup Nurse 1980;11(9):16–18.
22. Jacox A. Collective action: the basis for professionalism. Sup Nurse 1980;11(9):22–24.
23. Wilensky H. The professionalism of everyone? Am J Soc 1964;70(2):137–158.
24. Kerfoot K, Buckwalter K, Curry J. Nursing students' perceptions of a career in nursing administration (Unpublished paper). IA: University of Iowa, 1984, p. 83.
25. National Labor Relations Act, as amended, 29 USC, 49 Stat. 449 (1935); 61 Stat. 136 (1947); 73 Stat. 541 (1959); 88 Stat. 395 (1974).
26. Hobart C. Collective bargaining with professionals: conflict, containment, or accommodation? Health Care Manage Rev 1976;1(2):7–16.
27. Bryant Y. Labor relations in health care institutions: an analysis of Public Law 93-360. J Nurs Adm 1978;8(3):28–39.
28. Wandelt M, Pierce P, Widdowson R. Why nurses leave nursing and what can be done about it. Am J Nurs 1981;81(1):72–77.
29. Beletz E. Organized nurses view their collective bargaining agent. The J Nurs Lead Manage 1980;11(9):3946.
30. Dolan A. The legality of nursing associations serving as collective bargaining agents: the Arundel case. J Health Polit Policy Law 1980;5(1):25–54.
31. Zimmerman A. Collective actions by professional employees. In: Jaeger B, ed. The impact of collective action on hospitals. Durham: Duke University Press, 1975,24–29.
32. Rowland H, Rowland B. Hospital administration handbook. Rockville, MD: Aspen Systems Corporation, 1984.
33. Fralic M. The nursing director prepares for negotiations. J Nurs Adm 1977;7(6):4–8.
34. Claus R. The ins and outs of collective bargaining. J Nurs Adm 1980;10(9):18–21.
35. Walton R, McKessie R. A behavioral theory of labor negotiation. New York: McGraw-Hill, 1965.

48

Nursing Education—
Nursing Administration:
Collaboration in Research

Jean A. Kelley
Ellen T. Patterson

ALL TYPES of approaches to research are needed to achieve a level of nursing practice that is "supported by a knowledge base stemming from research."[1] Single investigator, team investigator, institutional, and interinstitutional approaches to research have been tried and tested as a means of advancing nursing knowledge. However, during the decade of the 1980s a concern for cost containment in both nursing education and nursing practice is causing administrators to look for more effective and efficient stategies for conducting nursing research. Approaches that utilize personnel, time, money, and resources in a more cost-effective manner, while producing added outcomes relevant to the further improvement of nursing care, education, and management practices are valued and are being sought by nurse administrators. Collaboration in research by nurse educators and nursing staffs is one approach that meets these criteria and is gaining favor with nurse administrators.[2]

Collaborative research is the bringing together of nurses from different settings, different areas of practice, and different agencies to work in groups for the purpose of designing research projects based on mutually agreed on, high-priority nursing problems.[3] It is an approach that musters multitalented workers to help with planning and conducting a study. Each member recruited is expected to make valued contributions to the research throughout its life span. Each member taken in owns and works on the project as a tenant-in-common, sacrificing some independence in decision making for the good of the group project.

Therefore, collaborative research is based on a philosophy of equal rights and ownership in which the goal is to provide a group product. What makes collaborative research unique is the opportunity its members have: (1) to debate and compromise while identifying and defining a common research issue; (2) to share and exchange ideas, knowledge, and experiences throughout the planning and implementation phases of the research; (3) to build on the diversity of talents in this group, and (4) to draw on a wider range of resources and support services available from a group of nurses who are brought together from different environments.[4] Collaborative research fosters peer review and provides more opportunities for group members to learn from each other. Additionally, participation in peer interaction, cooperation, and critique has the potential for increasing dissemination of research. Moreover, involving several nurses with varying talents in one study strengthens the probability for development and implementation of a sounder research design. While one member may have expertise in defining terms, another may be more skilled in developing hypotheses, another with data collection, and still another in writing for scientific publications. Further, it is through the cooperative exchange of ideas that collaborative research has the increased possibility of generating several offshoot studies related to the common study.

An analysis of the nature of collaborative research reveals it to be distinguishable from other types. Collaborative research differs from other approaches when its cooperating multitude of researchers becomes united—after much debate and compromise—around a common research cause, and when the group is successful in maintaining equality among its members while producing a group product. Group research, on the other hand, brings together multiple investigators who do not ordinarily achieve a strong feeling of equality and group ownership of the study. Nor are the broad range of resources available in a group needed for conducting the research; rather the resources from only one source may be necessary. In group research the division of labor is easily assigned to different members with little need for coordinating and integrating individual research activities into the final product of the group.[5]

Traditionally, nurses have tended to participate in group research rather than in collaborative research. Their usual role has been that of data collector, or implementor of an experimental intervention. Collaborative research, on the other hand, offers nurses unlimited opportunities to contribute their special expertise throughout the design and conduct of a cooperative endeavor that belongs to a group of investigators. Nurses who possess the best profile as potential collaborators in nursing research are those who are open to differing ideas and reliable in fulfilling commitments. They are self-starters who can work interdependently, individuals who are tolerant of ambiguity and group tension, creative thinkers and doers, and en-

thusiastic team builders who maintain a sense of humor in the face of vulnerability to a peer critique of their ideas. In the final analysis, collaborative research is the approach of choice when: there is mutual interest in a researchable issue, conduct of the research requires resources above and beyond those available from a single investigator, a structure exists to facilitate cooperative research activities, and a group of researchers are willing to work with each other as peers in a collegial relationship.[6]

FACTORS AFFECTING COLLABORATIVE RESEARCH

Nurse executives are in a unique position to create a work climate that encourages collaborative research and that will advance nursing knowledge and improve nursing care, education, and managerial practices. Although knowledge about the complex nature of collaborative research is not totally complete, there are several critical factors that influence its success.[7] In planning for collaborative research, the nurse executive needs to take into consideration each key variable in terms of its individual nature and its interrelationships with others. Consequently, the role of the nurse executive in facilitating collaborative research is affected by, and differs with, the interaction of several factors.

Environmental Factor

The first variable critical to success with collaborative research in nursing education and nursing practice is the environment. A nursing organization is affected by three different types of environments and in turn affects the environment in which it functions. There is an external, an internal, and a lateral environment. Nursing organizations exist in hospitals, home health-care agencies, nursing homes, and health departments. A hospital, for example, may exist in the environment of an academic health-science center that has a traditional triad of purposes related to teaching, research, and service; or it may be located in a for-profit corporation with the primary mission of a profit-generating service and a research purpose last. The external environment includes also the community, region, state, federal government with its rules and regulations governing research, and national nursing and health-care organizations. The mission and goal of the external environment in relation to research will influence to a great extent the attitude of the nurse executive toward the value, support, and use of collaborative research.

The internal environment, on the other hand, is the climate that is created and maintained toward research in the nursing organization. A nurse executive is expected to facilitate research on nursing care and administration practices.[8] Creating an internal atmosphere in which professional nurses are expected to perform using a research-based practice, and writing this into position descriptions is critical to facilitating research. Providing time for nurses away from routine responsibilities to collaborate in doing research with other interested nurses is also essential. Arranging for support services and necessary funds for nurses to carry out cooperative research ideas is fundamental. And allocating resources for the publication and disseminating of research results is basic to the success of collaborative research as well. The nurse executive who participates in all four of these activities will be the one who establishes an internal climate that fosters collaborative research.

The often overlooked environment affecting collaborative research in nursing education and nursing practice is the lateral one. This is the peer climate toward research. It involves the attitude of the chief executive officer and other department heads or administrators toward scientific inquiry. Providing leadership in moving the nursing or-

ganization in the direction of collaborative research with other departments and disciplines is uncharted territory that needs to be bridged by today's nurse executives.

Structure Factor

There is no one best model to guide the nurse executive in organizing a nursing department or school of nursing to facilitate collaborative research. The structure selected is influenced by its mission, goals, the people involved, the nature of work to be done, the health-care needs of consumers, and the resources available. The availability of both a school of nursing and hospital nursing department provides one of the richest resources for collaborative research. However, even with these entities present, the structure selected may vary. Potential structures for collaborative research may be viewed on a continuum with the unification model on one extreme, the collaborative model in the middle, and the separation model at the other end (Figure 48.1). At the University of Alabama at Bir-

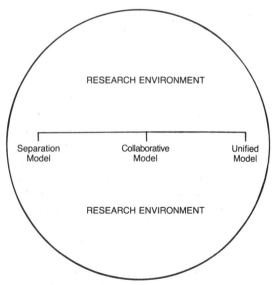

Figure 48.1. Continuum of Structural Models for Research in Nursing Education and Nursing Practice

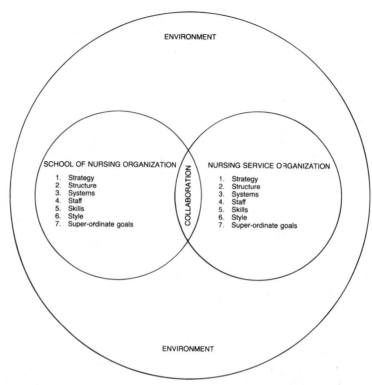

Figure 48.2. Collaborative Model for Nursing at the University of Alabama at Birmingham (UAB). (Adapted from McKinsey & Co. Organization design and development—enhancing organization capability and effectiveness: the never-ending juggling act. Unpublished discussion draft. San Francisco: McKinsey & Co., 1978; and Peters TJ, Waterman RH. In search of excellence: lessons from America's best-run companies. New York: Harper & Row, 1982).

mingham (UAB), for example, a collaborative model for nursing service and nursing education has existed since the spring of 1973. It has as its goal strengthening the quality of patient care, nursing education, and nursing research in an academic health-science center. Both the Nursing Service Organization and Nursing Education Organization maintain individual structures with separate administrative heads (Figure 48.2). But there are some dual and joint appointments along with many cross appointments to committees. An overall Joint Council on Nursing with representatives from all levels of administration (top, middle, and first) from both organizations meets quarterly to promote an exchange of information and to facilitate collaboration on mutually agreed on projects and issues facing nursing in an academic health-science setting.

Structural enablers for collaborative research, practice, and education were built into the Rules of the Joint Council on Nursing in the form of three standing committees—Research, Practice, and Education. Each standing committee is comprised of two representatives from service and two representatives from education. Annual objectives are developed by each standing committee and meetings are held throughout the year to monitor progress toward achievement of the objectives.

The Standing Committee on Nursing Research has been instrumental in stimulating collaborative research at the organizational and individual level. At the organizational level, the committee actively influenced change by proposing that a position for a nurse researcher be created in the hospital's Department of Nursing. The committee surveyed hospitals employing nurse researchers and from data gathered in this survey developed a position description and recommendations for the placement of it in the organization. Out of that effort, the Coordinator for Nursing Research position was created and filled by a doctorally prepared nurse. An integral component of that position is the facilitation of collaborative research between faculty, students, and nursing staff and liaison work with the school's Center for Nursing Research.

With the advent of more research being conducted by students, faculty, and staff, the Joint Council began to take a closer look at the costs, both hidden and manifest, of nursing research. Subsequently, the Standing Committee on Nursing Research was given the charge to look into the issue of the cost of conducting research. With the cooperation of one graduate student researcher and one staff nurse researcher, the committee collected detailed data on expenses incurred during the development, implementation, and completion of two research projects.

These findings were presented to the Joint Council and several outcomes emerged. There developed an increased awareness and understanding on the part of both nursing service and education of the cost of research and of the contributions each was making to the effort. Second, resources available to support research at both agencies were identified. This information was useful for planning and avoiding duplication. Third, dialogue surrounding this issue resulted in an enhanced spirit of sharing.

At the individual level, the Standing Committee on Nursing Research has worked actively to bring together nurses from service and education who share common research and clinical interests. A formal effort is presently underway to establish cluster study-groups by bringing together clinical nurse specialists from the Department of Nursing and faculty members from various clinical councils in the School of Nursing. It is anticipated that out of these discussions will emerge several cluster research "umbrellas" of high clinical relevancy to which individuals from both service and education will want to commit themselves. One such group will be discussed in more detail later.

Another unique feature in the UAB structure that facilitates collaborative research is the release time quarter (RTQ). The school operates on a calendar-year faculty appointment system, and the RTQ started in the summer of 1980 allows each faculty one quarter with annual pay for scholarly activities. The most common options selected by faculty for an RTQ are clinical practice, research, and other scholarly activities.

From the service perspective, the RTQ is an opportunity to receive intensive consultation and assistance from nursing faculty with particular research and educational expertise. The nature of the consultation has varied across time depending on departmental needs.

Initially, nursing faculty on RTQ were asked to consult on the development of the nursing research program in the hospital. The consultants worked closely with the newly employed coordinator of nursing research in developing departmental goals and objectives and in implementing strategies to meet those objectives. For example, a detailed plan for involving staff nurses in research was generated. One consultant assisted in planning and implementing an Introduction to Nursing Research workshop for the nursing staff. This faculty member also conducted a workshop for clinical nurse specialists on how to organize and lead a journal review group.

More recently, faculty on RTQ have been

asked to consult on research design and statistical analysis. The quantity and sophistication of the research projects generated by the nursing staff is increasing rapidly and the need for consultation from experts on the faculty continues to grow. Consequently, the consultants now work with staff nurses, head nurses, and clinical specialists in designing research projects and in planning data analysis. RTQ faculty have served also as mentors to this coordinator of nursing research as she develops further as a nurse researcher.

To summarize at this point, consultation from RTQ faculty is mutually beneficial and serves to enable quality nursing research. Faculty consultants receive remuneration for their efforts and the Department of Nursing is assured of quality input from experienced nurse researchers.

Human Factor

People need to, want to, and have to work together. For collaborative research to succeed, people need to want to work together on a problem of mutual concern. The role of the nurse executive is to provide a climate that motivates nurses to do and use research that will improve nursing practice, nursing education, or both. Nurses who do not work well together or who are coerced into working together can sabotage collaborative research, waste time and money, and produce little meaningful research. Nurse executives need to be cognizant of working relationships and foster those that are productive in terms of collaborative research. In addition, nurse executives need to provide leadership in integrating research based nursing practice into the professional value system of all nurses—novice, proficient, competent, and expert.

Most faculty have been acculturated into valuing research and research activities as critical to promotion and tenure. Staff nurses, however, are in environments where histori-

cally the production of services, not knowledge, has held the highest priority. How then, are practicing nurses motivated to become involved in collaborative research?

In some service settings, research activity is rewarded through a career ladder system. In others, the performance appraisal system incorporates research activities. Promotion in some settings may be contingent upon research activity. These external motivators have proven to generate only a lukewarm response, often not accompanied by a real commitment to the research process.

Practicing nurses who enthusiastically participate in collaborative research tend to do so out of self-initiative in an environment that actively supports research. Clinical interest and intellectual curiosity serve to motivate some practicing nurses. Research also provides variation on the routine of daily practice. Other nurses, with the support of nursing administration, have gingerly entered the research waters and found them stimulating and rewarding.

Encouragement from peers in other health professions has led some nurses to begin to consider research activity as part of their professional role. And last, conducting a research project can be a strategy for head nurses to create a more professional climate for practice.

In several ways collaborative research has been useful in helping nurses incorporate research into their professional value system. For example, R.N. baccalaureate students at the UAB are required to do a preceptorship in the last quarter of their program. Many opt for an administrative preceptorship instead of a clinical one because of their expert clinical proficiencies. Recently several R.N. baccalaureate students have opted for a research preceptorship. They work with the coordinator of nursing research in collecting data, reviewing the literature, and tabulating data. The students work on a variety of projects and complete the quarter with a new respect and enthusiasm for research.

Another way that collaborative research has been useful in helping nurses integrate research into their role has been through clinical nurse specialists working with faculty members on a project. Many clinical specialists have a working familiarity with research but are often hesitant to become involved because of their novice status and lack of confidence in their abilities. Collaborating with a faculty member experienced in research is one way for the clinical specialist to become clearer about what he or she knows and does not know, and to learn more about the process while under the tutelage of an expert researcher.

Work Factor

The work of a nursing organization in education or practice in relation to research is measured in terms of its output—the results of research and the extent to which it contributes to organizational effectiveness and efficiency. At the UAB, the Joint Council on Nursing through its collaborative model identified the research work that needed to be done in the cooperating structures and the mechanism or process through which it could be accomplished. Consequently, the Council and its Committee on Nursing Research delineated its goals and tasks for collaborative research and established timetables. Also addressed in their planning strategies was how these activities interrelated with the goals and tasks of the other two standing committees on nursing practice and nursing education. Subsequently, several major areas of work were emphasized: (1) development of a UAB nursing research directory, (2) implementation of collaborative research studies in nursing, (3) nurturing cluster studies, and (4) enhancing clinical research by graduate students in nursing.

Directory of Nursing Research

Fostering collaborative research in a large organization can be a challenging enterprise. With over 900 registered nurses practicing in the Department of Nursing and over 120 faculty members in the School of Nursing, establishing a formal mechanism for networking became essential. A RTQ faculty member, working with the coordinator of nursing research, developed this network in the form of a directory that lists nurse researchers in the university.

Permission was obtained from Sigma Theta Tau International to use the survey format developed for their research directory. This survey categorizes respondents in several ways including research topic, nursing model used, and population studied. The survey was distributed to all faculty in the School of Nursing and to clinical specialists, head nurses, directors, nursing staff development, and interested staff nurses in the Department of Nursing. The response rate was over 80%.

Data were coded and can be accessed through a computerized data base or from hard copies available in the Learning Resources Center in the School of Nursing or in the Nursing Staff Development Library in the hospital. The directory has proven useful in identifying nurses with similar interests or with expertise in a particular area. Graduate students new to the university community have found the directory helpful in identifying resource persons for their research.

Collaborative Studies

The first major collaborative study undertaken by the Joint Council was a five-year evaluation of the implementation of primary nursing at the UAB. Completed in the fall of 1981, the study involved the staff on 22 nursing units, nurse educators on RTQ, and an ad hoc committee of the Joint Council. Data were collected on the quality of care, nurse satisfaction, and patient satisfaction. A comparison of data from three nursing units revealed no significant difference in the quality of care, some frustration of nurses with the implementation of primary nursing, but belief in its benefits and higher patient-satisfaction scores. The evaluative study recommended that data continue to be collected and analyzed. Two important outcomes of the collaborative project were: (1) the involvement of many nurses in a research project affecting their practice as professional nurses, and (2) the inclusion of research activities in the job description and competency-based performance evaluation system for nursing staff.

The majority of the collaborative research taking place is in the area of clinical studies. Several authors[9,10,11] have written about the value of bringing together clinicians with practice expertise and researchers with theoretical and scientific expertise. Such a combination is more likely to generate research questions more relevant to practice, as well as quality studies. While the individuals collaborating on clinical studies usually have a primary area of expertise—clinical or research—often they move back and forth between roles. Many practicing nurses do not have a strong background in research methods but are able to identify pressing clinical issues, while faculty researchers are often able to help those nurses to define and delineate the clinical problems in need of investigation. The most effective collaborative teams are the ones where the members are conversant in both research and practice.

Collaborative research teams have come together in a variety of ways. In one of the first collaborative clinical projects at the UAB, a faculty member with students on a unit in the hospital began discussing the problems experienced by patients receiving tube feedings with the unit's clinical specialist. Out of that discussion came a study of 100 patients that described the side effects and weight

changes experienced while receiving tube feedings. The study was supported by an allocation from the hospital's Hazel Taylor Nurses Research Fund.

The coordinator of nursing research has been able also to help facilitate the development of collaborative teams. A head nurse concerned with the debilitating symptoms some patients experience following a myelogram asked for assistance in designing a study in that area. A faculty member on RTQ was asked by the coordinator of nursing research to assist the head nurse in designing the project. The unit's quality assurance committee generated the hypotheses for a correlational study, and the faculty member helped develop the hypotheses into a proposal. Following data collection, a statistician from the school assisted in data analysis and in publishing the findings. Side effects such as headache, nausea, and vomiting that are common following a myelogram appeared to be mitigated in patients who were well hydrated by mouth and IV, rather than by mouth only.

Collaborative efforts have also been initiated by nursing service administrators. In one situation, the director of rehabilitation nursing wanted to coordinate a quality assurance study of patient falls in the rehabilitation setting. She requested assistance from a RTQ faculty member, and subsequently a detailed analysis of incidence reports on patient falls was conducted. As a result of this study, patients at greatest risk for falling—those over age 60, those with cerebral-vascular accident, and those with a history of falling—are identified and carefully monitored.

Also graduate students have sparked the creation of several collaborative teams. One graduate student who worked also as a staff nurse planned to investigate the incidence of respiratory infection in patients being suctioned with a reusable tracheal suctioning device. Concurrently, a head nurse on another unit was interested in having the same data collected on her unit. Interest in the project mounted, and it became apparent that expert leadership was essential for a project of this scope. At that point, a faculty member who is a nurse epidemiologist volunteered to lead the collaborative team. The project generated broad interest, and the team grew to include the master's student, the faculty member, a doctoral student, two head nurses, the coordinator of nursing research, three infection control practitioners, and a respiratory therapist.

Cluster Study-Groups

As introduced earlier, the creation of several cluster study-groups is being facilitated through the Joint Council's Committee on Nursing Research. A cluster study-group is organized around a concept of common interest. The group serves to advise and support researchers who may be working together on a project or in a parallel fashion on a related project. Out of such a cluster group, an organized and sustained research effort in a specific area can be achieved.

The first cluster study-group was formed for the purpose of studying nursing documentation. Several factors served to stimulate the formation of the group—the need to improve quality monitoring scores on objectives related to nursing documentation, the need to develop a plan to evaluate documentation on bedside personal computers, and the desire of several members of the nursing staff and faculty to become more involved in research. The cluster group also provides a supportive environment for those nurses new to research or those not recently involved in research.

A 15-member collaborative research group was made up from undergraduate and graduate faculty, a master's student, a doctoral student, several nursing service administrators, a clinical specialist, a head nurse, a staff nurse, the quality monitoring coordinator, the nursing research coordinator, and two computer instructors. Initially, the group discussed and developed a philosophy of documentation that would give direction to their studies. Following the development and adoption of this philosophy, the group generated a list of research questions related to documentation. From this list, five project areas were identified of which group members committed themselves to working on one. Various roles served by the individuals include reviewing the literature, seeking funding for the projects, reviewing quality monitoring data to better define the problem, and writing the proposals.

The cluster study-group strategy has proven to be beneficial in sustaining a research effort. Because of the competing demands of clinical practice, research activities may be given low priority and lay fallow, often never to be continued. But with the cluster group concept, other team members are able to maintain the project's momentum, while one or more members of the team is occupied with other priorities. Additionally, a sense of commitment to the group serves to maintain researcher involvement and accountability.

Graduate Student Research

Master's of science in nursing (M.S.N.) degree students have been conducting clinical research studies at UAB since the mid-1950s, and doctor of science in nursing (D.S.N.) degree students since the mid-1970s. Although graduate students were required to have a peer review of their research proposal by a graduate committee and by an institutional review board, those selecting the use of patients or nurses as research subjects at the University Hospital did not go through a comprehensive review by the Department of Nursing. Consequently, a procedure for conducting research in the hospital's Department of Nursing was established collaboratively, critiqued, and refined by the Joint Council on Nursing. Inherent in the procedure is evaluation criteria for determining the feasibility for conducting the study. Categories reviewed include harmony of the research with the philosophy of the Department of Nursing; time commitment of nursing personnel in relation to the data collection procedure; and cost factors.

Reward Factor

Why nurses do not feel rewarded and motivated to do research is often related to a composite of external and internal factors. Nurse executives who are sensitive to the impact of these factors are more likely to create an enriched environment for collaborative research. Such a climate needs to be challenging; needs to nurture in nurse educators and nurse providers an attitude of enjoying research; and needs to make resources available for nurses to be more productive in conducting research and in applying findings to practice. Traditionally, external factors such as released time, financial assistance, technical expertise or consultation, computer time, and technology have been provided to nurses interested in conducting research, but these efforts have shown only short-term effects. Internal factors, on the other hand, that center on increasing a researcher's responsibility, personal achievement, recognition, growth, and learning have been shown to produce long-term effects.[12]

Collaborative research by its unique nature fosters internal motivation. A cooperating group of researchers committed to a common problem has considerable freedom and accountability for designing and carrying out a mutually agreed on study. A collaborative group taps into the individual talents of group members in order to master difficult tasks identified by the research team. Through the peer review mechanism inher-

ent in collaborative research, both individuals and the group grow, learn, and develop further expertise in research. In addition, the opportunity to disseminate research findings through poster sessions, presentations, and publications brings with it both professional recognition and a personal sense of achievement. The ultimate reward is to see research findings applied in practice, and to make a difference in the quality of nursing care.

For example, in the tracheal suctioning study described earlier, findings demonstrated no significant difference in respiratory infection rates in patients who were suctioned using the traditional one-time use sterile catheter and the newly developed, reusable sheathed catheter. Since there were no differences in infection rates, the decision was made to suction with the reusable catheters because of the considerable cost savings. Nursing staff that assisted as data collectors and the head nurses instrumental in conceiving the study idea have taken pride in the fact that their study had a direct and substantial impact on the quality and cost effectiveness of nursing.

Rewards from collaborative research come not only to an individual researcher or team, but also to the institution employing the investigators. Quality research conducted on pressing problems in nursing practice or education brings recognition to a health-care institution, the school of nursing, or both; this is particularly true when the application of research findings improves nursing care. Patients come to hospitals and nursing homes primarily for nursing care. Quality nursing care that is research based enhances the reputation of the institution. It is a critical marketing strategy that, in an era of declining occupancy rates and shorter lengths of study, attracts patients back repeatedly with the expectation of receiving the same high level of nursing care. In the final analysis, research-based nursing care gives the institution a competitive edge. Further, it provides a foundation on which external funding for additional or expanded research can be built. Nursing departments and schools of nursing should seek external support for research and projects that demonstrate the application of research-based nursing interventions, but with nurses in the role of the principal investigator.

ROLE OF THE NURSE EXECUTIVE IN FACILITATING COLLABORATIVE RESEARCH

It is generally accepted that the nurse executive in nursing education and practice is responsible for integrating nursing with other units of an institution to achieve organizational goals and make quality decisions that affect the department as a whole. Hospital-based nurse executives are concerned primarily with the achievement of goals related to patient care.[13] Facilitating the conduct of collaborative research in nursing, promoting the utilization of research findings into nursing practice and education, and encouraging staff development activities that integrate research into the professional value system of registered nurses will move the nursing departments more effectively toward accomplishing organizational goals related to quality patient care.

Multiple variables affect the role of the nurse executive in relation to collaborative research. Five factors—environmental, structural, human, work, and reward—influence the role of the nurse executive, causing it to be diversified and to differ with the unique nature of each variable. However, the overall expected role is that of facilitating research on nursing and management practices.[14] To do this, the nurse executive needs to possess a broad knowledge of the functions of a researcher. According to Drucker,[15] the nurse executive is a knowledge worker—an idea generator and information processor—who gets the right things done and produces re-

sults. To get the right thing done in relation to collaborative research, the nurse executive in education or practice skillfully exercises the functions of administration by:

conceptualizing why and what needs to be achieved in terms of collaborative research;

developing a strategic plan for when, where, how, and with whom the right things need to be done in relation to collaborative research;

setting appropriate priorities and reasonable deadlines for achieving collaborative research;

providing an enriched environment, organizational structure, and resources to support the conduct and utilization of research in nursing;

integrating research into the nursing organization and with other functional units in the institution; and

measuring the productivity and quality of research conducted and implemented into practice.

Nurses need the opportunity to engage in research and are expected to practice nursing from a knowledge base emanating from research.[16] The nurse executive plays a key role as a facilitator and supporter of collaborative research by creating the climate, providing collegial support, and allocating the human and technical resources needed to get things done in nursing research that will improve and further nursing practice, education, and administration.[17,18]

REFERENCES

1. Kruger J, Nelson A, Wolanin M. Nursing research: development, collaboration and utilization. Germantown, MD: Aspen Systems Corp, 1978, p. 4.
2. Williams C. Collaborative research: a commentary. Journal of Professional Nursing 1987;3(2):82, 124.
3. Kruger, pp. 8–10.
4. Mauger B. Characteristics of faculty and collaborative research. Nursing education research in the south. Atlanta: SREB, 1980, p. 61.

5. Williams, p. 82.
6. Williams, p. 82.
7. Schaefer M. Leadership and management styles for educational administrators. Roles, rights and responsibilities: the educational administrator's 3 R's. New York: NLN, 1978, pp. 1–9.
8. American Nurses Association. Roles, responsibilities and qualifications for nurse administrators. Kansas City: ANA, 1978, p. 13.
9. Bishop BE. A case for collaboration. Nursing Outlook 1981;29:110–111.
10. Engstrom JL. University, agency and collaborative models for nursing research: an overview. Image: the Journal of Nursing Scholarship 1984;16:76–80.
11. Smeltzer CH. Reflections of a decade. Research Bridge 1987;6:1–2.
12. Herzberg F. One more time: how do you motivate employees? Harv Bus R 1968;46(1):53–62.
13. American Nurses' Association. Roles, responsibilities and qualifications for nurse administrators. Kansas City: ANA, 1978, pp. 4–5.
14. American Nurses Association. Roles, responsibilities and qualifications for nurse administrators. Kansas City: ANA, 1978, p. 13.
15. Drucker P. The effective executive. NY: Harper and Row, 1976.
16. American Nurses Association. Human rights guidelines for nurses in clinical and other research. Kansas City: ANA, 1985.
17. McArt E. Research facilitation in academic and practice settings. Journal of Professional Nursing 1987; 3(2):84–91.
18. Henning E. Collaborative research by faculty: a dean's perspective. Nursing education research in the south. Atlanta: SREB, 1980, pp. 63–64.

49

The Changing Role of Administration in Home Health Care

Myrtis J. Snowden
Mary Lou Steedley

THIS CHAPTER explores the changing role of nursing administration in home health care. Critical issues related to nursing administration in rapidly changing home health-care practices are examined from a historical perspective. The examination focuses on and enumerates issues related to planning programs and evaluating services; documenting patients' needs and budgeting for nursing services; and the influence of legislation, federal regulations, and reimbursement services on agency survival and the administrator's role. The chapter concludes with discussion of selected theory and research useful to administrators, educators, and managers of home care services.

HISTORICAL INFLUENCES

The fields of medicine, nursing, and public health, each with a slightly different philosophy, make claims about the origins of home health care and each states basic reasons for becoming involved in it. All report concern about the health of people and have demonstrated concern about the ability of indigent persons' access to health care. There are, however, basic differences. Medical practitioners are concerned about disease and its cure, whereas nurses and public health workers are concerned about the prevention of disease and the promotion of health as well as the cure of disease. Thus, the genesis of home health care needs to be examined from the medical perspective—with the influence of the hospital-based model on home care, and from the perspectives of nursing and public health—with the influence of illness prevention and health promotion models of service delivery.

The first nurses providing home health care were employed in 1877 by the Women's Branch of the New York City Mission, a voluntary agency. These nurses carried out orders of medical inspectors, visited the homes of children enrolled in schools, instructed mothers in infant care, and transported children to the hospital. The improved health status of this select group in New York City was attributed, in part, to the nursing care provided through the Mission's services. The concept of providing services for indigent people spread to other communities, including Buffalo in 1885, and Boston and Philadelphia in 1886. The Buffalo and Philadelphia organizations were referred to as "societies," but the Boston organization was called the Boston Instructive District Nursing Association. Within a short time the pioneering organizations changed their names to Visiting Nurse Associations (VNAs). These organizations were administratively responsible to lay boards, and the nurses were supervised by lay persons. Because the Philadelphia organization hired a nurse supervisor it is credited with being the first to provide professional supervision for nurses.[1] Before the turn of the century the number of groups providing visiting nurse services to communities grew slowly, and such groups were mainly found in large urban areas, but Buhler-Wilkerson reported that by 1909 there were approximately 595 such organizations in this country.[2] From the beginning, nurses in these agencies served indigent populations, focusing on the needs of individuals and families rather than on diseases or conditions.

The Metropolitan and John Hancock Life Insurance companies contributed to home health-care program development. For example, in 1909, the Metropolitan Life Insurance Company initiated programs to improve conditions of the acutely ill and developed programs of disease prevention for newborns and their mothers. Overall, the programs were aimed at reducing claims from policy holders, while promoting health, preventing disease, and reducing hospital days consumed by policy holders. The insurance company hired nurses to carry out its programs, but increased work volume led to contractual agreements between the company and 850 VNAs.

The success of community nursing in other agencies was partially responsible for employment of nurses by local, state, and federal agencies. Whereas local health department nurses mainly provided direct services to communities, nurses in state and federal agencies were involved, sometimes with direct care, through demonstration projects and initiation of programs. Nurses at both federal and state levels, however, were mainly concerned with planning programs and providing assistance to nurses more directly involved with the day-to-day rendering of care in various localities.

As nursing defined its role more clearly and various governing bodies specified boundaries for the different levels at which tax-supported agencies would assume responsibility, an important issue arose. The debate was whether nurses with special, rather than generalized preparation were more useful in situations where skills were needed to address multiproblem families. Concern for the integrity of the family was at the center of the argument. A further concern was that nurse specialists would attend to problems only in their speciality and ignore other patients' problems. A realistic fear existed that families with several problems would be overwhelmed by "successive visits of a series of specialized nurses."[3] For example, a family with several problems could, conceivably, receive visits from nurses for each identified problem. Thus, families with multiple problems would be overwhelmed with multiple nurse visits, agencies would be overwhelmed scheduling the visits and financially exhausted by providing overlapping services. A standard of nursing practice emerged from the debate: Nurses with generalized preparation for community nursing, as evidenced by a baccalaureate degree, were sought for community health nursing jobs. Further, nurses were designated as community health nurses or public health nurses, based on the type of agency in which they worked. Therefore, nurses employed by official agencies such as health departments were designated public health nurses, and nurses employed by voluntary agencies such as VNA were designated community health nurses. Presently, early hospital discharge and patients' critical need for various types of nursing expertise in the home makes any equivocation over title designation somewhat meaningless. The important factor is to provide families with high quality nursing service.

At the turn of the century, private-duty nurses were employed in support of private medical care in the home. Employment in homes was sought because most graduate nurses had little chance for hospital employment. Further, because people chose to recover from illness at home rather than in the hospital, private duty nurses were in demand. The advent of antibiotic therapy, improved medical technology, and extended hospital stays, however, contributed to gradual decline in the use of private duty nurses and to the demise of such services by nurses in the home.

Nurses involved in home visiting and private-duty nursing shared a common concern. Roberts asserted that both private duty nurses and visiting nurses were troubled because they knew too little about foods patients needed and did not know how to deal with social, psychological, and physical conditions in patients' homes.[4] Later, as nursing curriculums improved, concerns about patients' nutritional needs and psychosocial nurse-patient interaction strategies were addressed. Moreover, by 1931 the National Organization for Public Health Nursing published functions, standards, and qualifications for public health nurses. Attention given to the functions statement influenced the content of inservice and field training programs. These programs focused on improving skills nurses needed for efficient community health nursing practice. By 1950 all baccalaureate nursing curriculums included content that prepared graduates for generalized nursing practice. Hanlon and Pickett reported that by 1962 most nurses in supervisory positions had one or more years of academic public health training.[1] Thus, the emergence of public health nursing standards of practice, enhanced curriculums, and planned inservice education programs contributed content beneficial to the preparation of nurses for practice in the community.

While community-based nursing services were developing positive images as providers of health care, physicians reasserted themselves in the care of the sick at home. The Montifiore Project, a physician directed hos-pital-based venture, launched in 1947, used principles of environmental medicine and advocated placing patients in their homes. In this instance, the project was a collaborative effort in which physicians, nurses, social workers, and various therapists provided a full range of home-care services.[5] Although patients admitted to the project had to meet eligibility requirements, other patients discharged from this hospital who needed home care were served by VNA nurses as a part of a contractual agreement. Presently, the model of home care for Medicare and Medicaid patients bears a striking resemblance to the Montifiore Project.

LEGISLATIVE INFLUENCES

Voluntary agencies such as VNAs and public agencies such as local health departments have traditionally provided home health care. VNAs traditionally supported themselves through philanthropic funds, endowments, and fees for services. Health department funds came from local and state taxes as well as from federal funds dedicated to specific health problems. For example, Title V of the Social Security Act, adopted in 1935, provided grants-in-aid to states for the development of maternal and child health programs. Enactment of this piece of legislation launched decades of health promotion and illness prevention programs that helped to improve the health of mothers, infants, and children. This model, which focuses on the prevention of disease, has contributed to lengthened life spans for Americans. The improved quality of life during one's younger years, however, sharply contrasts with the quality of life in later years. We now have an older population more vulnerable to disability and increasingly prone to chronic illnesses.

Society's concern about cost as well as barriers and access to care, led to congressional action that addressed some of the problems of acute and chronic illness among indigent populations. Federal funds, allocated according to specific legislative acts, contribute to an expanding home-care industry. Legislation influencing home health-care development and expansion of funded services are as follows:[6]

Title XX, Social Security Act (1975), supplements existing services for low-income groups. State administered funds are provided for eligible persons of all ages who receive care in the home. State administration may limit the scope of the programs,

Title III, Older American Act (1965), permits persons 60 years of age and older to receive services in the home. It is also a state administered program whose scope may be limited.

Title XIX, Social Security Act (1965), provides services for persons receiving categorical assistance such as welfare assistance, and for long-term care benefits such as end-stage renal disease. This legislation, which is state administered, is specifically supportive of individual care. Funds are not available for family health care. Individual coverage varies as well as reimbursement practices under this piece of legislation. Some states place a cap as low as 50 allowable visits whereas other states permit unlimited numbers of reimbursable visits.

Title XVIII, Social Security Act (1965), provides home health-care coverage through home health visits for persons aged 65 and over. Agency reimbursement is based on the patient's confinement at home with need for skilled care as determined by a physician. Services must be provided by a Medicare-certified agency. The Equity and Fiscal Responsibility Act (TEFRA) and Social Security Amendments (1983) led to development of prospective payment systems in hospitals in 1974. The institution of diagnosis related group (DRG)-based payments caused decreased hospital admissions and shorter lengths of hospital stays.

DEFINING CRITICAL ISSUES IN HOME HEALTH CARE

For this chapter, issue is defined as "a point of debate, point of controversy, point at which an unsettled matter may be ready for decision."[7] Issues discussed in this chapter are derived from the historical background of public and community health nursing practice, private medicine, and legislative influences on home health-care delivery.

The nurse administrators of home care agencies are faced with several critical issues including the following:

- Consideration of philosophic and humanistic underpinnings of nursing practice in conflict with an economically constraining and task-oriented system,
- Budget initiatives and barriers to access to home health-care services,
- Quality assurance
- Need for documentation of patient care needs, and
- Agency management and survival by means of diversification.

At the center of the issue, however, is the definition of home health care. The term is difficult to define. Speigel asserted that the designation of "health" in the title is misleading because the array of services brought into the home are not related to the concept of health, which in its broadest sense, disputes wellness.[8] The definition of home health-care as developed by a federal government Interdepartmental Work Group states:[9]

Home health care is that component of a continuum of comprehensive health care whereby health services are provided to individuals and families in their places of residence for the purpose of promoting, maintaining, or restoring health or of maximizing the level of independence, while minimizing the effects of disability and illness including terminal illness. Service appropriate to the needs of the individual patient and family are planned, coordinated, and made available by providers organized for the delivery of home health care through the use of employed staff, contractual arrangements, or a combination of the two patterns.

Nursing of the sick in the home was built on a tradition of caring for members of families and focused not only on carrying out recommended medical regimes but on using measures aimed at preventing further erosion of the human condition. Further, nursing activities outside the medical model became the bench mark from which all community nursing activities were patterned. Thus, community nursing ranged from focusing on patients with infectious diseases to caring for elderly and chronically ill patients. Formerly, these patients needed less intensive care than that provided in hospitals and their needs could be met less expensively in the home. Further, the advantages of being with their families probably helped patients recuperate more rapidly. It is out of this tradition that a humanistic philosophy of nursing in the community was derived. The current definition of home health care carefully addresses concepts of comprehensive care, health promotion, maintenance, and restoration of health, all of which conflict with reimbursement mechanisms that appear to hamper holistic approaches to care. Thus, a major issue with which the nurse administrator must deal is an agency's philosophy that may force differences between its objectives and its belief statement, and issues of holistic care versus task performance.

Ray asserted that the nursing profession is perplexed by the moral conflict between health care economics and human caring.[10] Ray's discussion centers around caring as a moral ideal in contrast to caring as a bureaucratic phenomenon. She stated:

For society, nurses must be not only loyal to caring as a moral ideal in health care, but also responsible to society by involvement in the search to formulate the means to preserve human caring in an increasingly economic health care delivery system.

The nurse administrator's role includes coordinating services and establishing close ties with community systems in order to interface with other agencies involved in the delivery of patient care services. Now, nursing in the community is undergoing radical change. Nursing service is extremely dependent on government funds for survival. Nursing service administrators realize that government agencies have subtly moved from the position of policymaker to that of partner in designing programs for the delivery of nursing care.

The complexion of home health-care agencies varies according to social, political, legislative, and economic situations. The nurse administrator needs to remain flexible and adapt to the changes created. In this era of change and dependency on tenuous funding sources, the administrator needs to be sure of the agency's philosophical position and determine whether that position allows the agency to fulfill human needs and still maintain an economically viable position. This warning is critical because most patients served by home health agencies are covered by Medicare, Medicaid, private insurance, or private payment.

Budgeting Methods

Results from a survey of home health-care agencies revealed that increasing numbers of Americans are not receiving the care they need. The increase is blamed, in part, on the DRG payment system to hospitals, which influences length of hospital stay. Thus, patients are being discharged from hospitals quicker and sicker. If additional care is needed, patients are generally referred to home health agencies. Not all patients referred, however, may be seen by the same health-care practitioner, and admission to service depends on eligibility for that service. Eligibility requirements and Medicare-Medicaid guidelines may cause denial of payment to the agency. Further, the commitment to reimbursement has not kept pace with the expanding need for health-care services. There is particular concern about care for patients discharged more quickly, as hospitals strive to demonstrate cost-effective health care.

Denial of expected reimbursement funds

places a home health agency in the position of providing care to those who need their services, only to have claims for payment denied for a number of reasons. From the agency's point of view denials result from Health Care Financing Administration (HCFA) suggestions to contracting insurance companies, yet these guidelines have been used as if they were laws or regulations rather than the suggestions they were meant to be. In essence, the agency may remain as a nursing care provider, living up to a commitment to provide care to the sick in their homes while not receiving reimbursement, thereby sustaining a loss in revenues.

Commitment to care can also cause revenue loss in another way in that agencies are reimbursed on a per visit basis rather than based on time needed to provide adequate care during the visit. For example, a patient who was formerly addicted to drugs was receiving intravenous antibiotic therapy and dressing changes at home as treatment for severe infection. The therapy was administered three times daily and usually required about one hour nursing time. The planned visits and therapeutic interventions occurred without incident except in one instance in which the nurse had to remain with the patient for about three hours. Thus, actual time needed for nursing care exceeded allotted time and therefore eroded funds budgeted for the visit.

This example is not dissimilar to common occurrences in providing care to more seriously ill patients. For example, sicker patients need more frequent home visits and longer periods of time for each visit. Meeting patient-care needs under these circumstances have a direct bearing on the budget. Any situation calling for staff to increase time spent in the home lowers productivity, thus causing lower revenues on a case-by-case basis. Loss of revenues are estimated to run from a low of $10,000 to a high of $7 million a year.[11]

Home health-care services represent a large and rapidly growing segment of the U.S. health-care market. For example, hospital-based agencies increased from 432 to 1312 in 1986. Chain or independently owned home-health agencies grew from 287 in 1981 to 1,942 in 1986. Veterans Administration agencies remained stable, whereas growth among VNAs and health department agencies was negligible.[12] Coleman and Smith report that federal expenditures alone have risen at an annual rate of 22% from 1969 through 1982, and current expenditures for home care exceed $1 billion annually.[13]

Although the number of home health-care programs in both the public and private sectors has burgeoned, this segment of the health-care industry is not as technologically sophisticated as hospital care. Competition for home health-care clients, however, is fierce and providers must compete with other entrepreneurs in the marketplace.

Documentation of Patient Care Needs

Proper documentation of patients' needs and services rendered are essential to the nurse administrator's strategy for maintaining or increasing revenues from federal sources. The documentation issue is related to the nurse's ability to describe a situation concisely, in sufficient detail, and in ordinary language. To document efficiently is to communicate effectively. Yet, the value of documentation as an adjunct to patient care management and its relevance to the financial stability or success in home health care has not been addressed. In order to receive reimbursement funds practitioners, regardless of discipline represented, must record the skill used in the patient's care. For example, the skill may be teaching the patient and family hands-on care in the case of nursing practice, or the manipulation of body parts in the case of physical therapy. Every home visit must be documented in terms of skills used. Skills used must be oriented toward goals established and based on the plan of care.

Inservice or continuing education programs are useful to nurses or case managers who have difficulties documenting patients' needs for services. Planned programs should help nurses become more proficient in: describing patients' needs for nursing care, developing objectives based on subjective as well as objective data, developing care plans based on data gathered, and using objectives to measure and validate patient care outcomes.

Documentation of service provided movement toward or attainment of goals; and the correlation between goals set and outcomes achieved are what the intermediary is looking for when reimbursement for funds is determined. Reward for more efficient documentation should be helpful to the administrator for several reasons. The administrator has more accurate data available for measuring quality and quantity of patient services. Further, reimbursement for services rendered may be achieved.

Quality Assurance

Nurse administrators must deal with quality assurance when managing home health-care agencies. The quality assurance concept relates to the desirable attributes of professional practice or qualities of excellence that administrator and staff believe exist among the professional care-givers. In turn, the professional care-givers are expected to be competent and are held accountable for the care provided. Confidence in professionals to consistently provide quality care is determined by using quality control measures. Quality control, the process of quality assurance, is a system that incorporates measuring the attainment of excellence according to predetermined criteria. Information gained from applying the process is used to signify, in some way, that excellence or high quality patient care has been provided.

The concept and process of quality assurance are workable, to some degree, in hospital settings. Quality assurance in home care is, for the most part, a carbon copy of programs designed for hospital settings. Yet, according to Mundinger, it is difficult to determine what constitutes "quality" in home health services.[14] Thus, improved quality assurance processes for use in the home health-care industry are critical. Part of the problem is that issues of quality and accountability are not clearly delineated in the home. Mundinger argued that accountability for services was split among various health providers, making it difficult to assign responsibility for decisions made about the care.[14] Moreover, assigning accountability to care givers who provide or assist with nursing care is elusive because care is often provided by aides who are nonprofessionals; therefore this concept is not applicable to them. Rather, the agency is wholly responsible for the levels of competence of its nonprofessional care-givers.

The National League for Nursing described the quality assurance problem as complex and warned that part of the problem was the delivery of service, concurrently, from several different professional practitioners and auxiliary caregivers.[15] Apparently, however, the American Hospital Association (AHA), expects hospital-based home health agencies to use hospital-oriented models of quality assurance and risk management.[16] Accordingly, the hospital board is ultimately responsible for the quality of care provided. The board is also expected to be provided data on patient care outcomes and other information such as instances of liability exposure, results of recruiting, and credentialing practices.

Nurse administrators of home health agencies recognize that Medicare certification and state approval or licensure to operate are acceptable quality assurance practices. The task is to move beyond meeting criteria that afford certification and licensure. The chal-

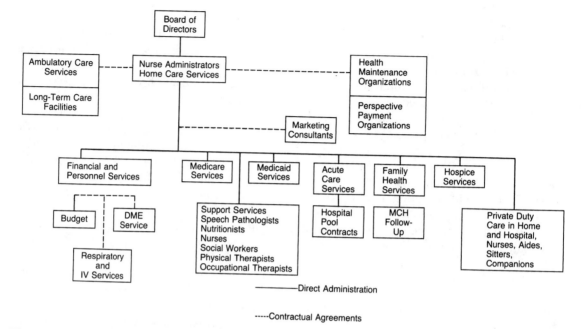

Figure 49.1 Sample Organizational Chart, Diversified Services. DME = disposable medical equipment; IV = intravenous services; MCH = maternal child health.

lenge is to create mechanisms that measure and evaluate consumer satisfaction with service received and implementation of a process that deals with individual visits by different health-care professionals in the home.

Agency Management and Diversification

Patient care will continue to shift from the hospital to the home. Nurse administrators need to use sound business practices if agencies are to survive in an intensely competitive market. Medium-size or large agencies may choose to diversify their services.

Diversification can be advantageous to an agency, but there are also disadvantages. Advantages of diversification include generating structural units that permit flexibility in providing a range of services to consumers. This flexibility also permits the agency to hire permanent staff in categories in which spe-

cific expertise is needed. Further, a corporate organizational structure permits administrative control of the total organization and proper allocation of resources (see Figure 49.1).

Disadvantages of diversification include the possibility of diminished consumer satisfaction and diminished service delivery. Further, there must be a careful balance among services to persons for whom no funding is available and those covered by third-party payers.

Whether an agency chooses to diversify its services or to maintain its present structure, competition for patients will continue to force administrators to seek and obtain contracts with viable markets. The agency that does not choose diversification may sustain itself by other means, including seeking contractual agreements with other health agencies or hospital facilities. For example, collaborative arrangements with hospitals or ambulatory care centers may prove to be advantageous. At one time health maintenance organizations (HMOs) were considered lucrative markets. HMOs are also competing, however, in the home health-care field and may no longer be open to persuasion.

Essential differences among home health-care agencies are minimal. Charitable funds, once contributed for indigent care, have diminished; and tax monies, once provided to official agencies, have been curtailed. Financial viability of an agency, regardless of type, depends on sound fiscal management and the judicious allocation of human and material resources.

SUGGESTED THEORY BASE FOR MEETING THE FUTURE OF HOME HEALTH CARE

Nurse administrators of home health-care agencies are witnessing the transformation of traditional agencies into new patterns and the conversion of standard agency units into new configurations. Whether single purpose or multipurpose, each organization must face challenges and meet current dynamic forces of change. Advice to nurse administrators includes emphasizing the need to analyze the environment in which the agency operates in order to: consider impending changes in reimbursement, meet organizational goals in the face of fiscal realities, and diversify activities in accordance with the current market place. Two theories appear well suited and relevant. One—change theory—delineates strategies that may be adopted by an organization in response to alterations in the organizations environment. The other, marketing theory, deals with marketing as organized rational innovation.

Gawthrop stated that organizational change was an extended interactive process, directed by sets of strategies that involved the organization's adaptive, relational, and re- sponsive mechanisms.[17] Accordingly, the administrator's view of several important variables reportedly influences assessment of the manner in which agencies adapt to change.

The first of these is viewing change in terms of the velocity. For example, one needs to determine whether the change process developed slowly or rapidly. Second, one determines manifestations of change in terms of whether it occurred instantaneously or evolved slowly. Last, the potential effect the change will have in the agency needs to be considered. That is, will the effect of change be major, minor, or have no influence at all? In addition, the administrator must assess a variable called perceived lead time. This assessment helps the administrator determine the length of time an agency has before the potential change becomes a reality.

After factors of perceived change have been weighed, response to potential change must be considered. Strategic responses to potential change can be categorized as reactive or anticipatory. Reactive strategy is change after the need for change has been fully manifested. Anticipatory strategy is adaptive in nature. It is future-oriented and designed to deal with change by adapting to it, or by acting on the perceived need before the need for change manifests itself. Response to change, before or after the fact, will be based on values held by leaders of the organization. Gawthrop contended that the extent to which managers viewed the future is a reflection of their value perceptions of change.[17] Value perceptions of change may reflect two different philosophical positions. One position involves viewing change as a projection of the present, based on the past. The other position is that patterns of the present can be changed and negatives of the past can be undone.

Whether to act or react after analyzing information relating to the organization and its environment must be decided. Change implies a new or different state of being. The process of change forces the administrator to focus on and make predictions about the future of the organization. For example, the administrator has to consider the organization's future in light of changes in the organization and the environment. The administrator's assessment of and ability and strength to act on the forces of change will relate directly to an organization's viability in the environment.

Marketing, according to Simmonds, is what marketers do to cause market changes. Simmonds's premise is that "marketing is fundamentally about change."[18] (p. 494) Further, marketing is of such importance that an agency's success depends on the administrator's correct assessment of the market and shaping of responsive actions accordingly.

Several marketing paradigms are specified in marketing theory. Simmonds suggested, however, a marketing paradigm using innovation concepts. This strategy, labeled the Eighth Paradigm, places emphasis on the process of change—a quality that is purportedly absent from other marketing paradigms.[18] (p. 480) The innovation paradigm has four process functions, as follows:[18] (p. 488)

1. Concern with the way any social unit organizes itself in order to identify necessary behavioral changes in light of the environment in which it exists.
2. Concern with how administrators view and recognize the need for change, and how information sources are evaluated.
3. Consideration and identification of strategies used by administrators to motivate the organization to accept responsibility for problem solving and the need for change.
4. Weighing decisions and plans that an organization uses to influence external environments.

Although nurse administrators are not experts in the field of marketing, their grasp of the discipline should be sufficient for quality decisions to be made about using marketing strategies. Further, services provided by the agency are its saleable products, and judicious action must be taken to inform and convince consumers about the products. In addition, the administrator must be able to determine the effectiveness of the marketing program as it relates to overall organization achievement and viability.

RESEARCH IN HOME HEALTH CARE

Research in relation to the health-care and illness service resources of home health care holds great promise of reward for consumers and professionals. Home health care is often called an alternative method of care. An immediate question is, alternative to what? While patients have been discharged from hospitals quicker, yet sicker, and hospitals document decreased costs for hospitalization, health professionals eagerly await results from research, already underway, on the effects of cost containment and early discharge on patient welfare.

The question of cost effectiveness in home care has been researched extensively. According to Vogel and Palmer, most of the studies were plagued by methodological problems.[19] The problems are related to attempts to compare institutional costs with home care costs although institutional data are usually expressed in terms of per diem, and home care costs are usually reported on a per visit basis. Other methodological issues include concern about differences in objectives for institution and home care programs, and the lack of a common costing unit for home health care and institutional care. Vogel and Palmer contended that other problems and issues related to home health-care analysis were "those related to client characteristics and need for service, equity in service provision, family-service agency cooperation, and mobilization of family and volunteer support.[19] (p. 353)

The home health-care industry and consumers of its services need research findings related to each issue discussed here, ranging from the influence of economic constraints on home health care to the influence of diversification on an agency's ability to deliver services that consumers need. Nurse administrators need both descriptive and experimental research in all areas. Descriptive research, designed on a sound methodological basis should generate clear hypotheses that can be used in experimental research. The heart of the problem for the administrator, however, is to locate funds to support demonstration programs where demographic factors, patient care needs, service provisions, and cost centers are comparable. Research aimed at determining the efficacy of the delivery of home care to consumers is also needed. What emerges from comparisons of care under controlled situations would be of tremendous benefit to providers and consumers of home health care.

REFERENCES

1. Hanlon JJ, Pickett GE. Public health administration and practice. 7th ed. St Louis: CV Mosby Co, 1979.
2. Buhler-Wilkerson K. Left carrying the bag: experiments in visiting nursing, 1877–1909. Nursing Research 1987;36:42–47.
3. Hanlon J. Principles of public health administration. 4th ed. St Louis: CV Mosby Co, 1964, p. 450.
4. Roberts MM. American nursing history and interpretation. New York: The Macmillan Company, 1954.
5. Bluestone EM. The principles and practice of home care. JAMA 1954;155:1379–1382.
6. Legislation related to home health care. Long-term Care Quarterly 1986;1:1–7. American Nurses Association, D-88C.
7. Models for health care delivery: now and for the future. American Academy of Nursing, Kansas City, MO, January 20–21, 1975.
8. Speigel AD. Home health care. Owings Mills, MD: National Health Publishing Ltd. Partnership, 1983.
9. USDHEW. Home health care. A discussion paper by the international HHC policy working group (unpublished). December 1976.
10. Ray MN. Home care economics and human caring in nursing: why the moral conflict must be resolved. Family and Community Health 1987;10:35–43.
11. Medicare: the broken promise. Caring 1986;5:4–7.
12. Department of Health and Human Services, Health Care Financing Administration, Office of Public Affairs, 1986.
13. Coleman JR, Smith DS. DRGs and the growth of home care. Nursing Economics 1984;2:391–395.
14. Mundinger MO. Home care controversy, too little, too late, too costly. Rockville, MD: Aspen Systems Corporation, 1983.
15. Position statement on ensuring quality in home health care. In: Public policy bulletin. New York: National League for Nursing, 1986.
16. Hospital Research and Educational Trusts. American Hospital Association, 1987.
17. Gawthrop LC. Public sector management, systems, and ethics. Bloomington: Indiana University Press, 1984.
18. Simmonds K. Marketing as innovation: the eighth paradigm. Journal of Management Studies 1986;23:479–501.
19. Vogel RJ, Palmer HC. Long-term care perspectives from research demonstrations. Washington, DC: Health Care Financing Administration, U.S. Department of Health and Human Services, 1983, pp. 337–389.

Contributions of Nursing Administration to the Development of Nursing as a Discipline

Barbara Stevens Barnum

NURSING administration is much maligned as the force responsible for impeding the development of nursing as a professional practice. "They" don't allow us to practice professionally; "they" work against us; "they" side with hospital management against the nurses. The cries are frequently heard and are part of the ritualized liturgy of the staff nurse. Nursing administration is a convenient scapegoat for all those failures on the part of nurses in direct clinical practice.

What is the truth of the matter? What has been the relationship between nursing management and nursing practice? As with most complex questions, the answer is not simple; but on the whole it is clear that nursing administration has done more to advance professional nursing practice than to inhibit it.

THE NEED FOR A SCAPEGOAT IN NURSING

Often nursing is not practiced at the level envisioned by its leadership. This is sad, but few of us would deny the fact. Those of us who are nurses and have had recent experience with our own families as patients report more blunders than heart-warming examples of the care delivered in even our prestigious institutions. Perhaps as nurses, we simply expect too much. Unfortunately, too little is delivered. There is frequently a large gap between the care expected—by the patient, by nurse educators, by nurse administrators—and the care delivered. The staff nurse and ideal professional nurse often are not the same people.

If there are gaps between the envisioned practice of the profession and its enactment, one is forced to seek causes. In this case, the causes are complex and multifold. Inadequate programs of education, less than ideal candidates for nursing education, stressful work environments, inadequate staffing, lack of mentors, infringements by other professions—the list can be as long as one can be creative in its production. And, yes, one source may be inadequate administration of nursing practice.

Yet, I would suggest that the excellent nurse seldom evinces poor practice. He or she may be rushed, harried, overworked; yet the good nurse continues to do what he or she does well. Even in the midst of too many activities the able nurse notes the status of her seriously-ill patients. Even in a depressing environment the excellent nurse gets to the essential things and lets the trivia hang. Sometimes the excellent nurse even makes judgments that shorten her work—perhaps letting the patient who needs sleep more than blood pressure monitoring sleep instead of being interrupted for that measure.

Excellent nurses are found all over. The last one I saw had just delivered a very reasoned plea to a physician for communication concerning a very sick patient. The physician answered that if he had anything to say to the nurse, he would put it in the form of an order on the chart. This excellent nurse didn't practice in an ideal setting, but that didn't stop him (yes, he was a man) from practicing at his highest level of capability.

I have also seen in 1987: (a) a nurse who wouldn't get a pillow for a patient with cervical arthritis because "that's housekeeping's job"—it didn't matter to the nurse that the patient who was exhausted from blood loss was unable to lie down on the flat bed without support of a pillow; (b) a nurse who placed a specially-ordered sheepskin between two rough sheets in spite of the patient's decubitus—after all, she said, the sheepskins get dirty if you let them touch the patients; and (c) a nurse who delivered "stretching" manipulations to a knee contracture by propping the patient's leg up and jumping with all her weight against the protruding knee. I could go on, but then so could any reader who has been immersed in observing day-to-day nursing practice.

I don't believe that the practice of these three far-from-exemplary nurses, or their thousands of peers, would be helped by nurse administrators supplying the Earth's best practice environment. I'm not sure that their practice could be helped except through extensive re-education.

I have a crude but simple yardstick by which to judge nursing practice: professional practice is the care delivered that makes best use of the available resources. These resources include the nurse's knowledge, intelligence, time, and creativity in making do with what other resources are at hand—material, intellectual, spatial, and spiritual.

Simply put, the quality of nursing can be judged separately from the quality of the management in the institution.

Why, then, is nursing administration so often the scapegoat for inadequate nursing practice? Scapegoating is surely not a new phenomenon. It is a common way to deal with inadequacies and embarrassment. The question is why nursing administration is selected as a prime target rather then the physicians, the dietary service, or even transportation services.

The nursing profession itself may have much to do with this displacement of blame. After all, we have long tried to make all nurses outside of those involved in hands-on practice feel guilty about their practice. "Those who can't, teach," is an example of imposing guilt on another group who lacks hands-on practice. Those of us with long memories recall when all nursing graduate programs went clinical. Nursing administration programs were shrunk to five or six nationwide, and most of those were inadequate. The message was loud and clear: if you're a good nurse, you belong at the bedside. Most of us who have been administrators of nursing practice have faced "the question" more than once. "Why did you leave the bedside?" Usually this is delivered with sonorous overtones. "Why did you leave nursing?" is the unexpressed yet barely veiled question-in-the-question.

My answer to that question was rapidly "canned" to make a liturgy of my own. "I left the bedside," I would respond, "in order that I might have an expanded effect on the conduct of practice. By functioning in a mediated role, one where I can influence the practice of many nurses, I can have more impact on patient care than were I to continue giving one-to-one care." In other words, I don't apologize for taking on a leadership role that is "away" from the bedside. Yet the question is always posed as if I should apologize.

The point is that nursing expects its leaders to apologize for taking on leadership roles. When we hold our leaders guilty just for being leaders, we are a profession in trouble. You may argue that the leadership of the profession should arise from our clinicians in one-to-one practice; but the very fact of their limited political and professional contacts makes that unlikely except in the case of a truly exceptional person. If we are uncomfortable with the notion of leadership, that makes the leadership vulnerable to unreasonable criticism. And it follows that all the problems will be laid at the door of those same leaders.

Hence, it isn't surprising that nurses blame their administrators for all that is wrong with nursing. Blaming the leaders is a well-established tactic in nursing. I am reminded of a meeting I once attended several years ago. It was a meeting suggesting strategies for political survival of community health nursing at an important historical juncture. Five speakers gave unprecedentedly good advice concerning what community health nurses should do politically in their neighborhoods and states. I listened from the back row, just behind that inevitable row of knitters and crewelers. When the envigorating speeches were finished and nurses were filing out of the room, one of the knitters turned to her peers. "That was wonderful," she said. "I certainly hope they follow through on their ideas." Her companions nodded their agreement. At that moment, I had a vision of the five speakers trying to organize in all the neighborhoods in all the states, all over the nation. Their brilliance had been lost on the group in the back; they failed to understand that the leadership was setting a course for the audience to follow. The leadership can't do it all, and that goes for nursing practice also. Leaders don't exist without followers.

Leaders aren't substitutes for followers; nurse administrators aren't substitutes for clinical nurses. The best administrators can

do is set a tone that calls for professional practice and structure care environments, be they resource-rich or -poor, for the best possible practice. Most nurse administrators are doing their best to make good practice possible—or better—in their institutions. That's their job; and few set out to make good practice impossible.

IMAGES AND REALITIES

Nursing administration consists of the strange activity of managing—not creating—the environments in which nursing takes place. There is an important difference. The environment is a given in many important ways. In 1988, for example, the economic aspects of the environment are foremost in the minds of many. Nursing didn't create that environment, but it has to manage in it.

Many nurses fail to differentiate between these subtle differences and hold the nurse administrator accountable for the whole scene, good or bad. It is true, however, that good or bad management can alter the environment in favorable—or disastrous—ways. But nurse administrators are not gods—not even the best of them. Few even carry magic wands. The best they can do is make the most of the world in which they find themselves, along with their nursing staffs. Nursing administration can, then, make the given workplace of an institution as open to good nursing practice as possible given the constraints of that world. But nursing administration, even if it is exquisite, cannot control and supplant the actions of all the nurses giving care to patients.

Many nurses are unrealistic concerning the limitations of nursing administration. They want administration to make everything all better, like their teachers promised it would be, or rather, said it ought to be. As a profession, we have done a remarkably effective job of rearing generation after generation of nurses to believe in a myth concerning the environment in which good nursing ought to be delivered—to believe in a world in which each nurse has only a few patients so that he or she may deliver ideal care; a world in which the best support services are available; a world in which peers and other professionals are supportive and excel in their own work; a world that doesn't exist.

Generation after generation of nurses reach the employment market, searching for that world where they can do perfect practice. A rare few find it, though they probably find it in themselves rather than in the "real" world. On the whole, the instilled myth of ideal nursing leads most nurses to bemoan their fate—that of working in a real institution, in the real world, with its real fallibilities. And, of course, since nursing administration failed to provide nirvana, the nurses aren't accountable for the fact that their practice has flaws. It is the fault of those administrators—those leaders who failed to make good on the promises of idealistic nurse educators, those educators who prepared their students for a world that ought to exist rather than for the one that does exist.

Some administrators, of course, are victims of the same idealism. Nurse administrators of that sort take one of two paths. The first group become disillusioned and leave nursing, either in fact or by turning their backs upon it. "I used to be a nurse," this sort of administrator will say when pressed to reveal his or her jaded past. The other group suffers a worse fate. They administer an ideal nursing service—at least in their minds. These administrators really believe that everything comes up roses. All their nurses practice in a most professional manner. All their patients are satisfied. Nobody ever makes a mistake. And they all live happily ever after. These administrators have a remarkable ability to selectively hear good news and drown out anything that might lead to a different interpretation of the reality. It's a toss-up as to which sort of nurse does the most damage.

Given the very real constraints of the situation, it is useful to ask what nursing administration really can do to encourage professional practice. What can management do to encourage quality in a service delivered on a one-to-one basis? A lot and a little, is the best answer. Administration can work to remove the obstacles that make good practice cost too much in terms of time and psychic energy for the nurse. Nursing administration can set up the systems that detect nurses who are incapable of professional practice, and devise systems to get rid of those who can't practice professionally and those who simply are not motivated to do so.

Nursing administration can act to set the tone, to be the cheering squad that encourages the right sort of practice. And that includes systematic dangling of the rewards, so that they go to the good guys, not the bad. Nursing administration deals with the macrocosmic, not the microcosmic. It deals with systems. Systems can be devised to control and encourage certain sorts of practice and to discourage others. But individuals will always find ways to subvert, go around, or crawl under the fence of the very best system. In other words, even the best nursing administration is fallible.

NURSING PRACTICE AND NURSING AS A DISCIPLINE

So far we have looked at the relationship of administration to professional practice—good practice in normative terms. It is easier to look at administration's relation to practice in that light. But is the practice of nursing identical to the discipline of nursing? Yes and no. When we think of excellent practice, we tend to think of what the nurse does in her care of an individual patient—or even a group of patients. But nursing as a discipline involves much more than direct care; it involves research into how best to deliver that care; it involves building track records of successful nursing therapies; and it involves the systematic testing of theories about how nursing can best be delivered. As a discipline nursing unites theory, practice, and research in a meaningful way; it also conveys how serious and scholarly all these activities are.

Nursing as a discipline (as opposed to a practice) is often as the domain of the professional educator, as the function of the university setting. This perception too is inaccurate. If the only place where nursing is practiced as a discipline is in the educational milieu, then we are just pretending. The real testing ground for a serious discipline is where the practice occurs. If nursing cannot be a discipline in our practice settings, then it isn't a discipline, no matter how much our schools pretend it is.

Nursing administration has had some remarkable successes in turning nursing practice into discipline. Sometimes we are too close to the phenomena to recognize them. I think first of our extensive quality control systems. Quality control is the first step in nursing research. It is the measurement of what is; it is the linking of outcomes to practices. And in this aspect of disciplined behavior—on the institutional level—researchers in nursing have taught those in medicine. I think next of our extensive measurement systems for sorting patients into acuity classifications—the magic link between quality and quantity of care. Again, we beat medicine to the punch. And in evaluating practitioners: nurses have evolved all sorts of employee performance appraisals—most with the intentions of actually judging the employee. Compare that to how persons in medicine evaluate their own practitioners.

In these and other managerial ways, nursing administration has done its best to help make nursing a discipline. In some cases, alas, it has not been achieved intentionally. We all know of cases where a nursing department has been forced into evaluation activities under the threat posed by various accrediting agencies. But who built the criteria into the accrediting agencies' protocols? Nurses—and more often than not, nurse administrators who understood how a system affects practice.

Our report card is less successful in other aspects of the discipline. Research has been an astounding failure. I am aware that individual nurse researchers have worked miracles. But they've usually worked those miracles against overwhelming odds. If you don't believe it, just try walking into any hospital or health-care agency and telling the medical staff that you want total control over all nursing judgments in the institution, that you are planning major research into the best nursing protocols of care.

Now, you may say I am talking about power and politics, not research. Of course I am, but what a pity that we don't control our own domain of practice. What a pity that a field as complex as ours has to have the additional burden of fighting the powers that be just to carry on the normative behavior of a discipline.

It is a lot easier for medicine. When is the last time you remember a nursing staff rebelling because some physician wanted to implement medical research that affected the ease or dis-ease of delivering nursing care? And guess what would happen if the nursing staff raised such a fuss? Like it or not, nursing mediates goals that are seen as secondary to those of medicine in our society. Is it right? Is it wrong? Regardless, that's just the way it is.

The amazing thing is that nursing administration has been as successful as it has been, given the nature of the social environment in which we find ourselves.

Now we come to the critical question of cause and effect. Is nursing administration, for example, the source of disciplinary nursing behaviors? Or are nurse administrators simply reacting to demands by nursing personnel that such procedures be instituted? When was the last time a nursing staff demanded that a recalcitrant administration put an evaluation system into effect? When was the last time that a nursing staff fought to establish quality control systems over the head of a nursing director who didn't want them? Personally, I can think of some situations where this is just what happened. But I can think of a lot more cases where the nurses grumbled and griped at having to carry out one more such project devised by administration.

Who is it that usually decides the institution needs a nurse researcher? Who is it that creates a quality control department instead of leaving that function to each head nurse? Who is it that institutes a full-time education department in nursing? Who structures in the disciplinary habits? The nursing administration? The nursing staff? Where the latter is the answer, it is an embarrassing situation. After all, the administrator should be the one with the greatest sense of profession. With any luck at all the administrator should have been appointed for his or her overall grasp of nursing as a discipline. And his or her subordinate administrative staff should have been picked for a similar advanced perspective.

SHOWING THE FLAG

If nursing administration has successfully implemented a disciplinary approach to nursing in an institution, with the nursing staff, it has still only done half its job. The other half conveys the image of nursing as a discipline beyond the nursing division. To the non-nurses in the organization and in the community, nursing is most often represented by its spokesperson, the nurse executive. Nursing is interpreted as he or she displays it. Rarely is nursing accepted as more advanced, more serious, or more scholarly than the picture painted of it by its leader. The nurse who is an equal among managerial peers in the organization does much to improve nursing's status. The nurse executive who is an equal

among professional peers in other health disciplines has done even more. Seldom is nursing able to compete on a disciplinary status if the nurse executive is not accepted as a true peer among the medical staff or its leaders. And that equity is not achieved easily; it is not an equal battle. The nurse and physician do not start out with equal advantages in this society, whatever their education.

Yet, as I sit here thinking about it, I am able to count at least 50 nurse executives whom I personally know, who are able to function in their upward and outward roles as peers with all comers. We have produced more remarkable leaders than the field gives itself credit for. And their numbers are increasing as we prepare our nurse administrators at doctoral levels, where research, scholarly work, and intertwining of theory and practice are normative behaviors. Perhaps our greatest danger is that our administrative leaders will so outstrip the field that it will bear little resemblance to the image being created of the clinical practice of nursing by the rank and file.

RESEARCH

Perhaps the sine qua non of a discipline is the research it produces. Has nursing administration contributed to this aspect of the discipline of nursing? Most students of nursing administration, at least those who study on the graduate level, sooner or later find that they are expected to do research relevant to their field. Now the tricky question is how the subfield of nursing administration relates to clinical nursing. Perhaps the best answer is to review some of the dissertations produced by administration students.

I did this task in the most perfunctory way, turning my swivel chair to the shelf of dissertations gathered behind my desk. I selected a handful of tomes produced exclusively by nursing administration students—not clinical students. Three or four of them dealt with managerial aspects of nursing management, but the rest clearly identified the interface of management and clinical nursing. Simply put, most nursing administration studies, one way or another, offer guidance for clinical practice as well as administrative insights. Even the titles of these remaining works illustrate the point:

1. A. Vautier, *The Nursing Executive's Power to Control Nursing Practice.*[1]
2. M. Wilsea, *Identification of Nonnursing Activities of Medical-Surgical Staff Nurses: An Observational Field Study.*[2]
3. A. Madea, *Organizational Climate for Professionalism in Nursing Service.*[3]
4. R. Alward, *Performance of Permanent Versus Rotating Night Nurses: Circadian-Related Factors.*[4]

If I had approached the task with any desire for comprehensiveness, the list could have grown to monumental proportions, without even leaving the boundaries of my own school's collection of research by would-be nurse administrators. Any school of nursing education that has a program for nurse administrators could easily add to the collection.

More important, of course, is the ability of practicing nurse administrators to facilitate clinical nursing research in their own institutions. Here again, the job is done by the administrator who structures his or her organization in ways that allow clinical research to happen. Alas, the nurse administrator often finds that creating a permissive environment is not enough. Often it is the encouragement—or design—of the nurse administrator that leads nurses to see research as part of their job. I could recite situation after situation in my years as a consultant in which nurse administrators were frustrated to find that research didn't just happen because they had set up the structures to allow for it. ·

Preparing the average nursing service organization for the enactment of nursing re-search, unfortunately, is remedial work. It is remedial work that many committed nurse administrators have undertaken. What does it involve from an administrative perspective? First, one runs the political gamut of objectors—those who don't think there is anything to research in nursing, those who don't want nursing to have the status of a research-based practice, those who just don't want to hear any more complaints from nursing, and those who don't want nursing to change—impose upon—their own practice in any way. If this category of outside opposition were the worst of it, nursing would long since have a well-established norm of research.

Once the external forces have been laid to rest—and they never quite are—then one can look internally at the nursing obstacles. The first is obvious; no matter what we say, the majority of our nurses, even in 1988, are not taught how to do research. Worse, they are not taught to function in a research-oriented environment. They are not taught to seek researchable care quandaries in the midst of their day-to-day practice. Nurses, on the whole, don't perceive research as having anything to do with them. They don't do it, they don't think of it, and they seldom even read it. If they do read it, they don't modify their practice according to what they read. That sounds like a heavy indictment, but it fairly, I believe, represents the sort of education that has been received by the majority of nurses in practice today.

Given that reality, what must the nurse administrator do to put a research impetus into effect? Usually the first step is to devise a nursing research department or hire a "nurse researcher" if cost is a factor. Sometimes this person or group are hired to do the research (the substitution tactic). Sometimes this person or group are to provide education for the masses, so that others—staff nurses—will begin a new behavior—research (the teaching tactic).

Often the new behavior of research is fostered by motivating encouragement: research conferences (demonstration models), nurse-researcher-of-the year awards (recognition), and attendance at free classes (skill upgrading that may hold salary implications). Appointment of a research committee is another structural support that is usually put in place.

Does nursing administration often take on such a massive reorganization of its resources so as to include a research arm? I have seen case after case where a nurse administrator has gone to this not-inconsiderable trouble in order to exemplify his or her concept of disciplinary nursing. I am sure there are also some instances where an advanced nursing staff have demanded such initiatives from their recalcitrant administrators. I just haven't happened to see one.

Of course, doing research is only part of the picture. The application, communication, and infiltration of a research approach to practice are other essential components of nursing as a discipline. It is probably not surprising that the nurse administrator, who had been exposed in most cases to scholarly pursuit, will be more appreciative of such an environment than will the average staff nurse. Whether nursing administration can be expected to substitute for this education deficit in our profession is a major question. Yet try they will. Administrator after administrator has taken on the task.

NURSING THEORY

What has been said of nursing research may be repeated for nursing theory. In my experience, it has been nursing administration that has been the key mover in the application of theory to practice. True again, an appreciation of theory and application of it to practice has always been done by some select staff nurses. But collective applications of nursing theories inevitably are started at the organizational level.

The primitive state of some of our nursing

theory may make its application more like the instillation of operational rules rather than a true theory-based practice, but it's a start. The fact that our theories are value laden instead of descriptive makes the task not wrong—but even more difficult.

The hardest task—the linkage of theory to research, with research feeding back to modify theory—is seldom achieved at this stage of nursing's development. Few instances of this necessary intertwining can be documented. But when we reach that stage, I think it is fair to assume that nursing administration will be at the forefront.

What has been the contribution of nursing administration to the development of nursing as a discipline? In summary, the thrust has been twofold. First, nurse administrators—not all of them, but many—have attempted to create the environments where disciplinary practice might take place. They have done so by making the structural modification requisite for disciplinary behaviors shine forth. Often they have put in place the remedial education programs and administrative rewards and punishments that support new behaviors. Frequently administrators have done so in spite of external pressures to conceptualize nursing in a different way. Overt signs of movement toward a disciplinary concept of nursing include: quality assurance systems, acuity measurement systems, personnel evaluation systems, inservice education departments, research organizations, organizational systems for care that are based on given nursing theory stances, nursing-care plan research, and implementation of structured patient reporting.

The second way that nurse administrators have supported a disciplinary approach to nursing is by themselves exemplifying the "nurse as professional" with disciplinary behaviors. This role modeling has only been partial; after all the nurse administrator has another job. But the tone that the nurse administrator sets as the leader, as the exemplar for his or her institution and department, can make a radical difference in how both nurses and others conceptualize nursing. Have nurse administrators served this function? I believe they have; certainly the best of them have. The truly effective nurse administrator does not achieve his or her goals by leaving nursing and becoming a "manager." The effective nurse administrator is first and foremost a nurse. Management becomes a tool to be used in the production of nursing care. Because the nurse administrator is in a mediated role, his or her actions can have more influence than can the actions of the average clinician. The administrator melds with the nursing organization. Sometimes it is hard to tell where one begins and the other leaves off. The nurse administrator is the nursing organization in many ways. Nurse administrators who set out to implement a disciplinary approach to nursing are halfway there because of the power of their office and the influence of their nursing perspective. Are there obstacles? More than have been mentioned in this short article. Are there successes? There must be if nursing is to become a discipline, and take its place among other fields of study and practice that have earned the title, discipline.

REFERENCES

1. Vautier AF. The nursing executive's power to control nursing practice. New York: Teachers College, Dissertation, 1988 (in progress).
2. Wilsea MJ. Identification of nonnursing activities of medical-surgical staff nurses: an observational field study. New York: Teachers College, Dissertation, 1987.
3. Madea AR. Organizational climate for professionalism in nursing service. New York: Teachers College, Dissertation, 1985.
4. Alward RR. Performance of permanent versus rotating night nurses: circadian-related factors. New York: Teachers College, Dissertation, 1986.

51
Quality Care
Barbara Donaho

ONE of the many changes in the health-care field is evidenced in the growth of the multihospital systems. American Hospital Association data indicates the evolutionary nature of the growth of systems. While the numbers of systems has stayed in a range of 240 to 270 the number of hospitals in systems has steadily increased to over 2400, representing over 43% of all the community hospitals in the United States. Other differentiating characteristics between the systems are organizational control, type of ownership and control, and nonprofit or investor ownership. Two hundred and sixteen of the existing systems in 1986 were nonprofit and more than half of that number were church related (see Table 51.1).

The number of hospitals with the corresponding number of beds illustrates the potential influence of "multis" on the health-care field (see Table 51.2). A study done by Arthur Anderson and Company and the American Hospital Association provides insight into the issues that the leadership in the "multis" will face if they are to remain successful. Anderson's report indicates that the success of multihospital systems will depend on their ability to

- Protect their profitability in the face of a growing indigent-care problem.
- Understand existing payment systems and position themselves competitively as new ones emerge.
- Acquire new medical technologies that positively affect patient care, offer a competitive advantage, and be cost justified.
- Acquire information systems that enhance communication between systems and their local units and accurately project and track the cost of care.
- Monitor quality of care and measure it in a meaningful way.
- Build management expertise and talent at both the corporate and local-unit levels.
- Assume a strong unified presence in political arenas in an effort to ensure that hospital's ability to provide high-quality care.

The diversity of the characteristics of the individual systems make it difficult to generalize, but there are some noteworthy generalizations that assist in understanding the nature of the health-care system as it is undergoing the often rapid or constant change.

The present existing systems are spread

Table 51.1 Multihospital Systems By Type of Organizational Control

Type of Control	Number of Systems
Catholic (Roman) church related	91
Other church related	20
Subtotal, church related	111
Other nonprofit	105
Subtotal, nonprofit	216
Investor owned	52
Total	268

Adapted from Directors of multihospital systems. 7th ed. Chicago: American Hospital Association, American Hospital Publishing, Inc, 1986.

653

Table 51.2 Hospitals and Beds in Multihospital Systems, By Type of Ownership and Control

Ownership	Catholic Church-Related (CC)		Other Church-Related (CO)		Total Church-Related (CC, CO)		Other Nonprofit (NP)		Total Nonprofit (CC, CO, + NP)		Investor Owned (IO)		All Systems	
	H	B	H	B	H	B	H	B	H	B	H	B	H	B
Owned, leased, or sponsored	480	130,352	119	25,888	599	156,240	448	98,953	1,047	255,193	835	109,638	1,882	364,831
Contract managed	73	8,592	26	2,870	99	11,462	123	11,386	222	22,848	373	41,688	595	64,536
Total:	553	138,944	145	28,758	698	167,702	571	110,339	1,269	278,041	1,208	151,326	2,477	429,367

H = hospitals B = beds
Adapted from Directory of multihospital systems. 7th ed. Chicago: American Hospital Association, American Hospital Publishing, Inc, 1986.

across the United States and vary enormously in size; they can be divided into two groups. About 80% of the multihospital systems are comprised of fewer than eight hospitals, with about one-half of all systems having either two or three member hospitals. The other group has twenty systems who have a range of 20 to 424 hospitals in their corporation.

Other identifying characteristics of "multis" are the type of ownership and control—nonprofit or investor owned; but when studying the quality of services offered, growth or effectiveness of services, it is difficult to differentiate the systems.

The growth of the multisystems is also exemplified by regionalization and by the redefining of hospitals as a managed health-care system. Therefore, under a corporate structure, a variety of subsidiary corporations to provide long-term care, home health, or medical equipment have been created. In fact, some "multis" have all the components needed to assist a patient to move through a defined system to receive care. This incorporation process represents the evolution from a sick-care system to a managed health-care system.

The complexities of organizational structures in the systems are evident when studying the variety. While each multihospital has a clearly identified corporate board and chief executive officer, as well as a chief financial officer, there are few other common structures present. Some have multiple layers of governance as well as varying levels of management. Each organization needs to be studied to determine how accountabilities have been assigned. The degree of centralized control also varies, often depending on the function. For instance, financial accounting may be standardized and centrally controlled, while the decision as to which service to offer is the prerogative of an individual hospital and its governing body.

All the "multis" focus on profitability since providing service is contingent on economic viability. In a consumer-driven market, providing cost-effective quality care is the critical element in being able to compete in the marketplace. Nurse executives have long identified the goal of cost-effective quality care as a primary accountability. The placement of a nurse executive in a corporate position is linked to the organization's valuing of nursing and the contribution nursing can make toward their success as a viable health-care system.

The importance of understanding the philosophy mission, goals, and objectives of the organization is particularly critical for the nurse who makes the decision to move into a corporate position. The corporate nurse executive is most commonly a staff position, thus influence on the organization is accomplished through the leadership skills using professional and personal power, establishing meaningful relationships and effective communications. The responsibilities include strategic planning, program development, policy development, and efficient use of resources.

There are at least seven functions or roles a corporate nurse executive may assume:

- Monitor
- Consultant
- Educator
- Coordinator
- Strategic planner
- Executive
- Governance (board member)

The first five are relatively clear since they involve common activities for nurse executives in all settings. The key difference in the corporate world is that the nurse executive may be reporting the results to a more varied forum such as the hospital vice-president of nursing, hospital chief executive officer, corporate officer, or corporate board. It is absolutely necessary to clarify expectations prior to undertaking any one of the functions since many audiences are being served. The corporate nurse executive may monitor cost, productivity, use of resources, fiscal bottom-lines, and environments that are established in a hospital. Consultation to evaluate quality of care rendered or competence of a vice-president of Nursing or the effectiveness of an organizational structure of a hospital or nursing department are common requests. The education role may include orienting corporate and divisional board members, as well as management and professionals throughout the system. The coordinating role requires the skills to facilitate the sharing of scarce clinical expertise, support systems, management expertise, or any other limited resources in order to strengthen components of the entire system and reduce the ever-present tendency of each hospital to "reinvent or create their own wheel." It provides an opportunity to facilitate interorganization collaboration. The availability of critical professional human resources is an important strategic planning issue that needs to be addressed at a corporate as well as institutional level. The necessity to set standards of practice, monitor quality of care, evaluate the outcomes of care, and determine the cost effectiveness of the service are all natural issues for a corporate nurse executive to address on a system basis.

In order for a corporate nurse executive to be successful in these roles, an understanding of both the national issues and the influence of these issues on each hospital and community in the system is essential. The conceptual skills to understand the complexity of the issues must be equal to the skills to evaluate and articulate the potential impact on each facility. The changes that organizations need to make in order to survive are dependent on corporate management being able to bring about responsive appropriate change in the way professionals deliver care under an often totally new environment.

The two functions just beginning to be evident for the corporate nurse executive are an executive with line-management responsi-bility and a governance role. As subsidiary corporations are being developed to provide long-term care, home health, or wellness centers, nurse executives are often being placed in a chief executive position or a governance position responsible for the new line of business. Both entail broader responsibilities with complex reporting relationships to corporate boards, multiple institutional boards, or both within the system. The commonly accepted organizational structures, and reporting relationships are constantly being challenged or often ignored. Corporate staff are expected to wear many hats; while it may cause some discomfort because there are no theories or few studies to describe this evolving world, the existence of multiple functional roles presents an exciting challenge and opportunity for growth for the strong and competent nurse executive.

The skills needed in the corporate role do not vary from a single institutional-base except in the degree of intensity and multiple variations on the theme. It is essential that facts and figures on multiple institutions and communities be kept separate. Since the various institutions in the system may have very different levels of service, productivity, and potential, it follows that strategic plans need to be developed for each of them as is appropriate for each to contribute to the corporate whole. The rapidity with which the health-care field is changing forces the corporate staff to provide a stabilizing force and at the same time be a facilitator of major change.

For the individual who desires to move into the corporate world, here are some pointers based on experience.

- Your calendar is a corporate calendar driven by the diverse needs of member institutions—often spread great distances apart. Therefore, travel commitments may be heavy and result in a great demand on personal time.
- Effectiveness is based on competence

and credibility, not line authority; therefore, you must deal with your perceptions of power.

- Be ready to deal with ambiguity. The role of corporate nurse executive is evolving in organizations that are undergoing continuous change, including the struggle to define the various lines of business to be included in the corporate structure.

- The position will be effective only if access to decision makers is available and appropriately utilized for the benefit of the public and the corporation.

The nurse executive in corporate or multisystems is a nurse leader critically positioned to influence the future role for nurse executives as well as for nursing. It requires a visionary, a risk taker, and one willing to commit the personal and professional sides of his- or herself to the evolution of the position.

BIBLIOGRAPHY

Beyers M. National Commission on Nursing, Source Book, Chicago: HRET, 1984.

Directory of multihospital systems. 7th ed. Chicago: American Hospital Association, American Hospital Publishing, Inc, 1986.

Longo DR, Hearle J. New frontiers in patient care assessment proceedings of multiinstitutional conferences. Chicago: Joint Commission On Accreditation, 1986.

Multihospital systems: perspective and trends. Chicago: Arthur Anderson & Co, American Hospital Association, 1987.

52

Nursing Administration in Long-Term Care

Sister Rose Therese Bahr
John McConnell

A CRITICAL issue facing nurse administrators in long-term care in contemporary society is the lack of and unavailability of professional nurses prepared to practice in that setting. Since gerontology and gerontologic nursing—the primary professional responsibility of long-term care nurses—are new specialities, it is not surprising that the bulk of the nursing professionals currently working with the elderly are not prepared to meet the new expectations of the public and the profession. The purpose of this chapter is to describe the dimensions of this critical issue, identify theoretical components in nursing and related fields that aid in the elucidation of the issue, and project mechanisms for future strategies that might be implemented to resolve it from the standpoint of nurse researchers, educators, and practitioners in nursing administration in long-term care.

HISTORICAL PERSPECTIVE

There was a time when society was satisfied with the custodial care of institutionalized elderly. That care was delegated to those nurses who were willing to work for less money, and accept the low prestige afforded them by their colleagues and other health professionals. With the changing demographics and shift to a growing elderly population came a new focus on the elderly and their health care. A new body of knowledge

was researched and developed. Along with that body of knowledge came higher standards and new expectations—standards and expectations that the majority of long-term care nurses have never been educated to meet. Robb and Malinzak[1] note that nurse administrators have been forced "to employ generalists or specialists in areas other than gerontology to deal with the complexity and multifaceted problems presented by increasing numbers and proportions of old people."[1] (p. 153) Studies by Robb and Malinzak[1] and Huckstadt[2] demonstrated a deficit in gerontologic nursing knowledge in nurses currently working with the elderly.

A survey of long-term care facilities by Eliopoulos[3] indicated that 69% of nurses working in the facilities were prepared in diploma programs; 11% were graduates of baccalaureate programs in nursing; and only 4% had master's degrees in nursing. There was little or no gerontologic nursing content in most basic nursing programs until the early 1980s. Currently, in the late 1980s, there continue to be many barriers to including gerontologic nursing content and experience in undergraduate nursing programs. Among them are: the historic focus on acute care in nursing programs; the lack of examination items on the nurse licensing examination related to gerontologic nursing; the complexities of changing curricular content in terms of faculty values and gerontologic nursing; and the dominance of the

Table 52.1 Number and Workplaces of Registered Nurses, 1984 (in thousands)

	Total Number		Full-Time Equivalents	
	No.	%	No.	%
Total	1,485.7	100	1,234.9	100
Hospitals	1,012.0	68	850.7	69
Nursing homes	115.1	8	91.6	7
Community/public health	167.5	11	144.1	12
Ambulatory care	97.4	7	74.4	6
Nursing education	40.3	2	35.0	3
Private duty	22.7	2	14.7	1
Other	30.9	2	24.5	2

Adapted from Third national sample survey of registered nurses. Division of Nursing, Health Resources and Services Administration, 1984.

traditional nursing specialties—for example, medical-surgical nursing, psychiatric-mental health nursing, community health nursing, and maternal-child health nursing. These barriers to resolving the problem of lack of professionally prepared gerontologic nurses available for employment in long-term care facilities were identified by nurse administrators in long-term care facilities.[3–5]

A recent study of the personnel for health needs of the elderly through the year 2020 identifies that nursing personnel are the largest segment of formal caregivers for older adults.[6] Data collected in the study are demonstrated in Tables 52.1–52.4. Future needs for nursing personnel were projected on the basis of two approaches: (1) A historical trend-based model that uses past and current trends in service and resource utilization, modified by assumptions regarding likely changes in these trends; and (2) A criteria-

based model that uses professional judgments about appropriate resources necessary to achieve health care goals. As noted in the tables, according to the latest projections utilizing the historical trend-based model, the estimated requirements for the year 2000 would be about 1.7 million full-time equivalent R.N.s and about 720,000 full-time equivalent L.P.N.s. These numbers of nursing personnel would be needed to provide services to persons 65 years of age and older in the year 2000.[6] (pp. 56A-57B) To qualify for provision of care to older adults the need for education in the speciality of gerontologic nursing is imperative.

CURRENT STATUS OF NURSING EDUCATION

In the 1980s, comprehensive gerontologic nursing education is occurring at the master's

Table 52.2 Number and Workplaces of Licensed Practical and Vocational Nurses, 1983 (in thousands)

	Total Number		Full-Time Equivalents	
	No.	%	No.	%
Total	539.5	100	472.8	100
Hospitals	310.8	58	274.5	58
Nursing homes	121.4	23	104.0	22
Community/public health	23.8	4	21.8	5
Ambulatory care	49.0	9	44.0	9
Private duty	20.0	4	15.4	3
Other	14.5	2	12.1	2

Adapted from First national sample survey of licensed practical and vocational nurses. Division of Nursing, Health Resources and Services Administration, 1983.

Table 52.3 Estimated Requirements (Full-Time Equivalents) for Registered Nurses in the Year 2000 (in thousands)

| | Historical Trend-Based Model | | Criteria-Based Model | | | |
| | | | Lower | | Upper | |
	No.	%	No.	%	No.	%
Total	1,683	100	2,328	100	2,958	100
Hospitals	872	52	897	39	1,208	41
Nursing homes	259	15	838	36	1,053	36
Community health	338	20	415	18	483	16
Physicians' offices	110	7	90	4	112	4
Nursing education	50	3	49	2	64	2
Other	54	3	38	2	38	1

level of education. There are approximately 25 graduate programs nationally with a major in gerontologic nursing.[7] Unfortunately, enrollment is small and recruitment of students for these programs continues to be a major problem.[8,9] According to Eliopoulos only 15% of the registered nurses practicing in long-term care have the capability of taking advantage of these graduate programs as matriculated students, primarily because of the availability of the programs near their site of employment.[3] Thus, over 70% of the registered professional nurses practicing in long-term care must rely on topical seminars and educational conferences for preparation in gerontologic nursing.

Two major obstacles preventing many nurses from attending these conferences to upgrade their knowledge of aging and care of older adults include: (1) Economics: it is not unusual for a long-term care facility of a major corporation, with over 300 beds, to have budgeted only $150 a month for training and education; and (2) Resource management: there is a scarcity of nurses available to free those nurses on tours of duty for educational activity by replacing them.[1] Hence, there is little or no incentive in long-term care for nurses to increase their formal education on their own time or at their own expense.

Because of the lack of prepared nurses in long-term care, most long-term care facility owners, administrators, and nurse administrators are not aware of the impact and substantial difference, both economically and in quality of care, that formally educated gerontologic nurses can make in the long-term care delivery system. Therefore, nurses are reimbursed primarily for their licensed status and not necessarily for their competence, educational background, or both.

Wage differentials in long-term care are sometimes provided for working weekends and evening or night tours of duty, but this is not a universal practice. In a system that is having difficulty recruiting the number of

Table 52.4 Estimated Requirements (Full-Time Equivalents) for Licensed Practical/Vocational Nurses in the Year 2000 (in thousands)

| | Historical Trend-Based Model | | Criteria-Based Model | | | |
| | | | Lower | | Upper | |
	No.	%	No.	%	No.	%
Total	720	100	423	100	494	100
Hospitals	246	34	82	19	54	11
Nursing homes	301	42	339	80	436	88
Community health	40	6	3	1	4	1
Physicians' offices	109	15	—	—	—	—
Other	24	3	—	—	—	—

nurses it needs, characteristics such as availability and reliability may take precedence over knowledge and performance. Although there has been a steady increase in nursing wages in long-term care, a short supply of nurses and the competition with hospitals and other care settings for the nurses to fill positions in the facilities remains a major problem for nurse administrators.[3,10–12] Nursing education has become a very expensive investment and nurses would like to believe they would profit by that investment or at least that they could count on a reasonable return. At issue here is the image of the professional nurses by administrators of long-term care facilities projected as the group that will work for whatever wage is offered regardless of the type of preparation they may possess. The image problem is also prevalent among the general nurse population nationally as well, in terms of long-term care.

CONTEMPORARY IMAGE AND PRACTICE OF NURSES EMPLOYED IN LONG-TERM CARE

The negative stereotype of the role of a nurse in long-term care as requiring less education and fewer skills may also be a barrier to increasing the educational level of professional nurses in gerontologic nursing. Many nurses come to long-term care from the hospital setting thinking that they are overqualified for the position.[2] After all, acute care has been the primary focus of nursing for years. Those skills, however, while valuable in long-term care, by themselves are not sufficient in caring for older adults. The superimposition of hospital skills on long-term care needs is a common occurrence; however, it is not an effective or efficient approach to long-term care.[13] For example, it is not uncommon for an acute care nursing text to begin a discussion of an illness or acute problem with the words "observing for the signs and symptoms

of that illness or problem" because they are usually evident when a patient presents himor herself to an acute care setting. Often it is the symptom itself that motivates the patient to go to the hospital or clinic.[14]

In the long-term care setting, however, the nurse must initiate and maintain an illness-prevention and health-promotion frame of mind and be adept at identification of potential problems in the long-term care environment and in the elderly population to prevent the signs and symptoms of illness from developing.[2,8,15] Focusing on the observation for signs and symptoms, in other words, waiting for a problem to occur can be a costly mistake not only in regard to quality of life but from the standpoint of health-care economics.[5,16,17] An acute problem such as a urinary tract infection will, minimally, cause discomfort to an elderly resident and may even lead to sepsis and an expensive hospitalization. With skillful nursing care the infection might have been prevented, if, for example, an excellent health-promotion plan were in effect. However, nurses coming into long-term care may bring with them common practices in acute care such as the use of foley catheters as an answer to incontinence and the use of bedpans, which can contribute to or increase the potential for infections of the urinary tract.[3,15,18]

In reviewing a list of common problems seen in long-term care such as constipation, impactions, contractures, urinary tract infections, skin breakdowns, respiratory infections, falls, incontinence, and dehydration, it becomes evident that the majority of these problems are amenable to preventive measures. Nurses, educationally and attitudinally prepared to prevent these problems in the institutionalized elderly, could easily influence positively and effectively the quality and cost of long-term care delivered across the country.[2,10,19]

The unavailability of prepared nurses in gerontologic nursing in long-term care settings has developed and fostered a task-oriented or functional model of nursing instead of promoting a professional nursing model. The functional model favors a central decision-maker and power source, usually the director of nursing.[1,3,11,15] This approach facilitates the efficient use of scarce resources, prepared nurses.[14] However, it can also focus overwhelming responsibility and accountability on a nurse in a situation or environment that he or she is not prepared for educationally. This director of nursing assumes the clinical and managerial leadership for the facility.[3,10] His or her responsibilities include a wide variety of administrative tasks and clinical programming in addition to the day-to-day supervision of the nursing operation. The centralization of decision making creates a dependency on that central figure, often making the quality of care as transient as that central figure. This phenomenon would explain the dynamics of a long-term care facility providing excellent care one year and poor quality the next, coinciding with the change in that central figure, the nurse administrator.[3,9]

Another characteristic of the functional model is that, when basic tasks are delegated to nurses to complete, there is little discernible difference between the educational background of the registered nurses—that is, those with diplomas, A.D.N.s, or B.S.N.s— nor is there much difference noticed between registered nurses and licensed practical nurses in terms of task completion.[1,14] If their time is filled with clerical responsibilities, passing medications, and delivering treatments, all are likely to perform equally; that is, all are likely to complete the tasks in an acceptable manner. Because there is often a substitution in long-term care nursing services of a registered nurse with a licensed practical nurse, due to the lack of professional nurses, many nursing positions have been brought down to the lowest or most basic common denominator, for example,

non-delineation of nursing tasks. Consequently, employers may ask, why not acquire the least expensive form of labor to do the job?[16,20] It will not be until professional nurses are utilized in long-term care in a professional nursing model that a significant difference will be appreciated in terms of educational preparation.[4,5,21] And, it will not be until registered nurses become prepared to practice with the elderly in long-term care that a professional model will evolve. Legislators and consumer groups are already preparing legislation requiring a certain ratio of registered nurses to residents in long-term care. This effort is an attempt to improve what the Heinz Report referred to as "inadequate nursing care."[12] More unprepared registered nurses may not make the quality difference expected by these groups.

Nursing staff inadequately educated in the care of the elderly significantly influence the care delivered. One of the major factors affecting quality of care and quality of life in nursing homes is "the number and quality of nursing staff in relation to the facilities requirements," a reference made in the recently published Report of the Institute of Medicine.[22] The complexity of the care required by the "confused resident," the "incontinent resident," or those severely debilitated after a stroke lends itself to catastrophic results when administered by educationally unprepared nurses. The lack of preparation of nurses in long-term care has led to their inability, in many instances, to meet the physiologic, psychologic, sociologic, and spiritual needs of their elderly clients.[4,20] Unfortunately, the issue of educational unpreparedness of nurses has often been misinterpreted as a result of malice or negligence and provided long-term care nursing with a negative image. The negative image continues to make recruitment of quality nurses into long-term care difficult and perpetuates the problem.[10,20,22]

The stress associated with attempting to

meet the expectations of nursing in long-term care without the necessary preparation takes its toll on staff and nurse administrators. Many long-term care facilities are experiencing difficulty meeting even minimal expectations of quality care. According to a report to the Special Committee on Aging chaired by Senator Heinz in May, 1986, titled *Nursing Home Care: The Unfinished Agenda,*[10] approximately one-third of the nation's skilled nursing facilities failed to meet at least one federal standard in assuring health and safety of residents in 1984. In addition, the report states that there has been a 61% increase in failure to provide 24-hour nursing care.[10]

Stress and burnout, often present in long-term care staff at all levels, are characterized by the following behaviors:

- Attendance problems—Tardiness and absenteeism are increased when staff are stressed. When calling in sick, staff may give symptoms associated with stress such as fatigue, backache, headache, insomnia, indigestion, and nausea.
- Poor morale—Staff may dread coming to work and spend most of the shift (tour of duty) watching the clock. Team spirit may be lost, and staff who enjoyed working together may begin bickering and arguing. Intershift conflict may arise, for example, between day tour-of-duty nurses and evening or night tour-of-duty staff.
- Depersonalization—Patients may come to be perceived as disease entities (the "bilateral amputee"), tasks (the "complete"), or room numbers ("301 wants a pain med") rather than as individuals.
- Avoidance—Staff may find every opportunity they can to decrease patient contact. Excessive cigarette smoking and coffee breaks or hurrying to complete

work so that they can congregate with coworkers are behaviors indicative of this problem.

- Inappropriate humor—Frequently, when people are under pressure they become sarcastic or laugh at situations that are not funny, for example, joking while doing postmortem care. Finding humor in the misfortunate situations of patients is symptomatic of a staff's emotional weariness.
- Withdrawal—Some staff may emotionally withdraw from interactions with patients and coworkers as a protective mechanism. Some may feel they must physically withdraw from the situation and resign from their positions. Several threatened or actual resignations may be signals of staff burnout.
- Rigidity—Staff who feel they must limit their emotional investment in their work may oppose deviating from standard routines that can lead to additional efforts from them. Comments associated with this symptom may include, "That's not in my job description," "I'm just following orders," "I can't make any exceptions for you," or, "I don't want any arguments, just do what I tell you."
- Substance abuse—In addition to excessive cigarette and coffee consumption, individuals who are experiencing burnout use drugs and alcohol more frequently.
- Family disruption—It is not unusual for work stress to affect one's emotional state at home. Arguments with children and spouse occur more frequently when one is under stress.
- Poor performance—The quality of services delivered may decline when staff is stressed. This factor can be detected through general observations, audits, and increased patient and visitors complaints.[3] (pp. 60–61)

Another characteristic of stress and burnout not mentioned above is a high turnover rate of nursing staff.[24] This prevalent problem in long-term care is an additional barrier to the nurses' educational preparation.[10,14,20] The high turnover rate in a facility often diminishes the benefits of any educational program in the facility. If the perceived benefits of a program are low, it follows that their importance or the value placed on them will also be low. Consequently, education departments in long-term care facilities are small and focus their attention primarily on orientation of new staff and in-service topics required by federal, state, and local regulations. A high turnover rate frustrates both the nurse educator and nurse administrator in the long-term care setting. The nurse administrator finds it difficult to make any progress when the staff oriented toward and educated for their positions choose to resign soon after employment and leave him or her to start over again in the cycle of hiring, orienting, and training new nursing staff for the facility.[3,10] A logical assumption to make, of course, is that turnover is more prevalent in areas of the country where other employment opportunities are available to nursing staff. In areas where those alternate employment opportunities do not exist one would expect a higher incidence of other symptoms of burnout instead.

The dimensions of the critical issue of insufficient numbers of prepared professional nurses in long-term care, can be demonstrated by a cyclic schema in which unprepared nurses attempt to provide specialized care to the elderly (see Figure 52.1). There is limited access to and motivation for nurses to obtain better preparation in gerontologic nursing through formal education because of stringent admission criteria. The result becomes an inefficient and ineffective nursing delivery system in the long-term care facility providing marginal or poor quality of care at high costs. These results add to an already

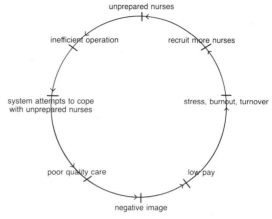

Figure 52.1 Cyclical Schemata of Frustration: Unprepared Nurses in Long-Term Care Attempting to Provide Specialized Care to Elderly. Moving counterclockwise beginning with unprepared nurses, the arrows move from inefficient operation from a nursing administration viewpoint through the cycle of frustration demonstrating the stress the total system is under when unprepared nurses attempt to provide specialized care to elderly in long-term care settings.

negative image of nurses working in long-term care, which further decreases any incentive for qualified nurses to seek employment in the long-term care setting. Meanwhile, wages remain as low as they can be and still attract enough registered nurses to fill the necessary positions in each facility. The job descriptions are often designed to accommodate registered professional nurses with all or any of the educational backgrounds (diploma, ADN, BSN) and even, if necessary, allow for a substitution of a registered nurse with a licensed practical nurse.

In an attempt to compensate for the small numbers of well-prepared nurses, long-term care maintains a functional or task-oriented model of nursing with a focus on centralization of decision making, responsibility, and accountability. This approach, combined with the stress already perceived by nurses trying to meet facility, resident, family, and nursing expectations they are unprepared to handle, contributes to burnout and staff turnover. The cycle then begins to repeat itself, that is, more nurses are recruited into a setting for which they are not prepared educationally to meet the needs of the aging individuals— their primary professional responsibility in the long-term care setting.

THEORETICAL ELUCIDATION OF THE CRITICAL ISSUE

With the critical issue of nonpreparedness of the professional nurse for long-term care nursing as a current reality, the practicing nurse administrator is bereft of a key source for implementation of nursing goals and evaluation of outcomes as delineated in the conceptual framework for quality nursing care. This missing link regarding the professional staff resources needed to promote and upgrade nursing care becomes a source of major difficulty for any delegation of responsibility for resident care and its continuity throughout the daily routine. The multidimensional difficulties posed by this major lack of prepared professional nursing personnel stymie the nurse administrator in achieving nursing's major goal—that is, the optimum functioning of the elderly residents who seek care within the long-term care setting or facility.[25] Currently it is estimated that only 0.001% of all nurses have specialized skills to care for elderly patients.[26]

Nursing personnel who seek positions in the long-term care facility are ill-prepared for the realities of providing care from the long-term care framework. They are unfamiliar with the approach used with older adults whose aging processes may not allow them to respond to treatments or activities as quickly as persons of a younger age-group, and utilize those procedures the nurse may be familiar with when practicing nursing in an acute, medical-model environment.[5]

Consequently, one dimension of this critical issue is professional accountability for care expected by the nurse executive in promoting the well-being of older residents in the long-term care facility. Porter-O'Grady notes that professional accountability in providing quality care is intermeshed with nursing knowledge and competency.[27] Without the knowledge a nurse cannot be expected to provide care as measured against professional standards of practice.

In this regard, without the key resource of prepared, qualified gerontologic nurses to assume responsibility and accountability for nursing care, a flaw in the health-care delivery system becomes evident. System models, if in place, aid in the identification of the organization, interaction, interdependency, and integration of parts and elements.[28] Through the system-model actual or potential problems of function in the system can be identified and appropriate interventions strategized to overcome inefficient methods of operation.

The system and its environment are the major features of systems models. A system is described as incorporating specified objectives and relationships between the objectives, their attributes, and desired outcomes.[28] Environment is described as all objects a change in whose attributes affect the system, and also those objects whose attributes are changed by the behavior of the system.[28] The system then could be a person, whose environment is the family; a community with families whose environment is the county in which the community is located; or, it could be the nurse whose environment is the long-term care facility in which practice of nursing takes place.

Systems may be open or closed. An open system is maintained by a continuous input and output of energy, and a closed system is isolated from its environment.[28] When the open energy is continuously present, differentiation, complexity, and ordering of the system become more evident; whereas, in the closed system, energy is stifled and more disorder of the system occurs.

Characteristics important in the systems models are boundary, or a closed circle around selected variables, where there is less interchange of energy, tension, stress, and conflict—forces that alter the system structure; equilibrium and steady state—the balance between internal and external forces and the parts—are not dependent on any fixed equilibrium point or level; and finally, feedback—the flow of energy between a system and its environment.[28] These characteristics allow for a systems model to function and provide a system in which productivity, motivation, and control are evident. What, then, is the system in place for long-term care? Is there a system to the care given to elderly in the long-term care modality?

LONG-TERM CARE: A NONSYSTEM

Long-term care is comprised of nursing, medical, and allied health-care needs of individuals who are dependent on professionals for meeting their health needs.[29] As the older population of the United States increases in numbers and age, 28.5 million over 65 years of age in 1985 with projections of 64.8 million over 65 in the year 2030,[30] the need for such care becomes a pervasive part of society. Many of the components of the approach to long-term care remain ill-defined, including who are the individuals who truly need long-term care. Since society has not identified the recipients of care, what care is needed and who is to administer it is a major dilemma facing the health-care administrators in nursing.

Long-term care arises from injury, disease, and processes of growing old that increase the degree of vulnerability for older adults.[29] A variety of supports are needed to provide adequately for persons dependent on long-term care facilities, ranging from provision of personal care to acute high-technology med-

ical interventions. With the acuity of the individual in long-term care settings increasing, the difficulty of adequately providing necessary professional nursing care becomes more pronounced.

Grimaldi and Sullivan suggested a classification of vulnerable individuals into four dependency categories:[31]

1. The independent—those having infrequent contact with the health-care professional.
2. The independence threatened—individuals who are vulnerable and require high levels of self-care with bouts of episodic intensive care.
3. The independence delegated—individuals who depend on others to provide care to accomplish most of the activities of daily living (ADL). Intensive care is needed which must be provided by others.
4. The dependent—individuals in poor health and unable to provide self-care. These individuals are usually the old-old (85 plus) and have complex health needs with accompanying self-care deficits.

These four categories of individuals needing assistance from long-term care are coupled with their personal goals, families' goals, and health-professionals' goals and outcomes. Services needed and services given are distinct from each other based on resources available and prepared personnel available in the settings providing the multidimensional services. However, few health-care planners of long-term care consider services across a variety of settings when providing long-term care. Planners assess only their own setting independently without providing for an interrelated, interagency, intercommunity approach to the system of care provided.

Consequently, it could be argued that no system of long-term care is provided in the United States at the present time. Many ele-

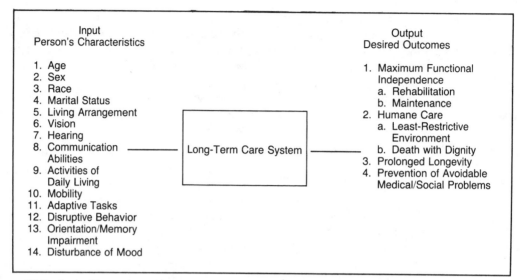

Input
Person's Characteristics

1. Age
2. Sex
3. Race
4. Marital Status
5. Living Arrangement
6. Vision
7. Hearing
8. Communication Abilities
9. Activities of Daily Living
10. Mobility
11. Adaptive Tasks
12. Disruptive Behavior
13. Orientation/Memory Impairment
14. Disturbance of Mood

Long-Term Care System

Output
Desired Outcomes

1. Maximum Functional Independence
   a. Rehabilitation
   b. Maintenance
2. Humane Care
   a. Least-Restrictive Environment
   b. Death with Dignity
3. Prolonged Longevity
4. Prevention of Avoidable Medical/Social Problems

Figure 52.2   Long-Term Care System Input-Output Overview. The input-output overview demonstrates the older person's characteristics in the long-term care setting in which the nurse provides care and the projected and desired outcomes of professional care when a well-functioning, efficient long-term care system exists. (Used with permission from Callahan J, Wallack P. Reforming the Long-Term Care System. Lexington, MA: Lexington Books, 1979.)

ments and structures exist but there is no linkage in any systematic fashion at the local, state, or national level. To project the dilemma further there is an evident lack of a system in each agency providing long-term care because of the missing link of professional gerontologic nurses needed to provide care to aging persons.

Callahan and Wallack proposed a Long-Term Care System input-output overview.[32] They identified the characteristics of the long-term care dependent person and the desired outcomes as suggested in the model (see Figure 52.2). When reviewing the desired outcomes in Callahan's model, each outcome requires nurses who possess up-to-date knowledge and skills in the fields of psychology, sociology, humanities, ethics, communications, and gerontologic nursing to promote the level of well-being identified as crucial to the health and maintenance of older adults seeking long-term care. Management science is incorporating more and more of the content of behavior modification and

assessment to motivate personnel to execute the goals and mission of long-term care facilities. When such personnel are highly motivated and perceive the importance of their work, the commitment to providing high-level care becomes a source of high morale and satisfaction with the position they hold.[27] With the system properly in place the professional nursing model of care becomes the norm and replaces the industrial model where one clocks in at the beginning of the "shift" and performs at the minimal level.[19] Custodial care, the result of a nonsystem of health care in long-term care facilities, would be replaced and a systematic orientation to true professional nursing with its focus on health at the optimal level would prevail. But many problems need to be addressed in the realm of education, practice, and research to elucidate the issues inherent in the long-term care nonsystem in the late 1980s.

Another dimension of the unpreparedness of professional gerontologic nursing staff for long-term care is clinical documentation. The legalities and ethical issues facing older adults who seek long-term care are mammoth.[5] When the professional nursing staff is not well prepared in the knowledge base of gerontology and gerontologic nursing, nursing care difficulties can abound, for example, when early detection is neglected due to lack of knowledge regarding such nursing processes as assessment, diagnosis, planning, and implementing the plan and evaluation of outcomes.[33] It is then that documentation of care is critical to the total system of care. Yet, in long-term care facilities, home health-care agencies, and other settings in which long-term care is delivered, insufficient recording of the care in detail to furnish adequate data is the norm.[33] Little use of the problem-oriented method of charting is in evidence; only the narrative form is used, for example, in such statements as "noncompliance with medication regime" and "failure to eat properly" without further details of what might be causing the difficulty. When documentation is inadequate, insufficient data are available for evaluating and analyzing how to further plan for nursing intervention to resolve the difficulty.

In addition, when documentation in the clinical setting is inadequate, difficulty in determining the breakdown of communication between staff, client, medical, and ancillary personnel and the nurse executive becomes a major obstacle in providing safe and professional care. Documentation is a legal responsibility of the professionals giving the care. When such charting is not accomplished, the client is not provided the opportunity to demand better performance from those who profess expertise in gerontologic nursing care. The importance of appropriate clinical documentation in the long-term care system is highly crucial in the promotion of the client's well-being and continuity of care. An example of poor-quality care when insufficient documentation is present is demonstrated in the transferring of a 78-year-old gentleman from an intermediate care unit in a long-term care setting to a unit for persons afflicted with Alzheimer's disease. This gentleman had dentures but this datum was not recorded on the chart. In his adjustment to the new unit the nurse in charge automatically ordered a pureed diet for him assuming he had no teeth and consequently not wanting to be bothered with attempting to feed him regular foods. It was the spouse of the man who informed the nurse of his use of dentures and wanted the dentures kept in the mouth. By keeping the dentures in the man's mouth the musculature remained firm, which facilitated jaw movement when chewing and aided in the act of swallowing. In this way the man continued to be independent of feeding assistance and his self-image and self-esteem were positively reinforced. The nurse in this situation did not appreciate the "interference" of the spouse in what she deemed "the nurse's responsibility." A simple act of recording information could have saved the gentleman's spouse some embarrassing moments and promoted a sense of well-being of the man through continuous wearing of the dentures.

Nursing theories or models are beginning to aid the understanding of complex nursing phenomena. The models of Self-Care by Orem[34] and Adaptation by Roy[35] provide a framework for appreciating the critical issues facing long-term care nurse administrators.

NURSING THEORISTS AND LONG-TERM CARE

One approach to the critical issues related to nursing administration in long-term care for the elderly—such as the paucity of professional nurses—is to briefly overview relevant nursing theories. Two theorists who have analyzed the phenomena facing nursing are Roy, in the Adaptation Theory, and Orem, who formulated the Self-Care Theory. Each theorist presents an approach that provides insight into the difficulties faced by long-term care administrators in provision of quality care to elderly residents.

Roy, in analyzing the adaptation of the individual to the environment, notes that stressors in the environment can hinder the performance of the individual. She describes the human being as an open, living system with exchange of energy and information that permits the individual to adapt to internal and external environmental changes in his or her own personhood and the physical environment in which work is accomplished. When barriers, such as stressors, to this open system are perceived the individual becomes maladaptive and problems arise.[35]

For the nurse administrator in the long-term care facility, the stressor most experienced is the lack of prepared gerontologic nurses who can operate with high levels of motivation and energy to promote the systemwide operation with nursing interventions-strategies applicable to elderly clients. The environment then becomes the stressor as well, resulting in a cyclic orientation that fails to upgrade the lowest level of performance simply because the prepared nurses are not available to facilitate a higher-level performance. Earlier the dilemma facing the nurse when unqualified for the position he or she holds was noted. The same dilemma faces the nurse administrator when stressors are such that goals and objectives formulated for the mission of the Nursing Division in the long-term care facility cannot be accomplished due to lack of qualified personnel.

Orem, in her Self-Care Theory, describes the necessity of prerequisites for self-care to take place in the individual or in an organizational structure. She noted that the universal regulations for health must be delineated and maintained in order to enjoy wellness. If all universal regulations for health factors are not evident, then a self-deficit model is in place.[34]

In analyzing the situation in long-term care administration in the 1980s, a self-care deficit model is apparent. There is a lack of motivation among nursing personnel with the consequence of minimal levels of care administered by the nursing personnel. There is a lack of perspective from a professional orientation; that is, priorities of care based on a conceptual framework of nursing care are not being accomplished. The task oriented, or functional, role of nursing with complete control over care and decision making ascribed to the nurse administrator rather than the nursing staff is in vogue. Consequently, instead of a professional nursing model being implemented in long-term care there is an industrial model in which the workers are concerned with punching time clocks and accomplishing only tasks assigned without being motivated to achieve a higher level of performance. In this mode the self-care universal needs of elderly residents are avoided or neglected. In such circumstances the elderly persons in the long-term care setting are the victims because the system is only as effective as the workers prepared to function in such organizations.

What, then, are some proposals in the areas of nursing education, practice, and research to overcome this critical issue of unprepared nursing staff in long-term care nursing administration? What mechanisms should be addressed and further researched to alleviate the dilemma in long-term care administration? Each of these arenas will be reviewed with a futuristic orientation toward the nursing professionals and their priorities.

FUTURISTIC MECHANISMS IN GERONTOLOGIC EDUCATION, PRACTICE, AND RESEARCH

Gerontologic Education

The key factor to overcoming the dilemma in long-term care nursing administration and the critical need for prepared gerontologic nurses lies in the realm of nursing education. Nursing education programs assume responsibility for preparing nurses to meet the challenges of the twentieth and twenty-first centuries in light of increasing aging populations. In this structure nurse faculty who control the curricular offerings in a nursing program must be encouraged strongly to address the needs of older adults in the course offerings for undergraduate and graduate nursing programs. What can be done to facilitate this?

1. Placement of gerontologic nursing content on the state board examinations testing clinical decision-making for nurses in settings where older adults are cared for by nursing personnel.
2. Establishment by the National League for Nursing of a strong and enforceable statement regarding content and clinical experience for all nursing students in all programs (A.D.N., B.S.N., and M.S.N.) as an accreditation criterion.
3. Facilitation of preparation of nurse faculty in the area of gerontologic nursing through a tuition reimbursement plan to encourage such preparation.
4. Establishment of liaison relationships between nursing educators and nursing service administration-personnel in community, hospital, and long-term care facilities to encourage staff nurses to pursue educational preparation in gerontologic nursing.
5. Establishment of advisory committees between nursing education and nursing service administrators in long-term care administration to bridge these two entities.[21,36]

With this approach a larger group of nurses who presently staff the long-term care facilities would be accessed into nursing education more easily, and would bring about the preparation needed to care for older clients who need and deserve the best possible preparation of nursing staff. The pyramid shown

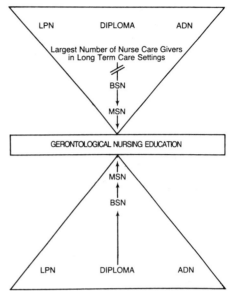

Figure 52.3 Gerontologic Nursing Education: Inverted Pyramid of Inaccessibility for Largest Nurse Population Serving the Elderly to Pyramid of Accessibility and Career Ladder to Elder Care in Long-Term Care Settings. The top pyramid, which is inverted, shows the largest number of nonprepared nurses—in terms of gerontologic background—are providing the majority of care for older adults in long-term care settings and that formal gerontologic nursing programs are inaccessible to the L.P.N., diploma, and A.D.N. group because of barriers to the mainstream of professional education. This is shown by the broken line in the top pyramid (inverted). The lower, correctly placed pyramid demonstrates a smooth transition from the various levels of preparation to a career-ladder approach to education in gerontologic nursing programs.

in Figure 52.3 could slowly turn from an inverted structure where the largest group of nurses are unprepared yet deliver care to the older adults, to that of a pyramid where all nurses have preparation in gerontologic nursing and can serve the elderly according to a professional nursing model in long-term care settings. The challenge for nursing education is to become innovative and creative in its approach to admission of students who make up the largest group of unprepared personnel and allow for larger numbers to obtain educational preparedness in gerontologic nursing with an emphasis on long-term care. The barriers, many of which are artificial and cumbersome, must be eliminated by admission officers who perceive the "ivory tower" of education unattainable for many nurses who started their nursing preparation in the community-based institutions of learning, not in the traditional mode. The assumption has been that if the individual is less prepared than at the registered-nurse level, he or she is less worthy of the attention of nurse-education personnel at the traditional baccalaureate level of education. When this assumption is challenged it is realized how difficult it has been for the mass numbers of nurses to move from one level of education to the other or to even obtain entrance into a nursing program of their choice.

Nurse educators, who now face student shortages, should aggressively promote education in the long-term care sector as a major purpose of their mission. It is precisely because the field of gerontologic nursing has been neglected that there are fewer prepared nurses in the field currently to meet the demands for nursing care of older adults. Because of this neglect, the nursing profession is taking a second seat to the organizations of service to elderly who have lobbied for increased preparation and numbers of nurses to staff long-term care facilities.[12] Legislation stemming from the Institute of Medicine study *Improving the Quality of Care in Nursing Homes*[11] recommends that nurse staffing be a major factor for nursing home regulation, which is being debated in the 100th Congress in 1988. It is hoped that a positive result from this legislative effort will occur. The ratio being proposed is for 1 registered nurse to every 30 older residents on the day tour-of-duty, 1 registered nurse to every 45 older adults on the evening tour-of-duty, and 1 registered nurse to every 60 older adult residents in the long-term care facility

on the night tour-of-duty. The rationale for this ratio is to meet the changing and unique health-care needs of older adults on a 24-hour basis.[12] Other personnel such as licensed practical nurses and nursing assistants would be utilized in proportional ratios as necessary to provide adequate coverage for nursing task completion under the direct supervision of the registered nurse. As noted earlier, a concern arises regarding the regulation if the emphasis is not inclusive of educational preparation of the registered nurse coverage. This attempt at more adequate coverage of nursing staff must be coupled with the aggressive stance that the nursing staff be prepared in the area of gerontologic nursing. Using this creative mechanism the nurse administrator in long-term care would have sufficient resources available to bring about a professional nursing model in the facility and upgrade the nursing care to a high professional standard. If nursing education accepts the challenge the greatest advocates for nursing will be the older persons who will be recipients of excellent nursing care under the competent administration of a nurse executive in the long-term care facility.

Mechanisms for nursing education, then, include: removal of barriers for access of candidates into nursing programs in schools of nursing across the country; education of nurse faculty in gerontologic nursing; integration of gerontologic nursing content and clinical experiences in long-term care; assurance of clinical knowledge and competence of nurses graduating from nursing programs in terms of older adults and long-term care; greater effort to enhance the attractiveness of gerontologic nursing as a career choice of nursing students entering nursing programs at all levels; greater interaction and supportive avenues to be pursued between nursing education and long-term care administrators and personnel; and, finally, a more aggressive stance by nurse educators in legislative activities for promotion of political activity to better the world of older adults in our society who need excellent nursing care in whatever setting they are found.

Gerontologic Nursing Practice

In the area of practice of gerontologic nursing, challenges must be faced with courage, determination, and creativity. The mode of custodial care must be eliminated entirely from the philosophic stance of care delivered to elderly residents in the long-term care setting. Nurse administrators must address the need for a professional model of nursing care to be incorporated in a philosophic statement of care so that the guidelines are available for all nursing personnel to implement. This philosophy of care statement projects the clinical framework of the nurse administrator, who presents a leadership style that motivates nurses to follow a professional nursing model rather than the traditional medical model currently implemented in long-term care facilities.

Nursing staff should be encouraged to continue their educational preparation. If their preparation is at the licensed practical-nurse level the nurse administrator should facilitate access to the associate degree program to assist the licensed practical nurse into the mainstream of nursing education at the technical level. If the nurse possesses the diploma-program level of preparation incentives should be initiated to encourage the nurse to seek further preparation in either the associate degree or baccalaureate-R.N. completion program. Nurse administrators should be in close communication with faculty of schools of nursing to insist that gerontologic nursing be an integral part of the education of these nursing personnel. Only when the nursing practice is based in the knowledge of gerontologic nursing will the practice of nursing involving older adults be improved. Not only will the preparation of nurses in gerontologic

nursing assist in the upgrading of care for older persons but the attitudes of the nurses will be more positive toward aging individuals. Attitudes control behaviors of nurses, and a positive attitude can only improve the current situation where nurses often perceive their role from a "job" orientation rather than from a professional perspective.

The nurse administrator who encourages a climate of professional growth in the practice setting of the long-term care setting or facility will be rewarded with highly motivated nurses who feel pride and satisfaction in caring for older adults. When a climate of participative management is present the nurses will feel an integral part of all decision making regarding the older adults and the facility in general, and will become more responsive and responsible for the needs of the residents and nursing in general. A strong nurse executive will then have the resources needed to implement a health promotion and health maintenance model of nursing that prevents health problems from becoming major difficulties. This approach will be more satisfying to the nursing personnel and will encourage even greater improvement of nursing care. Reward systems in place by the nurse administrator such as recognition ceremonies, vertical promotion demonstrating greater responsibility for clinical care, and other such mechanisms that reward the nurse who tries harder because he or she has more knowledge will only promote better nursing care for the older adults in the long-term care facility.

Primary nursing-care models have slowly been implemented in several long-term care facilities around the country. This model should be encouraged in all long-term care facilities based on sound gerontologic nursing knowledge. Aging persons do not adapt easily to frequent personnel changes. When the primary-care nursing model is instituted the aging person does not have to invest so much physical and emotional energy in adjusting to various systems of care by a great number of nursing personnel. Documentation of information on admission by the professional nurse completing the history and health examination will facilitate knowledge about the individual and promote a greater trust relationship between the older adult and that individual's primary nurse. This approach promotes great satisfaction among the older adults and the nurses. Thus, turnover of staff could be reduced, producing greater stability of staff for the nurse administrator. When such a practice model is implemented, then experimentation of finer points of nursing care can be tried with the focus on always improving the care and bringing greater satisfaction to the nursing staff.

When nursing staff are prepared, the practice of gerontologic nursing becomes a joy rather than a burden to both the nursing personnel and the nurse administrator. Only then can a true system of nursing care be identified with adequate and well-educated nurses who deliver high-quality care. Only then can the nurse administrator demonstrate to all components of the long-term care facility—for example, families, older adults, administrators, and the community-at-large —that the long-term care system is operating at high levels of efficiency and quality. Nursing practice in long-term care facilities has a long way to go to obtain this type of recognition; however, an initial step is being taken by legislative bodies in Congress who perceive the necessity of nursing care of older adults in the country. We in nursing must do our part by upholding our tradition that professional nursing care does make a difference where knowledgeable and intelligent care is ministered by nurses with a scientific knowledge-base on which their nursing care and clinical judgments rest. The standards of nursing practice need to be implemented so that there is clear evidence that nursing is the

responsibility of persons in the facility who are educated in nursing.

Mechanisms, then, in the area of nursing practice include: utilizing a philosophic statement of nursing care as guideline for improved nursing care in long-term care facilities; implementation of a professional nursing model to replace the traditional medical model; experimentation with the primary nurse model to facilitate continuity of care for elderly residents; institution of incentives to motivate nursing personnel and reward them for excellent nursing care; utilization of nursing standards as an evaluative tool for measuring quality of nursing care; and promoting a climate for growth professionally through participative management and decision making in a collaboration between nursing personnel and nurse administrator.

Gerontologic Nursing Research

Finally, the arena in which change will need to be implemented most drastically is gerontologic research. Long-term care for older adults has been sparsely researched because there are so few gerontologic nurses with research skills at the master's and doctoral levels. Yet the vast number of researchable questions make this setting a rich environment for research. It is through research that improvement of care can be demonstrated for older adults in various stages of illness and changes in the aging process in the four dimensions of the physiologic, psychologic, sociologic, and spiritual components of the individuals. Numerous areas of research need to be explored that will be valuable to nurses prepared in gerontologic nursing. Such areas of research include the "impact of nursing interventions as they relate to cost containment, health promotion, and disease prevention in long-term care."[37] In addition, studies that could assist in long-term care staffing requirements, employee motivation, leadership, participative-management styles, patient classification, nursing diagnoses with defining characteristics and etiologies particular to older adults in long-term care facilities, life satisfaction of older residents, and primary-care nursing model implementation are needed for upgrading gerontologic nursing and long-term care facilities in the United States.

It is also important that major focus be on the dissemination of research findings through presentations at local, regional, and national meetings and in publications of various journals with the reading audience of gerontologic nurses. Nurse administrators of long-term care facilities should be active participants in research studies that give visibility to excellent nursing care and its improvement in the facility. A nurse executive who demonstrates a strong commitment to improvement of nursing care and to the nursing staff through encouragement of their preparation in gerontologic nursing and continued educational opportunities will be the recipient of loyalty and dedication on the part of the nursing staff in the Department of Nursing. A major commitment, then, is the creating of opportunities for research to promote the well-being of the older adults and their care, and of the nursing staff, family, and friends of the long-term care facility. Research is the key to the upgrading of long-term care and its administration.

In summary, this discussion has focused on the emergent and critical need for prepared gerontologic nurses to staff the long-term care facilities in the nation. Because this major resource is insufficient to meet the demands of the increasing aging population in long-term care facilities, the nursing administration of these facilities is greatly hampered and is in need of great attention by the nursing world. Only through educated gerontologic nursing personnel-staff who are the major resources for the nurse administra-

tor can the long-term care facility enjoy the opportunity for implementing a philosophy of care built on a professional nursing model, with the resultant rejection of the current custodial-care–medical model. Nursing theories that form the framework for professional nursing are slowly being introduced into the clinical settings of long-term care but much more needs to be accomplished in this area to undergird the nursing care of older adults.

Finally, the improvement of long-term care administration will come through the triple arenas of education, practice, and research where critical issues facing administration can be tested and implemented in appropriate settings. Much greater attention needs to be given to the critical issue of insufficient numbers of nurses employed in long-term care settings with adequate preparation of gerontologic nursing knowledge and standards of care. The nursing professionals and the nursing profession cannot allow this area of responsibility to be addressed in a haphazard approach any longer. Older persons deserve our full attention to their health-care needs. They are the individuals who put their energies to work for us in the past and have passed on to us vital information regarding life. Are we to abandon them now by not providing nurse professionals who have expertise about the aging and their unique health-care needs? The American Nurses' Association Code of Ethics and Interpretative Statements will not allow the profession to avoid addressing this issue. Professionally, the elderly have the right to receive excellent nursing care when they approach a facility such as the long-term care setting, and the profession will not avoid its responsibility to them in the future. Education, practice, and research in gerontologic nursing are the key factors in promoting full acceptance of that responsibility by the nursing profession. Gerontologic nursing is a respected nursing specialty both in terms of clinical practice and nursing administration approaches. Together these two components will make a difference in the long-term care setting in the future.

REFERENCES

1. Robb S, Malinzak M. Knowledge levels of personnel in gerontological nursing. J Geron Nsg 1981;7(3):153–158.
2. Huckstadt A. Do nurses know enough about gerontology? J Geron Nsg 1983;9(7):392–397.
3. Eliopoulos C. Nursing administration of long-term care. Rockville, MD: Aspen Publications, 1983.
4. Bahr RT, Spencer M. Opportunities for geriatric education in nursing education. Geriatric education-new knowledge, new settings, new curricula. Conference report. Bethesda, MD: Bureau of Health Professions, Health Resources and Service Administration, U.S. Dept of Health and Human Services, 2–4 June 1986.
5. Bahr RT. Ethicolegal issues in gerontological nursing curriculum. J Geron Nsg 1987;13(3):7–10.
6. Hatch TD, Williams TF. Personnel for health needs of the elderly through year 2020. Washington, DC: National Institute on Aging Administrative Document, September, 1987.
7. American Nurses' Association. Facts about nursing—1985. Kansas City: ANA, 1986.
8. Nodhturft VL, Banks DO, MacMullen JS. Training the geriatric nurse. J Geron Nsg 1986;12(5):24–29.
9. Schneider E, Wendlend C, Zinner AW, List N, Ory M. The teaching nursing home. New York: Raven Press, 1985.
10. Special Committee on Aging, United States Senate. Nursing home care: the unfinished agenda. Washington, DC, May 21, 1986.
11. Improving the quality of care in nursing homes. Washington, DC: Institute of Medicine, National Academy Press, 1986.
12. Special Committee on Aging. Senator Heinz personal communication. July 17, 1987.
13. Tollett S, Adamson C. The need for gerontologic content within nursing curriculum. J Geron Nsg 1982;8(10):576–580.
14. Hogstel M. Management of personnel in long-term care. Bowie, MD: Robert J. Brady Co, 1983.
15. Gray P. Gerontological nurse specialist, luxury or necessity? AJN 1982;31(1):82–85.
16. Feldstein P. Healthcare economics. New York: John Wiley & Sons, 1983.
17. Brower T. The nursing curriculum for long-term institutional care. Creating a career choice for nurses: long-term care. New York: National League for Nursing, 1983.
18. Davis B. The gerontological specialty. J Geron Nsg 1983;9(10):527–532.
19. American Nurses Association. Position statement on nursing personnel for long-term care. Oasis 1986;3(2):2.
20. Mitty E. Institutional long-term care: nursing roles and responsibilities. Community-based initiatives in long term care. New York: National League of Nursing, 1986.
21. Bahr RT. Professional and public initiatives: addressing health and related needs of elderly persons. New York: National League for Nursing, 1986.
22. Nursing and nursing education: public policies and private actions. Washington, DC: Institute of Medicine, National Academy Press, 1983.
23. Rankin B, Burggraf V. Aging in the 80s. J Geron Nsg 1983;9(5):272–308.
24. Rowland HS, Rowland BL. Nursing administration handbook. Germantown, MD: Aspen Systems Corporation, 1980.
25. American Nurses Association. Scope and standards of gerontological nursing practice. Kansas City, MO: Council of Gerontological Nursing Practice, 1988.
26. Kent VC, Canton DS. An interview: Senator Daniel K. Inouye: a champion for nursing in Congress. Nur Prac 1986;11(4):66.
27. Porter-O'Grady T. Creative nursing administration: participative management into the twenty-first century. Rockville, MD: Aspen Systems Corporation, 1986.
28. Hersey P, Blanchard K. Management of organizational behavior utilizing human resources. Englewood Cliffs, NJ: Prentice-Hall, Inc, 1982.
29. American Association of Retired Persons. Long-term care statement. Washington, DC: Long-Term Care Task Force, 1986.
30. American Association of Retired Persons. A profile of older Americans, 1986. Washington, DC: Administration on Aging, Dept. of Health and Human Services, 1987.
31. Grimaldi P, Sullivan T. Broadening federal coverage of non-institutionalized long-term care. Washington, DC: American Health Care Association, 1981.
32. Callahan J, Wallack P. Reforming the long-term care system. Lexington, MA: Lexington Books, 1979.
33. Yura H, Walsh M. Nursing process: Assessing planning, implementing, evaluating. 5th ed. Norwalk, CT: Appleton-Lange, 1987.
34. Orem D. Nursing: concepts of practice. 2nd ed. Norwalk, CT: Appleton-Century-Crofts, 1981.
35. Roy SC. Adaptation: a model for nursing. Philadelphia: WB Saunders, 1979.
36. Anderson L. National forum on health personnel needs for care of the aged. Unpublished paper. Washington, DC: American Association of Colleges of Nursing. 23 October 1986.
37. Gunter LM, Estes CA. Education for gerontic nursing. New York: Springer Publishing Co, 1979.

53

Consultation and the Nurse Executive

Lois C. Malkemes
Sandy Wisener

CONSULTATION to health-care organizations has become a significant activity in providing guidance and support to executives primarily in the areas of management, finance, planning, and corporate restructuring. Requests for consultation come from large multihospital systems; small, rural hospitals; for profit, as well as nonprofit institutions; and community, as well as tertiary and teaching centers. Consultation is less readily thought about by nurse executives, yet where it has occurred successfully, consultants have had a major influence on the organization and nursing practice.

The nursing division and ancillary areas have acquired consultation primarily in the development of systems to support staffing. We have recently seen changes in the need for consultation including the integration of financial and clinical consultation to determine the most effective and efficient ways to provide care. Organizations are asking questions about their internal organizational structure regarding how to best align operations. Roles and practices are being questioned as to whether or not traditions and accepted methods are any longer appropriate. Longer-term strategies are not as important as short-term tactics in positioning organizations to compete effectively. Nursing is an integral and essential component in each of these issues and considerations, and the nurse executive should be a participant in the consideration of effective change in the organization.

In today's health-care institutions, the nurse executive is responsible and accountable for the operations of the division of nursing. As the environment changes and institutions respond, nurse executives are faced with the need to change the operational mode of the nursing division. The time frame for accommodating the magnitude of change necessary has shortened significantly with increased pressures and threats to organizational viability. Given the demands on nurse executives and the need to facilitate change quickly and effectively, consultation is a mechanism for assisting the organization and the nurse executive in providing necessary changes and minimal risk. Issues related to the use of consultants by nurse executives, modes of consultation, some focal issues, the role of the consultant, and the benefits of consultation will be addressed.

The role of the consultant as defined by Blake and Mouton (1983) is "to aid a person, a group, an organization, or a larger social system by helping the client identify and break out of . . . damaging kinds of cycles . . ."[1] (p. 6). Consultation involves intervention designed to produce specific change in a deliberate and controlled manner. Change is the goal of consultation, and intervention is the many-faceted tool used to achieve the desired change. Intervention occurs when the consultant does something with a client in the context of a cycle-breaking endeavor.

Blake and Mouton define the consultant as the person who is intervening,[1] (p. 8). The recipient of the intervention is called the client and may be an individual, or a group. The problem to be solved revolves around the interaction of the consultant and client regarding the focal issue.

EXAMPLES OF FOCAL ISSUES

As census declines in hospitals and competition intensifies for populations to serve, health-care institutions are faced with increasing pressures for enhanced revenues and reduced costs. In the past, institutions made the assumption that the means to improve their quality and competitive position was to expend dollars. Those dollars were frequently allocated to improve access, increase technology, and balance equity. The approach to success was "more is better." Indeed, we are now realizing that the relationship between more costs and improved quality is not necessarily linear. Instead, we are learning that higher costs may mean inappropriate care, ineffective use of resources, and inefficient protocols and treatment. The focus is on quality and competition, while managing diminishing resources versus succeeding through spending.

As the viability of health-care institutions is more dependent on the performance of professionals who practice, nursing is experiencing a decline in the quantity and quality of readily available providers of care. The interface of this dichotomous phenomenon provides the framework for the dominant issues faced by the nurse executive and the consultant to nurse executives. The issues for nurse executives fall into two categories as they manage the operations of the nursing division, technical issues, and process issues. The consultative issues likewise fall into two categories, technical and process issues. The two

categories of need and consultation are not mutually exclusive, but it is necessary to understand and differentiate the categories to address them successfully. The approach to addressing the two categories of need are unique and require different levels of skills, both from the nurse executive and the consultant.

Health-care organizations frequently express their interest in consultative services as one of the following issues: cost reduction or cost management, improved productivity, recruitment and retention of qualified staff, or information to support decisions. The impact of changes in any of these areas will significantly affect nursing and the nurse executive's ability to fulfill responsibilities of the role.

COST REDUCTION

Cost reduction is frequently approached with the assumption that the organization will remain essentially the same structurally and functionally after the implementation of efforts to reduce costs. This approach is derived primarily from an engineering, productivity viewpoint that attempts to reduce the costs by "across-the-board" reductions, and uses fairness and equity as its rationale. Taking an "across-the-board" approach or even a pie-shaped approach to cost reductions does not accommodate the emphasis required for clinical services or the need of specific patient populations. This approach has proven disastrous to the quality of care in many health-care institutions, as is particularly the case when cuts have been made previously and the cushion in patient care divisions is gone. Although it is necessary for organizations to set criteria for the extent of cost reductions necessary to achieve financial viability and to have the resources available to pursue organizational strategies, the approach must include an understanding of the needs of patients, the services required to support clinical programs, and the quality of resources available to achieve the outcomes required.

In considering reductions, the integration of costs and revenues is an essential part of the planning process. Most important, the organizational changes necessary to drive the cost reductions must be put into effect. It is evident from this discussion that both technical and process issues are involved in addressing the reduction of costs in health-care institutions. We believe that process consultation for cost reductions should be provided by individuals who have an understanding of the impact of changes in clinical services and the delivery of patient care. The need for technical assistance flows from process consultation and should be supportive to the process. From our experience in the changing health-care environment, assumptions regarding the level of reductions that can be accommodated in each department need to be analyzed individually and collectively to provide the appropriate resources and synergy to support the clinical programs of the institution. It has also been our experience that the alignment and functionality of the organizational design should be challenged when reductions are made to assure that the reduced organization can operate effectively.

COST MANAGEMENT

The management of costs is addressed once the costs have been reduced to the most efficient level that can be achieved by the organization. Cost management involves the selection, development, and implementation of systems that reflect the philosophy, alignment, and production levels of the new organization. For example, a nursing organization may have previously operated from a framework of team nursing but may have implemented a change to primary nursing. Information regarding the cost of nursing care on a unit-specific basis may now be needed on a nurse-specific basis. The implementation of a clinical career ladder may require other kinds of nurse-specific information to support the evaluation process of individuals.

The need for integrated charting or documentation may no longer support a patient classification system expressed in terms of nursing tasks but require a system expressed in terms of nursing diagnoses that can be used as the basis for planning care and interfacing with quality monitoring information. Quality monitoring may not be adequate as an indicator of unit performance, but may be needed by patient and nurse.

Because of a focus on products versus traditional clinical services, reporting relationships and report formats may need to be changed. As volumes rise in one product line and decline in another, systems should be in place to make corresponding adjustments in staffing and other resource requirements. In product lines an organization can utilize nurses as case managers and will need information to evaluate the effectiveness of each case manager's performance as to cost management and outcomes of care.

Process consultation supports the evaluation and selection of approaches and assists in the design criteria of systems to support cost management. Technical consultation provides methodologies necessary to support the implementation and installation of systems for ongoing monitoring and control.

PRODUCTIVITY IMPROVEMENT

Productivity improvement is often understood as "doing the same things in the same way with fewer resources." Although the idea may seem intriguing as a method of cost management, the expectation may be unrealistic and even detrimental when applied to patient care. Improving productivity in clinical areas often involves the challenge of "doing some of the same things in different ways with fewer resources *and* achieving desired outcomes." Quality, along with cost, can often be the deciding factor in winners and losers in health-care providers.

Comparative information for evaluating productivity can be helpful in identifying ranges and providing bench marks. Standards that are developed to measure and control productivity in an individual hospital should be developed with an understanding of the philosophy and components of care being measured when applied to nursing. For example, a neonatal intensive care standard for nursing care that captures all the direct and indirect care components required by acutely ill infants may seem appropriate. However, if the philosophy of care and care model conceptualizes the care unit as the infant and family, the standard may not be an adequate measure. Consultation in the development of productivity standards for nursing has a process component that requires an understanding of the framework of care delivery for each clinical area. The framework, once defined, is supported technically with methodologies to adequately measure resource utilization.

The development of cost-center specific productivity standards that reflect efficient and effective care delivery are an undergirding of cost-management efforts. Those standards can serve as the basis for determining costs of care on a case-by-case basis. Cost information by case type will be increasingly important as managed care continues to expand and health-care institutions are more involved in prospective bidding for patient groups. Costs-by-case types are also important in evaluating the management and profitability of case types in general and planning for new or expanded services.

RECRUITMENT AND RETENTION

Nursing has experienced cycles of inadequate resources to meet staffing requirements throughout its history. We believe that the inadequate supply of proficient nurses will

extend into future years. Staffing, therefore, needs to be considered from a new perspective. Although creative approaches to recruitment and retention need to be thoroughly analyzed and evaluated, it is important that organizational designs that will minimize health-care organizations' dependency on professional nurses and provide consistent safeguards for desired outcomes be considered. Consultation in consideration of new care models is a very specialized process and must be provided by consultants with an in-depth understanding of nursing, care delivery, organizational design, and change theory. This highly specialized level and focus of consultative services for nursing can be supported with methodologies and technologies for allocating staff in the most efficient and effective manner within the model criteria and role expectations. Patient classification systems provide the basis for determining the number of staff required for patients with varying acuities. Staffing and scheduling systems allocate care givers efficiently to match required resources with available resources. The greatest challenge to nurse executives in the near future will be the development of new models that respond to the demands for cost reduction, cost management, and quality outcomes with limited and unpredictable resources.

INFORMATION TO SUPPORT DECISION MAKING

Nurse executives as a group are not afraid to make decisions. Nurse executives as a group are not unwilling to make unpopular decisions. Nurse executives, like many other executives in health-care organizations, do not have the right information to make necessary decisions in today's environment. If a financial executive makes a bad decision, it can affect the bottom line. If a nurse executive makes a bad decision, it has the potential to affect patient care as well as the bottom line. The types of information that the nurse executive needs along with information about cost and productivity is information about the quality of care being provided on a patient-specific and nurse-specific basis.

The issues that we have discussed up to this point need to be analyzed, evaluated, and need to have new models implemented prior to determining the type and format of information required. For example, the framework implemented for a patient classification system may indicate criteria for outcomes of care that demonstrate quality. It may be possible to link the two systems—patient classification and quality monitoring—to provide a basis for determining how variances in nursing processes affect outcomes. The model of care delivery and role of care givers may determine how information is made available. The need for information to support decision making is indisputable. Nurse executives need information just as do other executives, but the information needed by nurse executives must provide support for decision making regarding care delivery as well. The process of understanding the environment and identifying what types of information are needed to support decisions is critical to having the right information. Methodologies and technologies can then be appropriately applied to provide information on a timely basis to support clinical and organizational decision making.

THE ROLE OF THE CONSULTANT

The consultant as problem solver is the most common conception of the role of the consultant; in actuality, consulting takes on a much broader perspective. Consultants act as an objective third party who can identify ways in which resources can be utilized more effectively and efficiently, opportunities can be maximized, and change can be managed. Consultants, therefore, should bring special knowledge, experience, and skills necessary to assist the client.

Consultants, because of their involvement

with many organizations, bring a fresh perspective in helping clients identify opportunities and ways in which change can take place. Since consultants are not tied to the exigencies or culture of the organization, they can observe, process information, and identify approaches and opportunities without bias. This is the basis for suggesting strategies, tactics, and approaches that are practical, workable, and effective.

How does a nurse executive select a consultant? The most effective consultative process for the nurse executive client is provided by a nurse consultant with both academic- and experience-based preparation for addressing issues of importance to the nurse executive and health-care institution. The interventions are determined through a process that is based on theory and understanding of nursing practice, patient care, and organizations. The implementation of the interventions is based on experience in managing planned change in health-care institutions. Technical support, integrated appropriately into the consultative process, can be provided by a variety of disciplines to support the desired outcome.

The challenges of effectively managing a dynamic nursing practice in an evolving health-care system require resources and skills that stretch the brightest and the best among nurse executives. Accessing and utilizing the assistance of appropriate support will be essential to success in this complex environment. Process and technical consultation is necessary and must be provided by consultants who have a first-hand knowledge of nursing practice and patient care and are able to interface with the methodologies and technologies necessary to provide information on a timely basis to support clinical and organizational change.

REFERENCE

Blake RR, Mouton, JS. Consultation. Reading, MA: Addison-Wesley Publishing Co, 1983.

54

Executive Succession

Barbara Fuszard
Linda Tilby

SELECTION of the top nurse executive in a health-care organization is generally considered to be one of the most important "man-power" decisions made. Existing research offers general information regarding executive succession, but has been extremely limited in the area of succession of nurse executives. It seems incongruent that while health-care literature has thoroughly documented the need for qualified nurse executives,[1-4] information that would assist in determining the characteristics of the person likely to be successful in the position is not available. The incongruency is increased when one recognizes that the primary goal to be accomplished when an organization selects a nurse executive is the selection of someone who will be effective in that specific organization.

Health-care organizations are complex, dynamic systems requiring sophistication on the part of those who manage them. The role of the director of nursing has changed over the years in response to the changing needs of the health-care market. Educational demands, technology, consumer activism, and government regulations all have prompted directors of nursing to re-examine and redefine their role continually.[5] According to del Bueno, "It is unrealistic . . . to think that managerial success in these organizations can be predicted or predicated by any single factor or theory. One perspective, however, that seems to be both practical and relevant, is a symbolic, or cultural view that emphasizes the importance of shared values and norms rather than the structural or rational variables stressed in traditional theories."[6]

Organizations of the health-care system traditionally have been bureaucracies noted for a slowness to change and oftentimes, immobility and obsolescence.[7] Health-care institutions that survive in the future will be those that are fiscally viable and operated as efficiently as any multimillion dollar business, yet without compromising patient care. The efficiency and effectiveness of the management team will determine the continued success of the organization.[8] The traditional bureaucratic organization of the health-care system will change and become a mobile organization "characterized by coordination, communication, integration, flexibility, complexity, dynamics interrelated with professional values, and autonomy."[9]

MODEL FOR STUDYING MANAGERIAL SUCCESS

Managerial success and subsequent organizational success depend on the characteristics of the individual circumstances, practical realities, and an understanding of the organization's culture. "Culture is the combination of the symbols, language, assumptions, and behaviors that overtly manifest an organization's norms and values. It is the taken-for-granted and shared meanings people assign to their social surroundings that can have a profound effect on an organization's decision making and performance."[10] Values are the basic element of an organization's culture—

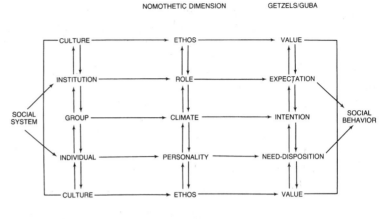

Figure 54.1 General Model of the Major Dimensions of Behavior in a Social System. From Getzels JW, Lipham JM, Campbell RF. Educational administration as a social process: theory, research, practice. New York: Harper & Row, 1968, p. 105. Used with permission.

"the way we do things here"—and are a predictor of organizational behavior.[11] Changes such as those that have been described in health-care and business literature may threaten the basic values of the organization. Executives in general, and nurse executives in particular, who understand organizational culture concepts will be crucial in accomplishing the necessary change.

Fiedler's Theory of Leadership Effectiveness has been studied by researchers for over 30 years. This theory, contingency theory, states that leadership qualities needed by an executive depend on the situation and the organization, and therefore do not form a constant constellation.[12] Fiedler's theory fits the premise of this chapter that successful behaviors of the executive are dependent on negotiation between personality and position, and individual versus organizational needs, all within the cultures of the individual and the organization.

A conflict of culture, values, and needs between institutions and employees is illustrated in the Getzels-Guba model (see Figure 54.1). This model identifies the interrelation of goal achievement for the institution and the goals of the individuals employed by that institution. The goals of the institution are met mainly through the actions of the em-

ployees; however, administration's responsibility is to direct the actions of the employees so that the goals of the institution will be achieved. At the same time administration needs to permit and assist individuals to attain their personal goals.

Characteristics of the model can be applied to the administrator as well as other personnel of the institution in relation to goal attainment. The institution establishes roles and expectations (based on institutional values) for the executive that are intended to fulfill the goals of the system. Simultaneously the executives, as individuals in the system, bring their own culture, personality, values, and need goals with them to the position. Institution, role, and expectations constitute the nomothetic, or normative dimension of the social system of the institution; and individual, personality, and needs constitute the idiographic, or personal dimension of activity. The successful "fit" between institutional and executive needs will determine the behavioral outcomes of the executive in his or her role.

A difficulty in identifying the proper executive for an institution is compounded by the changing nature of an institution. Institutions pass through developmental phases that necessitate different emphases being placed on the particular tasks of the organization. Perrow, in a widely quoted case study, demonstrated that a health-care institution requires varying leadership approaches over time.[13] The various dimensions of executive succession, then, need to be identified and quantified as to their relative importance to an institution over varying cycles of growth and development.

Existing research offers some indications of the dimensions of executive succession. All of the following are important variables: tenure (mobility), leadership style, origin of successor, cosmopolitan versus local, organizational-individual need fit, executive development programs, academic preparation, gender, and age. Also available in the literature are various instruments for assessing executive potential. This review will cover the dimensions of tenure, origin of successor, leadership style, and organizational-individual need fit.

The reader is advised to accept the following research findings with caution. Succession research is in its infancy. Few studies have been replicated; terminology is not always consistent or discriminatory. Especially noteworthy is the difference between subjects in the nonnursing studies and the nursing studies.

The organizational "subject" analyzed in the literature on succession typically is a white male; married; with children; in a business, manufacturing, or engineering organization. This literature review speaks to such subjects except when addressing nursing literature. A 1985 survey conducted by the American Organization of Nurse Executives (AONE), formerly the American Society for Nursing Service Administrators, indicated that the nurse executive typically is a married female between the ages of 40 and 49, and has a master's degree with a nursing major.[14]

TENURE

Tenure in a management position includes the number of years spent in one position in the same organization. Tenure ends when the incumbent takes another position in that organization, or transfers to another organization.

Kirschenbaum and Goldberg identify from the literature four broad categories encountered by professionals that may influence their propensity to move. The first category encompasses job satisfaction factors, such as autonomy and participation in decision making. A second category relates to a cosmopolitan versus local orientation, with the cosmopolitan more likely to move than the local. A third is that of incongruent values. Incongruent occupational values are defined chiefly as requirements of the institution that are at variance with personal values, especially regarding a "people versus things" orientation. The last category identified from the literature is that of career cycle stages.[15]

Veiga has identified a matrix of career cycles or situations that he found in the job histories of 1300 managers. A main finding of his study revealed a significant relationship between age and the situational factors of organizational, family, and individual needs (see Figure 54.2).[16]

As can be seen in Figure 54.2, the typical manager spends an extended learning time in one or two positions, usually managing a technical function. At about age 38 this manager has a series of job changes intraorganizationally that expose him or her to various aspects of the organization. About age 45 to 47 this manager is ready for the executive suite. The manager's family is also relatively stable, with children raised, so that the employee is free to move interorganizationally. This is the age also at which the manager is able to assess personal strengths and weaknesses. He or she not only can contemplate a new organization, but may even choose to enter a new career. The matrix illustrates that persons who fail to make the transitions mentioned above remain with their organization, enjoying job security, until "gold watch" time.

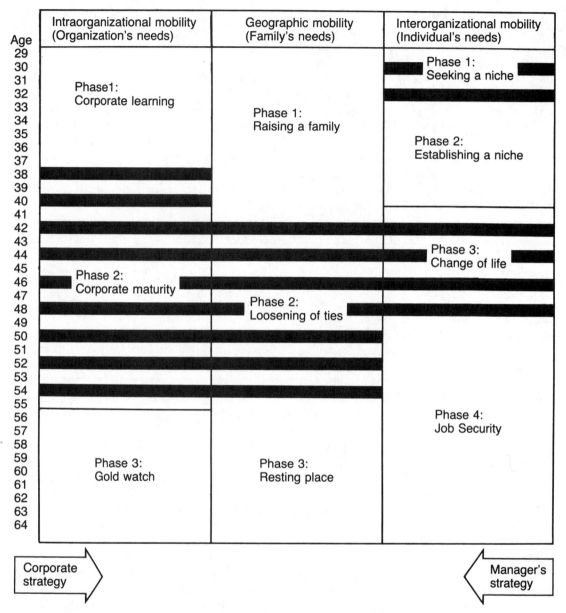

Figure 54.2 The Career-Mobility Phase Matrix. From Veiga JF. The mobile manager at mid- career. Harvard Business Review 1973;51(1):117. Used with permission.

In a later reported study, Veiga identified newer influences on the matrix categories, particularly that of family changes. He found that up to age 50, managers face close to a 50-50 chance that every change of jobs will require relocation.[17] This impediment to mobility becomes more significant as the number of dual-career families increases. The changes in the family career roles of corporate men and women may alter their mobility characteristics in the future to patterns more similar to those of nurse executives, who have consistently faced the problem of dual-career alliances.

The answer to the question of length of tenure of the nurse administrator varies according to whom the question is addressed. In many instances nurses, administrators, and physicians will cite examples of rapid succession of nurse administrators, while a different group will give illustrations of nurse administrators who have been in their positions for many years.[18] Data to support either group's perceptions are limited. A study conducted by Freund in the early 1980s failed to confirm or deny either position on tenure. His sample was divided equally between nurse administrators with five or more years and less than five years tenure in their positions.[19] Generally in management sectors, appropriate tenure for executive positions has been considered to be five to seven years. There have not been any supporting data for this impression, and with the recent emphasis on the Japanese style of management, which stresses the value of lifelong employment with the same organization, this impression is becoming somewhat altered.

Reasons for nurse executive turnover may give more insight into the managerial succession process than actual tenure. Although studies in this area are also limited, currently available information suggests that the greatest percentage of turnover is due to termination and requested resignation—both involuntary turnovers. Frequent reasons given for termination and requested resignations are changes in administrative staff, that is, the chief executive officer (CEO), lack of support from administrative staff, limited educational credentials, assumption of the position without a true understanding of its implications, and inability to change with the changing needs of the organization.[20–23]

ORIGIN OF SUCCESSOR

The successor can be identified as either promoted from within or recruited from outside the organization. It appears that the ratio of chief executive officers recruited from outside to those promoted from within is increasing in the last decades. A study of 9000 CEOs in manufacturing organizations in the early 1950s showed only 17% were "outsiders."[24] By the 1980s that percent was found to be 38.[25]

Brady and Helmich hypothesize some reasons for the increase in selection of outsiders for executive positions. They see the increase in complexity of business organizations, high technology, and a rapidly changing environment calling for persons with visions larger than the single organization. They suggest that by the time a CEO has internalized the values of an organization and learned its traditional strategies, that person is a liability. "Tough-minded leaders" are words that repeatedly appear in the literature, as are terms such as executives willing to cut, remove, condense, and take risks. Organizational leaders are required to be quickly observant of needed changes, and adaptive to changing situations.[26]

Katz and Kahn hypothesize the differences between insider and outsider promotion in the following words:

The advantages of staying within the system are greater motivation and morale among the members in the long run, greater stability of direction and operation, greater familiarity with the candidates, lower cost than in the comprehensive outside search. The increased morale resulting from promotion from within is accentuated if the vacancy is at a high level in a large organization, so that the promotion creates a string of vacancies down the line. The advantages of outside recruiting are the influx of new ideas and practices, greater range of experience and ability among candidates, the breakdown of institutional discrimination against minority groups and the possibility of less conflict, politics, rivalry, and resentment among people on the inside. These factors take on different weightings for various organizations confronting different situations. Stability may be more important for one organization at a certain point in its history, and new direction more important for another organization. It is not always true that going outside opens up a wider range of capable candidates, and the intraorganizational variance among candidates needs to be compared with interorganizational variance.[27]

The relation between insider and outsider promotion has been studied in relation to organizational effectiveness. Helmich and Brown found significant differences in organizational change between organizations headed by outsiders and insiders. Insiders headed 23% of organizations that were graded above average in change, whereas outsiders headed 41% of such organizations.[28] Helmich's later study titled organizations headed by outsiders as "adaptive," and those with insider executives as "nonadaptive," with the findings that only 21% nonadaptive organizations indicated subsidiary growth compared to 27% of the adaptive organizations.[29] Pfeffer and Salancik also found a correlation between growth in industry sales and outsider executives.[30] Brady and Helmich caution about interpreting results of published studies regarding organizational effectiveness and origin of executives. They suggest further study is needed on changes and achievements over time, rather than in the early period of succession.[31]

Outsiders are seen as needed by organizations reaching maturity. A time of plateauing, or even a downturning of sales, can come to the mature organization that does not continue to tap its environment and seek growth or change.[32]

Size of organization and inside versus outside succession have shown significant relationships in several studies.[33-35] Larger organizations appear to have more inside promotions than smaller ones. Larger organizations, of course, have a larger well of candidates from which to draw, and ostensibly more finances for executive development. Pfeffer and Salancik in their study of 100 hospitals found, for example, that inside succession was more common the greater the number of beds in a hospital and the larger the annual operating budget. These researchers hypothesized that the larger hospitals had more administrative positions from which to draw top executives. They also surmised that the complexity of a large hospital, with its rules and procedures to be learned, would make acquaintance with the institution an especially important criterion for the position.[36] Size of organization appeared to be the one criterion for promoting an insider to the top executive position, although recruitment firms have advocated looking in one's own organization for leadership potential.[37-38]

A final consideration in the insider-outsider executive question is the length of tenure. Early writings and theories described the insider as one loyal to the organization, bound to it through tradition and dedication. The outsider was seen as a change agent who came to meet changing goals of an organization, and then moved on to another challenge. Some researchers have indeed found such patterns.[39-40] Brady and Helmich caution against the generalizations that such data have generated. They quote research that indicates less simplistic relationships.[41] Some of the possible influencing variables they identify are age of the organization, ability of the executive to meet the needs of the organization, achievement goals of the executive, cosmopolitan versus local orientation, pressure from boards of trustees, and environmental changes.

At this point, there are no data that consistently support either promotion from within or recruiting from outside as the right answer to a hospital's nursing management needs. According to McConnell, several criteria that may be considered when comparing promotion from within versus outside recruitment are:

1.   recruitment costs
2.   significance of change
3.   capability
4.   credibility
5.   interpersonal relationships
6.   length of time required to become fully effective
7.   trouble in the department

A comparison using these criteria may help give an organization a sense of direction and a beginning basis for making the crucial decision of "within or outside."[42]

LEADERSHIP STYLE-PERSONALITY

Leadership style refers to task-oriented versus people-oriented leadership. Leadership behavior is a composite of specific perceived actions performed by the leader. Both aspects of leadership will be addressed here.

McKenney and Keen found that executives have different cognitive styles. Some are seen as systematic thinkers, others as intuitive; some are seen as receptive, and others as perceptive. The authors believed these styles to be inherent, fairly fixed at time of maturity, and probably all workable, depending on the situation.[43]

Heisler asked 100 chief executives what characteristics were most important for "promotability" of a manager to top positions. The chief executives named both task and interpersonal criteria as highly important leadership styles. They also agreed on the importance of behaviors such as finding new ways to handle problems, meeting deadlines, needing a minimum of direction, winning the respect of subordinates and colleagues, and understanding of others.[44]

The trait theory of leadership has been tested by various researchers without conclusive findings. Data do suggest that frequent turnover in the executive position tends to result in authoritative, task-oriented leadership in a successor's initial period.[45]

Heisler compared responses of top corporate executives and Master of Business Administration (M.B.A.) students as to trait importance. Executives felt task orientation and interpersonal skills were equally important, whereas M.B.A. students rated the interpersonal abilities higher than task orientation.[46]

Harvard Business Review over 20 years ago surveyed almost 2000 businessmen from all levels of management to get opinions as to what type of person is successful in getting promoted. The description that evolved for the top executive position was one of almost a superhuman individual. The top executive would be expected to absorb masses of data and then set long-range goals that would profit the company and also meet the needs of society. He or she was expected to be dynamic, a self-starter, and a motivator. Qualities rated necessary by over 90% of the businessmen were: ability to communicate, ambition (drive), college education, making sound decisions, self-confidence, good appearance, getting things done with and through people, capacity for hard work, and conscientiousness.[47]

A more recent study of "promotability" surveyed 11,000 executives at the time they were promoted to top positions in their organization. Findings revealed the new entrants were better educated than their predecessors, but about the same age at the time of promotion as them. Those reaching the top position were usually group vice-presidents in the same company, having spent four years or less at the vice-president level. A final consistent finding was the high mobility of the new generation of top executives, compared to their forebears.[48]

In the nursing literature, Price's study indicated that the nurse executive must have knowledge and skill in the areas of:

administration and management
financial management and budgeting
organizational theory
labor relations and human relations
economic and political aspects of
    management
research
a generalist approach to clinical subject
    matter[49]

Price's study concluded that "graduate programs in nursing need to prepare administrators who are creative and can function at the executive level in a collegial relationship with other health administrators. Such administrators will promote organizational restructuring for the delivery of nursing services, define nursing's role and responsibility in interdisciplinary endeavors, and critique and utilize research findings."[50] When the educational backgrounds of nurse administrators were reviewed, surveys published by the American Nurses' Association (ANA) and the American Society of Nursing Service Administrators (ASNSA) found that from 1977 to 1978 almost half of the nurse executives (50% and 48%, respectively) were either diploma or associate degree graduates. Approximately 25% of the nurse executives held a baccalaureate degree and 25% held a master's degree or higher. Increasing changes occurring in, and the importance placed on the nurse executive's position are reflected in a 1985 survey completed by AONE. This source showed that 3% of nurse executives held a diploma or associate degrees, 28% held baccalaureate degrees, 60% held master's degrees, 3% held doctoral degrees, and 6% held graduate degrees in another field. These percentages represent a tremendous

change between 1977 and 1985 and lend additional support to the recognition, at least by nursing, of the importance of additional educational preparation for nurse executives.[51–53]

In an effort to determine what makes an effective nurse executive, Freund, as part of a larger study, administered questionnaires to directors of nursing (DONs) and CEOs that elicited characteristics associated with DON effectiveness. Both DONs and CEOs credited DON effectiveness to knowledge of general management, health, and nursing (81% of CEOs as well as 81% of DONs).[54] This category included finance, accounting, computer literacy, as well as content in the health-care field and nursing. The second highest credit, both from DONs and CEOs was human management.[55] The human management skill referred to the importance of the people-oriented aspect of the role. A third characteristic cited by both groups was possession of a total organizational view; that is, the DON kept the well-being of the entire organization in mind when making decisions. Other characteristics were: CEO support, medical staff relations, flexibility, political "savvy," and being a positive role-model. This particular study pointed out that neither DONs nor CEOs perceived knowledge of advanced clinical practice as important to effectiveness. As seen above, they valued general knowledge of the practice of nursing, the nursing profession, and the health-care field.[56]

Using a random sample of 150 hospitals in California, Friss studied organizational commitment, job involvement, and background characteristics of nurse administrators to provide data for developing a career perspective for this group.[57] Predictors utilized were hospital size, location, ownership, sociodemographics, personal values-motives, and work experience. Sociodemographic predictors were education and salary; work experiences included tenure and balance between personal and material rewards for effort expended; motives-values included service career anchor, management career anchor, and professional commitment; and a moderating variable included ease of leaving. Findings showed that the higher the professional commitment, the higher the organizational commitment. Tenure and salary also showed a positive correlation with organizational commitment.

Friss found a positive, statistically significant relationship between positive job involvement and the variables of management career anchor and professional commitment.[58] The variables of hospital location, hospital ownership, hospital size, or size of community in which the director was raised did not show significant relationships with organizational commitment or job involvement.[59]

For purposes of analysis, the leadership style-personality characteristics have been reviewed in isolation from the organizational component of the Getzels-Guba model. The final section of this chapter reunites the leader and the organization in a study of organizational-individual "fit."

ORGANIZATIONAL-INDIVIDUAL NEED FIT

This section deals with selection of an executive based on a "fit" between the organization's culture and goals and the individual's personal needs and goals. Sellery states that the first action of a search plan should be

to define carefully the future direction and character of the organization. This requires a review of current and anticipated status with regard to the organization's structure, positioning within its competitive peer group, finances, and anticipated additional personnel needs. In short, the desired direction and character of the organization and what must be done to achieve these two goals must be determined. Logically, the next questions to be answered are: Who can set the organization on its desired course? What kind of experience, education, and personal qualities should he or she have?[60]

As reported earlier, Helmich found executives hired from the outside more able than insiders to adapt to the environment of the organization. The inside-promoted executive showed a lack of concern for the organization's desire to "co-opt" its environment.[61]

Pfeffer and Salancik found that succession to and tenure in leadership positions were related to the executive's ability to cope with organizational contingencies and uncertainties.[62] Salancik and colleagues also hypothesized that tenure of the executive was related to organizational difficulties and the ability of the executive to cope with these difficulties.[63] Pfeffer and Salancik offer numerous anecdotes as evidence that organizational context determines the selection of executives appropriate for coping with that context. For example, at one time production was the greatest problem in organizations, and executives were drawn from inside production managers. When production became routinized and mechanized, executives became concerned with sales, and marketing executives were selected for top management. In the 1960s, financial concerns became the critical organizational contingency, and financial executives were sought. In the 1980s, corporations face legal and regulatory problems and consequently value attorneys who can deal with this present contingency.[64]

Levitt suggests that the prospective successor be carefully studied not only for beliefs about management activities, but more importantly, for style, attitude, personality, and philosophy, and to ascertain whether a particular applicant will fit with the company situation and the people who work in the company.[65]

Writers agree that executive succession causes organizational disruption, at least temporarily. However, Carroll and Reinganum demonstrated that the effect of succession is related to the organizational context of the firm.[66–67] Brady and Helmich include research that indicates those organizational contingencies that have demonstrated importance at time of succession: "stage of organizational maturity, state of employed technology, the predecessor's style, past loyalties, the nature of required changes, professionalism of staff, and personality of the successor."[68]

Organizational needs, as listed above, must be "fit" to the individual prospective executive's own need constellation. A statistically significant problem of "fit" has been identified as the task versus people orientation among professionals. If the organization requires one orientation and the executive has need for the other, turnover will occur.[69]

Helmich found that executives in mature, large organizations demonstrate a need for self-actualization, as measured by opportunity for personal growth and development. He found that the lack of need fulfillment leads the new successor to a task form of leadership. Inability to meet one's needs quickly tends to lead the successor to further mobility behavior.[70]

Outside successors have repeatedly been shown to be more success oriented than inside successors.[71] High achievers have also been found to have strong drives toward self-actualization.[72] Task-oriented executives will fit better into small, immature firms, whereas those executives who function best interpersonally will find a better fit with large and mature companies.[73]

Helmich and Erzen report different needs of men and women corporate successors. The male respondents' leadership style was seen as a function of prestige and personal growth needs. The female respondents' leadership style appeared as a function of the opportunity to develop close friendships. Using Maslow's terminology, they stated that behavior of men seems more closely related to esteem and self-actualization needs, whereas women appear to be reaching chiefly for satisfaction of social needs.[74]

Compensation and fringe benefits are also covered in the literature, although not in the form of studies. Compensation for the exec-

utive often includes shares of stock in one's own company, and a parachute clause to provide extra remuneration in case of severance. Fringe benefits may include such perks as private dining rooms, first-class air travel, and free financial counseling.

Gerstein and Reisman offer an extensive analysis of personal characteristics of the leader needed as the organization is experiencing different contingencies. They list seven organizational situations, the needed major job thrusts, and specific characteristics of ideal candidates related to the situations (Tables 54.1 and 54.2).[75]

Gordon and Rosen, in analyzing the literature on succession, agree with so-called contingency theory, that regardless of personality and leadership style, the new executive will be at least partially influenced by how his or her superiors, colleagues, and subordinates expect him or her to function; and expectations of those groups are at least partially influenced by the behavior of the new executive's predecessor.[76]

In summary, replacing the nurse executive is seen as an extremely important event for an organization, yet little has been studied regarding the succession of the nurse executive. Perhaps no one organizational contingency or personal characteristic makes the difference between the successful and the unsuccessful successor. Yet it appears that a match between the organization's and the individual's values, and consequent needs, offer an opportunity for a "fit" between organization and executive.

Health-care organizations are highly complex and rapidly changing. Therefore, one could anticipate an individually tailored decision, rather than a pat prescription, would be needed for every succession event. Managers, too, have been shown to change over time in their own career and personal needs.

Tenure of an executive is influenced by job satisfaction, cosmopolitan versus local orientation, conflict between organizational and

Table 54.1   Characteristics of Various Strategic Situations

I. Start-up	—High Financial Risk; —Limited Management Team Cohesiveness; —No Organization, Systems, or Procedures in Place; —No Operational Experience Base; —Endless Workload: Multiple Priorities; —Generally Insufficient Resources to Satisfy All Demands; —Limited Relationship with Suppliers, Customers, & Environment.
II. Turnaround	—Time Pressure for "Results": Need for Rapid Situational Assessment and Decision Making; —Poor Results, but Business Is Worth Saving; —Weak Competitive Position; —Eroded Morale; Low Esteem & Cohesion; —Inadequate Systems: Possible Weak or Bureaucratic Organizational Infrastructure; —Strained and Eroded Relationships with Suppliers, Customers & Environment; —Lack of Appropriate Leadership: Period of Neglect; —Limited Resources: Skills Shortages; Some Incompetent Personnel.
III. Extract Profit-Rationalize Existing Business	—"Controlled" Financial Risk; —Unattractive Industry in Long Term: Possible Need to Invest Selectively, but Major New Investments Not likely to Be Worthwhile; —Internal Organizational Stability; —Moderate-to-High Managerial/Technical Competence; —Adequate Systems and Administrative Infrastructure; —Acceptable to Excellent Relationships with Suppliers, Customers, & Environment.
IV. Dynamic Growth in Existing Business	—Moderate-to-High Financial Risk; —New Markets, Products, Technology; —Multiple Demands and Conflicting Priorities; —Rapidly Expanding Organization in Certain Sectors; —Inadequate Managerial/Technical/Financial Resources to Meet All Demands; —Unequal Growth across Sectors of Organization; —Likely Shifting Power Bases as Growth Occurs; —Constant Dilemma between Doing Current Work & Building Support Systems for the Future.
V. Redeployment of Efforts in Existing Business	—Low-Moderate, Short-Term Risk/High Long-Term Risk; —Resistance to Change: Likely Bureaucracy in Some Sections; —High Mismatch between Some Organization Skill Sets, Technology, People vs. Needs Created by Redefining Strategy; —Likelihood of Lack of Strategic Planning for Some Historical Period—Highly Operational Orientation to Executive Team.
VI. Liquidation/Divestiture of Poorly Performing Business	—Weak Competitive Position, Unattractive Industry, or Both; —Likely Continuance of Poor Returns; —Possible Morale Problems and Skills Shortages; —Little Opportunity for Turnaround or Redeployment Due to Unsatisfactory "Payback"; —Need to Cut Losses and Make Tough Decisions.
VII. New Acquisitions	Acquisitions may be classified into one of the above situations. In addition, the following conditions characterize a recent acquisition situation: —Pressure on New Management to "Prove Themselves"; —Existing Management Ambivalent/Defensive about Change; —Fundamental Need to Integrate Acquired Company with Parent at Some Levels.

Reprinted by permission from Gerstein M, Reisman H. Strategic selection: matching executives to business conditions. *Sloan Management Review* 1983;24(2):36.

Table 54.2 General Management Requirements for Various Strategic Situations

Situation	Major Job Thrusts	Specific Characteristics of Ideal Candidates
I. Start-up	—Creating Vision of Business: —Establishing Core Technical & Marketing Expertise; —Building Management Team.	—Vision of Finished Business; —Hands-on Orientation: A "Doer"; —In-depth Knowledge in Critical Technical Areas; —Organizing Ability; —Staffing Skills; —Team-Building Capabilities; —High-Energy Level and Stamina; —Personal Magnetism: Charisma; —Broad Knowledge of All Key Functions.
II. Turnaround	—Rapid, Accurate Problem Diagnosis; —Fixing Short-Term and, Ultimately, Long-Term Problems.	—"Take Charge" Orientation: Strong Leader; —Strong Analytical and Diagnostic Skills, Especially Financial; —Excellent Business Strategist; —High-Energy Level; —Risk Taker; —Handles Pressure Well; —Good Crisis Management Skills; —Good Negotiator.
III. Extract Profit/Rationalize Existing Business	—Efficiency; —Stability; —Succession; —Sensing Signs of Change.	—Technically Knowledgeable: "Knows the Business"; —Sensitive to Changes: "Ear-to-the-Ground"; —Anticipates Problems: "Problem Finder"; —Strong Administrative Skills; —Oriented to "Systems"; —Strong "Relationship Orientation"; —Recognizes Need for Management Succession & Development; —Oriented to Getting Out the Most: Efficiency, Not Growth.
IV. Dynamic Growth in Existing Business	—Increasing Market Share in Key Sectors; —Managing Rapid Change; —Building Long-Term Health toward Clear Vision of the Future.	—Excellent Strategic & Financial Planning Skills; —Clear Vision of the Future; —Ability to Balance Priorities, i.e., Stability vs. Growth; —Organizational & Team-Building Skills; —Good Crisis Management Skills; —Moderate-High Risk Taker; —High-Energy Level; —Excellent Staffing Skills.
V. Redeployment of Efforts in Existing Business	—Establishing Effectiveness in Limited Business Sphere; —Managing Change; —Supporting the "Dispossessed."	—Good Politician/Manager of Change; —Highly Persuasive: High "Interpersonal Influence"; —Moderate Risk Taker; —Highly Supportive, Sensitive to People: Not "Bull in a China Shop"; —Excellent "Systems Thinker": Understands How Complex Systems Work; —Good Organizing & Executive Staffing Skills.
VI. Liquidation/Divestiture of Poorly Performing Business	—Cutting Losses; —Making Tough Decisions; —Making Best Deal.	—"Callousness": Tough-Minded, Determined—Willing to Be the Bad Guy; —Highly Analytical re: Costs/Benefits—Does Not Easily Accept Current Ways of Doing Things; —Risk Taker; —Low-Glory Seeking: Willing to Do Dirty Jobs—Does Not Want Glamour; —Wants to Be Respected, Not Necessarily Liked.
VII. New Acquisitions	—Integration; —Establishing Sources of Information & Control.	—Analytical Ability; —Relationship Building Skills; —Interpersonal Influence; —Good Communication Skills; —Personal Magnetism—Some Basis to Establish "Instant Credibility."

Reprinted by permission from Gerstein M, Reisman H. Strategic selection: matching executives to business conditions. *Sloan Management Review* 1983;24(2):37.

personal values, and career-cycle stages. Tenure among nurse executives chiefly depends on termination and requested resignation, both involuntary turnovers.

Succession to the executive level occurs in one of two ways—promotion from within or recruitment from outside the organization. An increase in "outsiders" has become more prevalent in recent years. Some research indicates greater organizational effectiveness with outside successors, openness of outside executives to change and especially to environmental needs and pressures. No data were found that support a clear benefit of one origin of succession over another.

Leadership style-personality characteristics are described in the literature either through reported surveys or conjectures. Trait, education, experience, and age are addressed without validation of controlled studies in the general literature or in nursing literature.

Studies of organizational-individual need fit appear to offer some direction for executive successor identification. Succession and tenure were found to be positively correlated with the executive's ability to cope with organizational difficulties. History confirms that Perrow's findings of changing needs in hospitals are paralleled in business organizations as well. Organizational-individual fit is shown to determine the level of organizational turmoil at time of succession, effect on individual needs, and subsequent retention or tenure of the executive. A possible difference between men's and women's needs in executive positions has been postulated, but the overriding determination of leadership behavior appears to be moderated by subordinates, superiors, and peers.

In conclusion, selection of the new nurse executive has received little attention in the literature. Nurses seeking executive positions are offered little guidance as to the type of organization best suited to them. Lacking available research findings, the nurse executives are advised to analyze the prospective organization's culture, values, and needs and their own, to seek a "fit" between position openings and their own characteristics. Instruments for personal analysis, unfortunately, are more plentiful than organizational-analysis instruments.

Researchers can identify a fertile field in the study of succession. Psychology and administrative reviews reveal small samples, circumscribed populations, nonreplicated studies, and inconclusive or contradictory findings. Cosmopolitan versus local studies have been confused with inside versus outside successors, and manager data with that of top executives. "Therapeutic turnover" has not been differentiated from harmful turnover, nor voluntary from involuntary turnover.

It would appear that nurse executives are a very different population from business executives, and perhaps the general succession literature has no value whatever for nurse executives. Carroll's study of nurse managers, although not of nurse executives, offers a possible pattern for comparing characteristics of the two groups of women executives. She identified characteristics of women in business from the literature, and then using the same instruments as those used in the businesswomen's studies, tested a small group of nurse managers.[77] With the appearance of more literature on women executives, a similar comparison with nurse executives may soon be possible.

Functioning nurse executives, wishing to be open to change, can no longer trust that the traditional roles and values of their institutions will survive. With the numerous changes occurring, value conflicts are likely to arise in all facets of the patient care environment. Filerman, president of the Association of the University Program in Health Administration, states that "through the increasing pace of organizational change, role redefinition, and conflicting values, it is the caring and compassion that nursing services embody which keeps the focus on the patient. The new common ground where values will advance and retreat is the management process. Nursing practice in the future will be effective in direct relation to the effectiveness of role enactment by the nurse executive."[78]

As nurse executives develop goals and objectives for the future, a careful analysis to determine whether the plans fit the organization's values, or whether a change in values will be necessary, may be crucial. The nurse executive needs to be able to meet multiple goals and consumers' needs, changing values in life-styles and personal expectations. "Success as a manager in any organization is deliberate, not happenstance and is conscious, not only intuitive. The successful nurse administrator will be professionally competent, politically savvy, and organizationally acculturated."[79]

REFERENCES

1. Knollmueller R. What happened to the PHN supervisors? Nurs Outlook 1979;27(10):666–667.
2. Fine RB. The supply and demand of nursing administrators. Nursing and Healthcare 1983;4(1):10–15.
3. Price S. Master's program preparing nursing administrators: what are the essential components. J Nurs Adm 1984;14(1):11–17.
4. Stevens B. Improving nurses' managerial skills. Nurs Outlook 1979;27(12):774–777.
5. Schofield V. Orientation of nurse executives. J Nurs Adm 1986;16(11):13–17.
6. del Bueno D. Organizational culture: how important is it? J Nurs Adm 1986;16(10):15–20.
7. Poulin M. Future directions of nursing administration. J Nurs Adm 1984;14(3):37–41.
8. Browdy J. Career planning for the newly appointed health care supervisor. The Health Care Supervisor 1985;3(4):31–41.
9. Poulin. Future directions of nursing administration.
10. del Bueno. Organizational culture: how important is it?
11. Bowen M. The will to manage. New York: McGraw-Hill, 1966.
12. Fiedler F. A theory of leadership effectiveness. New York: McGraw-Hill, 1967.
13. Perrow C. Goals and power structures: a historical case study. In: Friedson E, ed. The hospital in modern society. New York: The Free Press of Glencoe, 1963, pp. 112–146.
14. American Organization of Nurse Executives. The

15. 1985 survey of American Organization of Nurse Executive members. Chicago, 1985, unpublished.
15. Kirschenbaum AB, Goldberg AI. Organizational behavior, career orientations, and the propensity to move among professionals. Sociology of Work and Occupations 1976;3(3):357–372.
16. Veiga JF. The mobile manager at mid-career. Harv Bus R 1973;51(1):115–119.
17. Veiga JF. Do managers on the move get anywhere? Harv Bus R 1981;59(2):20–28.
18. Freund C. The tenure of directors of nursing. J Nurs Adm 1985;15(2):11–15.
19. Ibid.
20. Freund C, Fagin C. Firings, unhappiness main reasons for job shifts by nurse heads. Modern Healthcare 1984;14(16):94–96.
21. Fine. The supply and demand of nursing administrators.
22. Sredl D. Administrative turnover. Nursing management 1982;13(11):24–30.
23. Freund. The tenure of directors of nursing.
24. Newcomer M. The big business executive. New York: Columbia University Press, 1955.
25. Brady GF, Fulmer RM, Helmich DL. Planning executive succession: the effect of recruitment source and organizational problems on anticipated tenure. Strategic Management Journal 1982;3(3):269–75.
26. Brady GF, Helmich DL. Executive succession: toward excellence in corporate leadership. Englewood Cliffs, NJ: Prentice-Hall, 1984.
27. Katz D, Kahn R. The social psychology of organizations. New York: John Wiley and Sons, 1978.
28. Helmich DL, Brown WB. Successor type and organizational change in the corporate enterprise. Adm Sci Q 1972;7:371–81.
29. Helmich DL. Organizational growth and succession patterns. Academy of Management Journal 1974; 17(4):771–775.
30. Pfeffer J, Salancik GR. The external control of organizations: a resource dependence perspective. New York: Harper & Row, 1978.
31. Brady, Helmich. Executive Succession.
32. Ibid.
33. Helmich, Brown, Successor type and organizational change in the corporate enterprise.
34. Pfeffer J, Salancik GR. Organizational context and the characteristics and tenure of hospital administrators. Academy of Management Journal 1977;20(1): 74–88.
35. Brady, Helmich. Executive succession: toward excellence in corporate leadership.
36. Pfeffer, Salancik. Organizational context and the characteristics and tenure of hospital administrators.
37. Graney CM. How to recruit, select, educate and train credit executives. Credit and Financial Management 1978;Mar:12–13+.
38. Meade TM. Executive promotions: does familiarity breed oversight? Personnel Journal 1972;51(8):45–49.
39. Gordan G, Becker S. Organization size and manage-

ment succession: a reexamination. American Journal of Sociology 1964;70(2):215–23.

40. Carlson RO. Executive succession and organizational change. Danville, IL: Interstate Printers and Publishers, Inc, 1962.
41. Brady, Helmich. Executive succession: toward excellence in corporate leadership.
42. McConnell C. Finding the new supervisor: inside or outside? The Health Care Supervisor 1984;3(1):69–79.
43. McKenney JL, Keen PGW. How managers' minds work. Harv Bus R 1974;52(3):79.
44. Heisler WJ. Promotion: what does it take to get ahead? Business Horizons 1978;21(4):57–63.
45. Helmich D. Predecessor turnover and successor characteristics. Cornell Journal of Social Relations 1974;9:249–260.
46. Heisler WJ. Promotion: what does it take to get ahead? Business Horizons 1978;21(4):57–63.
47. Bowman BW. What helps or harms promotability? Harv Bus R 1964;42(1):6–26.
48. Swinyard AW, Bond FA. Who gets promoted? Harv Bus R 1980;58(5):6–18.
49. Price. Master's program preparing nursing administrators: what are the essential components?
50. Ibid.
51. American Nurses Association. 1977 national sample survey of registered nurses. Kansas City, MO: American Nurses' Association, 1980.
52. American Society for Nursing Service Administrators. Report of 1977 survey of nursing service administrators. Chicago: ASNSA, 1977.
53. AONE, 1985 American Organization of Nurse Executives, 1985.
54. Freund C. Director of nursing effectiveness: DON and CEO perspectives and implications for education. J Nurs Adm 1985;15(6):25–30.
55. Ibid.
56. Ibid.
57. Friss L. Organizational commitment and job involvement of directors of nursing services. Nurs Adm Q 1982;Winter:1–10.
58. Ibid.
59. Ibid.
60. Sellery RA, Jr. How to hire an executive. Business Horizons 1976;19(4):26–32.

61. Helmich DL. Organizational growth and succession patterns. Academy of Management Journal 1974; 17(4):771–775.
62. Pfeffer J, Salancik GR. Organizational context and the characteristics and tenure of hospital administrators.
63. Pfeffer J, Salancik GR. The external control of organizations: a resource dependence perspective.
64. Ibid.
65. Levitt T. The managerial merry-go-round. Harv Bus R 1974;52(4):120–128.
66. Carroll GR. Dynamics of publisher succession in newspaper organizations. Adm Sci Q 1984;29(1):93–113.
67. Reinbanum MR. The effect of executive succession on stockholder wealth. Adm Sci Q 1985;30(1):46–60.
68. Brady, Helmich. Executive succession: toward excellence in corporate leadership, p. 247.
69. Kirschenbaum AB, Goldberg AI. Organizational behavior, career orientations, and the propensity to move among professionals. Sociology of Work and Occupations 1976;3(3):357–373.
70. Helmich D. Executive succession in the corporate organization: a current integration. Academy of Management Review 1977;20(2):252–266.
71. Brady, Helmich. Executive succession: toward excellence in corporate leadership.
72. Richards M, Greenlaw P. Management decisions and behavior. Homewood, IL: Richard D. Irwin, Inc, 1972.
73. Brady, Helmich. Executive succession: toward excellence in corporate leadership.
74. Helmich D, Erzen P. Leadership style and leader needs. Academy of Management Journal 1977;18:397–402.
75. Gerstein M, Reisman H. Strategic selection: matching executives to business conditions. Sloan Management Review 1983;24(2):33–49.
76. Gordon GE, Rosen N. Critical factors in leadership succession. Org Beh Hum Perf 1981;27:227–254.
77. Carroll TL. Characteristics of nurse managers. The Facilitator 1986;12(2):4.
78. Filerman G. Nursing managers preparing for the future. Nursing and Health Care 1985;6(2)
79. del Bueno. Organizational culture: how important is it?

55

Issues in Financial Management

Gaye W. Poteet
Nannette L. Goddard

IN 1932, the United States was spending 4.5 percent of its gross national product for health and medical services.[1] Most authorities of the day believed that the expenditure was reasonable and adequate, if only the total expenditure were distributed rationally and equitably. At that time no one was able to predict the sweeping changes in medical technology, societal expectations, and utilization of health services that were to take place over the next 50 years and result in an ever-increasing share of the gross national product being devoted to health care.

For the past 30 years, since employee health plans became widely available, Americans have clung to the notion that when it comes to health care, money is no object. For the most part, an insurance company or the government paid the bill. By the late 1970s, during the Carter administration, politicians and economists were starting to panic. The nation's bill for health care, $41.7 billion in 1965 (the year before the advent of Medicare and Medicaid), was on a rise that took it to $387.4 billion by 1984. Health-care costs have risen rapidly and presently approach 12 percent of our nation's gross national product, up from 6.4 percent in 1967.[1]

Corporations were blanching at the price of their employees' health benefits. In 1982, Lee Iacocca found that employee health-care expenditures accounted for 10 percent of the costs of Chrysler automobiles.[2] Plainly, health-care costs were soaring, and some-

thing had to be done. Reasons generally given for the increases in health care costs included inflation, use of expensive new technologies and intensive care units, growing medical needs of an aging population, rising costs of malpractice insurance, provision of unnecessary care, and payment policies of insurance plans and other coverage, especially Medicare and Medicaid. Over the past seven years government and other insurers have concocted various programs designed to trim the fat from the health-care system. The different approaches have one underlying theme: to control and reduce costs.

The health-care industry is in the throes of major change. The revolution in health-care financing is just beginning. It is likely that hospitals will continue to experience decreased utilization and lengths of stay in their acute care operations, as well as more financial pressure. Years of spending and capacity building in hospitals have produced a "hangover" resulting from the industry's many indulgences. The effects of this hangover are felt in the financial drain produced by empty beds, underutilized and/or duplicated services, and the oversupply of physicians. "Cures" in the form of changes in financial climate and reimbursement methodologies have brought about a sobering effect and caused uncertainty in nearly every health-care market in the country.

Excess capacity is a major issue presently facing the industry, for excess capacity exists both in hospitals and among physicians. Buyers are seeking and getting price concessions. All the elements are in place to bring about even more price competition; and the situation will not go away under any socially acceptable public policy, outside of nationalization of the health-care industry. Therefore, the industry must adapt to the changing economic environment. Hospitals in general have reached a point where they will operate, if they survive, at much lower occupancy rates than most thought possible. Certainly, as hospitals pare down their number of acute care beds, the nationwide total of occupied beds will be dramatically lower than the expectations of the past.

Criticism of rapidly increasing health-care costs led to the passage of the prospective payment legislation and the subsequent awareness of the necessity for health-care executives, including nursing administrators, to possess financial management skills. However, the legacy of nursing education at the undergraduate and graduate levels has produced almost 3 decades of nurses with little or no theoretical basis for sound financial management. Part of the blame for this deficiency in the curricula may rest with the health-care industry's tendency to discourage the involvement of nurses in the financial arena. Many experienced nurse managers have encountered a long line of fiscal officers who communicated that nurses need not worry about these matters.

Traditionally, undergraduate nursing educators have largely ignored financial management and budgeting content. The study of nursing administration at the graduate level was almost abandoned during the 1960s and 1970s in favor of graduate education that focused on advanced clinical content. Mounting recognition in the profession of the necessity for prepared nursing service administrators has led to the reestablishment of graduate programs focusing on nursing service administration. The emphasis and

course content related to financial management principles and budgeting skills have varied from school to school. The rapid proliferation of graduate programs in nursing administration created an imbalance in the supply and demand ratio of qualified faculty to teach in these programs. In 1983, Poteet offered the following introductory remarks for an issue of *Nursing Clinics of North America* devoted to the topic of nursing administration:

After almost two decades of disinterest, the academic world of nursing has rediscovered nursing administration as a field of study. This renewed interest is documented by the establishment of approximately 50 new programs in nursing administration since 1974. Early graduate programs in nursing were focused on preparing the nursing student for the role of teacher or administrator. In the late fifties, the emphasis shifted to advanced clinical preparation and nursing specialization. Nurses who were interested in preparing themselves for higher-management positions were forced to choose graduate programs outside of nursing in areas such as business and public administration. The nursing administrator had the task of applying and adapting the content to the practice of nursing administration. Lack of systematic graduate study or nursing research into the real or potential problems of nursing administration added to the limitations of graduate study for nurses in administrative roles[3] (p. 425).

For almost 20 years, nurses entered the practice of nursing administration with an insufficient educational basis. Compounding the problem is the fact that approximately 70 percent of all nursing service administrators presently possess only the baccalaureate degree, diploma, or associate degree in nursing.

During the golden years of health-care financing, fewer pressures—including financial ones—were placed on nursing service administrators. The advent of lower reimbursement levels, prospective payment, declining patient days, and patient census figures have combined to create a mandate for competent financial management skills for the nursing manager and executive. Yet there is a dearth of information and knowledge about the financial competencies necessary for the successful practice of nursing administration.

COMPONENTS OF FINANCIAL MANAGEMENT

In nursing, as in the larger arena of hospital management, financial activities and fiscal affairs are becoming less separate and distinct functions. Monitoring of dollars and other resources is more integrated into the overall management function at each level in the organizational structure. Competent financial management is necessary in all departments, including nursing and clinical areas, if efficient and effective management is to be achieved. According to Berman and Weeks, financial management is rapidly becoming an integral component of total operational management (in hospitals).[4]

The budgeting process is one of the most important aspects of financial management in the nursing department. The budget is defined as a plan for allocation and utilization of financial resources. Typically an institution has personnel and supply-expense budgets as well as a plan for purchase of capital items.

Covaleski and Dirsmith described budgets and the budgeting function in a clear and concise manner: "Budgets may be considered a quantitative or financial expression of a plan of action that provides a basis for directing and assessing the performance of individuals and subunits within an organization. Thus, budgets have been widely conceived as fulfilling management control needs of organizations[5] (p. 17)." In most institutions, the chief financial officer has ultimate responsibility for the budgeting process. However, the nurse executive is increasingly acquiring both the authority and the accountability for generating and monitoring the nursing budget.

Accounting, like nursing, is both an art and a science. Accounting data derived from the nursing and related departments provides a historical record of the department's finances. The prudent nurse executive recognizes that accounting practices, including the process of budgeting, serve to enhance—not replace—sound management judgment. Basic concepts of accounting, such as fixed assets, depreciation, and inventory have been described by numerous authors and are one set of financial management skills thought to be essential to the nurse executive.

Management is often defined as getting the work done through others. Drucker defined management's basic purpose to be the management and utilization of human resources to solve problems and accomplish work.[6] Financial management can be seen as evolving from the more comprehensive overall management function.

According to Neumann, Suver, and Zelman, financial management has its origins in three academic disciplines: financial accounting, managerial accounting, and managerial finance.[7] These three disciplines have contributed a separate body of knowledge along with a specific set of behaviors, tools, and techniques that can be used to improve administrative decision-making regarding the institution's acquisition, utilization, and control of resources.

Although definitions and concepts vary to some degree according to the source, the following definitions have been found to be applicable in a wide variety of health-care settings:

Financial management—The body of knowledge and activities involved in obtaining funds that the institution needs, optimizing the use of those funds to support operations, and ensuring that outcomes are in line with goals.
Accounting—The art of collecting, summarizing, analyzing, reporting, and inter-

preting, in monetary terms, information about the institution.[4]

Budget—A plan for the acquisition, allocation, and utilization of financial resources.

Resources—The human labor, physical plant, and raw materials available for use in implementing institutional goals.

Financial management competencies—
Those job behaviors or skills that establish the control and effective use of budgetary resources, including personnel, supplies, and capital equipment expenditures.

Nursing administrators direct the provision of a major component of care and services in the health-care system of the United States and manage huge amounts of the system's resources in terms of personnel, supplies, and equipment. At this time the cost of the health-care industry to the American population represents approximately 12 percent of the nation's gross national product and an ever-increasing total price tag. In this climate nursing faces the challenge of adapting its traditional quality of care standards to significantly more demanding cost of care standards. It is clear that the profession needs to identify those specific activities that are essential to the role of the nurse executive in the financial management of today's institutions.

ROLE OF THE NURSING ADMINISTRATOR

A review of nursing and related health-care literature provides some insight into the determination of the appropriate role of the nurse executive in financial planning. The ultimate purpose of a department of nursing is to provide sufficient amounts of nursing care of the appropriate quality to all patients and clients. A realistic statement of the philosophy of nursing, along with workable objectives, can be used as the framework for guiding the work of the department. These documents can serve to provide direction and

guidance for the day-to-day operations of the department, in addition to those necessary functions of financial planning and control. According to Cantor, these documents serve the following goals: "Thoroughly prepared statements of purpose, philosophy, and objectives based on reality, understood and used by those responsible for implementation, can promote efficiency and effectiveness in the operation of institutions, departments, and programs [including departments of nursing]"[8] (p. 9).

Nurse executives have many reasons for their involvement in the financial management and budgeting process. First, other nursing employees depend on nurse administrators to acquire and control financial resources. Second, participation in the political negotiation process surrounding budgeting provides the opportunity for the nurse executive to represent and voice the needs of the patient population and the nursing department. Third, control of the budgeting process permits the nurse executive to respond to mandates for fiscal responsibility.[5,9]

Determining the appropriate and prudent role of the nursing service administrator in the financial management of the nursing department and the overall institution is a major challenge within each unique health-care setting. The framework for a departmental philosophy of financial management and the plan of action or involvement for each nursing staff member are drawn from sources on management, financial management, financial management of health-care institutions, accounting, budgeting, negotiating, and diplomacy skills.

Beyond understanding the global processes of budgeting, standards of accounting, and principles of financial planning, the nurse executive is responsible for performing the task of developing a workable methodology of nursing finance and budgeting. The nurse executive needs to be able to translate the desired components of nursing practice and the chosen modality of care delivery into logical requests for staff and other resources. In short, nursing needs to be translated into the language of the fiscal officer, so that nursing departmental requests may be understood and compared equitably to those submitted by other departments.

The competition for the shrinking resources within each health-care institution is examined by Covaleski and Dirsmith with the following insights:

In particular, issues related to allocating scarce resources within the hospital have the potential for generating many social-psychological hurdles for its personnel—administrator and health-care professional alike. . . . Organizations in a period of decline are unique in comparison with stable or growing systems. It is in such organizations that politics, interdepartmental disputes, power struggles, and battles for resources are likely to be in evidence. It is in such organizations that anxiety is likely to be high and where readily transferable, non-disputable—objective, quantitative—information is likely to be dominant[5] (pp. 18, 20).

In many instances, the nurse executive may be the only member of the uppermost administrative team with a clinical background and an ability to continually focus on the needs of the patient or client being served by the organization. It is often the nurse executive who has the most frequent and largest number of contacts with the consumers themselves. Unless the chief financial officer and other executives are also making patient rounds in clinical areas, the nursing administrative team may be required to spend much of their time interpreting even the most basic clinical issues and educating the other executives about priorities of patient care.

A clear vision of the contributions of all members of the health-care team is an essential ingredient in developing a financial plan that will suit the entire organization. Finkler emphasized the importance of "interactive communication" among all the managers of the institution: "Managers must know the basic assumptions upon which the budget is

to be based. They must know the overall goals and directions of the organization, as well as the specific measurable goals for the coming year. They must be able to coordinate their plans with those of the other departments of the organization"[10] (p. xv).

Each department has a direct or indirect contribution to make to the provision of patient care and services. The patient has to rely on everyone to perform their interrelated functions correctly and in a timely manner. Nurses providing direct patient care are often the employees who coordinate the activities of all others involved, so as to ensure that the treatment plan is being carried out completely and the patient is satisfied with the process.

In a study performed by Arthur D. Little consultants and some of their client hospitals, the productivity of nursing personnel was found to be affected dramatically by the performance of the support services:

A well-organized materials management department can cut an average of 1.5 nursing hours per patient day. That means, for a hospital with a daily census of 150 patients, a savings of 39.5 full-time equivalent personnel. With support service instead of nursing personnel performing logistics and transportation activities, potential salary savings can run $118,500 annually if the salary difference between the two personnel groups averages only $3,000. . . .

In a suburban hospital with an average daily census of 200 patients, 46 nursing service hours per day were devoted to transport: 26 in "unnecessary" patient transport and 20 in the transport of supplies, equipment and papers—clearly not nursing tasks, although necessary in providing patient care. About three-fourths of the trips, none requiring nursing participation, had been made by registered nurses, including head nurses and supervisors[11] (p. 101).

The involvement of the nurse executive in the financial management process of the entire organization is also necessary if the institution is to plan appropriate job assignments to higher paid, more versatile workers. The two situations described above illustrate the urgent need for close collaboration, within the executive team, which will yield higher productivity and better financial planning across all departments.

As predictions of declining nursing school enrollments and increasingly severe shortages of nurses continue to appear in the literature, the nurse executive is also required to remain as informed about the nursing staff as all executives must be about the consumers. It is one thing to lobby effectively for the needed complement of staff positions, and quite another task to fill all the approved positions with qualified employees. Appropriate budgets that support the long-term strategies for building the essential recruitment, retention, and staff development programs need to be factored into the financial plans of the institution.

Other writers offer more specific suggestions in the area of financial management for the nursing department. According to Stevens, appropriate charges should be designated for nursing services.[12] In many institutions, nursing is not viewed as a source of revenue. If specific charges were billed to the patient for nursing care, this image would change. Two methods are possible. In some settings, patients can be billed for each separate nursing procedure or skill performed with the patient. In more complex situations, billing can be based on a patient classification system. The number of nursing hours and type of care, required and then provided, may be measured and charged to the individual patients who receive varying levels of services.

Some work has been reported in the literature concerning the management competencies necessary for the successful practice of nursing administration.[13–16] Among the personnel functions identified were development and dissemination of human resources policy, along with development of budget and salary scales. Educational activities were

seen as an important part of the nurse executive role. Delegation was described as a pivotal skill necessary for success as a nurse executive, cost-effective utilization of administrative time, and avoidance of a constant crisis management style that prevents strategic planning. The grooming of competent nursing administration colleagues and head nurses who function well within the financial arena is the ultimate responsibility of the chief nurse executive.

SOCIAL FORCES AND TRENDS: IMPACT ON NURSING FINANCES

Because of the ever-increasing cost of health care, economists, policymakers, and financial planners have been asked to find ways to reduce the nation's health-care costs. Since the 1980 election of Ronald Reagan, governmental policies have been designed to decrease the cost of health care for all Americans.

While many providers of health care continue to lament the loss of the golden years of health-care financing, the reality of the situation is that there are major economic and societal changes taking place in the U.S. culture that will prevent any possibility of a return to unlimited financing for health care. These include major demographic changes in the United States's population, increased ethnic and cultural diversity of the population, technological advancements, and the country's status and problems associated with being the largest debtor nation on earth.

Population Demographics

The United States's population is getting older and more ethnically diverse. By the year 2000, there will be 35 million residents of the United States who are 65 years of age or older. These elderly citizens will make up more than 13 percent of the entire population. A class of citizens, termed the frail elderly, will number an estimated 4.9 million by the year 2000.[17] These elderly citizens can be expected to consume a far greater percentage of the health-care services than their numbers in the population would suggest. For example, in 1980 those over 65 composed approximately 11 percent of the population, yet they were responsible for 31 percent of the health-care expenditures. If health-care programs for the elderly are continued at the present rate of funding, it has been estimated that these programs have the potential to consume up to 50 percent of the federal budget.[17]

Increased Ethnic Diversity

At the same time that the nurse administrator is striving to cope with decreased health-care funding and an older patient population, the challenges and problems associated with rapid changes in the ethnic population of Americans are presenting themselves. The immigrants of the 1980s have been predominantly Asian and Hispanic, not European. By 1990, the Hispanic population is projected to outnumber the Black population in the United States, making Hispanics the largest minority group.[18]

Nurse administrators face a twofold challenge in responding to this diversity. First, the health-care needs and expectations of these ethnically diverse citizens are likely to be more difficult to meet. Languages and cultural barriers are not easily overcome in the health-care environment. Second, it can be expected that large numbers of these citizens will seek employment in the industry. Employee development departments at this time rarely include programs specifically designed for the new American. The situations from both perspectives combine on a collision course between patient, employer, and employee abilities and expectations.

Anthropologist Gould-Stuart recently described the scene identified and the solution proposed for one long-term care facility in New York City:

People working in nursing homes frequently must deal with residents who are culturally and racially different from themselves. Stereotypes held by carers about ethnically different residents can have a negative effect on the quality of care. . . .

The administration recognized that if residents' behavior and desires were judged negatively, from an ethnocentric standpoint, then trust would be thwarted and kindness diminished. Thus, a seminar dealing with cross-cultural issues was particularly relevant in this institutional setting. . . .

Over a 10-week period [for 90 minutes each week], the participants in a seminar on cross-cultural perspectives in aging began to question some of their assumptions about "good" and "bad" behavior, as well as reflect on their own belief systems. They learned to look at the nursing home residents as products of their cultural, historical, and generational backgrounds and gained more appreciation of them as people[19] (pp. 319, 321).

In the near future, similar cross-cultural educational programs, highlighting information about each of the many possible cultures of clients and employees, will be recommended as ongoing in most health-care facilities. The time and expense of such vital offerings will be a growing portion of human resource, education, and nursing departmental budgets.

Technological Advancements

The demand and necessity for computer utilization in health-care institutions have unfortunately preceded and exceeded the present abilities of health-care workers at all levels. Nursing administrators, ward secretaries, and numerous other health-care employees are all scrambling to acquire the necessary knowledge and skills to perform at the desired and acceptable technological levels within their institutions.

Like it or not, this most recent wave of computer mania is just a precursor of things to come. In a small article that appeared in January 1985, a reporter from a leading U.S. news magazine provided readers with the following provocative glimpse of the future:

Visionary researchers are pursuing a tantalizing goal: to devise an electronic chip from organic products.

American scientists, looking to 1985 and beyond, are working feverishly to enhance the usefulness of computers in everyday life.

The goal is a dramatic one: To grow computer circuitry in biology labs from living bacteria, producing micro-processors with 10 million times the memory of today's most powerful machines. . . .

In theory, such tiny supercomputers would find a virtually endless list of applications. They could connect with the human nervous system, serving as artificial eyes, ears, and voice boxes.

. . . man-made "organic" computers might be able to detect their own internal-design flaws and even repair and replicate themselves.

Minuscule computers implanted in the blood-stream could monitor body chemistry and correct imbalances.[20] (p. 50)

News flashes such as this might remind us of the genius of Roddenberry's *Star Trek* television series and cause us to recollect the familiar scene of Dr. "Bones" McCoy scanning his patients, from several feet away, with something called a "tricorder." With the availability of the "living computer" technology described in the above quotation, it seems feasible that each crew member of the Starship Enterprise could have had multiple computers floating in their bloodstreams, constantly supplying the good doctor and nurses with all the read-outs they needed to diagnose and monitor their patients' untoward responses to space travel and occasional onslaughts from alien beings.

Within the next twenty years, nurses will be trying to write the care plans for just these types of patients—patients who will rely on increasingly sophisticated levels of technology for their health care and maintenance of life. The demand for adequately prepared staff nurses and the demands placed on inhouse nursing education departments for continual in-service updates will pose an even greater challenge to the nurse executive who attempts to negotiate appropriate financial resources.

Economic Status

Economics is the study of the efficient allocation of scarce resources among competing uses. Currently, the United States ranks as the world's largest debtor nation. The country's leaders are scrambling to identify possible products for export.

It would seem that two scenarios are possible for the health-care industry. In the first, hospitals continue to experience financial losses and declining censuses. More and more of them will close, thus reducing the size of the industry and the number of jobs available to U.S. workers.

In the second scenario, espoused by Kaiser, the health-care facilities of the United States become the centers of excellence for the entire globe and begin attracting larger numbers of patients to this country for their health care. Advances in research, care, and technology in the United States may establish its hospital system as the "transplant, implant, and replant capital of the world."[21] This possibility forecasts the opposite of the doom-and-gloom picture only for those institutions that survive the current financial climate and respond well to the pressures of change by embracing innovation.

The nurse executive who is able to do more with fewer resources will be the survivor in either of the scenarios presented. Willis cautions her staff and colleagues by using her own modification of a familiar saying: "We can't do more with less, unless we've got the best."[22] Nursing needs to develop the best systems, the managers, the tools, and financial support possible within each health-care facility; complacency and mediocrity will not be tolerated in the business of health care.

AREAS OF PRESENT AND FUTURE RESEARCH

Research in nursing administration and the financial management of nursing departments is focusing on a variety of research questions and management issues. A small sample of pertinent studies draws attention to the need for more research endeavors that will assist the nurse executive in strategic and financial planning.

In one research effort, currently in progress, the nursing administrator members of the American organization of Nurse Executives are asked to participate in a study designed to determine the financial competencies essential to the successful practice of nursing administration. The study seeks to answer the following research questions:

1. What financial resources are nurse executives presently accountable for in their institutions?
2. What kind of process is used for budget preparation?
3. What kind of financial management competencies do nurse executives identify as expectations in their jobs?[23]

Another group of researchers reported the results of a study designed to identify the nursing care hours and costs associated with the nursing patient classification groups and the diagnosis related groups (DRGs) constituting the study hospital's case-mix. Sovie and colleagues provided a significant leap forward in their newsworthy results:

> The findings in this study are instructive as they relate to the percentage of direct nursing costs that are included in the room costs of patients in the DRGs. When the extremes are removed (i.e., DRGs with limited numbers of patients), the most common percentage of average direct nursing costs in the average room costs fall within the range of 18 to 24 percent. . . . These data surprise many individuals involved directly in hospital health care, including practicing nurses and physicians, as well as observers of the hospital health scene. The assumption has been that nurses ac-

counted for a much larger share of the room costs[24] (p. 34).

Another recent study linking the costs of nursing care to the federal prospective payment-system categories is the research conducted by Medicus System Corporation, a health-care consulting and information system firm. This study collected data from 22 Medicus client hospitals, ranging in size from 202 to 1,181 beds. More than 80,000 patient records were collected and, of these, 24,000 representing 40 DRGs were analyzed. The analysis revealed the following important findings:

- That the data reveal which DRGs require the most nursing resources (see Table 55.1)
- That nursing costs represent 17.8 percent of Medicare reimbursement—a smaller percentage than many expected
- That sharp differences exist between surgical and medical DRGs in patient-to-patient variations of nursing care costs
- That the data fail to reveal a correlation between nursing staffs with high percentages of RNs and lower costs[25] (p. 50)

The findings of this study prompted many favorable reactions from a number of key nurse leaders. There is an obvious need to pursue similar research projects as nurse executives attempt to identify the true costs and contribution margins of individual nursing departments.

Nurse managers are often interested in comparing their units' specific productivity standards to those of similar units in other settings. In an effort to seek uniform performance measures across the industry, chief financial officers often ask the nurse executive to identify the "normal standards" for target nursing hours per patient-day values. The nurse administrator, confronted with these requests, is usually hard pressed to offer many well-documented guidelines. The difficulties in attempting nursing research in

Table 55.1 The Most Expensive DRGs in Terms of Variable Nursing Labor Costs per Case

DRG #	Description	Nursing labor cost per case	RN cost component	Average LOS (days)
106	Coronary bypass with cardiac catheterization	$1,547.80	82.6%	15.7
110	Major reconstructive vascular procedures without pump (patient over 70)	$1,497.68	78.6%	15.8
1	Craniotomy (patient over 17), except for trauma	$1,492.18	75.0%	15.1
148	Major small and large bowel procedures (patient over 69)	$1,263.49	70.4%	14.8
462	Rehabilitation	$1,262.19	55.2%	21.7
121	Circulatory disorders with acute myocardial infarction and complications	$1,204.51	82.2%	11.6
210	Hip and femur procedures, except major joints (patient over 90)	$1,195.70	65.0%	14.2
14	Specific cerebrovascular disorders, except transient ischemic attacks	$1,018.76	67.8%	11.0
416	Septicemia (patient over 17)	$981.61	67.1%	10.1
430	Psychoses	$917.97	58.4%	16.6
209	Major joint and limb reattachment procedures	$865.85	63.7%	13.2
89	Simple pneumonia or pleurisy (patient over 69)	$780.05	66.9%	9.2
122	Circulatory disorders with acute myocardial infarction and without complications	$748.93	83.1%	8.2
320	Kidney/urinary tract infections (patient over 69)	$728.60	64.9%	8.1
82	Respiratory neoplasms	$720.86	68.5%	9.4
108	Other cardiovascular or thoracic procedures	$710.31	79.6%	7.4
296	Nutritional/miscellaneous metabolic disorders (patient over 69)	$670.13	66.9%	7.7
127	Heart failure/shock	$665.33	70.5%	8.2
88	Chronic obstructive pulmonary disease	$569.97	66.0%	8.0
174	Gastrointestinal hemorrhage (patient over 69)	$565.75	68.6%	6.9

From McCormick B. What's the cost of nursing care? *Hospitals* 1986;60(21):49. Reprinted by permission of the publisher.

this area are many; even the best of studies indicate such a wide variation in practice that "standards" are almost impossible to identify.

In 1982, the National Association of Children's Hospitals and Related Institutions (NACHRI) attempted to discover the patterns of nursing hours per patient-day standards between like units caring for like pediatric patients. In an extensive study, the NACHRI Nurse Staffing Data Program was used to amass detailed staffing information, along with a hospital profile and an individual patient care unit profile, from a total of forty-eight units from seven different institutions. The results did not lead to conclusions about what figures to recommend as appropriate nursing hour standards. Instead, the results of this highly sophisticated study served to document the diversity of staffing standards that exist across the country:

The monthly staffing and utilization data submitted by each of the seven hospitals were compiled. Unit-specific and total hospital annual averages for nursing hours per patient day (required, worked, and paid) and occupancy rates were then reviewed by comparison group. . . .

The total hospital median of worked nursing hours per patient day was 11.8 hours. Individual hospital values ranged from 8.2 to 14 hours. The median of worked hours per patient day for the medical-surgical units was 9.3 with the intensive-care units recording a median value of 22.6 hours. The ranges in worked hours per patient day for the medical-surgical units and intensive-care units were 5.9 to 14.7 and 16.2 to 30 hours respectively[26] (p. 148).

Years of inattention, misdirection, or simply lack of serious concern about the funding for and costs of delivering patient care have left many nurse and health-care administrators with a significant knowledge gap regarding the management of fiscal resources. Understandably the nurse executive wants to preserve nursing's major influence in decisions about how patient care is accomplished and how nursing is practiced in every venue of health care. For that purpose, the chief nurse executive must participate as a full member of the organization's administrative team and be able to demonstrate how nursing staff and nursing contributions may enhance the entire organization and its goals.

The nurse administrator best prepared for this role is proficient in financial management and related skills, cognizant of future societal and economic trends, and aware and supportive of innovative research in nursing administration. Beyond the institutional or corporate setting, the expert nurse executive also needs to be able to establish nursing's value, effectiveness, and productivity within an industry that must seek out the best, in order to do more with less.

REFERENCES

1. Arthur Anderson and Company, American College of Hospital Administrators. Health care in the 1990s: Trends and strategies. Chicago: Arthur Anderson and Company, 1985.
2. Iacocca L, Novak W. Iacocca: An autobiography. New York: Bauhaus, 1984.
3. Poteet GW. Forward to symposium of nursing administration. Nursing Clinics of North America 1983;18(3):425.
4. Berman HJ, Weeks LE. The financial management of hospitals. 5th ed. Ann Arbor: University of Michigan Health Administration Press, 1982.
5. Covaleski MA, Dirsmith MW. Budgeting in the nursing services area: Management, control, political and witchcraft uses. Health Care Management Review 1981;6(2):17–24.
6. Drucker PF. Management: Tasks, responsibilities, practices. New York: Harper & Row Publishers, 1973, pp. 39–42, 182, 184.
7. Neumann BR, Suver JD, Zelman WN. Financial management: Concepts and applications for health care providers. Owings Mills, Maryland: Rynd Communications, 1984, pp. 11–14.
8. Cantor MM. Philosophy, purpose and objectives: Why do we have them: J Nur Admin 1971;1(3):9–13.
9. Sovie MD. Managing nursing resources in a constrained economic environment. Nursing Economic$ 1985;3(2):85–94.
10. Finkler SA. Budgeting concepts for nurse managers. Orlando, Florida: Grune & Stratton, Inc., 1984.
11. Swenson B, Wolfe HB, Schroeder, R. Effectively employing support services the key for increasing nursing personnel productivity. Modern Healthcare 1984;14(16):101–104.
12. Stevens BJ. What is the executive's role in budgeting for her department? J Nurs Adm 1981;11(7):22–24.
13. Poulin MA. The Nurse executive role: A structural and functional analysis. J Nurs Admin 1984;14(2):9–14.
14. Cleland V. An articulated model for preparing nursing administrators. J Nurs Admin 1984;14(10):23–31.
15. Zander K. Management training won't work . . . unless administration provides it. Nursing Administration Quarterly 1983;7(2):77–87.
16. Poteet GW. Delegation strategies: A must for the nurse executive. J Nurs Adm 1984;14(9):18–21.
17. Harrington C. Crisis in long-term care: Part 1, the problems. Nursing Economic$ 1985;3(1):15–20.
18. Hodgkinson HL. Guess who's coming to college: A demographic portrait of students in the 1990's. In: Gutek GL, Tatum R, eds. Standard education almanac 1984–1985, 17th ed. Chicago: Professional Publications, 1984.
19. Gould-Stuart J. Bridging the cultural gap between residents and staff. Geriatric Nursing 1986;7(6):319–321.
20. Wellborn SN. Race to create A "living computer." U.S. News and World Report 1985;97(27):50.
21. Kaiser L. Affirming an executive balance. Lecture to the American Organization of Nurse Executives. Denver, Colorado: November 14, 1985.
22. Willis KK. Resources consumption or cost effective delivery. Lecture to the Texas Nurses' Association. Houston, Texas: March 21, 1986.
23. Poteet GW, Hodges LC, Goddard NL. Financial competencies study. (In progress.)
24. Sovie MD, Tarcinale MA, Vanputee AW, Stunden AE. Amalgam of nursing acuity, DRGs and costs. Nursing Management 1985;16(3):22–28, 32–34, 38, 40, 42.
25. McCormick B. What's the cost of nursing care? Hospitals 1986;60(21):48–52.
26. Gorman M, Borovies DL. Comparative nursing hours in tertiary pediatric facilities. Nursing Economic$ 1985;3(3):146–151.

56

Application of the Neuman Model in Nursing Administration and Practice

Patricia Hinton-Walker
Mona Raborn

THE APPLICATION of nursing theoretical models to nursing practice settings is not new. However, the use of one conceptual nursing model as a basis for *both* nursing administration and nursing practice within an acute care setting is infrequently described. Wood, when discussing implementation of a nursing model to nursing administration states "nursing administration has had a difficult time maintaining goals congruent with professional nursing practice. The patient is not always the focus of nursing practice in hospitals."[1] (p. 357) She suggests a new approach, the use of conceptual models as a basis for nursing practice and the delivery of nursing services.[1]

Meleis describes the evolution of nursing theory, and the subsequent concern that one nursing theory could not address all aspects of nursing care. She states that, in the past, nurse practitioners avoided the use of nursing theory in nursing practice settings. Meleis traces the use of theory in education (1966–75), and then traces the beginning of attempts to bridge the gap between theory and research and theory and practice (1976–80). She characterizes the years 1981 to 1985 as a time when theory was accepted as a useful tool for practice and research.[2]

In 1984, the nurse administrator at Jefferson Davis Memorial Hospital, in Natchez, Mississippi, began the process of adopting the Neuman Health-Care Systems Model as an organizing conceptual model for nursing administration and delivery of nursing care. This major step came as a result of a need for a unifying approach to the delivery of nursing care, reorganization of nursing administration structure, and a need to provide the nursing staff with opportunities for scholarly inquiry. Neuman and Wyatt suggest that the role of the nurse administrator is to provide optimal health care, improve practice, and refine nursing theory.[1]

In this chapter, the use of the Neuman model in the reorganization of the structure and function of nursing administration, and the delivery of nursing care in an acute care setting will be presented. Impetus for the use of a nursing model and reasons and critera for selection of a particular theoretical model are discussed. Administrative issues and problems involved in the integration of a conceptual model as an organizing framework for the structure and function of administration, as well as nursing practice will be described. Additionally, future ideas for use of this particular model in the changing health-care delivery system will be explored.

REASONS FOR USE OF A THEORETICAL MODEL

Deciding to use a theoretical nursing model was a major decision for the nursing staff at Jefferson Davis Memorial Hospital. The nurse administrator, Mona Raborn, R.N., believed that staff nurses needed a framework to provide a focus for nursing practice. A clear direction for the nursing department was needed to enhance interfacing within the department and with other departments. A nursing model would also provide a common language and conceptual frame of reference for charting, care plans, and so forth. Meaningful definitions could be adopted that would promote clarification of purpose and unification of the nursing department.

Head nurses had identified a need for revision of charting forms such as the history and physical assessment, discharge planning, and nursing care plan. An objective patient classification system was desired rather than the current subjective criterion used. In order to prevent fragmentation of committee work, problems with the education of staff nurses with numerous changes in nursing care documentation, it seemed important to establish one approach, define common terms, and find an organizing framework for the delivery of nursing care.

These reasons for use of a nursing model are consistent with those in the literature. Brink indicates that a model simplifies and diagrammatically presents parts of an interaction.[1] Meleis, when discussing the use of theories in practice, states that they provide common labels and definitions for phenomena, which assist with comunication. In addition theory provides the nurse with goals for use of the nursing process, particularly assessment, nursing diagnosis, and intervention.[2]

Nursing theory can suggest a framework for research as well as practice. Opportunities for research and scholarly development were of prime consideration to the nurse administrator. The nurse administrator was concerned about retention of nurses seeking higher education, since neither the organizational structure, nor the budget allowed for clinical nurse specialist positions. Establishing an environment that would encourage scholarly development, opportunities for inquiry, publishing, and testing theoretical phenomena in nursing practice was an important consideration in adopting a nursing theoretical model for nursing service. Meleis describes scholarliness as the combining of "theory, research, philosophy, and in disciplines such as nursing, practice."[2] (p. 300) She further states that theory is evolving from practice and being tested in practice.[2]

In addition to utilizing a nursing model as a focus for clinical practice and scholarly inquiry, another goal of the nurse administrator was to use a model as an organizing framework for the structuring and functioning of nursing administration. Fawcett supports this idea stating that conceptual models can guide the construction and implementation of nursing education programs, and can assist in planning organizational structures in health care delivery agencies.[3] Once the idea of using a theoretical nursing model was explored, the next step was to select the appropriate model for use at Jefferson Davis Memorial Hospital.

SELECTION OF THE APPROPRIATE MODEL

Selection of an appropriate conceptual model involves both objective and subjective processes.[2] Although there are a number of methods for evaluating and critiquing a theory, Fawcett's writings regarding selection of a theory closely describe the process used at Jefferson Davis Memorial Hospital. Of primary importance is the necessity for congruence of a model with one's philosophical beliefs.[3] The Neuman model was congruent with the total patient care approach already philosophically accepted by the nursing staff. Also, the Neuman model as a systems approach to care, can be used in very complex organizations, which are composed of many subsystems. The model can be applied to patients, employees, groups, organizations, and committees. Leddy and Pepper describe systems theory as one that can be useful to "understand, predict, and control the possible effects of nursing care on the client system and the concurrent effects of the interaction on the nurse system."[4] (p. 118) Since changes, at Jefferson Davis Memorial Hospital, were needed in both the nursing system (administration) and the client system (delivery of nursing care), the Neuman model seemed most appropriate.

The aim of the Neuman model is to provide a unifying focus for approaching varied nursing problems, and understanding mankind and its environment. It is based on an individual's reaction to stress, and factors of reconstitution are thought of as dynamic in nature.[1] Since the nursing department at Jefferson Davis Memorial Hospital was experiencing increasing stress, this aspect of the model could be used to identify stress factors in the environment, create effective stress reduction measures, and facilitate problem solving for nursing leadership and staff. Purposeful interventions aimed at stress reduction and elimination of adverse conditions would assist individuals and groups in maintaining optimal functioning and productivity. Neuman and Wyatt state that it is the responsibility of nurse administrators to respond to and initiate changes necessary for the health of individual employees, clients, and the organization as a whole.[1]

The nursing department was also looking for a model that would provide flexibility, yet stability. With the rapid and dramatic changes taking place in the health care system and society, it was important to have a structure and processes that facilitated creative decision making and flexibility. Arndt states that "the traditional bureaucratic model is not appropriate when applied to nonroutine, 'creative' decisions and activities."[5] (p. 110) She further describes the functions of nursing service administration as facilitating achievement of overall goals, diagnosing problems that stress organizational members, initiating interventions for the best interest of all members of the organization.[5]

When analyzing the usefulness of a theory, it is necessary to explore its use in practice, research, education, and administration. In nursing administration, use of a theory is considered both in terms of the organizational structure and in the delivery of care.[2] Arndt discusses the use of nursing theory, particularly the Neuman model, as a way of bringing together diverse functions into an integrated, organized whole, with all parts of the system working to achieve organizational goals.[5]

Evaluation of a model for its social congruence is another criterion for selection. "Critical assessment of societal values and theory values is an integral part of a thorough theory critique."[2] (p. 163) In a critique of the Neuman model, Fawcett indicates that the Neuman model is congruent with societal expectations of needs for secondary and tertiary care. She discusses the primary prevention aspects of the model and identifies roles of nurses in ambulatory care settings, in promotion of wellness and prevention of illness as important in the evaluation of the model.[3] The Neuman model is adaptable for all types of clinical settings and for the broad scope of nursing interventions. In addition to traditional health care services offered at Jefferson Davis Memorial Hospital, the nurse administrator anticipated starting community outreach programs, as well as increased ambulatory and one-day surgical services. These changing trends in health-care delivery affirmed the use of the Neuman model for patient care in a variety of settings.

Assessment of variables affecting the individual client was also important in the selection of an appropriate nursing theoretical model. The multidimensional approach in the Neuman model assists the nurse in obtaining the patient's perceptions of illness as well as the nurse's own perception of the patient's problems.[1] Nurses at Jefferson Davis Memorial Hospital expressed frustration at not being able to teach and influence patients to improve their own care. Also, in the Natchez community, there were frequent readmissions of some of the patients due to apparent noncompliance with the treatment plan. Traditional approaches of assessment based on nurses' perceptions can influence the lack of patient motivation for wellness, and lack of compliance with medical regimen.[1] This characteristic of the Neuman model, with "emphasis on negotiation between client and nurse . . . may lead to greater client adherence to health care measures than when goals are dictated by the health care worker."[3] (p. 161)

In addition to the congruence of Neuman's definition of person, health, nursing, and environment with the nurse administrators' philosophy, there were other reasons for selection of the Neuman model for Jefferson Davis Memorial Hospital. Although a number of staff nurses were educated locally at Alcorn State University, where Orem's self-care model was used, most nurses were educationally prepared at the associate-degree level. At the time of the selection of the model, seven nurses, (five baccalaureate and two master's degree nurses) had experience with the Neuman model in their educational programs. Also, the management consultant, Patricia Hinton-Walker, Ph.D., R.N., of Hinton Associates had worked with the Neuman model and assisted with its implementation in nursing administration and practice. The reasons mentioned previously were consistent with Meleis' reporting of the most cited reasons for selection of a model, "knowledge

of the theorist, mentorship by others who have used a particular theory, and being part of an education program."[2] (p. 146)

APPLICATION OF THE MODEL IN NURSING ADMINISTRATION

Application of the Neuman model to the reorganization of structure and function of the nursing department at Jefferson Davis Memorial Hospital began in 1984, and is still a major project of the nursing leadership in that institution. Prior to 1980, a traditional bureaucratic organizational structure was in place in nursing service, which maintained roles of house supervisors and head nurses over the units. In an initial attempt to decentralize, the house supervisor position on the 7 AM–3 PM shift was eliminated, clinical coordinators were established, and a new plan for decentralization and management development was explored.

When the nursing service department decentralized and removed traditional middle management, the head nurse role was maintained as the key or pivotal point of nursing practice decisions. There were however, concerns regarding the administrator's span of control—26 positions, including head nurses, support services of education, patient teaching, operating room, recovery, and so on. Head nurses and staff on their units were placed in subgroups. These groups consisted of subsystems of head nurses and other services with similarities of delivery of nursing care or support functions.

When considering the restructuring of the organization and the decision-making process, the Neuman model provided not only a mechanism for analysis, but the potential for a new type of organizational structure with the patient at the center, or focal point. The organizational structure was subsequently revised with the Neuman model in mind. The committee working on organizational structure believed that the organizational chart for

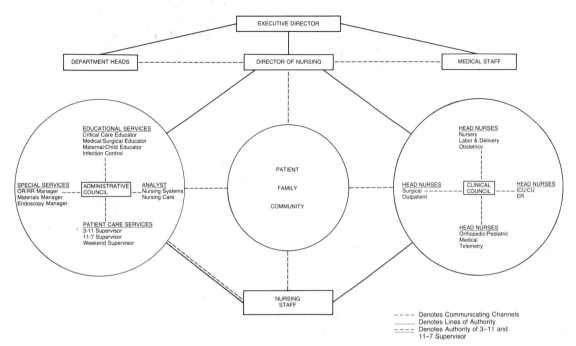

Figure 56.1 Organizational Chart of Nursing Services at Jefferson Davis Memorial Hospital. Administrative council is composed of support and supervisory personnel. Clinical council is composed of all direct patient care services. Each council is further subdivided into work groups of similar characteristics.

nursing service clarified not only the decision-making process and communication channels, but moreover, the reason for the existence of any nursing department: the patient. The patient is not depicted on most organizational charts for nursing service departments. The reasons for depicting the organizational chart in a creative new way (see Figure 56.1) is supported by a statement in the Magnet Hospitals publication "the organizational structure provides the framework in which nurses practice and appears to contribute significantly to the total ambience of the hospital."[6] (p. 20)

It was important that an organizational structure allow for participative decision-making, and facilitate goal setting with individuals and units. Head nurses and their staff were placed in subgroups for the purpose of goal setting, cross-training for staffing

changes due to rapid fluctuations in inpatient census, and staffing. Early in the reorganization, the nursing service administrator conducted regular meetings with these subgroups to assist with problem solving and to help with communication in a developing new structure. These meetings encouraged nurses to explore portions of the decision-making process where staff nurse influence was possible, and to share in the management decisions when appropriate.[7]

Head nurses rotated the leadership position within the subgroup quarterly. Although this concept was not true job sharing as described in the literature, this approach in most cases decreased frustration and stress through peer support.[8] The leader facilitated the submitting of reports, establishing of goals, identification of educational needs, and the exploring of financial and staffing needs for the subgroup as well as for individual units. This approach was consistent with the participative management style as well as with the emphasis on the importance of shared perceptions and needs in the Neuman model. The individual unit or subgroup participated in assessment of needs, and worked with the administrator implementing the management plan of action. Later, the subgroups of head nurses and their staff comprised a clinical council, which recommended creation of or changes in policy, procedure, and services, and participated in problem solving.

Although the input of the clinical council was vital to the organization, of equal importance to quality patient care are support services such as the evening and night supervisors, staff development, infection control, quality assurance, nursing systems analyst, and the nursing care analyst. An administrative council was also established which included these support functions. After much discussion about the appropriate place for surgery and recovery staff, they were placed in the support services, because they did not have staffing needs or functions in common with patient care units. Operating room and recovery had some responsibilities in common with other support groups: the need for communication with patient care units, and problems coordinating activities with more than one unit.

The administrative council was designed to complement the clinical council and balance decision making between clinical and administrative functions. New policies, procedures, problem solving, and recommendations could be generated from either council, and then would have to be presented to the other council for approval or endorsement. Decisions or recommendations made by the clinical and administrative councils required the approval or endorsement of the nursing service administrator prior to implementation.

Communication between and among different clinical areas and administrative support systems (such as evening and night supervisors) was another area for consideration. To facilitate communication and decision making that considered appropriate factors, most committees had membership from each council in addition to staff nurses. Any task-force appointments included membership from each council. This method of committee assignments enhanced communication and problem solving between and among groups.

Consistent with the Neuman model, intrapersonal stressors, interpersonal stressors, and extrapersonal stressors were identified and analyzed by the nursing staff and nurse administrator. Flexible lines of defense from the Neuman model were used as a part of the strategy for planned change. These lines of defense "act as a buffer against stressors that can break through and invade the normal line of defense."[9] (p. 132) They were used to assist particularly with extrapersonal stressors to the nursing department.

Interpersonal stressors were analyzed and discussed by subgroups of head nurses and support services. Differences in behavioral styles in communication and problem solving were explored in management training workshops with Hicks of Carl Hicks Associates. Other interpersonal stressors involved periodic misunderstandings and communication problems between head nurses and the evening and night supervisors. These concerns were consistent with problems identified in the literature between the head nurse and the evening and night supervisor.[6] In order to address these interpersonal stressors, a communication and problem identification form (with multiple carbons) was designed and implemented. This facilitated communication about employees, patient care problems, and administrative or clinical concerns between head nurses, supervisors, and the nursing service administrator. This method of communication continues to be most helpful.

Intrapersonal stressors included the difficulty that nursing staff had in adjusting to staffing changes, being moved from one unit to another when census fluctuated, and educational or training needs of the nurses. Additionally, intrapersonal stressors were caused by some staffing inequities, where different head nurses would prioritize differently, set different expectations for holiday and vacation requests, and so forth. Changes in the administration of scheduling and staffing addressed this problem.

The nursing service department staffing had previously been decentralized. Although maintaining this would seem to be consistent with decentralization, it was determined that staffing should be centralized. Benge reports regarding decentralization, that "it may not be wise to decentralize all functions, many times there is a need to maintain centralized functions for the improved functioning of the total organization."[10] (p. 128) This allowed for participative decision making regarding vacations, holidays, and so on, at the unit level. These decisions were coordinated with other head nurses in the subgroup, and were more consistent across units because of newly established policies. Centralization allowed some control across the nursing department of the total number of staff nurses present for staffing readjustment according to changes in the patient classification. Also, a rotation schedule for head nurses allowed them to function in a supervisory capacity (when needed) and to experience the planning, staffing, and coordinating concerns of middle management for the entire organization.

Job descriptions were revised and clarified, addressing managerial functions and clinical functions. The nurse administrator facilitated scheduling of head nurses to be present in the managerial function on certain days for meetings, decision making, and planning purposes. Head nurses, however, continued to have some flexibility of their own scheduling for staffing needs of the unit. This rein-

forced commitment to both practice and management in the key pivotal decision-making role of head nurses.

An example of extrapersonal stressors was resistance of the medical staff when patient teaching plans and new charting forms were designed. Attempts were initiated to take these new charting forms through appropriate hospital committees. A plan of action was chosen to strengthen flexible lines of defense (according to the Neuman model), and to persuade key physicians of the usefulness of the nursing history and assessment. Although the nursing assessment form was not adopted, a new nursing history form was accepted that reflected the Neuman model.

Other extrapersonal stressors periodically occurred between nursing and other hospital departments. Improved relationships with other departments were facilitated with the establishment of two new positions. A nursing systems analyst coordinated staffing, scheduling, financial planning, budgeting, and purchasing. This position began in 1985, and has subsequently been valuable in improving relationships with patient accounts, medical records, and purchasing. Recently, a new supply distribution system was implemented in conjunction with purchasing and the nursing departments. The smooth transition was due to the nursing systems analyst's work with the purchasing department.

In 1986 another position, a nursing care analyst, was created. Although the initial purpose was to develop and assist in maintaining nursing standards, this role has been expanded. The nurse in this position has been instrumental in improving guest relations throughout the entire hospital. A nursing inservice program, initiated to respond to patient complaints, was requested to be presented to employees throughout the organization. Through changes in administrative structure and function, the nursing department was able to decrease stress, thus strengthening the flexible lines of defense, and improving communications between nursing service, physicians, and other departments in the organization.

APPLICATION OF THE MODEL TO NURSING PRACTICE

The need for revision of nursing forms and processes was identified as part of the overall change needed in nursing to improve quality and documentation of patient care. In early 1984, when the idea of using a conceptual model was explored, one of the planned changes was to incorporate the terms and scope of the model in nursing practice at Jefferson Davis Memorial Hospital. The head nurses met and began developing a long range plan for revision of forms and improving quality and documentation of nursing care. Among the charting forms discussed were the physical assessment form, an interview tool for admission assessment, a discharge planning form, and a new nursing care plan system. There were also concerns shared about the use and reliability of the patient classification system.

Subcommittees were established to work on job descriptions, organizational structure, the assessment forms, staffing issues, and the patient classification system; organizational structure, job descriptions, and staffing have already been discussed in this chapter.

The revision of the nursing history and assessment form began with nursing staff in the critical care area. The major focus of revisions in the nursing history portion of the form included information related to developmental, sociocultural, and psychological factors as described in the Neuman model. As this was the first form to be revised after the adoption of the model as an organizing framework, the nursing history and assessment form did not reflect as much Neuman model terminology as subsequent forms. One section of the history was a social history, which addressed sociocultural factors; an-

other section had a question regarding recent changes or stress in life-style. The daily assessment, which was largely a physical assessment form, was not accepted by the medical staff even after several revisions. The nursing department now incorporates a detailed physical admission assessment in the nurses' notes.

Another application of the Neuman model was the development of a nursing admission assessment interview tool similar to the published Neuman assessment-intervention format.[1] This was revised by a staff nurse as a part of a staff development project. Staff nurses enrolled in Staff Nurse Action Program (SNAP) completed projects of interest that could be useful to the department. The Neuman tool was revised to be more consistent with lay terms and language particular to the regional area of Mississippi. The admission interview is currently being used by staff nurses as a guide, and it is hoped that the nursing department will be working in collaboration with the admissions department to incorporate this assessment into the interview process.

A new patient classification system developed specifically for use at Jefferson Davis Memorial Hospital reflected the Neuman model in principle and application. The previous patient classification system consisted of subjective categorization of patients with a formula for unit staffing. A more objective method was desired by head nurses. In the summer of 1984, a weighted system was introduced where actual minutes and hours were computed for different nursing activities. The new system was needed particularly for determining staff mix, future costing out of nursing services, and increasing confidence in objective data.

The patient classification form for data collection (see Figure 56.2) reflects Neuman terminology, which included physiologic, psychologic, sociocultural, and developmental factors in the assessment of patients.

PATIENT CLASSIFICATION WORKSHEET

DRG #: _____

DIAGNOSIS: _____   (Circle Appropriate Numbers)

SURGICAL PROCEDURE: _____

DOCUMENTATION FOCUS — BETTY NEUMAN MODEL

	DATE							
SECTION A (Aides, LPN's and/or RN's)								
TRANSFER		8	8	8	8	8	8	8
ASSISTANCE: MINIMAL		11	11	11	11	11	11	11
MODERATE		19	19	19	19	19	19	19
TOTAL		29	29	29	29	29	29	29
TREATMENTS: NON COMPLICATED		8	8	8	8	8	8	8
VS: q 2-4 HOURS OR WHILE AWAKE		6	6	6	6	6	6	6
q 1 HOUR OR MORE FREQUENTLY		25	25	25	25	25	25	25
TRACTION		2	2	2	2	2	2	2
SCORE								
SECTION B (LPN's and/or RN's)								
TREATMENTS: SIMPLE		2	2	2	2	2	2	2
COMPLEX		7	7	7	7	7	7	7
TRACTION		19	19	19	19	19	19	19
MEDICATIONS: SIMPLE - IM, PO, SC		5	5	5	5	5	5	5
REQUIRE EVALUATION OF EFFECTIVENESS		6	6	6	6	6	6	6
OBSERVATION: q 4-8 HOURS		7	7	7	7	7	7	7
q 2-3 HOURS		13	13	13	13	13	13	13
TEACHING/DISCHARGE PLANNING: 0-14 MINUTES		3	3	3	3	3	3	3
15-29 MINUTES		8	8	8	8	8	8	8
SOCIO/EMOTIONAL CARE: 0-14 MINUTES		6	6	6	6	6	6	6
15-29 MINUTES		13	13	13	13	13	13	13
SCORE								
SECTION C (RN's)								
TREATMENTS: COMPLEX		15	15	15	15	15	15	15
INTENSE		20	20	20	20	20	20	20
TRACTION		20	20	20	20	20	20	20
SPECIAL PROCEDURES: ASSIST		3	3	3	3	3	3	3
MAINTAIN		7	7	7	7	7	7	7
INTRAVENOUS THERAPY: WITHOUT MEDS		6	6	6	6	6	6	6
WITH MEDS		11	11	11	11	11	11	11
1 OR 2 SEPARATE IV'S		17	17	17	17	17	17	17
q 2 HOURS OR MORE FREQUENTLY		31	31	31	31	31	31	31
REQUIRE ON-GOING ASSESSMENT		5	5	5	5	5	5	5
OBSERVATION: q 30 MINUTES - 2 HOURS		23	23	23	23	23	23	23
q 0-29 MINUTES		40	40	40	40	40	40	40
TEACHING/DISCHARGE PLANNING: 30-59 MINUTES		15	15	15	15	15	15	15
60 MINUTES OR MORE		25	25	25	25	25	25	25
SOCIO/EMOTIONAL CARE: 30-59 MINUTES		32	32	32	32	32	32	32
60 MINUTES OR MORE		53	53	53	53	53	53	53
ADMISSION ASSESSMENT		6	6	6	6	6	6	6
SCORE								
TOTAL SCORE								
CATEGORY								
INITIALS								

TOTAL SCORE/ CATEGORY GUIDE
- PRIMARY - Category I - 0 - 60
- TERTIARY - Category II - 61 - 120
- SECONDARY - Category III -121 - 180
- SECONDARY - Category IV -181 - 240
- SECONDARY - Category V -241 - 340

Figure 56.2 Patient Classification Worksheet.

Forms and processes for classifying patients have been revised since the first use in 1984, to more accurately assess and classify patients for primary and tertiary interventions.

An increase in outpatient census and a concurrent fluctuation in inpatient census was another reason for use of the Neuman model as a framework for the patient classification system. Grouping of patients followed the Neuman model according to primary, secondary, and tertiary interventions. As would be expected, patients in acute and critical care units were classified in the secondary intervention approach in the Neuman model. Outpatient and ambulatory surgery services for patients have rapidly increased. Census in ambulatory care alone increased from approximately 20 patients in November, 1983, to 160 plus in 1986.

Other primary interventions have included activity by the education services, such as cardiopulmonary resuscitation for groups in the community, and blood pressure and diabetic screening in local shopping malls. In addition, a program of preoperative teaching by appointment and other health teaching by appointment have been initiated. These latest primary interventions have not yet been incorporated into the patient classification for staffing and budgeting purposes.

Recently (1986), two programs were initiated that fall in the area of tertiary care. A respite care program allowed families in the community to bring their elderly into the hospital to a particular unit for short stays (weekends, vacations, or both). This tertiary care service was offered to families with elderly individuals in their homes, who require supervision and care. A nurse was assigned to visit the home and make a health assessment, and evaluate the client to determine if he or she met the criteria for the respite care program. Another purpose was to establish rapport with the elderly person prior to coming into the hospital. Staffing in this area was

included as part of the tertiary care section of the patient classification system.

Another type of tertiary intervention is a new program of cardiac rehabilitation. After teaching patients about coronary artery disease in the critical care unit, the patient and family are further instructed on the cardiac step-down unit. Goals of the cardiac rehabilitation program include: education of patients and families with individualized instruction, a planned exercise program, the fostering of emotional and social support, dietary instruction, and stress management. Of particular interest are the social support groups, which meet for weekly sessions. Patients and families meet with members of the nursing staff and social service. Issues related to life changes are discussed, and patients and families are encouraged to share concerns and feelings with each other. Patients who have been discharged, as well as their families, may return for these weekly sessions in the next phase of implementation. This tertiary intervention is consistent with the Neuman model where interventions focus on re-education, readaptation, and stability after treatment.[1]

ISSUES AND FUTURE DIRECTIONS

There are a number of issues to be addressed when implementing a conceptual model to nursing administration and practice. Education of staff, the planning and implementation process, preparation of nurses in middle management, and use of nurse consultants are issues recommended for exploration.[11] Identification of resources is mentioned by these authors; however, cost is a major consideration that was not explored in detail.

The costs and benefits of adopting a nursing conceptual model for nursing administration and practice are issues that are difficult to accurately measure. One major factor to consider is the cost of education of staff. Budget increases for staff development departments may result from an overall plan for education of staff to a nursing model. Also, costs of replacement for staff, changes in scheduling of key leaders for planning and implementation of the nursing model, and release time (away from normal managerial and clinical responsibilities) for meetings related to the nursing model can be anticipated. In addition, major revisions of nursing documentation forms require extensive education of staff for proper implementation.

Development of new nursing documentation forms, particularly if there is an attempt to incorporate the nursing model into charting and documentation, is costly. Another issue related to the revision of forms is the process of getting these new charting forms through hospital and medical staff committees that may have input in changes on the chart. The importance of sharing ideas and obtaining support from various groups in the hospital is addressed by Capers and colleagues.[11] Explanation of the importance of the use of a nursing model to individuals outside nursing is sometimes difficult; however, the language and terms of the Neuman model are common terms and do not require a new vocabulary. This makes the model attractive to nurses and other health care professionals.[3]

Communication and the development of a planned change process for use of a nursing model is another issue. The approach taken at Jefferson Davis Memorial Hospital was consistent with recommendations made by nurses at Mercy Catholic Medical Center. Middle managers were involved early in planning for use of a nursing model. Also, a nursing consultant was used to assist with education, planning sessions, problem solving, and group discussions with nursing leaders.

The use of consultants can be beneficial but very costly. Whether facilitating development of nurses as middle managers, as was important for the changes in nursing administra-

tion at Jefferson Davis Memorial Hospital, or educating them in the use of a nursing model, the use of outside consultants may be considered. Consultants can offer in-house staff development, which may be better than sending a number of nurses to workshops away from the agency. Zander points out that "the cost would have to be weighed against the nondollar benefits, which result in a cohesive, participative, confident management group."[12] (p. 82)

When facilitating planned change, even change that allows participative management, one potential cost is staff turnover. Adequate planning and communication can help in eliminating unnecessary staff changes. However, this factor must be considered: at Jefferson Davis Memorial Hospital, there was more turnover of nursing staff with less educational preparation. Retention of nurses with baccalaureate or higher degrees remained fairly constant. Job satisfaction is considered a positive benefit in decreasing turnover when a traditional organization moves to a more decentralized structure.[13]

For nurse administrators considering the use of a nursing model for changes in organizational structure there are a number of questions that need to be explored. Does the nursing department have the time and resources to facilitate the change? Does the nursing leadership (middle management) have the interest and ability to facilitate and support staff nurses as they go through the change process? Is the climate in the entire organization conducive to major changes in the nursing organization and nursing documentation? Will there be adequate support and/or cooperation with hospital administrators and medical staff? Are there ways to improve or revise reward systems in nursing service to reward scholarly inquiry, publication, and other nontraditional areas of professional growth? How much education regarding a nursing conceptual model does the nursing staff need at all levels? Do staff nurses need to completely understand the philosophy and processes of the model, or do they just need a good orientation with a focus on the revision of the documentation forms? Are there resources available for the research and theory exploration possibilities that can come from adopting a nursing conceptual model?

Research and theory exploration are inherent in the future possibilities for use of the Neuman model at Jefferson Davis Memorial Hospital. There are a number of potential research projects for nursing leadership and staff that can be explored relating the Neuman Health-Care Systems Model with other models used as a basis for research and practice. The stress coping model[14] has potential to be linked in a creative way to the different stressors and the multidimensional approach to the patient in the Neuman model. Patterns in the study of human and environmental characteristics are a conceptual way to study relationships.[15] This could be related to the Neuman model, particularly with the social support group in cardiac rehabilitation program previously mentioned.

Other factors that would allow for potential research projects are in the community environment in the Natchez area. Studies using the stressors in the Neuman model could be explored in relation to unemployment. Two major industries, International Paper and Armstrong Tire Company, have experienced changes that affect both clients and staff members at the hospital. Also, studies comparing perceptions of stressors and response to nursing interventions by clients of different races could be explored from a sociocultural perspective. These projects are consistent with comments in the literature related to the Neuman model. "Questions generated by the model would best lend themselves to descriptive and correlative research studies."[16] (p. 122)

In conclusion, the use of a conceptual model such as the Neuman Health-Care Systems Model in nursing administration and practice presents a challenge. A major result of using this model is a difference in attitude and professional growth of nurses, particularly those in middle management at Jefferson Davis Memorial Hospital. The nursing administrator reports that nursing leaders are more creative, have grown clinically, and have increased in confidence in their abilities. The organizational climate has allowed for growth and pursuit of knowledge. Since implementing the Neuman model, nurses at Jefferson Davis Memorial Hospital are experiencing opportunities for integrating theory, practice, and research. Implementation of the model is still in early stages, but a window of opportunity has been created. "Time and sociocultural conditions are right for the development of theoretical nursing, which in turn is significant for patient care, and nurses are 'going for it.' "[2] (p. 52)

REFERENCES

1. Riehl JP, Roy SC. Conceptual models for nursing practice. 2nd ed. New York: Appleton-Century-Crofts, 1980.
2. Meleis AI. Theoretical nursing: development and progress. Philadelphia: J. B. Lippincott Company, 1985.
3. Fawcett J. Analysis and evaluation of conceptual models of nursing. Philadelphia: F. A. Davis Company, 1984.
4. Leddy S, Pepper JM. Conceptual bases of professional nursing. Philadelphia: J. B. Lippincott Company, 1985.
5. Neuman B. The Neuman systems model. Norwalk: Appleton-Century-Crofts, 1982.
6. American Academy of Nursing. Magnet hospitals. Kansas City: American Nurses' Association, 1983.
7. Peterson ME. Motivating staff to participate in decision making. Nurs Admin Q 1983;7(2):63–68.
8. Hyndman C, Personius J. Job sharing in the head nurse role—decreased stress. Nurs Admin Q 1983; 7(2):35–41.
9. Winstead-Fry P, ed. Case studies in nursing theory. New York: National League for Nursing, 1986.
10. Benge EJ, Editors of the Alexander Hamilton Institute. Elements of modern management. New York: Amacom Publishing Company, 1976.

11. Capers CF, O'Brien C, Quinn R, Kelly R, Fenerty A. The Neuman systems model in practice. J Nurs Admin 1985;29–39.
12. Zander K. Management training won't work ... unless nursing administration provides it. Nurs Admin Q 1983;7(2):77–86.
13. Shoemaker, H, El-Ahraf A. Decentralization of nursing service management and its impact on job satisfaction. Nurs Admin Q 1983;7(2):69–76.
14. Scott DW, Oberst MT, Dropkin MJ. A stress-coping model. Adv Nurs Sci 1980;3(1):9–24.
15. Crawford G. The concept of pattern in nursing: conceptual development and measurement. Adv Nurs Sci 1982;5(1):1–6.
16. Thibodeau JA. Nursing models: analysis and evaluation. Monterey: Wadsworth Health Sciences Division, 1983.
17. McLaughlin JS. Toward a theoretical model for community health programs. Adv Nurs Sci 1982; 5(1):7–28.
18. Salmond SW. Supporting staff through decentralization. Nursing Economics 1985;3:295–300.

Afterword

THE PRIMARY market for *Dimensions of Nursing Administration* is master's and doctoral students in nursing administration. There is no doubt in my mind that they will find in this volume a rich source of information about the field of nursing administration, especially in relation to concerns about the importance of theory and research, and about questions relative to nursing and nursing administration.

Readers will be stimulated to wonder to what extent, if at all, research and theory in nursing administration should arise from, or be related to, research and theory in clinical nursing. And they will question whether the orientation for nursing administration should not be closer to theory and research in management.

If theory building in nursing administration depends on an understanding of nursing, on what is theory building in hospital administration dependent? Is not the understanding of the total organization in which nursing administration takes place of greater consequence than understanding the one activity—nursing—which takes place in the single department of nursing? Knowledge of what nursing is, and what a total organization is and does, are two vastly different fields.

I agree with Fawcett, who states that because the theories from nursing models have not been sufficiently developed, the conceptual-theoretical system of knowledge for nursing administration must begin with management science. Nurse administrators cannot wait, nor have they waited, until nursing models are well established. They should proceed in their exploration by starting with the good theories that exist in management science. Educators, however, especially those who operate master's and doctoral programs, need to be constantly alert to the development of nursing concepts and theories that can be used in nursing administration—its practice and its research.

A second audience for the book is faculty in undergraduate and graduate programs. I suspect, however, that faculty primarily involved in graduate education will be the largest group to find the readings useful. For them it will be a valuable resource.

Education for nursing administration is important and a topic of great significance for any discussion of where we are heading. The discussions of the management component of all levels of nursing education should prove useful.

But I wondered as I read these sections whether or not we have come to an agreement yet about what the responsibility of nursing education and nursing administration is with respect to the employment and practice of new graduates. My position is that students completing undergraduate programs in nursing certainly should not be expected to move into more than the simplest of nursing management positions without further formal preparation. I believe this: Nursing service administration is responsible for aiding nurses to develop the knowledge and skill required by both nursing and management. Based on these statements, one might then ask, what is the role of formal nursing education in this responsibility? Isn't nursing education responsible for providing basic knowledge, and nursing service for developing the needed skills through supervisory practices in a goal-directed, supportive environment?

Is any other premise viable for nursing administration other than that the nurse administrator should know what clinical nursing is, what is essential to the attainment of organization objectives, and what is not? But to what extent those who practice clinical nursing need to know what nursing administration is in its fullest complexity has *not* been established. To the extent that clinical nurses are responsible for managing or directing the activities of others, they need to know what performance is expected of them and what the criteria are for competence and acceptable performance.

A third audience for the book is practicing nurse administrators. The assumption the editors and authors make is that nurse administrators are, and ought to be, fundamentally interested and involved in research. It is good to see that the chapter on research in nursing administration differentiates methods for basic research from methods that may be more useful for problem solving. I, for one, am delighted to see these two sections.

Using research for theory building is different than using research approaches to solve immediate problems in the workplace. When the differentiation is clear, the guilt imposed on nurse administrators for *not* doing basic research may be relieved. And the enormous importance of the evaluation studies done in practice to assure quality will be given the recognition by academics that these investigations so justly deserve.

Just how many nurses in faculty positions in education settings, where the search for knowledge is as important as imparting knowledge, are involved in research that seeks to build theory? It may well be that practicing nurse administrators, many of whom have made such significant strides in

measuring performance, the quality of programs, and the outcomes of care are well ahead of most educators with respect to empirical investigation.

Just what is the responsibility of nursing administration in regard to research? Are nurse managers as individuals expected to do basic, theory-building research? Can they not be recognized and respected because their problem solving is based on sound investigative technique? And what is the responsibility of graduate faculty in institutions of higher education for doing basic research and building and testing theories of nursing administration? Do we not still have dichotomies that need resolution before both nursing and nursing administration can improve and become more effective in attaining their individual and joint goals?

This may sound like heresy: but neither intellectually nor in the workplace have we resolved our ideas about what we think nursing administration—and therefore the nurse administrator—really is. Nurse executives, especially those in hospitals, are still faced with the dilemma of determining whether they are or are not members of the nursing profession. To a large extent, our professional organization, the American Nurses' Association, counts nurses in management out because of the realities of the U.S. labor market, assigning them to management's side in collective bargaining where important compensation and working conditions for employed nurses are debated.

So, even if one reaches for clinical nursing theories—even those that have been substantiated to some extent through research—to integrate them into nursing administration research and practice, is the dichotomy eliminated between clinical and administrative nurses in the practice setting? I think not.

Perhaps this particular aspect of practice in nursing administration isn't of all that much concern to master's and doctoral students. But the editors describe the book as a set of discussions of problems in the field. And this dual nursing-management orientation of nurse executives is a real problem for many, one that deserves to be addressed in discussions of where we are heading with respect to theory, research, and practice, today and for the future.

Many points of view about nursing administration are presented in the wide-ranging discussions found in this book. In this brief Afterword, I have raised some questions for which all defendable points of view may not have been addressed. But how could they be in just one collection? I recognize that this is more than can be expected and am pleased that the editors and publisher have provided a forum for the expression of ideas about nursing administration that have not been heard or disseminated widely until now.

Eva H. Erickson
Professor Emeritus
University of Iowa
Iowa City, Iowa

Index

t = table; *f* = figure.